DAVID Z. LEVINE, M.D.

Professor of Medicine
Division of Nephrology
University of Ottawa
Faculty of Medicine
Head
Division of Nephrology
Ottawa General Hospital
Department of Medicine
Ottawa, Ontario
Canada

CARE OF THE RENAL PATIENT

SECOND EDITION

1991

W.B. SAUNDERS COMPANY
Harcourt Brace Jovanovich, Inc.

Philadelphia London Toronto Montreal Sydney Tokyo

W. B. SAUNDERS COMPANY
Harcourt Brace Jovanovich, Inc.

The Curtis Center
Independence Square West
Philadelphia, PA 19106

Library of Congress Cataloging-in-Publication Data

Care of the renal patient / [edited by] David Z. Levine.—
2nd ed.
p. cm.

Includes bibliographical references.
Includes index.

ISBN 0–7216–3056–1

1. Kidneys—Diseases—Treatment. I. Levine, David Z. [DNLM: 1. Kidney Diseases—diagnosis. 2. Kidney Diseases—therapy. WJ 300 C271]

RC902.A2C37 1991 616.6′106—dc20

DNLM/DLC 90–8954

Editor: John Dyson
Designer: Maureen Sweeney
Production Manager: Bill Preston
Manuscript Editor: Wendy Andresen
Illustration Coordinator: Brett MacNaughton
Indexer: David Prout

Listed here are the latest translated editions of this book together with the language of the translation and the publisher.

Portuguese (*1st Edition*)–Livraria Roca, Ltda., São Paulo, Brazil
Japanese (*1st Edition*)–Igaku Shoin/Saunders Ltd., Tokyo, Japan
Spanish (*1st Edition*)–NEISA, Mexico City, Mexico

Care of the Renal Patient ISBN 0–7216–3056–1

Printed in the United States of America.

Last digit is the print number: 9 8 7 6 5 4 3 2 1

*To our patients—in the hope that
we may serve them better*

CONTRIBUTORS

Sharon G. Adler, M.D.
Adjunct Associate Professor
University of California at Los Angeles School of Medicine
Los Angeles, California
Assistant Professor of Medicine
Department of Medicine
Division of Nephrology and Hypertension
Harbor-UCLA Medical Center
Torrance, California
Diabetic Nephropathy

Robert J. Alpern, M.D.
Professor of Medicine
Division of Nephrology
Department of Internal Medicine
University of Texas Southwestern Medical Center
Chief of Nephrology
Parkland Memorial Hospital
Zale-Lipshy University Hospital
Dallas, Texas
Sodium and Potassium Disturbances in Renal Patients

John Badalamenti, M.D.
Assistant Professor of Medicine
University of Texas Medical Branch at Galveston
Galveston, Texas
Chronic Renal Failure

Norman Bank, M.D.
Professor of Medicine
Albert Einstein College of Medicine
Bronx, New York

Director
Renal, Electrolyte and Hypertension Division
Montefiore Medical Center
North Central Bronx Hospital
Bronx, New York
Assessment of Patients with Renal Disease

William M. Bennett, M.D.
Professor of Medicine and Pharmacology
Division of Nephrology and Hypertension
Oregon Health Sciences University School of Medicine
Co-Head, Division of Nephrology and Hypertension
Oregon Health Sciences University Hospital
Portland, Oregon
Drug Use in Renal Patients and the Extracorporeal Treatment of Poisonings

Kevin D. Burns, M.D.
Research Fellow
Division of Nephrology
Vanderbilt University
Nashville, Tennessee
Acid-Base Disturbances in Azotemic Patients
Urgent Problems in the Renal Patient

Daniel C. Cattran, M.D., FRCP(C)
Professor of Medicine
University of Toronto
Active Staff
Toronto General Hospital and Women's College Hospital
Toronto, Ontario
Canada
Acute Nephritic Syndrome

Jack W. Coburn, M.D.
Adjunct Professor of Medicine
University of California at Los Angeles School of Medicine
Staff Physician
West Los Angeles Veterans Administration Medical Center (Wadsworth Division)
Attending Physician
Cedars-Sinai Medical Center
Visiting Physician
UCLA Center for the Health Sciences
Los Angeles, California
Renal Bone Diseases and Aluminum Toxicity in Renal Patients

Cecil H. Coggins, M.D.
Associate Professor of Medicine
Harvard Medical School
Cambridge, Massachusetts
Clinical Director
Renal Unit
Massachusetts General Hospital
Boston, Massachusetts
Hematuria, Proteinuria, and Nephrotic Syndrome

Thomas D. DuBose, Jr., M.D.
Professor of Medicine, Physiology and Biophysics
University of Texas Medical Branch at Galveston
Chief of Nephrology
Department of Internal Medicine
University of Texas Branch
Galveston, Texas
Chronic Renal Failure

Alfred J. Fish, M.D.
Professor of Pediatrics
University of Minnesota
Department of Pediatrics
University of Minnesota Hospitals
Minneapolis, Minnesota
Pediatric Nephrology

Richard J. Glassock, M.D.
Professor of Medicine
University of California at Los Angeles School of Medicine
Los Angeles, California
Chairman
Department of Medicine
Harbor-UCLA Medical Center
Torrance, California
Diabetic Nephropathy

Marc B. Goldstein, M.D., M.Sc., FRCP(C)
Professor of Medicine
University of Toronto
Director
Hemodialysis Program
St. Michael's Hospital
Toronto, Ontario
Canada
Acid-Base Disturbances in Azotemic Patients

William G. Goodman, M.D.
Associate Professor of Medicine
University of California at Los Angeles School of Medicine
Los Angeles, California
Staff Physician
Chief, Dialysis Unit
Sepulveda Veterans Administration Medical Center
Sepulveda, California
Renal Bone Diseases and Aluminum Toxicity in Renal Patients

Raymond Hakim, M.D., Ph.D.
Associate Professor of Medicine
Division of Nephrology
Vanderbilt University
Director, Clinical Services
Vanderbilt University Hospital
Nashville, Tennessee
Hemodialysis
Urgent Problems in the Renal Patient

J. Harold Helderman, M.D.
Professor of Medicine
Vanderbilt University
Medical Director
Vanderbilt Transplant Center
Vanderbilt Medical Center
Nashville, Tennessee
Urgent Problems in the Renal Patient

Raimund R. Hirschberg, M.D.
Assistant Professor of Medicine
University of California at Los Angeles School of Medicine
Los Angeles, California
Attending Physician
Division of Nephrology and Hypertension
Harbor-UCLA Medical Center
Torrance, California
Nutritional Therapy in Patients with Renal Failure

Nuhad Ismail, M.D.
Clinical Instructor in Medicine
Division of Nephrology
Vanderbilt University
Nashville, Tennessee
Hemodialysis
Urgent Problems in the Renal Patient

Randy Kaplan, M.D.
Medical Staff
Meadville Medical Center
Meadville, Pennsylvania
Assessment of Patients with Renal Disease

Ramesh Khanna, M.D.
Professor of Medicine
Director of In Hospital Peritoneal Dialysis
University of Missouri Health Sciences Center
Columbia, Missouri
Peritoneal Dialysis

Saulo Klahr, M.D.
Joseph Friedman Professor of Renal Disease
Director, Renal Division
Washington University School of Medicine
Physician
Barnes Hospital
St. Louis, Missouri
Obstructive Uropathy

Joel D. Kopple, M.D.
Professor of Medicine and Public Health
University of California at Los Angeles Schools of Medicine and Public Health
Los Angeles, California
Chief of Nephrology
Harbor-UCLA Medical Center
Torrance, California
Nutritional Therapy in Patients with Renal Failure

David Z. Levine, M.D.
Professor of Medicine
Division of Nephrology
University of Ottawa
Faculty of Medicine
Head
Division of Nephrology
Ottawa General Hospital
Department of Medicine
Ottawa, Ontario
Canada
Acid-Base Disturbances in Azotemic Patients

Mortimer Levy, M.D., FRCP(C)
Professor of Medicine and Physiology
McGill University

Senior Physician and Director, Nephrology
Royal Victoria Hospital
Montreal, Quebec
Canada
Edematous States and Hepatorenal Syndrome

Norman B. Levy, M.D.
Director
Liaison Psychiatry Division
Professor of Psychiatry, Medicine, and Surgery
New York Medical College
Valhalla, New York
Psychiatric Aspects of Renal Care

Marshall D. Lindheimer, M.D.
Professor of Medicine and of Obstetrics and Gynecology
University of Chicago
Attending Physician
University of Chicago Hospitals and Clinics
Director
Medical High Risk Clinic
Chicago Lying-In Hospital
Chicago, Illinois
Renal Disease and Hypertension in Pregnancy

Douglas J. Norman, M.D.
Professor of Medicine
Oregon Health Sciences University
Director
Transplant Medicine
Director
Laboratory of Immunogenetics and Transplantation
University of Oregon Health Sciences Center
Portland, Oregon
Renal Transplantation

Dimitrios G. Oreopoulos, M.D., Ph.D., FRCP(C)
Professor of Medicine
Director
Peritoneal Dialysis Unit
Toronto Western Hospital
Toronto, Ontario
Canada
Peritoneal Dialysis

Biff F. Palmer, M.D.
Assistant Professor of Internal Medicine
University of Texas Southwestern Medical Center
Division of Nephrology
Department of Internal Medicine
Assistant Professor of Internal Medicine
Parkland Memorial Hospital
Zale-Lipshy University Hospital
Dallas, Texas
Sodium and Potassium Disturbances in Renal Patients

Rhonda Rubin, M.D.
Nephrology Fellow
Montefiore Hospital
Bronx, New York
Assessment of Patients with Renal Disease

Isidro B. Salusky, M.D.
Associate Professor of Pediatrics
University of California at Los Angeles School of Medicine
Staff Physician
Director
Pediatric Dialysis Program
UCLA Center for the Health Sciences
Los Angeles, California
Renal Bone Diseases and Aluminum Toxicity in Renal Patients

Roger A. L. Sutton, D.M., FRCP, FRCP(C)
Professor and Head
Division of Nephrology
Department of Medicine
University of British Columbia
Head
Department of Medicine
Vancouver General Hospital
Vancouver, British Columbia
Canada
Stone Disease

Suzanne K. Swan, M.D.
Clinical Instructor
Division of Nephrology
Oregon Health Sciences University School of Medicine
Staff Doctor

Division of Nephrology
Oregon Health Sciences University Hospital
Portland, Oregon
Drug Use in Renal Patients and the Extracorporeal Treatment of Poisonings

Robert D. Toto, M.D.
Associate Professor of Medicine
University of Texas Southwestern Medical Center
Division of Nephrology
Department of Internal Medicine
Clinical Director of Nephrology
Parkland Memorial Hospital
Zale-Lipshy University Hospital
Dallas, Texas
Sodium and Potassium Disturbances in Renal Patients

Jason G. Umans, M.D.
Assistant Professor of Medicine
University of Chicago
Attending Physician
University of Chicago Hospitals and Clinics
Chicago, Illinois
Renal Disease and Hypertension in Pregnancy

Norman M. Wolfish, M.D., FRCP(C), FAAP
Professor of Pediatrics
Faculty of Medicine
University of Ottawa
Head
Nephrology Service
Pediatric Nephrologist
Children's Hospital of Eastern Ontario
Ottawa, Ontario
Canada
Pediatric Nephrology

PREFACE

On four of five weekday mornings, a special tutorial session lasting about 40 minutes is held in the conference room of the renal ward at the Ottawa General Hospital. One staffperson presents a topic to a group of trainees consisting, usually, of one or two medical students, a "straight" or family medicine intern, a more senior resident in internal medicine, and, often, a trainee in the Royal College Nephrology Program.

Seems preposterous, doesn't it? How can one present a topic effectively to a group with such diverse needs? The medical student needs to learn how to perform the initial assessment of the renal patient and what dialysis machines do; the more senior residents have to decide which of our 25 in-patients need dialysis today; and the nephrology trainee needs to learn the indications for parathyroidectomy in dialysis patients, which membranes are best, how to assess adequacy of dialysis, and whether a fungal infection is an absolute indication to remove a CAPD catheter. The first edition of *Care of the Renal Patient*, a tutorial course in itself, provided in an easily accessible format the information that our students and trainees told us they wanted—information we could not cover in our small group sessions. This second edition, completely restructured, aims to be better in every way.

My experience using this book as a complement to our sessions goes something like this: When every trainee has recognized that ECF volume overload indicates the need for dialysis in an anuric patient, I might ask the senior resident how much weight we take off, how we know it's enough, and what orders need to be written. After a brief discussion, I refer the group to the chapter on hemodialysis (Chapter 18). In the same chapter, the nephrology trainee can review details of catheter placement and how to formulate the dialysis prescription. When we discuss double acid-base disturbances in dialysis patients, the residents are told that Chapter 5 has instructive case histories. When I am asked to guide a house officer about modification of drug use in renal failure, I say, without embarrassment, that I look it up in the tables in Chapter 12. In discussing how to use fractional excretion of sodium to distinguish between azotemia caused by ECF volume depletion and intrinsic renal disease, I advise students and interns to review the basic principles given in Chapters 1 and 4. We expect our senior residents to appreciate the altered pathophysiology in the hepatorenal syndrome (Chapter 11) and thereby learn not to rely on the FE_{Na} in this situation.

For this new edition, I have succeeded in persuading a number of remarkably talented nephrologists to provide chapters. Not only have they covered areas of nephrology to which they have made significant original contributions, but they have accepted the extra burden of presenting the material in a way that facilitates learning. Throughout the book, all authors have made a special effort to provide case studies illustrating key issues, algorithms to clarify approaches to complex problems, boxes and boldface sections for emphasis, and detailed therapy including drug dosages. The last chapter is devoted to the management of emergency situations associated with electrolyte and acid-base disturbances, hypertensive crises, hemodialysis, and transplantation.

This sounds as though we have tried to write a "Washington Manual of Nephrology." It should, because we did. When the senior editors at Saunders saw the three lengthy chapters on CAPD, hemodialysis, and transplantation and asked "Whom is this book really written for?," I told them that it was written primarily for the trainee but that practicing nephrologists also would find it useful. For example, because one member of our group does most of the CAPD work, the rest of us will be happy to have at hand the algorithms for treatment of infection provided in Chapter 17. (I noted him sneaking a look at them also.) Other topics of interest to the practicing nephrologist include an approach to the once-psychotic patient who requires transplantation, how to dialyze pregnant patients, and an update of cyclosporine interactions with other drugs.

Here are additional examples of some of the subjects covered.

For the student

- the history and physical examination in adult and pediatric renal patients
- laboratory assessment of renal function
- overview of dialysis and transplantation
- disturbances of acid-base balance and electrolytes
- obstruction and stone disease

For the trainee

- emergencies in dialysis and transplantation patients
- presentation and treatment of primary nephritis
- management of diabetic nephropathy, renal disease in pregnancy, hepatorenal syndrome, etc.
- drug use and nutritional therapy
- bedside insertion of Tenckhoff's catheter for CAPD, establishing hemodialysis access

For the nephrologist

- approach to digitalis-related arrhythmias in dialysis patients
- management of frequent dialysis hypotension
- alternative antibiotic dosing for CAPD peritonitis
- different immuno-suppression guidelines for living related, living unrelated, and cadaver donor transplantations
- prophylaxis of CMV infection in transplant recipients

I am very indebted to my colleagues who have provided the superb chapters following a specific format. I am most grateful to Saunders, and in particular to my friend John Dyson, who supported the project in every way. It was a delight to negotiate boxes and boldface text with Amy Norwitz, who, along with Bill Preston, produced a book that reflects the excellence of the contributors.

DAVID Z. LEVINE, M.D.

CONTENTS

CHAPTER 1

ASSESSMENT OF PATIENTS WITH RENAL DISEASE

Rhonda Rubin, Randy Kaplan, and Norman Bank

House staff officers and medical students are frequently confronted with laboratory data showing an elevated blood urea nitrogen (BUN) concentration and serum creatinine (S_{cr}), often before they have had an opportunity to examine the patient or to take a medical history. Abnormal BUN and S_{cr} levels may be accompanied by several other disturbing laboratory findings, such as elevated serum potassium and phosphorus levels, low bicarbonate and calcium levels, and marked anemia as revealed by a complete blood count. Although renal disease is not a common illness in the general population or in office practice, it is encountered daily in large city hospital emergency rooms and in hospitalized patients. Most often, house staff physicians are the first to evaluate such patients, and in teaching institutions they may become the primary care physicians. If a hospital is affiliated with an outpatient dialysis center, patients who have end-stage renal disease and are undergoing chronic dialysis treatment are admitted for any of a wide variety of intercurrent illnesses and complications. The house staff frequently have important responsibility for the care of these patients as well. How does one begin the process of evaluating a patient with such laboratory findings? The purpose of this chapter is to provide junior house officers and medical students who are new to nephrology with a method for evaluating this type of patient over the first few days. During this time, most of the critical aspects needed to establish a diagnosis and to formulate a treatment plan can be defined. More detailed consideration of most of the issues surveyed can be found in other chapters of this book.

HISTORY

Medical History

As with the workups of all patients, the history (Table 1–1), physical examination, and appropriate laboratory tests constitute the cornerstone of the initial evaluation. In patients with renal disease, taking a medical history is often the most important step in making a diagnosis. Several questions should be addressed.

History Suggesting Previous Renal Disease

Directly questioning a patient about the presence of previous renal disease (see Table 1–1) may provide essential information, such as urine test results that were positive for albumin and/or blood or serum chemistries revealing elevated levels of BUN and S_{cr}. In many cases, however, renal disease is relatively silent and patients may not have sought medical attention. Therefore, questions need to focus on symptoms that might indicate the presence of chronic renal disease. A poor appetite, weight loss, weakness, and fatigue may be caused by chronic renal disease. Other uremic symptoms include nausea, vomiting, metallic or ammonia taste in the mouth, pruritus, and insomnia. A history of edema, not only of the legs but also of the face and periorbital region, unexplained by other causes, may be evidence of fluid retention due to renal failure. Hypertension often may be the first abnormality discovered in a patient

Table 1–1. MEDICAL HISTORY

A. *Previous evidence of renal disease*
   1. Elevated BUN or creatinine in the past
   2. History of albuminuria or foamy urine, hematuria or dark urine, edema, or urinary tract infections
   3. Previous medical examinations (clinic, private physician, insurance, employment, military, incarceration)
   4. History of hypertension
   5. Lower urinary tract symptoms: urgency, burning, frequency, hesitancy
   6. Oliguria, polyuria, nocturia
   7. History of infections (throat, skin)
   8. Family history of renal disease: polycystic, Alport's (deafness)

B. *History of systemic diseases*
   1. Diabetes mellitus
   2. Collagen vascular diseases: systemic lupus erythematosus, scleroderma, polyarteritis, Sjögren's, Wegener's granulomatosis, Henoch-Schönlein purpura
   3. Malignancy: myeloma, breast, lung, colon, lymphoma
   4. Essential hypertension
   5. Sickle cell disease
   6. Primary or secondary amyloidosis

C. *History of drug exposure*
   1. Nonsteroidal antiinflammatory drugs
   2. Penicillin family drugs
   3. Aminoglycoside therapy
   4. Chemotherapeutic drugs
   5. Narcotic abuse
   6. Recent intake of any new drug that may be temporally associated with renal failure (e.g., angiotensin-converting enzyme inhibitors)
   7. Heavy metal exposure: lead, gold, cadmium

D. *History of factors contributing to prerenal or postrenal azotemia*
   1. Congestive heart failure
   2. Diuretic use
   3. Nausea with vomiting, diarrhea, high fever, gastrointestinal bleeding
   4. Salt-restricted diet
   5. Liver cirrhosis
   6. Lower urinary tract symptoms
   7. Pelvic disease

E. *Uremic symptoms*
   1. Nausea, anorexia, vomiting
   2. Weight loss
   3. Pruritus
   4. Weakness, fatigability
   5. Lethargy, drowsiness

with underlying renal disease. Alternatively, long-standing primary hypertension can be the cause of eventual renal damage, especially in black patients. Therefore, a detailed history about previously observed hypertension, including its severity and duration, is important.

Urologic disease may lead to renal damage; therefore, a history of dysuria, bladder infections, stones, and difficulty initiating urination is important information. Changes in urine volume perceived by a patient, such as oliguria, polyuria, or alternating volumes, can also provide important clues to the diagnosis. Nocturia can be a symptom of loss of concentrating ability due to intrinsic renal disease, whereas partial urinary tract obstruction may cause polyuria alternating with oliguria.

Certain hereditary forms of renal disease (polycystic kidney disease) are common, whereas others are rare. Autosomal dominant polycystic kidney disease (ADPCKD) afflicts males and females equally. It is usually recognized clinically in the fourth or fifth decades of life, although its presentation can be quite variable. Approximately half of all ADPCKD patients progress to renal failure. Patients have an increased risk of occult intracranial aneurysm. The most common and often presenting complaint is intermittent abdominal pain, which is often associated with gross or microscopic hematuria. Hypertension occurs frequently, as do renal infection and lithiasis. Calcifications can develop within both the kidney parenchyma and the urinary collecting system. Anemia, however, is less common than in other types of renal failure. If the history reveals that members of a patient's family have had renal disease, the diagnosis, age of onset, course, gender, and relationship to the patient should be recorded.

History of Systemic Diseases that May Cause Renal Abnormalities

The most common systemic diseases that can lead to renal failure are listed in Table 1–1, part B. In the medical history, special attention should be placed on any evidence of underlying systemic diseases that may affect the kidneys. An example is type 1 or type 2 diabetes mellitus, which can result in diabetic nephropathy. Systemic lupus erythematosus, systemic sclerosis, and various vasculitides including periarteritis nodosa and Henoch-Schönlein purpura can also cause intrinsic renal disease. **In elderly patients, an occult malignancy may be the cause of an immunologically mediated glomerulopathy.** The most common tumors associated with glomerulopathy are those of the breast, lung, and colon. Hodgkin's disease and non-Hodgkin's lymphomas may be associated with obstruction of the ureters. Less frequently, a nephrotic syndrome occurs in the course of lymphomas. Rarely, lymphomas cause renal failure by direct invasion of the kidneys. Multiple myeloma not infrequently first presents with signs and symptoms of recent-onset renal insufficiency.

Drug Exposure

Three major categories of drugs that commonly cause renal insufficiency are non-steroidal antiinflammatory drugs (NSAIDs), the penicillin family of antibiotics, and illicit narcotics (see Table 1–1). NSAIDs can lead to several patterns of renal dysfunction. The most common adverse effects are related to their pharmacologic action (*i.e.*, inhibition of cyclooxygenase-mediated arachidonic acid metabolism). **Acute renal failure can occur with the use of NSAIDs, especially in high-risk groups, including persons with hemodynamic compromise (*e.g.*, volume depletion, congestive heart failure, cirrhosis, and nephrosis) or those with previous renal insufficiency.** The mechanism is decreased levels of vasodilatory prostaglandins, leaving vasoconstrictor hormones unopposed. The course is notable for its rapid onset and frequent hyperkalemia out of proportion to the level of BUN or S_{cr} as a result of hypoaldosteronism. Interstitial nephritis can also occur with prolonged use of these agents, one of the most notable clinical features being heavy albuminuria and the nephrotic syndrome. Now that some NSAIDs can be purchased without a prescription, renal complications will likely be encountered more frequently. Penicillin-related drugs may cause an allergic clinical syndrome that includes rash, eosinophilia, fever, and evidence of acute interstitial nephritis, including pyruria with eosinophils and rising BUN and S_{cr} levels. Intravenous aminoglycosides and certain chemotherapeutic agents are a very common cause of acute renal failure in hospitalized patients. Illicit narcotics taken intravenously or subcutaneously can lead to infectious endocarditis and subsequently to glomerulonephritis. Heroin nephropathy, renal amyloidosis, and nephropathy associated with the acquired immunodeficiency syndrome (AIDS) also can occur from drug abuse. These nephropathies are characterized by nephrotic-range albuminuria. In contrast, cocaine can cause rhabdomyolysis and acute renal failure.

Patients with renal artery stenosis from either atheromatous lesions or fibromuscular hyperplasia involving both renal arteries are at risk for developing acute renal failure when started on angiotensin-converting enzyme (ACE) inhibitors. Renal glomerular filtration, especially in bilaterally stenotic kidneys, depends on high renin-angiotensin levels, which preferentially increase resistance of the efferent arterioles and maintain or raise glomerular hydraulic pressure. ACE inhibitors decrease angiotensin II levels and cause an acute decline in intraglomerular pressure resulting in reduced filtration rate. This can also be noted in patients with atheromatous disease of a solitary kidney or of a transplanted kidney. In most cases, glomerular filtration rate (GFR) is restored after the ACE inhibitor has been discontinued.

History of Conditions that Predispose to Prerenal or Postrenal Azotemia

Abnormal renal function may result from prerenal or postrenal conditions, in either the presence or the absence of intrinsic renal disease (see Table 1–1). The most common prerenal factors are congestive heart failure, diuretic use, diarrhea, vomiting, liver cirrhosis, and a severely salt-restricted diet. Lower urinary tract disease or other postrenal conditions might be suspected if a patient gives a history of dysuria, difficulty in starting urination, frequency, passing blood in the urine, and recurrent urinary tract infections. Previous urologic surgery should also be ascertained.

Uremic Symptoms

Severe renal failure causes anorexia, nausea, and vomiting (see Table 1–1). Weight loss may be related to decreased food intake or to increased catabolism. In some cases, weight gain due to edema may be noted. Generalized weakness and easy fatigability are often associated with azotemia and are largely related to the accompanying anemia. If renal failure is chronic and slowly progressive, patients tend to tolerate the chemical changes and have few symptoms until renal function is severely impaired. On the other hand, rapid development of renal failure causes more severe gastrointestinal and neurologic symptoms. Patients who have markedly elevated BUN and S_{cr} levels and are relatively asymptomatic invariably have long-standing renal impairment.

PHYSICAL EXAMINATION

Physical examination can reveal further clues to the cause and duration of renal functional impairment. Those aspects of the physical examination that should receive special attention are listed in Table 1–2. In particular, evaluating a patient's effective blood volume through determinations of orthostatic changes in blood

Table 1–2. PHYSICAL EXAMINATION

Vital signs
Fever
Blood pressure (hypertension, hypotension)
Volume status
Volume depleted: orthostatic changes in blood pressure and pulse, skin tenting
Fluid overload: jugular venous distension, rales, ascites, edema
Evidence suggesting systemic illness
Skin: malar rash (lupus), purpura (vasculitis, Henoch-Schönlein purpura), macular rash (acute interstitial nephritis), scleroderma
HEENT: alopecia (lupus), uveitis (sarcoid, vasculitis), papilledema (malignant hypertension), icterus, funduscopic examination (diabetic retinopathy, arteriovenous nicking of hypertension), throat infections, hearing loss (Alport's)
Lungs: consolidation (glomerulonephritis secondary to pneumonia)
Heart: murmurs (endocarditis)
Abdomen: bruits (renal artery stenosis), palpable organs (kidneys—polycystic kidney disease)
Extremities: livedo reticulitis (vasculitis), blue-toe syndrome (embolic events), Janeway lesions, Osler's nodes, angiokeratomas
Signs of uremia
Skin: uremic frost, ecchymoses
Heart: pericardial rub
Extremities: asterixis, Trousseau's or Chvostek's signs (Ca^{2+} disorders)
Vital signs: pulsus paradoxus (tamponade)
Lungs: Kussmaul's respirations (metabolic acidosis)
Signs of obstruction
Percussible bladder, enlarged prostate, phimosis

pressure and pulse (decrease in systolic blood pressure >20 mm Hg and/or a rise in pulse ≥10 beats per minute supine vs. upright position) can provide useful information. The skin should be examined for rashes or purpura that might provide evidence of collagen vascular disease or vasculitis. The optic fundi should be examined for lesions resulting from hypertension or diabetic retinopathy. The lung examination may reveal signs of fluid overload. Cardiac evaluation should include listening for the rub of pericarditis. The abdominal examination should include palpation of the kidneys (for polycystic kidney disease) and percussion of the bladder (for obstruction). Auscultating for bruits in the epigastrium and both dorsal flanks is important for the diagnosis of renal artery stenosis, and rectal and pelvic examinations are critical in evaluating possible obstructive disease. Extremities should be examined for signs of edema, vascular insufficiency, embolization, or vasculitis (blue toes, livedo reticularis). Asterixis and Trousseau's or Chvostek's signs should be tested, and the presence of a half-and-half (Lindsay) nail (*i.e.*, the proximal half of the nail is white while the distal half is pink, red, or brown secondary to constriction of venous return) should be sought. A patient's general appearance may also reveal evidence of uremia (uremic frost, ecchymosis, Kussmaul's respiration) and the need for acute intervention. Neurologic examination may reveal mental confusion, drowsiness, or impending coma.

SYMPTOMS AND SIGNS OF RENAL FAILURE

Chronic renal failure can affect many organ systems. The most common signs and symptoms are listed in Table 1–3. Pruritus is one of the most common symptoms of renal failure. It may remit and recur, and its causes are multifactorial, including elevated levels of parathyroid hormone, abnormal calcium and phosphate metabolism, and sebaceous and sweat gland atrophy. Uremia can change skin color to a yellow or yellowish-brown as a result of urochrome or pigmented metabolite accumulation.

The metallic taste and odor of ammonia on the breath are likely due to ammonia liberated from urea by urease-producing bacteria of the mouth. Ammonia may also contribute to esophagitis and gastritis. Gastrointestinal lesions include angiodysplasia, peptic ulcer disease, gastritis, and hemorrhage. The bleeding is further complicated by a coagulopathy owing to platelet dysfunction.

Cardiovascular disease is a major factor contributing to mortality in chronic renal failure. Uremic cardiomyopathy is not a specific or solitary disease but is thought to be multifactorial. These factors include hypertension, hyperlipidemia, uremic toxins, hypervolemia, myocardial calcium deposits, iron overload, electrolyte disturbances, hormone disturbances, and anemia.

Table 1–3. SPECIFIC ORGAN SYMPTOMS AND SIGNS OF CHRONIC RENAL FAILURE

Skin
Pruritus
Soft-tissue calcification
Uremic frost
Gastrointestinal
Stomatitis, parotitis
Metallic or ammonia taste
Upper or lower gastrointestinal hemorrhage (angiodysplasia, peptic ulcer disease, gastritis, coagulopathy)
Cardiovascular (accounts for >50% chronic renal failure-related deaths)
Hypertension
Accelerated atherosclerosis
Cardiomyopathy
Pericarditis
Calcification of medium-sized arteries
Pulmonary
Pulmonary edema
Pulmonary calcification
Pleural effusion (exudative, serosanguineous, or hemorrhagic), pleuritis
Neurologic
Encephalopathy (symptoms include fatigue, drowsiness, insomnia, cognitive changes, asterixis, hiccups, disorientation, and coma)
Subdural hematoma
Muscle cramps
Peripheral neuropathy, sensory and motor
Autonomic: central nervous system dysfunction
Skeletal (renal osteodystrophy)
Osteomalacia (defective mineralization), aluminum related
Osteosclerosis
Osteitis fibrosa: parathyroid hormone related
Growth retardation
Osteoporosis (osteopenia): reduced bone density
Spontaneous tendon rupture (quadriceps, triceps, extensors of the fingers)
Extraskeletal calcification
Corneal and conjunctival
Visceral (heart, lungs, kidneys)
Periarticular

Pericarditis occurs in patients with predialysis renal failure and in patients already receiving maintenance dialysis. It presents clinically as a combination of chest pain, a pericardial friction rub, and/or electrocardiographic (ECG) signs. The chest pain is either constant or pleuritic in character, often relieved by leaning forward. The rub is a rasping, grating, or scratching sound (likened to two pieces of leather rubbing together) most commonly auscultated between the left sternal border and the apex of the heart. It may be heard throughout the cardiac cycle or only during systole. The rub usually disappears with the formation of significant pericardial effusion. The ECG signs of pericarditis may be absent or may be fairly diagnostic, showing elevation of the ST segments in some leads without reciprocal depression in others. This may be followed by temporary or permanent inversion of T waves. The pericardial fluid can be serous, fibrinous, serosanguineous, or hemorrhagic.

Patients who have not previously undergone dialysis usually respond well to aggressive dialysis (*i.e.*, the pericarditis improves significantly or completely resolves). On the other hand, pericarditis developing in a patient undergoing chronic dialysis is less likely to resolve with dialysis alone. In either situation, large pericardial effusions are less likely to resolve with dialysis and may require other intervention. In patients undergoing chronic dialysis, the fluid is often hemorrhagic, possibly from heparin anticoagulation used during hemodialysis. The rate of pericardial fluid accumulation is crucial in determining whether cardiac tamponade will occur. **One must be vigilant in suspecting cardiac tamponade in dialysis patients because the usual clinical signs, such as pulsus paradoxus, distant heart sounds, and hypotension, may not be apparent because of long-standing hypertension and a hypertrophic cardiomyopathy.** Development of hypotension while a patient is being dialyzed may be the initial presenting sign of incipient tamponade. Findings on diagnostic tests, such as the cardiac silhouette on chest radiograph, two-dimensional echocardiogram showing large effusions or right ventricular collapse, and right heart catheterization demonstrating equalization of pressure of the right and left sides of the heart, remain essential for the diagnosis of cardiac tamponade in dialysis patients.

Pulmonary edema is also a common complication in patients with chronic and acute renal failure, both before and while on maintenance hemodialysis. It not only results from salt and water retention, but it also may involve increased pulmonary capillary permeability along with increased transcapillary pressure. Fluid overload must be suspected in patients who have end-stage renal disease and who present with a pulmonary infiltrate on chest radiograph, shortness of breath, or a chronic cough. Fluid removal by dialysis is needed to correct the condition.

Pleural effusions can also occur in patients with chronic renal failure. These are often serosanguineous or hemorrhagic. If thoracentesis is performed, one commonly finds lymphocytosis and elevated levels of lactate dehydrogenase and proteins, consistent with an exudate.

These effusions may decrease with aggressive dialysis, but other causes need to be considered.

Neurologic abnormalities, termed uremic encephalopathy, can occur with either chronic or acute renal failure, and symptoms include sluggishness, drowsiness, fatigue, asterixis, hiccups, disorientation, confusion, slurring of speech, restlessness, memory or cognitive changes, hallucinations, and convulsions or coma. Patients with chronic renal failure are also prone to develop subdural hematomas, likely as a result of their bleeding tendency. Patients may present with sudden headache, nausea, vomiting, loss of consciousness, seizures, or other mental status changes, but in some cases neurologic symptoms may be rather subtle. Any change in mental status in a patient undergoing chronic dialysis should raise the suspicion of a subdural hematoma. A special attempt should be made to identify an initiating factor, such as recent head trauma or excessive anticoagulation during dialysis.

Autonomic and peripheral nerve dysfunction may be another component of uremic neuropathy. Some findings include postural hypotension, peripheral neuropathy (sensory and motor functions), cerebral eighth nerve abnormalities (auditory and vestibular), vision loss, nystagmus, vertigo, and Valsalva's maneuver disturbance.

LABORATORY EVALUATION

Laboratory studies should include a complete chemistry and hematology profile (Table 1–4). Chronic renal failure is suggested by a constellation of findings, including elevated BUN and S_{cr} levels, hypocalcemia, hyperphosphatemia, hyperkalemia, hyperuricemia, acidemia, hypoalbuminuria, anemia, and hyperlipidemia. Because these serum abnormalities can also occur in acute renal failure, it is essential to combine the laboratory data with a concise medical history, physical examination, microscopic urinalysis, and, at times, a renal biopsy to determine if a patient has chronic or acute renal failure.

Urinalysis. A urinalysis performed by a physician can provide essential information. A specific gravity of $\leq$1.010 is consistent with a concentrating defect. A urinary pH >6.5 raises the question of urinary tract infection with a urea-splitting organism or an acidification defect. Heavy proteinuria determined by dipstick usually represents an abnormality in the glomerular filtration barrier, because the dipstick predominantly measures albumin. The sulfosalicylic acid test detects all types of proteins. Proteinuria may also result from excretion of protein present in distal tubules (Tamm-Horsfall protein), reduced tubular absorption of normally filtered low-molecular-weight proteins, or overwhelming filtration of light-chain proteins (kappa and lambda). In normal individuals, albumin constitutes only a fraction of the total protein measured in a 24-hour urine collection.

Microscopic examination should be carried out on freshly voided urine (*i.e.*, within 30 minutes after voiding). Casts deteriorate when urine is stored, especially if the pH is alkaline, and important diagnostic information can be missed. Ten milliliters of urine should be centrifuged for 5 minutes, and the supernatant poured off into another tube that is sent to the laboratory for analysis of protein, sodium, creatinine, and osmolality. The sediment is resuspended, transferred to a slide, and covered with a coverslip. The presence of urinary casts, although often nonspecific, can provide evidence of intrinsic renal disease, as opposed to prerenal or postrenal failure. These casts include granular (representing cellular debris), waxy (derived from tubular epithelial cells), hyaline (predominantly albumin), and broad casts (secondary to tubular hypertrophy from nephron loss). Fat may occur in the urine as oval fat bodies, free droplets, or in casts and is characteristic of the nephrotic syndrome. Fat exhibits birefringence under polarized light (Maltese crosses). Hematuria and especially dysmorphic red blood cells (RBCs) suggest glomerular inflammation, and RBC casts are definite evidence of active glomerulonephritis. Crystals can also be found in the urine and may give insight into congenital or acquired disorders. These include calcium oxalate (most common), calcium phosphate, uric acid, cystine, and tyrosine crystals.

There are certain pitfalls to be alert for when using dipsticks for urinalysis. These are outlined in the paragraphs that follow.

Albuminuria. In general, a dipstick reading of 1+ = 30 mg/dl, 2+ = 100 mg/dl, 3+ = 300 mg/dl, and 4+ = >2 g/dl. However, the specific gravity is very important in interpreting the dipstick value, because 1+ in dilute urine represents a greater absolute amount of protein than 1+ in highly concentrated urine. False-positive readings may occur with highly buffered or alkaline urine, or with urine contaminated with quaternary ammonium compounds or chlorhexidine (as found in antiseptics and

Table 1–4. LABORATORY TESTS

	Prerenal	Acute tubular necrosis
Urinalysis		
Specific gravity		
Proteinuria		
Hematuria		
Pyuria		
Sediment—casts, crystals		
Chemistry profile		
Electrolytes, BUN, creatinine, total protein, albumin, glucose, liver function tests, creatine phosphokinase, cholesterol, calcium, phosphorus		
Hematology profile		
White blood cell count		
Hematocrit		
Platelets		
Urine electrolyte profile	*Prerenal*	*Acute tubular necrosis*
$Fe_{Na} = (U/P_{Na} \div U/P_{cr}) \times 100$	<1%	>3%
Renal failure index = $U_{Na} \div U/P_{cr}$	<1	>1
U_{osm}	>500	<320
Urine specific gravity	>1.015	<1.010
BUN/creatinine ratio of plasma	>15/1	<10/1
Ultrasonography of kidneys and ureters		
Size of kidneys		
Cysts		
Obstruction		
Postvoiding sonogram of bladder		

certain skin cleansers, respectively). Dissociation between the 24-hour protein excretion and the dipstick reading (*i.e.*, higher excretion than expected from the dipstick) raises the suspicion of light-chain proteins in the urine. Immunoelectrophoresis of the urine and plasma should be carried out if myeloma or other light-chain disorders are suspected.

Specific Gravity. A measurement of specific gravity by dipstick has recently been introduced. This test is based on the pKa change of pretreated polyelectrolytes in relation to ionic concentrations of the urine. Dipsticks can show falsely low specific gravity with highly buffered alkaline urine and falsely elevated specific gravity readings in the presence of moderate amounts (100 to 750 mg/dl) of protein. Although dipstick evaluation generally agrees with a refractometer or hygrometer, these latter instruments are preferred. The specific gravity of the urine is increased by the presence of large amounts of glucose or by radiocontrast agents. The intrinsic ability of the kidneys to concentrate urine is obscured under these conditions.

pH. It is important to be aware that if a dipstick is left in the urine too long, runover may occur (*i.e.*, acid buffer from the protein reagent will run onto the pH area, causing a false lowering of the pH). Thus, the dipstick should be removed quickly. Also, bilirubin in the urine can obscure the color reaction of various tests on the dipstick.

Prerenal and Postrenal Failure. Urine examination is also important in diagnosing prerenal and postrenal failure. Prerenal failure is most often due to a decrease in renal perfusion, encountered in patients with volume contraction, congestive heart failure, cirrhosis with ascites, or systemic vascular dilatation as in sepsis. Urinalysis may show a specific gravity of 1.020 or higher and U_{osm} above 500 mOsm, with at most a few cells and little or no protein. Thus, an essentially negative urinalysis in a patient with azotemia is an important piece of diagnostic information. Urinary sodium concentration is often <10 mEq/L and FE_{Na} is <1%. FE_{Na} is easily calculated from the following equation:

$$FE_{Na} = [U/P_{Na}/U/P_{cr}] \times 100$$

That is, fractional excretion of sodium, expressed as a percent, is the quotient of urine and plasma sodium concentration divided by the quotient of urine and plasma creatinine concentration, **in the same units,** all multiplied by 100.

Careful fluid administration with appropriate monitoring may be all that is needed to restore BUN and S_{cr} levels to normal.

Postrenal failure is caused by obstruction anywhere along the urinary tract, but to result in azotemia it must be bilateral, or the contralateral kidney must be diseased. Common causes are prostatic enlargement, neurogenic bladder (functional obstruction), retroperitoneal fibrosis, and pelvic or retroperitoneal malignancies.

Acute tubular necrosis can be caused by a large number of drugs and clinical conditions. Urinalysis is often helpful in establishing the diagnosis. In the typical case, urine sodium concentration is >40 mEq/L, U_{osm} is isosmotic, and the urine sediment may reveal renal tubular cells. In acute renal failure due to myoglobinuria or hemoglobinuria, muddy brown casts may be seen in the urine, the heme test is positive, but few or no RBCs are seen in the spun sediment. Thus, a positive heme test result in the absence of RBCs in the urine is very suggestive of acute myoglobinuria or hemoglobinuria.

Imaging Techniques

Noninvasive imaging techniques can be used to evaluate renal morphology and to determine the cause of the renal disease. Renal sonography that shows small kidneys is consistent with chronic parenchymal renal disease. Increased echogenicity can be seen with either chronic or acute renal failure. Large or normal-size kidneys (>11 cm) may denote acute renal failure or chronic renal failure due to certain systemic diseases such as diabetes, amyloidosis, AIDS, or infiltrative diseases (lymphoma or leukemia). Acute renal failure is often associated with normal-size kidneys. Hydronephrosis is usually apparent on ultrasound examination. Asymmetry can be a clue to atherosclerotic disease of a renal artery (renal artery stenosis) or previous infection of the kidneys that was more severe on one side than the other. Ultrasonography is the initial test of choice for diagnosis of cystic disease of the kidneys and for obstruction, but it is also useful for detecting renal calculi (radiopaque and radiolucent).

Renal radionuclide scan using either radioisotope-labeled diethylenetriamene pentaacetic acid (DTPA) or hippurate can assess glomerular filtration (DTPA), renal plasma flow (hippurate), arterial occlusion, and outflow obstruction. In contrast to ultrasonography, radionuclide scan is a functional test that allows comparison of the function of the two kidneys as well as overall function. Differences in function may be due to vascular occlusion, intrinsic parenchymal disease, or unilateral outflow obstruction.

Invasive angiography can be used to assess the anatomy of the renal vasculature if ultrasonography, computed tomography (CT), or radionuclide scan suggests renal artery stenosis or a renal neoplasm. Since the advent of noninvasive ultrasonography, noncontrast CT, and radionuclide studies, intravenous pyelography (IVP) is being used less often because of the potential risk of dye-induced contrast nephropathy. The risk is quite small, however, and IVP is still very useful in detecting anatomic abnormalities of the renal calyces, collecting ducts (medullary sponge kidney), and papillary necrosis. The most direct diagnostic test in determining the cause of intrinsic parenchymal disease is a renal biopsy, which is usually performed only if the kidneys are normal size or large, rather than shrunken.

PATIENT MANAGEMENT

Many patients with chronic renal disease are relatively asymptomatic in spite of significantly reduced GFR (<25 to 30 ml/min). They can be managed by dietary modification and specific medications to deal with metabolic disturbances, fluid balance, blood pressure control, and hematologic abnormalities. This management may slow the progression of renal disease or at least prevent some of the complications of chronic renal failure. Dietary modifications include restriction of protein, phosphate, potassium, magnesium, sodium, and water, as outlined in Table 1–5.

Medical therapy can also assist in the management of hypocalcemia, hyperphosphatemia, fluid overload, elevated blood pressure, acidemia, renal osteodystrophy, and anemia. Calcium supplements increase the serum calcium concentration when taken *between* meals, elevate serum bicarbonate (if given as $CaCO_3$), and lower the serum phosphate concentration when taken *with* meals. Aluminum-containing antacids bind phosphorus in the gut and lower serum phosphate when taken *with* meals. Their use is decreasing in practice because with prolonged ingestion there is increased risk of bone and central nervous system aluminum toxicity. The vitamin D metabolite 1,25 $(OH)_2$ D_3, when given intravenously, can help in the treatment of hyperparathyroidism secondary to renal disease, as it acts directly on the parathyroid glands to inhibit parathyroid hormone synthesis.

Fluid retention due to diminished GFR can contribute to hypertension and life-threatening fluid overload (congestive heart failure, acute pulmonary edema). Diuretics such as furosemide, ethacrynic acid, bumetanide, and metolazone can increase urine output even when the GFR is <25 ml/min. Much higher doses than usual may be required and are more effective when given in single rather than divided doses.

Table 1–5. MANAGEMENT OF CHRONIC RENAL FAILURE (RECOMMENDATIONS)

Dietary modification
- Protein restriction: 0.6–0.8 g/kg/day (long-term effects under investigation)
- Phosphate restriction
- Potassium: 2 g/day
- Magnesium restriction: avoid magnesium-containing antacids
- Sodium restriction: not absolute and depends on individual case, usually 2–4 g/day.
- Water restriction: individualize—1000 ml plus urine output.

Medical therapy
- Calcium replacement (Tums, Os-cal) calcium carbonate tablets
  - Starting dose: 650 mg t.i.d.–q.i.d.
  - To ↑ Ca^{2+}: take between meals
  - To ↓ PO_4: take with meals (binds PO_4)

Aluminum-containing antacids (Amphojel, Basaljel)
- Starting dose: 15–30 ml orally t.i.d.–q.i.d., take with meals

Vitamin D analogue (Rocaltrol, Calcijex in intravenous form)
- Starting oral dose: 0.125 μg–0.250 μg

Diuretics
- Furosemide (Lasix 80–400 mg orally)
- Ethacrynic acid (Edecrin 25–200 mg orally)
- Bumetanide (Bumex 0.5–2.0 mg orally)
- Metolazone (2.5–10 mg orally)

Antihypertensive therapy
- Angiotensin-converting enzyme inhibitors
- Calcium channel blockers
- α-blockers
- β-blockers
- α_2 agonists

Anemia
- Iron: replacement therapy once dialysis is started
- Folate: replacement therapy once dialysis is started
- Recombinant erythropoietin: drug of choice

Additional blood pressure control is often needed, but the specific drugs used depend on the individual patient. Drugs that tend to decrease potassium excretion, such as potassium-sparing diuretics and ACE inhibitors, should be avoided because severe hyperkalemia may develop. If an ACE inhibitor is given to treat hypertension, a loop diuretic should also be prescribed and serum potassium should be carefully monitored.

Metabolic acidosis is also common in chronic renal failure, and serum bicarbonate levels <20 mEq/L can be treated with either $NaHCO_3$ or $CaCO_3$ tablets. Caution is advised, because elevating the blood pH may increase calcium binding to serum albumin and decrease the free ionized calcium level, thus exacerbating hypocalcemia and possibly precipitating tetany.

The anemia of chronic renal failure has been of much concern to nephrologists and patients because of its consequences: weakness, fatigue, exacerbation of angina and arrhythmias, and risks from multiple transfusions (hepatitis, human immunodeficiency virus infection, and transfusion reaction). Iron, folate, and vitamin B_{12} deficiency should be looked for, but in predialysis patients, unless previous deficiency existed, replacement of these factors does little to improve the anemia. Iron and folate supplements are prescribed after a patient has been started on hemodialysis treatment, to replace losses due to this therapy. Human recombinant erythropoietin (r-hEPO) has been shown in numerous trials to completely correct the anemia of renal failure in a dose-dependent fashion and will certainly make a major contribution to patient well-being in the near future. However, the rising hematocrit may exacerbate hypertension, presumably as a result of increased blood viscosity. Other side effects of the rise in hematocrit are clotting of an arteriovenous fistula, need for increased time on dialysis because less plasma flows through the dialyzer per unit time, and development of iron deficiency as iron is utilized for new RBC production.

INDICATIONS FOR DIALYSIS

There comes a time when conservative measures will no longer be sufficient to maintain adequate well-being. At some point, renal replacement therapy becomes necessary. The choices are hemodialysis, peritoneal dialysis, or transplantation. **The major nonurgent indications for starting dialysis** (Table 1–6) in patients with slowly progressing disease are as follows:

1. **Uremic symptoms.** These are most often manifested as anorexia and vomiting, but cognitive changes are also common although more subtle. One should consider other causes of changing mental status before attributing them to uremia. Intrinsic bowel disease should be considered in the differential diagnosis of uremic vomiting, especially diabetic gastropathy.
2. **Difficult-to-control hypertension.** In many

Table 1–6. INDICATIONS FOR DIALYSIS

Nonurgent indications
- Uremic symptoms
- Difficult to control hypertension
- Fluid overload, congestive heart failure
- Preoperative preparation

Urgent indications
- Pericarditis
- Hyperkalemia with ECG changes
- Pulmonary edema
- Severe metabolic acidosis
- Drug overdose

patients with chronic renal failure, salt and water retention is an important factor contributing to their hypertension. Instituting dialysis therapy often reduces blood pressure and lessens or eliminates the need for antihypertensive drugs.

In addition to these, **urgent indications** (see Table 1–6) **for dialysis** arise in patients who have or have not been previously dialyzed:

1. **Pericarditis.** When this occurs in a patient who has not previously been dialyzed, it is an indication for instituting hemodialysis. Accumulation of a large pericardial effusion in a patient already on dialysis may not respond to more intensive dialysis, although this is usually tried first. Other therapeutic interventions such as needle aspiration, drug instillation, and surgery may be required.
2. **Hyperkalemia.** Especially when it occurs in patients unresponsive to conservative measures, such as diuretics, $NaHCO_3$, insulin plus glucose, and cation-exchange resins, hyperkalemia is an indication for prompt hemodialysis. ECG changes, progressing from peaked and narrowed T waves to widening QRS complex, loss of P waves or sine wave pattern, are even more urgent indications for hemodialysis.
3. **Fluid overload** leading to cardiac compromise and pulmonary edema.
4. **Severe metabolic acidosis.** In oliguric or anuric patients, bicarbonate administration may not be possible because of the threat of pulmonary edema. Hemodialysis can both remove fluid and restore serum bicarbonate levels in a short time.
5. **Drug overdose.** Dialysis is used as therapy for certain drug overdoses depending on their protein binding and water/lipid solubility. Hemodialysis has been used for lithium, salicylate, methanol, ethylene glycol, and bromide overdose that is unresponsive to other therapy. Charcoal filter hemoperfusion is more effective than hemodialysis for theophylline and barbiturate overdose.

CHOICE OF DIALYSIS MODALITY

The choice of the mode of dialysis depends on multiple factors (Table 1–7). In the acute situation, if rapid fluid removal or electrolyte correction is needed and a patient is hemodynamically stable, hemodialysis is preferred. On the other hand, if a patient is hemodynamically unstable or the time factor is less crucial, peritoneal dialysis may be an appropriate choice.

Table 1–7. CHOICE OF MODE OF DIALYSIS

Hemodialysis
Rapid fluid removal
Rapid electrolyte correction
Risks: hemodynamic instability, initial electrolyte disequilibrium, bleeding from heparin, catheter-induced sepsis, thrombosis
Peritoneal dialysis
Fluid and electrolyte correction is slower
Most useful in hemodynamically unstable patients
Risks: peritonitis, tunnel infections
Continuous arteriovenous hemofiltration
Dependent on adequate blood pressure (systolic > 80–90 mm Hg)
Useful in hemodynamically unstable patients who have contraindications to both hemodialysis and peritoneal dialysis
Difficult to set up and maintain without clotting of filter
Risks: clotting, infection, thrombosis, and bleeding

Either an acute stylet catheter or chronic Tenckhoff's catheter can be placed to initiate peritoneal dialysis. An acute stylet catheter is very useful in patients with acute renal failure that is expected to resolve, whereas a surgically introduced Tenckhoff's catheter is used when more prolonged peritoneal dialysis is anticipated. An acute catheter should be replaced or removed after approximately 3 days. Peritoneal dialysis is an effective means of dialysis for clearance and ultrafiltration, although fluid and electrolyte correction is slower than with hemodialysis. Continuous arteriovenous hemofiltration (CAVH) is a relatively new type of dialysis that has generally been used for short-term problems in hemodynamically unstable patients who have contraindications to, or failure with, use of hemodialysis or peritoneal dialysis. CAVH has been used mostly for removal of large amounts of fluid in patients with fluid overload and renal insufficiency. The procedure can be carried out by trained personnel in an intensive care unit. This process involves diverting arterial blood through a small artificial kidney filter. The filter has both arterial and venous ports, located on opposite sides, for connection to a large artery (*i.e.*, femoral, subclavian) and a major vein (*i.e.*, femoral, subclavian, jugular). The blood flows through the kidney filter and back through the venous system. The ultrafiltrate is removed through a drain port. This mode of dialysis is predominantly flow dependent. Systolic blood pressure of at least 80 to 90 mm Hg is usually required for its function; otherwise the system will clot, even with heparin used locally or systemically. If adequate blood pressure is maintained, large amounts of fluid can be removed by ultrafiltration. Because serum protein concentrations rise during CAVH, intravascular volume is maintained by their colloid oncotic pressure effect. Thus, fluid is drawn into the vascular compartment as ultrafiltrate is being removed by the kidney filter.

In the case of nonurgent dialysis, patients should play a central role in the choice of therapy, although practical considerations often limit the choice. Self-care treatment by continuous ambulatory peritoneal dialysis (CAPD) is a satisfactory method for many patients, as it allows a more liberal diet and fluid intake than is possible with in-center hemodialysis. Patients also have greater flexibility of private time and movement than is possible with in-center hemodialysis.

For eligible patients, renal transplantation is believed by many to be the treatment of choice, because not only the excretory function of the kidneys is replaced, but also the endocrine function.

The pros and cons of each of the modalities of replacement therapy are complex and beyond the scope of this brief introductory chapter. Each type of treatment has its advocates, but each can be highly successful or can fail miserably in individual patients.

COMPLICATIONS OF DIALYSIS

Complications related to the mode of dialysis must be considered. Peritoneal dialysis-associated complications include peritonitis, tunnel and exit site infections, fibrin clots in the catheter, blockage against the peritoneal wall, and external catheter cracking. Chemical peritonitis may also occur, characterized by abdominal pain, ileus, and high white blood cell count, with increased numbers of eosinophils in the dialysis fluid but sterile cultures.

Hemodialysis-associated complications are diverse, but commonly encountered ones include muscle cramps, infected access with or without bacteremia, clotted access, stenosis of the arteriovenous fistula, hemodynamic instability, and disequilibrium syndrome.

CASE SUMMARY 1

A 73-year-old black man with a past medical history of chronic renal insufficiency, diabetes mellitus (type 2), hypertension, diabetic retinopathy, and coronary artery disease presented to the emergency room with complaints of increasing shortness of breath, nausea, vomiting, and reduced urine output noted during the past week. Physical examination revealed moderate respiratory distress, blood pressure of 180/100 mm Hg, jugular vein distention, bilateral rales, and 3+ leg edema. Chest radiography revealed congestive heart failure, and the ECG showed peaked T waves. The arterial blood gases were pH 7.22, pCO_2 28 mm Hg, pO_2 60 mm Hg. SMA 6 results were as follows: sodium 135 mM/L, potassium 6.8 mM/L, chloride 100 mM/L, HCO_3 10 mM/L, BUN 120 mg/dl, creatinine 9.8 mg/dl, and glucose 400 mg/dl. Urinalysis showed 4+ proteinuria and some granular casts.

The patient presented with congestive heart failure, which was most likely due to progressive renal failure and fluid overload from diabetes mellitus. This is suggested by the hyperglycemia, diabetic retinopathy, 4+ proteinuria, and long-standing renal disease. The heart failure was treated with increasing doses of intravenous furosemide, oxygen, and nitrates. Because of the ECG changes, the hyperkalemia was treated with intravenous calcium gluconate, insulin, glucose, and $NaHCO_3$. Kayexalate was given by retention enema. Subsequent hemodialysis was performed to remove fluid, relieve respiratory distress, and improve oxygenation. Workup in the hospital confirmed irreversible end-stage renal disease, and the patient was prepared for chronic maintenance hemodialysis.

CASE SUMMARY 2

A 30-year-old white woman who was a jogger and had previously been in good health presented to the emergency room with confusion, hypotension, and brownish-red urine. She had just completed a 6-mile run on a hot, humid summer day. Physical examination revealed anhidrosis, hyperpyrexia (40.6°C, 105°F), hypotension (blood pressure 80/50 mm Hg), tachycardia, and altered mental status. Laboratory data revealed sodium 145 mM/L, chloride 105 mM/L, potassium 6 mM/L, HCO_3 19 mM/L, Ca^{2+} 8 mg/dl, PO_4 6 mg/dl, uric acid 10 mg/dl, BUN 50 mg/dl, creatinine 3 mg/dl, and creatine phosphokinase 20,000 units. Urinalysis showed 4+ heme, 1+ protein, 3 to 5 RBCs per high-power field, and muddy brown pigmented casts. CBC showed a white blood cell count of 12,000 mm^3, hematocrit of 42%, and platelet count of 50,000 mm^3. The FE_{Na} was 3%.

The patient had rhabdomyolysis and myoglobinuria, as suggested by the history and the findings of 4+ heme in the urine but only a few RBCs and the markedly elevated creatine phosphokinase. Although previous medical records were not available, it was assumed that she had been healthy until the day of admission and that the elevated BUN, creatinine, uric acid, potassium, and phosphorus levels represented rapid changes due to skeletal muscle release as well as impaired renal function. The low plasma bicarbonate concentration was most likely due to metabolic acidosis secondary to increased lactic acid production (anion gap was 21 mEq/L), but because blood gases were not obtained, a respiratory alkalosis component could not be excluded. Thrombocytopenia is frequently encountered in these patients, being a component of a coagulopathy. The patient was treated promptly with fluid replacement (0.9% NaCl intravenously, then 5% dextrose plus three to four ampules of $NaHCO_3$ at a rate of 200 ml/hr). The renal sonogram revealed normal-appearing kidneys, and the renal scan showed reduced uptake and slowed excretion bilaterally. She remained oliguric for the next several days despite correction of hypotension and adequate hydration. Her BUN and creatinine levels continued to rise, indicating that acute renal failure had resulted from the rhabdomyolysis. She received hemodialysis treatments by femoral catheterization on two occasions for acute tubular necrosis. After 6 days, urine output increased, and during the following 4 days, the BUN and creatinine levels declined toward normal. She made a complete recovery of renal function.

Suggested Readings

Eknoyan G, Knochel JP: The Systemic Consequences of Renal Failure. Grune & Stratton, Orlando, 1984.

Lippman RW: Urine and the Urinary Sediment—A Practical Manual and Atlas. Springfield, IL, Charles C Thomas, 1957.

CHAPTER 2

HEMATURIA, PROTEINURIA, AND NEPHROTIC SYNDROME

Cecil H. Coggins

DETECTION OF HEMATURIA OR PROTEINURIA

Hematuria or proteinuria is generally detected through urinalysis. The dipsticks most frequently used for this purpose detect blood by a pseudoperoxidase reaction. A positive reaction reflects the presence of the heme structure and does not differentiate clearly among red blood cells (RBCs), free hemoglobin, and myoglobin. Examination of the urine sediment will detect the presence of abnormal numbers of RBCs. Variability in a patient's urine flow rate, the volume centrifuged, the time and speed of the centrifugation, the volume used to suspend the sediment, and the magnification of the microscope objective and eyepiece make the measurement imprecise, but presence of more than three to four RBCs per high-power field is considered abnormal.

The proteinuria test square on the dipstick contains a pH color indicator dye buffered by citric acid at pH 3.5. Albumin influences the dye to show a color, falsely indicating a higher pH, which can be read as +, + +, or + + + proteinuria. Errors are possible in this measurement. Globulins and light chains have a much weaker effect in changing the indicator color and may not be detected by dipstick measurement.

Prolonged immersion of the dipstick in the urine sample, or its use in strongly alkaline urine, might overcome the buffering ability of the citric acid. An alkaline color would register on the dipstick and be erroneously interpreted as proteinuria. The dipstick should be dipped just long enough to wet it thoroughly.

HEMATURIA

CASE SUMMARY 1 (introduction)

A 32-year-old physician finishes the Boston marathon and soon after comes to the aid station reporting he has just passed dark red urine. He is unusually muscular for a distance runner and has finished well back in the pack. The day is rather warm. You are the aid station physician. How will you investigate his problem?

Gross and Microscopic Hematuria

Gross hematuria may appear pink, red, or the color of tea or cola. A few drops of blood will color a liter of urine distinctly red, and hematuria ordinarily does not represent serious blood loss. With smaller quantities of RBCs, the urine looks normal grossly, and only microscopic hematuria is present. Urine may also occasionally appear reddish from precipitated urate crystals, from the ingestion of beets, from porphyria, or from certain drug metabolites. The urinalysis dipstick registers positive for blood, hemoglobin, or myoglobin.

Approach to the Patient

When the dipstick examination is positive for blood, it is first necessary to differentiate among hematuria, hemoglobinuria, and myoglobinuria. The presence of large numbers of RBCs in the urine sediment establishes the diagnosis of hematuria. If only small numbers are present or if the dipstick is more strongly positive than would be expected from the number of RBCs per high-power field, then the possibility of hemoglobinuria or myoglobinuria should be considered.

Hemoglobinuria

Free hemoglobin results from rupture or leakage of RBCs. This may happen in the urinary tract when bleeding occurs into very dilute urine and the cells rupture osmotically. The hemolysis may occur intravascularly from trauma (*e.g.*, aortic valve replacement), immunologic factors, or other causes. A low serum haptoglobin level and the presence of free serum hemoglobin will aid in the diagnosis. The intact hemoglobin tetramer is too large to be easily filtered at the glomeruli. The dimer and monomer components are filtered and reassembled in the urine.

Myoglobinuria

Myoglobin is released into the blood after muscle damage. Comparable to the hemoglobin monomer, it is quickly filtered and is not found circulating in the blood, even with massive rhabdomyolysis. Serum elevations of muscle enzymes such as creatine phosphokinase and aldolase will be clues to the diagnosis. Differentiating myoglobin from hemoglobin in the urine is difficult but can be done by radioimmunoassay or enzyme-linked immunoassay (ELISA).

Glomerular vs. Nonglomerular Hematuria

When the presence of RBCs in the urine has been established, it is extremely useful to distinguish glomerular from nonglomerular sources. If the origin can confidently be assigned to the glomeruli or to a location high in the renal tubules, lower tract workup (*e.g.*, cystoscopy, intravenous urogram, computed tomography scans, ultrasonography studies, arteriography) need not be performed. Four clues help in this determination. A physician must look at the urine sediment and be skillful in its interpretation. Laboratory technicians are unable to give to a single specimen the time and attention necessary to search for RBC casts (Table 2–1).

Red Blood Cell Casts. The presence of RBCs in casts formed in the renal tubules establishes a glomerular or proximal tubular source. The significance of the finding is great enough that an observer must be absolutely sure that (1) the structure seen is a cast, not a clump or streak of mucus and (2) that the RBCs are within the cast and not simply stuck on its surface. Although not as specific as RBC casts, epithelial cell or leukocyte casts or numerous granular casts would suggest renal disease and a probable renal source for the RBCs.

Dysmorphic Red Blood Cells. When hematuria results from glomerular disease, a large fraction of the cells in the urine are smaller than circulating RBCs and have visible defects in their membranes, often with irregular protrusions. These are visible under high power by light microscopy but are more clearly evident by phase-contrast microscopy. The passage of such cells through the glomerular membrane and through the changes in osmolarity, pH, and enzymatic environment in different portions of the nephron apparently produces these effects, which are not seen when the bleeding source is the prostate, bladder, ureter, or renal pelvis.

Accompanying Proteinuria. If a dipstick shows more than trace or 1+ proteinuria, probably renal disease is present and is the source of the hematuria.

Three-Glass Test (particularly for males). Three urine collection containers are labeled "1," "2," and "3." A patient is asked to collect

Table 2–1. INVESTIGATING HEMATURIA FLOW SHEET

If positive "blood" on urinalysis dipstick test, then centrifuge with examination of sediment by *physician*
If numerous red blood cells (RBCs) appear in the sediment, then hematuria is present. Check for RBC casts, other cellular casts, dysmorphic RBCs, and accompanying proteinuria. Consider performing the three-glass test.
If cells are of renal origin, check glomerular diseases (Table 2–5). Although less likely, interstitial diseases (Table 2–4) are also possible causes.
If cells are of lower urinary tract origin, check for infection, stone, tumor.
If few or no RBCs are present in the sediment, then consider hemoglobinuria, myoglobinuria, or the hemolysis of RBCs in dilute urine (look for RBC "ghosts"). Differentiate hemoglobinuria from myoglobinuria by history, physical examination, serum creatine phosphokinase, aldolase, haptoglobin, and free hemoglobin or urine radioimmunoassay for myoglobin.

during a single continuous voiding the first few milliliters in container 1, then the bulk in 2, and the last few milliliters in 3. If the concentration of RBCs in glass 1 or 3 is considerably higher than in 2, a bleeding source in the urethra or prostate is suspected.

Nonglomerular Hematuria

If the careful urinalysis just described suggests a nonglomerular source of the RBCs, the causes listed in Table 2–2 should be considered.

Approach to the Patient. Obtain a urine culture. If history and physical examination do not strongly suggest the cause, obtain renal imaging. Although ultrasonography and abdominal CT can be helpful, in patients with normal renal function an intravenous urogram is likely to give more useful information about structure *and* function. Urologic consultation may be required for further diagnosis and therapy. A careful search for malignancies is particularly important for patients older than 50 years.

Massive Hematuria. Massive hematuria occasionally produces anemia or shock due to blood loss. The urine registers significant hemoglobin or hematocrit levels and usually contains clots. The cause is found in the lower tract (often tumor) or in a vascular malformation in the kidney. An immediate urologic consultation is usually indicated. Patients sometimes have recurrent massive bleeding that stops suddenly before the source can be found. In such cases, prearranging for immediate renal arteriography to be done at the time of the next bleeding episode is wise.

Glomerular Hematuria

With Accompanying Proteinuria. If proteinuria accompanies the hematuria, the diseases listed in Table 2–5 should be considered; investigation and treatment are discussed in the section on proteinuria.

With Little or No Proteinuria. The following types of glomerular disease should be considered:

IgA nephropathy (Berger's disease)

Hereditary nephritis (including Alport's disease, with associated nerve deafness and cataract formation)

Poststreptococcal or other postinfectious glomerulonephritis

Systemic vasculitis, infection, or connective tissue disease such as lupus, Henoch-Schönlein purpura, bacterial endocarditis, hepatitis B

These diseases can also present in more severe forms with substantial proteinuria.

Approach to the Patient. A carefully taken history should include inquiries about streptococcal or other infection and family history of renal disease, cataracts, or deafness. Physical examination should devote particular attention to the eyes and ears, nails, patellae, rashes, and spots. Laboratory studies might include, as appropriate, antinuclear antibody, anti-DNase B, hepatitis B surface antigen, blood culture, complement, circulating immune complexes, and antineutrophil cytoplasmic antibodies.

Management. In general, when both hematuria and proteinuria are present, the prognosis of the glomerular disease correlates most closely with the quantity of proteinuria. Thus, patients with normal serum creatinine and with hematuria and 0, trace, or 1+ proteinuria (corresponding to <1 g/day), no matter which underlying pathology is present, tend to remain stable for long periods. No specific therapy is generally recommended for this group.

Periodic urinalysis for hematuria and proteinuria, blood pressure assessment, and serum creatinine determinations will provide warning of advancing disease. (Note that minimal change nephrotic syndrome may have a favorable prognosis despite large quantities of proteinuria. It rarely has much hematuria, however.)

Despite careful examination, a significant fraction of cases of hematuria remain unexplained.

Table 2–2. SOURCES OF NONGLOMERULAR HEMATURIA

Infection: cystitis, pyelonephritis (including tuberculosis), urethritis, prostatitis. Pyuria is usually present.
Tumor: of bladder, ureter, renal pelvis, prostrate, or kidney.
Stone: of kidney or bladder.
Kidney disease: polycystic kidney or sickle cell nephropathy.
Trauma to kidney or bladder.
Bleeding diathesis; disease or iatrogenic. Note that anticoagulation may provoke bleeding from an organic lesion in the urinary tract.
Vascular malformation/arteriovenous aneurysm of kidney or collecting system.

CASE SUMMARY 1 (continued)

As you examine the runner, you consider myoglobinuria from anterior tibial compartment ischemia or rhabdomyolysis from heat stroke; hemoglobinuria from traumatic hemolysis of RBCs in the feet; and hematuria from the anterior and posterior bladder walls rubbing against each other during the run, among other causes. Investigation discloses no fever, positive dipstick for blood, no RBCs in the sediment, normal serum muscle enzymes, and abnormally low levels of serum haptoglobin. You diagnose hemolysis, prescribe running shoes with more generous metatarsal and heel padding, and arrange a follow-up appointment.

PROTEINURIA AND THE NEPHROTIC SYNDROME

CASE SUMMARY 2 (introduction)

A 65-year-old woman comes to you because of fatigue, weight loss, bone pain, and ankle swelling. She is pale and edematous on examination, and the urinalysis dipstick is strongly positive for protein. How will you proceed?

When proteinuria is detected on dipstick urinalysis (see the section on urinalysis, above), it is wise to check the finding with a heat and acetic acid test or a sulfosalicylic acid test for protein. These tests are better in estimating quantities of proteinuria and also detect Bence Jones protein more accurately. The sulfosalicylic acid test may give false-positive results with metabolites of the penicillins, aspirin, oral hypoglycemia agents, or other drugs.

Glomerular Proteinuria

Glomerular proteinuria occurs when glomerular capillary walls are damaged and become permeable to serum proteins. In some types of glomerulonephritis, the membrane disruption allows albumin, serum globulins, and even RBCs to pass into the urine. In others, a more limited and specific loss of fixed negative electrical charges on membrane surfaces allows a more selective loss of negatively charged albumin molecules. (When proteinuria consists almost exclusively of albumin, it is called *selective* and is particularly characteristic of minimal change nephropathy.)

Nephrotic Syndrome

Nephrotic syndrome (or nephrosis) is a term used to describe clinical situations in which there is loss of large amounts of albumin. The loss of albumin leads to hypoalbuminemia, which is followed by edema, hyperlipidemia, and lipiduria. The combination of these elements constitutes nephrotic syndrome. The presence of the entire syndrome probably has no more diagnostic specificity than that of massive albuminuria itself. Proteinuria (predominantly albumin) of >3 or 3.5 g/day (or 2 g/day/m^2) will suffice for the diagnosis.

Tubular Proteinuria

Tubular proteinuria describes a pattern frequently found in tubular and interstitial renal disease. Many small proteins and peptides circulating in the blood are filtered by normal glomeruli. β_2-Microglobulin and amylase are two examples. These proteins are not normally found in urine because they are actively reabsorbed during their passage through the nephron. With tubular disease, they escape reabsorption and appear in the urine as one component of tubular proteinuria. A second component consists of brush border and cellular enzymes and other cellular proteins released from damaged renal tubular cells. A third component is the very high-molecular-weight Tamm-Horsfall protein. This polymer is secreted by cells of the ascending limb of Henle's loop and distal nephron and forms the matrix of most urinary casts. It appears to be secreted in larger quantities in renal disease. Thus, tubular proteinuria is a mix of heterogeneous large and small proteins and does not consist predominantly of albumin. Tubular proteinuria is most frequently found in the range of 1 to 1.5 g/day, although occasionally it may reach 2 g. When 3 g/day or more protein is found, the type will almost certainly be glomerular (nephrotic) or monoclonal Bence Jones proteinuria.

Monoclonal Overflow Proteinuria

In monoclonal overflow proteinuria, kidneys may be normal but an abnormal small protein circulates in the blood and is filtered by the glomeruli in quantities exceeding the tubules' capacity for reabsorption. This occurs with the production by myeloma or other hematologic malignancies of monoclonal globulin fragments. These usually consist of light chains and in the urine are called Bence Jones proteins. As noted earlier, they may not be sensitively detected by dipstick urinalysis. Heat and acetic or sulfosalicyclic acid tests are more accurate in their detection. Bence Jones proteinuria may be present in quantities ranging from <1 g to 30, 40, or more g per day.

Approach to Patients with Proteinuria

The objective of the initial evaluation of a proteinuric patient is to identify the quantity, the type, and the reproducibility of the proteinuria.

Quantity of Proteinuria. The quantity of proteinuria can most directly be determined by collecting all the urine produced during a 24-hour period. Provide patients with a suitable bottle (at least 2 L). A preservative such as a cup of vinegar may be used if refrigeration is not possible. Pick a time, such as on arising in the morning, to begin the collection period.

At that time, patients should empty the bladder and *discard* the urine. All urine output during the next 24 hours should be added to the bottle, and the next morning, at precisely the same time, patients should again empty the bladder, adding the urine to the collection. Starting and finishing times and dates should be recorded on the bottle.

Another method to approximate the quantity of proteinuria is to collect a single voiding specimen (preferably the first morning void) and measure both total protein and creatinine in the sample. Assuming that protein and creatinine are excreted in parallel during the day (not an entirely correct assumption) and that daily creatinine excretion remains relatively constant in an individual (also not entirely correct), the ratio of protein to creatinine will be an index of proteinuria that can be monitored to mark changes with treatment or disease progression.

Type of Proteinuria. Proteinuria can be categorized as glomerular, tubular, and monoclonal overflow types most easily by sending urine samples for protein electrophoresis and immunoelectrophoresis. Standard protein electrophoresis (*e.g.*, paper or cellulose acetate) shows a predominant albumin peak in glomerular proteinurias, a broad grouping of nonalbumin proteins in tubular disease, and often an "M spike" demonstrating Bence Jones proteins in myeloma. Immunoelectrophoresis is more sensitive in picking up monoclonal light chains and globulins.

Reproducibility of Proteinuria. Small amounts of proteinuria normally follow severe exertion or accompany high fever without indicating any serious renal abnormality. In those settings, workup might only include repeating the dipstick test on a later occasion. Proteinuria occasionally occurs only in the erect position and disappears completely with recumbency. This *orthostatic proteinuria* has a generally benign prognosis. It is best evaluated with 24-hour urine collection as described earlier, but divided into daytime ambulatory and nighttime recumbent portions. The bedtime void completes the daytime collection. Patients then remain recumbent until morning. The morning urine sample (plus any urine that may have been voided during the night) constitutes the nighttime specimen. If the nighttime collection has no more than 50 mg/8 hr (or is completely negative by dipstick test) and the day's sample has more than 150 mg/16 hr (or is positive by the dipstick test), orthostatic proteinuria may be diagnosed. It is important to remember that proteinuria of *any* origin will be excreted at higher rates during standing and ambulation, so a *completely* normal nighttime protein level is necessary for this diagnosis. The investigation of proteinuria is summarized in Table 2–3.

Management of Monoclonal Overflow Proteinuria

Management involves the evaluation and treatment of myeloma or occasionally lymphoma and often begins with bone marrow examination including search for clones of

Table 2–3. INVESTIGATING PROTEINURIA FLOWSHEET

If urine is Bence Jones positive, consider myeloma or lymphoproliferative disease.

If 24-hour collection contains less than 3 g/day, check protein electrophoresis.
- If a tubular pattern is noted, consider interstitial disease (see Table 2–4).
- If a glomerular pattern (mostly albumin) is noted, check for orthostatic proteinuria and consider mild forms of nephrotic diseases (see Table 2–5).

If 24-hour collection contains more than 3 g/day, consider nephrotic diseases (see Table 2–5). Check for infections, offending drugs, glucose, antinuclear antibody, and other pertinent laboratory studies and consider *biopsy*.

Be alert for renal vein thrombosis, particularly if symptoms suggest pulmonary emboli or if histology shows membranous nephropathy.

Consider searching for malignancy if the histology is membranous and the patient is elderly and has weight loss or other signs suggesting underlying malignancy.

plasma cells expressing exclusively kappa or lambda immunoglobulins. It should be noted that monoclonal "gammopathies" may be associated with amyloid, a cause of nephrotic syndrome. Thus, large amounts of albuminuria together with evidence of a monoclonal serum or urine protein may suggest renal amyloid.

Management of Tubular Proteinuria

A wide variety of tubular and interstitial renal diseases may demonstrate tubular proteinuria. They may be divided into toxic, congenital, immunologic, infectious, metabolic, and vascular categories, as indicated in Table 2–4.

Diagnostic workup includes careful history of familial renal disease, polyuria, headaches, backaches or other chronic pain requiring analgesics, and exposure to any of the drugs or substances listed in Table 2–4. Physical findings might include band keratopathy or Kayser-Fleischer rings, lead line on the gums, enlarged kidneys, or gouty arthritis. Laboratory studies might include determinations of serum calcium, potassium, bicarbonate, phosphate, and uric acid, and hemoglobin electrophoresis. Hypercalcemia may be a cause, and Fanconi's syndrome, renal tubular acidosis, or nephrogenic diabetes insipidus may result from tubulointerstitial nephritis. Blood and urine samples may be evaluted for heavy metals as appropriate, and if lead poisoning is a strong possibility, lead excretion after EDTA injection may help establish the diagnosis.

Table 2–4. CAUSES OF INTERSTITIAL NEPHRITIS

Drug toxicity
Analgesic abuse
Nonsteroidal antiinflammatory drugs
Lithium
Cyclosporine
Cisplatin
Heavy metal toxicity
Lead (may present as gouty nephropathy)
Cadmium, uranium, mercury
Hereditary/developmental
Polycystic kidney disease
Medullary cystic disease
Medullary sponge kidney
Immune diseases
Drug allergy (penicillins, sulfonamides, rifampin, others) (These are more likely to cause *acute* interstitial nephritis)
Collagen/vasculitis group (lupus, Sjögren's)
IgA nephropathy
Transplant rejection
Sarcoid
Infection, "pyelonephritis"
Bacterial infection: especially in a kidney with obstruction, reflux, diabetes mellitus, sickle disease
Tuberculosis, leprosy, viral, fungal parasitic infection
Metabolic
Hyperuricemia, uricosuria
Hypercalcemia
Oxalosis
Cystinosis
Amyloid
Vascular
Diabetes mellitus
Hypertension and nephrosclerosis
Atheroemboli
Sickle cell disease
Radiation nephritis
Obstruction/reflux especially if combined with infection

The urine sediment usually contains increased numbers of leukocytes and often tubular epithelial cells as well. Granular and cellular casts (neutrophils or epithelial cells) are frequent. Staining for urinary eosinophils may help in the diagnosis of allergic interstitial nephritis, usually due to drugs such as the penicillins. If a high percentage of numerous white blood cells in the sediment are eosinophils, the test has fair diagnostic specificity. If only small absolute numbers of eosinophils are present, it is much less specific.

The urine should be cultured whether or not bacteria are visible in the sediment. If pyuria is marked but routine culture is negative, a culture for mycobacteria should be considered. An acute infection can cause interstitial nephritis, and chronic or repeated infections when combined with reflux, obstruction, diabetes, or sickle cell disease can cause severe renal damage.

Management of Glomerular Proteinuria (Table 2–5)

If the proteinuria is relatively mild the first investigations should be done to show whether it is reproducible and whether it is orthostatic, as described earlier. **Transient mild proteinuria is generally of little significance and need not be intensively investigated.** Proteinuria that is truly orthostatic generally also has no symptoms and a good prognosis and need not be pursued to the point of kidney biopsy or treatment.

Asymptomatic Proteinuria. Mild glomerular proteinuria that is reproducible, not orthostatic, and in the range of 1 to 2 g/day usually occurs without accompanying symptoms, although edema may occasionally be present. Investigation of underlying systemic disease is appropri-

Table 2–5. CAUSES OF NEPHROTIC SYNDROME

	Approx. Relative Incidence	
	Adults (%)	*Children (%)*
Primary glomerular disease	(75)	(90)
Membranous nephropathy	30	
Minimal change (lipoid) nephrosis	15	80-90
Focal glomerular sclerosis	15	
Membranoproliferative GN, including dense deposit disease	7	
Mesangial proliferative GN, including IgA nephropathy	5	
Rapidly progressive GN	3	
Acute poststreptococcal GN	—	
Systemic conditions	(25)	
Relatively common		
Diabetes mellitus		
Systemic lupus erythematosus (SLE)		
Amyloid (including multiple myeloma)		
Less common causes		
Other immunologic diseases (in addition to SLE): Polyarteritis (small-vessel form), Wegener's, dermatomyositis, scleroderma, Takayasu's disease, Sjögren's disease, Henoch-Schönlein purpura, serum sickness, transplant rejection, sarcoid, mixed cryoglobulinemia		
Associated with malignancy		
Hodgkin's lymphoma (usually minimal change)		
Other tumors (usually membranous)		
Heavy metals, drugs, allergens: gold, mercury, probenecid, penicillamine, angiotensin-converting enzyme inhibitors, "street" heroin, nonsteroidal antiinflammatory drugs		
Infections		
Bacterial endocarditis and shunt infections, acquired immunodeficiency syndrome, malaria, hepatitis, secondary and congenital syphilis, schistosomiasis		
Congenital or familial: including Fabry's, Alport's, nail-patella		
Pregnancy associated		

GN, glomerulonephritis.

ate as described later for nephrotic syndrome. Because the prognosis of asymptomatic proteinuria is often good, it is reasonable to follow patients without biopsy or specific treatment until the proteinuria becomes nephrotic or evidence of deterioration in overall renal function (rise in serum creatinine level) occurs.

Pathophysiology of Nephrotic Syndrome. Nephrotic levels of proteinuria may occur in many different glomerular diseases, with different histologic appearances (see Table 2–5). They all share, however, an abnormality of the glomerular capillary wall, allowing increased passage of plasma proteins.

The urinary loss of protein together with increased rates of catabolism of albumin in the body (including the renal tubular reabsorption and degradation of filtered protein) lead to hypoproteinemia. The renal retention of salt and water leading to edema is caused in some nephrotic patients by the hypoproteinemia and reduced plasma volume. In others, the plasma volume is normal and the glomerular change appears to lead directly to fluid retention.

Hyperlipidemia results largely from overproduction of apolipoproteins by the liver. This synthesis, like that of albumin, appears to be stimulated by reductions in plasma oncotic pressure. Lipiduria follows from the hyperlipidemia and increased glomerular permeability.

Nephrotic patients have varying degrees of hypoalbuminemia and lipid abnormalities, not always proportional to the amount of proteinuria. These differences no doubt reflect differences in nutrition, in the hepatic capacity to synthesize albumin and apolipoproteins, and in genetic predisposition.

General Management of Patients with Nephrotic Syndrome

Edema and Hypoproteinemia

Management of edema is considered in detail in Chapter 11. Nephrotic patients with hypoalbuminemia treated with diuretics generally have contracted plasma volumes. Further attempts to reduce edema with powerful diuretics or diuretic combinations may reduce plasma volume to the point of circulatory impairment, prerenal azotemia, and intractable diuretic resistance. The temporary use of albumin infusions may be considered to reestablish the circulation in such cases. Although albumin administration is fruitless in the long run because of its short life in the circulation of nephrotic patients, it may help in alleviating anasarca (especially in patients without really massive proteinuria). Infusing perhaps 50 g of albumin followed by a large dose of a diuretic combination each day for 2 or 3 days may temporarily provide relief for patients in whom edema and ascites are truly threatening.

It is important that nephrotic patients have adequate dietary protein to allow for hepatic synthesis of albumin. Raising protein intake above normal, however, seems only to increase the proteinuria without raising serum albumin. Protein intakes of 0.8 to 1 g/kg of lean body weight supplemented 1 g for each gram of proteinuria would seem appropriate. Proteins of high biologic value should be emphasized. A managment summary is indicated in Table 2–6.

Hyperlipidemia

When the nephrotic syndrome is responsive to therapy and lasts only a few weeks or months, treatment of hyperlipidemia is probably not indicated. Even when nephrotic hyperlipidemia is of longer duration, its risk of causing atherogenesis is controversial. It seems likely, however, that sustained extreme elevations of low-density lipoprotein cholesterol such as occur in many nephrotic patients merit attempts at treatment. Clofibrate frequently leads to muscle injury in nephrotic individuals, perhaps because of reduced binding to plasma proteins. Lovastatin is better tolerated but may also have to be used in reduced doses to avoid creatine phosphokinase elevations from skeletal muscle. Lovastatin most frequently is insufficient by itself, and even when combined with a bile acid-binding resin, or with gemfibrozil, it accomplishes only moderate lipid reductions.

Table 2–6. SUMMARY OF MANAGEMENT OF NEPHROTIC SYNDROME

1. Treat the underlying glomerular disease if effective specific treatment is available.
2. Prescribe a low-sodium, liberal-potassium, low-saturated-fat diet. The protein content should not be high, but about 0.8 to 1 g/kg/day, emphasizing high-biologic-quality protein. Meals should be small and frequent if ascites is present. If hyponatremia occurs, fluid may be restricted; but if there is a sudden diuresis, more salt and water may be needed.
3. Provide a multivitamin supplement with vitamin D and iron (e.g., prenatal formula).
4. Diuretics should be cautiously administered with or without temporary albumin infusion when hypoalbuminemia is severe. Watch for serious reduction in plasma volume with "prerenal" or acute renal failure.
5. Be alert for thromboses and infection.
6. If the proteinuria is very severe and debilitating, consider cautious indomethacin/furosemide or angiotensin-converting enzyme inhibitor/furosemide therapy to reduce the glomerular filtration rate and proteinuria.
7. Treat hyperlipidemia if it is severe and prolonged.

Treatment of Specific Glomerular Diseases

This chapter provides only a brief outline. (See also Chapter 3.) Referral to a nephrologist is appropriate for treatment for conditions other than minimal change disease.

Minimal Change Disease. Minimal change disease (lipoid nephrosis) responds to 3 or 4 weeks of corticosteroid therapy in at least 80 to 90% of cases. One regimen is to give prednisone, 2 mg/kg/day (maximum 80 mg/day). If no response occurs, stop at 4 weeks. If a patient responds with diuresis and almost complete disappearance of proteinuria by dipstick test, then continue for 2 additional weeks, followed by a slow taper (ideally with alternate-day dosage) over 4 to 6 months. Relapses can be treated the same way or with a more prolonged taper. Cyclophosphamide and chlorambucil can prolong remissions but have considerable toxicity, which may not be justified unless the disease is severe.

Focal Segmental Glomerular Sclerosis. Focal segmental glomerular sclerosis is less likely to respond than minimal change disease. Responses do occur on occasion, however, particularly in children and particularly when therapy with prednisone is combined with cyclophosphamide or chlorambucil. Although treatment is controversial, in patients with fairly severe edema and proteinuria, but without marked elevation of serum creatinine levels, a vigorous but short (4 to 6 weeks) trial of combined therapy might be undertaken. If no marked improvement occurs, one would then stop treatment to avoid the toxicity, which is much greater with prolonged therapy.

IgA Nephropathy. IgA nephropathy (Berger's disease) has not been convincingly shown to respond to any therapy.

Membranoproliferative Glomerulonephritis. The treatment of membranoproliferative glomerulonephritis (MPGN, mesangiocapillary GN) is controversial, and no present treatment leads to clear-cut total remission. Some patients with type I MPGN benefit from prolonged courses of alternate-day prednisone (40 mg/m^2 every other day). If serious hypertension results, prolonged daily aspirin and dipyridamole treatment is an alternative.

Membranous Nephropathy. Many patients do well without treatment. For those with risk factors for progressive disease (very high levels of proteinuria, serum creatinine levels beginning to rise above normal, male gender, resistant hypertension), prednisone therapy may help, particularly when combined with cyclophosphamide or chlorambucil in a prolonged program.

Role of Renal Biopsy in Management of Nephrotic Syndrome

In childhood nephrotic syndrome, the cause in 90% of cases is minimal change disease, so prednisone treatment is often appropriate without a biopsy-proven diagnosis. In adults, however, various underlying diseases requiring specific treatments occur. It has been argued that a uniform, 2-month alternate-day prednisone treatment given to all adult nephrotic patients would be helpful to many and harmful to few. In the author's opinion, however, the small risk of percutaneous renal biopsy is outweighed by the guidance for specific treatment, general management, and knowledge of prognosis that a histologic diagnosis provides.

CASE SUMMARY 2 (continued)

You initially consider myeloma but are puzzled about how Bence Jones proteinuria might be associated with edema and surprised that it registers so strongly on the dipstick test. Further study shows hypoalbuminemia, urine immunoelectrophoresis demonstrating monoclonal light chains (Bence Jones protein), and cellulose acetate protein electrophoresis showing an M spike *and* a much larger peak of albumin. The patient is found to have myeloma with renal amyloid causing nephrotic syndrome.

Suggested Readings

Coe FL: Clinical and laboratory assessment of the patient with renal disease. *In* Brenner BM, Rector FC Jr (eds): The Kidney. Philadelphia, WB Saunders, 1986.

Coggins CH: Membranous nephropathy. *In* Schrier RW, Gottschalk CW (eds): Disease of the Kidney, 4th ed, Chapter 65, section 10. Boston, Little, Brown & Co, 1979.

Coggins CH: Nephrotic syndrome. *In* Flamenbaum W, Hamburger RJ (eds): Nephrology—An Approach to the Patient with Renal Disease. Philadelphia, JB Lippincott, 1982.

Coggins CH: Glomerulonephritis and nephrotic syndrome. *In* Rubinstein E, Federman DD (eds): Scientific American Medicine. New York, Scientific American, 1989.

Rose BD: Clinical approach to glomerular disease. *In* Rubenstein E, Federman DD: Scientific American Medicine. New York, Scientific American, 1989.

Schapner HW, Robson AM: Nephrotic syndrome: Minimal change disease, focal glomerulosclerosis, and related disorders. *In* Schrier RW, Gottschalk CW (eds): Disease of the Kidney, 4th ed, Chapter 64, section 10. Boston, Little, Brown & Co, 1979.

CHAPTER 3

ACUTE NEPHRITIC SYNDROME

Daniel C. Cattran

Acute nephritic syndrome (ANS) is the most serious and potentially devastating form of the various renal syndromes. It consists of two components. One element reflects the structural change with active proliferation of both intrinsic glomerular cells and invasion of extrinsic mononuclear and polymorphonuclear leukocytes into both the interstitium and the glomeruli. The second element reflects the functional parallel of this activity, with proteinuria, a reduction in glomerular filtration rate (GFR), and an active urine sediment with red blood cells (RBCs) and RBC casts. This pathology results in sodium and water retention, expansion of intravascular volume, edema, and frequently systemic hypertension.

Although the broad definition of ANS may be generic, categorization into primary and secondary forms based on histology and etiology is mandatory because their prognosis and therapy differ markedly.

INCIDENCE

Glomerulonephritis (GN) represents 25 to 30% of all cases of end-stage renal disease. Approximately one fourth of affected patients will present with ANS. Most cases that do progress do so relatively quickly, and end-stage renal failure may occur within weeks or months of an ANS presentation.

CLINICAL FEATURES OF ACUTE NEPHRITIC SYNDROME

Clinical features are edema; decreased volume and frequency of urination; systemic hypertension; uremic symptoms (see Chapter 13); rarely, costovertebral tenderness (enlarged kidneys); and gross hematuria.

GENERAL EVALUATIONS

Historical information is important and serves four purposes: to date the onset of the disease; to identify possible etiologic agents (*e.g.*, streptococcal throat infection); to identify any systemic disease features (*e.g.*, arthralgias); and to assess the consequences of the disease process (*e.g.*, uremic symptoms).

In the primary or idiopathic form of this syndrome, often no features or only nonspecific flulike symptoms date the onset. When a secondary (systemic) disease process is responsible, the renal symptoms may be preceded by other features such as skin rash or arthritis in disseminated lupus erythematosus, or by arthralgia and purpura in anaphylactoid purpura. Other sources of information that may help to date the onset include previous urinalysis or other laboratory investigations done for insurance purposes or as part of a family physician's general monitoring. The effects of the disease on renal function may vary from minor changes, such as a change in the pattern of urination or vague backache, to gross changes such as frothy urine, gross hematuria, or manifestations of salt and water retention such as periorbital edema in the morning or ankle edema by evening. The more common etiologic agents and their clinical manifestations will be discussed later in this chapter.

The physical examination should include an estimate of size and degree of tenderness of the kidneys, intravascular volume status, blood pressure, and the presence of peripheral or pulmonary edema. A search for a systemic disease should include an examination of the skin for features of rash or purpura, of the joints for arthritis, of the lymph system for adenopathy or splenomegaly, of the cardiovascular system for features of subacute bacterial endocarditis or other infections, and of the respiratory system for findings suggestive of vasculitis or infection. The general features associated with renal failure (see Chapter 13) should also be considered.

> Urinalysis by a physician is crucial in the evaluation of patients with the ANS.

Microscopic examination of the urine frequently shows RBCs, white blood cells (WBCs), and cellular casts. The finding of RBC casts is almost pathognomonic of glomerulitis and reflects the ongoing active cellular proliferation within the glomerular tuft.

Although rare, it is possible in patients with acute and severe renal failure to have a benign urine sediment, perhaps because of the very poor glomerular permeability.

LABORATORY INVESTIGATION

Radiologic evaluation is of limited value. A radioisotope scan to assess renal perfusion is appropriate and should replace the standard intravenous pyelogram because the latter can be both noninformative (no dye uptake) and dangerous (osmotic load) when used in this type of patient. Ultrasonography is noninvasive and is useful for several reasons. It can confirm that there are two kidneys, and by estimating their size it may help determine disease duration (*i.e.*, normal or large kidneys implies acute and small kidneys suggests chronic disease). Ultrasonography can help rule out obstruction and other abnormal anatomy and is also useful in defining position and depth of the kidneys in preparation for a closed biopsy.

Laboratory estimates of serum creatinine and urea nitrogen levels and a 24-hour urine collection for creatinine clearance and proteinuria determine the severity of the renal disease. **Both creatinine clearance and proteinuria may not reveal the severity of renal failure in patients with an ANS presentation, because both poorly reflect renal function under conditions of rapid change.** The delta of serum creatinine levels determined serially most clearly and simply reflects rate of change in function.

RENAL BIOPSY

Clinical and laboratory evaluations cannot establish the histologic type of ANS.

A renal biopsy is essential in most cases because histology will guide both prognosis and therapy. Although the risk of bleeding after a closed biopsy is increased in the presence of renal failure, proper coverage of the coagulation defect with material such as desamino-D-arginine vasopressin (DDAVP) permits the great majority to be done safely. In most cases with this presentation, the kidneys are large and readily assessed by this technique although an open biopsy occasionally is required. The tissue obtained should be examined by light, immunofluorescent, and electron microscopy.

PATHOLOGIC CLASSIFICATION

The light microscopic findings determine the major histologic groupings. Immunofluorescence microscopy has allowed additional categorization such as IgA nephritis, and electron microscopy has permitted further definitions such as type I and type II membranoproliferative GN (MPGN). The classification is based largely on a description of the activity of the three intrinsic glomerular components (*i.e.*, epithelial, endothelial, and mesangial cells), the presence of extrinsic cells such as polymorphonuclear leukocytes, and the secondary effects of this activity on the glomerular basement membrane. For example, mesangial and endothelial cell proliferation typifies the diffuse proliferative varieties, but with rupture of the basement membrane and leakage of both cells and plasma into Bowman's space, extracapillary proliferation occurs and crescents are produced. The presence of polymorphonuclear leukocytes in either variant is indicated by the additional designation "exudative" and reflects a heightened disease activity. A vasculitic process is suspected when focal and segmental necrotizing lesions are noted (Fig. 3–1).

PATHOGENESIS

Immunofluorescence microscopy adds a pathogenetic dimension to classic pathology. Three major immunofluorescent patterns are seen in patients with ANS: immune complex disease (granular deposits); antibody-mediated (linear deposits); and nonimmune mediated (no deposits).

The immune complexes are usually formed in the circulation and deposit secondarily in the glomeruli. These complexes may occasionally form *in situ* (*i.e.*, a circulating antibody attaches

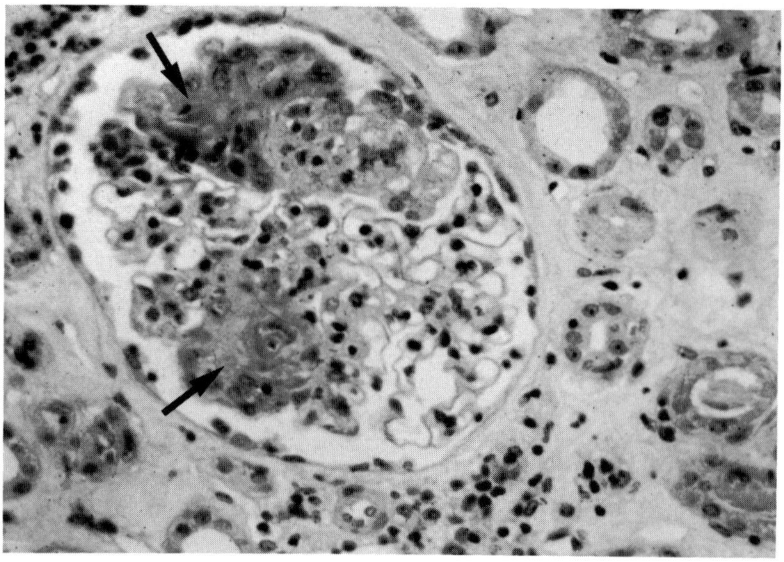

Figure 3–1. Segmental necrotizing glomerulonephritis. This glomerulus shows two areas of segmental proliferation surrounding two areas of necrosis (arrows). This lesion is commonly associated with vasculitis.

to a fixed antigen either planted or primarily located within one of the cellular or membrane elements of the glomerulus).

Primary antibody-mediated disease is largely limited to Goodpasture's syndrome, in which the antigen is known to be located within the basement membrane substrate of both the kidneys and lungs. The antibody binds to the antigen and produces a smooth, linear pattern along this membrane.

The third category (*i.e.*, no immunofluorescence reaction) is most commonly associated with vasculitis. In diseases with this finding (i.e., polyarteritis nodosa and Wegener's granulomatosis), it is presumed either that the inflammation, thrombosis, and necrosis occur without a primary immune insult, or that the vasculitis is transient or below the level of resolution of our present techniques. Figure 3–2 illustrates the relationships of the elements of the glomerulus and the possible positions of immune deposits.

A description of additional factors activated by the primary immune process is beyond the scope of this textbook but is important when considering present (and future) treatment regimens. These factors include known mediators of vascular damage and repair such as endothelial growth factor, platelet-derived growth factor, lysozymes of the polymorphonuclear leukocytes, and the complement cascade and its attack complex, and the coagulation cascade.

PRIMARY (IDIOPATHIC) FORMS OF ACUTE NEPHRITIS

The term *primary* is used to refer to diseases in which only the kidneys are involved. In secondary forms, the renal involvement is part

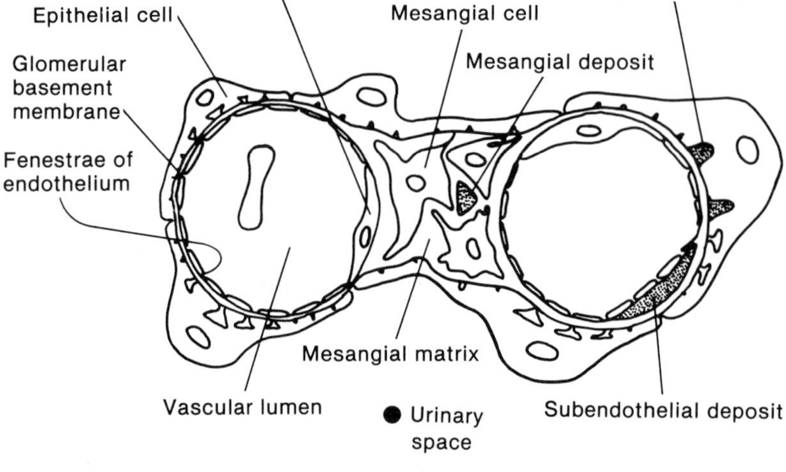

Figure 3–2. Glomerular unit showing the positions of the major cellular elements and their orientation to the vascular lumen, the urinary space, and the supporting mesangium and the basement membrane.

Table 3–1. RENAL PATHOLOGY OF THE VARIANTS THAT COMMONLY PRESENT WITH ACUTE NEPHRITIC SYNDROME

Type of Glomerulonephritis	Light Microscopy	Immunofluorescence	Electron Microscopy
Crescentic	Cellular or fibrocellular elements within Bowman's space with additional endocapillary proliferation within the glomerular tuft	Granular peripheral and mesangial IgG and C3 55%; no deposits 35%; linear deposits of IgG, C3 along the basement membrane 10%	Deposits present or absent depending on type
Diffuse proliferative	Diffuse hypercellularity of mesangial ± endothelial cells ± polymorphonuclear leukocytes	Coarse granular peripheral and mesangial IgG, C3	Subepithelial variable-size deposits
Membranoproliferative			
Type I	Mesangial cell proliferation and increased mesangial matrix, classic double contouring of basement membrane	Peripheral C3 ± IgG ± mesangial deposits	Subedothelial ± paramesangial deposits with mesangial matrix interposition and basement membrane splitting
Type II	Mesangial cell proliferation; apparent basement membrane thickening, which tends to be segmental	C3 interrupted peripheral deposits ± "mesangial rings"	Intramembranous diffuse dense "deposits" in the capillary loops ± mesangium rarely in Bowman's capsule and proximal tubule membrane
IgA/IgG nephropathy (Berger's syndrome)	Diffuse mesangial cell and matrix proliferation	Mesangial IgA (100%) ± IgG (65%) IgM (20%), segmental crescents	Mesangial and paramesangial deposits

of a systemic disease process. The primary forms are classified by the renal pathology, and hence our discussion focuses first on the pathologic description (Table 3–1) and then on the associated clinical and laboratory characteristics of each type (Table 3–2).

Subtypes

Crescentic Glomerulonephritis

Pathology. Crescents are formed by a proliferation of cells within Bowman's space (Fig. 3–3). In their most active phase they are cellular, but with time they become fibrocellular then acellular. There may be associated endocapillary proliferation, but this is often obscured by the crescent as it expands and compresses the glomerular tuft. Immunofluorescence often shows fibrin-related products within the crescent, and the idiopathic variants may show granular (55%), linear (10%), or no deposits (35%) when tested against specific immune probes. Electron microscopy confirms these findings and also may reveal breaks in the glomerular basement membrane. These breaks are an important factor in the generation of the crescents, as the escape of plasma proteins into Bowman's space probably produces the cellular reaction and the crescent formation. A common feature in the most severe varieties is an interstitial mononuclear cell infiltrate, which may indicate an underlying T-cell–mediated process.

Clinical Presentation and Treatment. Although more than 50% of patients with crescentic GN present with ANS and rapidly deteriorating renal function, other modes do occur (i.e., asymptomatic, 15%; nephrotic, 10%; chronic renal failure, 25%). Rapid deterioration is classically defined as a doubling of the presenting serum creatinine level within 3 months. Features at presentation include an active urine sediment (90%), edema (50 to 60%), and systemic hypertension (35%). In the elderly, congestive cardiac failure is not uncommon, and the primary renal process can be missed if the urine is not examined. Secondary forms make up more than 40% of this category and will be discussed in more detail later in this chapter.

Abnormal laboratory features are usually limited to renal function tests. Complement levels are normal. Poor prognostic factors include large crescents in >80% of glomeruli (especially if fibrocellular or acellular), an initial serum creatinine level >600 μmol/L, and oliguria. Crescentic GN is a relatively rare histologic type and represents <4% of cases in large renal biopsy series. In general, the prognosis is poor

Table 3–2. CLINICAL FEATURES ASSOCIATED WITH THE COMMON PATHOLOGIC VARIANTS

Pathologic Classification	Age (yr) Range	Sex (m/f)	BP	Urinalysis	24-Hour Protein	Creatinine Clearance	C3	Renal Survival %* 5 yr	10 yr	Treatment
Crescentic glomerulonephritis	55 10–80+	2/1	N/↑	Active	<2 g	Markedly ↓	N	50	30	Pulse steroid, cytotoxic therapy
Diffuse proliferative	20 10–80+	m>f	N/↑	Active	0.5–5 g	↓	↓	95	90	None necessary
Membranoproliferative disease										
Type I	18 5–60	1/1	N/↑	Active	0.1–5 g	↓	N/↓	75	50	See text
Type II	12 3–35	1/1	N/↑	Active	0.1–5 g	↓	↓↓	80	50	See text
IgA/IgG nephropathy (Berger's syndrome)	25 10–70	m>f	N/↑	Active	0.1–5 g	↓	N	65	45	See text

*This prognosis refers only to patients in these categories who present with the acute nephritic syndrome; not all patients with these histologic patterns present this way (see text).

and aggressive therapy is warranted. Although unproven in randomized clinical trials, studies have suggested that methylprednisolone (Solu-Medrol) (5 to 20 mg/kg) on alternate days for two to three courses followed by high-dose alternate-day prednisone (2 mg/kg) for 2 to 3 months has improved the 1-year renal survival from 40 to 70%. The addition of cytotoxic agents such as pulse cyclophosphamide (500 mg/m^2 on a monthly basis over 2 to 4 months) and/or the addition of 4-L plasma exchanges given every second day for 2 weeks have been advocated, but their justification in the idiopathic variant is poor, and they should not be used when a patient's life risk is heightened (*i.e.*, age >60 or in the presence of factors such as infection or concomitant serious disease). In the absence of any response within 3 to 5 weeks, acceptance of end-stage renal disease is preferable to death secondary to iatrogenic causes. The prednisone and cytotoxic drugs should be tapered and discontinued and dialysis or transplantation planned if required.

Diffuse Proliferative Glomerulonephritis

Pathology. Glomerular tufts are expanded by the proliferation of both mesangial and endothelial cells. This proliferation, plus the presence of neutrophils in the capillary loops, gives a glomerulus a solid-looking appearance (Fig. 3–4). Immunofluorescence microscopy usually shows coarsely granular peripheral deposits of IgG and complement component C3. Mesangial deposits are seen less frequently. Electron microscopy usually reveals both large and small

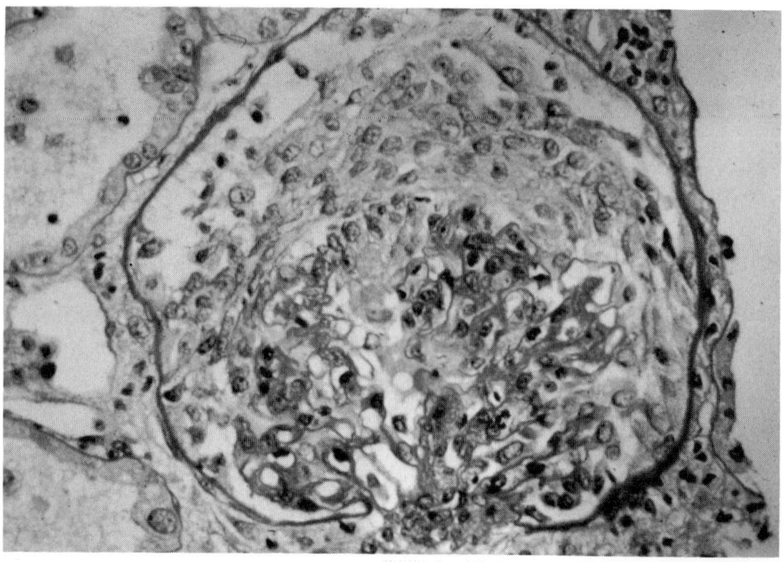

Figure 3–3. Crescentic glomerulonephritis. A large fibrocellular crescent occupies Bowman's space and compresses the glomerular tuft.

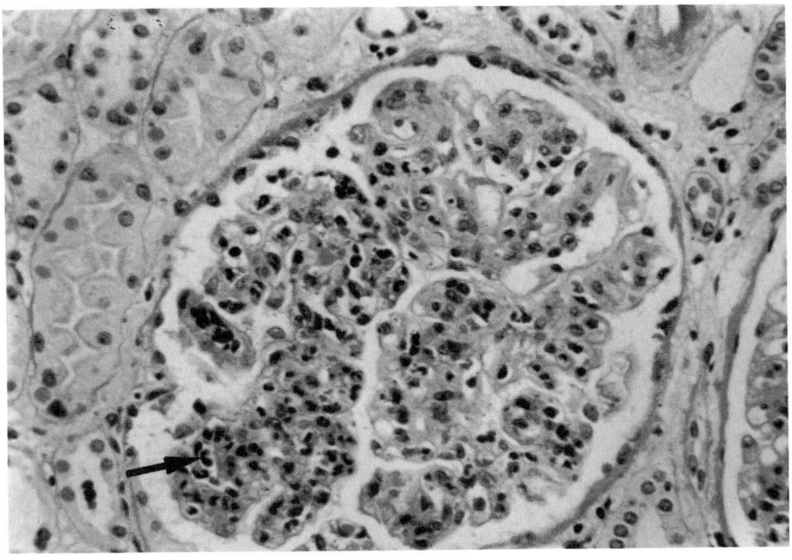

Figure 3–4. Diffuse proliferative glomerulonephritis. Endocapillary and mesangial cell proliferation associated with exudated polymorphs (arrow) produce an expansion of the glomerular tuft, with a concomitant reduction in Bowman's space and compression of the capillary loops.

subepithelial deposits. Rarely, mesangial and subendothelial deposits are also seen.

Clinical Presentation and Treatment. This lesion classically presents 2 to 4 weeks after a streptococcal infection of the skin or pharynx, although it may follow many different bacterial, protozoal, or viral infections. Although more common in children, it may occur at any age. There is a 2:1 male dominance. The typical case presents with cola-colored urine, peripheral and periorbital edema, and hypertension. The urine often shows RBCs and RBC casts and a variable degree of proteinuria, usually in the range of 1 to 3 g/day. The serum creatinine level is typically elevated at presentation and may rise rapidly into the same range as in crescentic GN. Throat swabs and acute and convalescent serum titers may reveal a poststreptococcal infectious etiology, but treatment with antibiotics does not modify the renal outcome.

Therapy is symptomatic only. Fluid, potassium, and hypertension control, as well as treatment of the complications that may ensue if uremia becomes severe, are all that is required. Although some reports have suggested that the long-term prognosis is not favorable, the great majority of studies in both adults and children with pure diffuse endocapillary proliferative GN have been excellent, with 20-year survival of >90%. Therefore, no "specific" therapy is warranted.

Membranoproliferative Glomerulonephritis

Pathology. A lobular pattern caused by the accentuation of the segmental nature of the glomerulus by the proliferation of the mesangial cells and the expansion of their matrix into the capillary loops is seen in both types of MPGN. The extensive mesangial expansion extending out around the capillary loops, combined with the laying down of new basement membrane, produces a double-layered appearance and the classic "tram tracks" on light microscopy (Fig. 3–5). Two major variants are distinguished by electron microscopy. Type I is characterized by subendothelial deposits, and type II by a ribbonlike continuous deposit of electron-dense material within the basement membrane. There is a less well recognized type III, which is associated with the features of type I combined with subepithelial deposits.

Clinical Presentation and Treatment. MPGN can present with ANS (30%), asymptomatic proteinuria (30%), the nephrotic syndrome (30%), or a mixed picture (10%). Type II is most commonly encountered in patients between the ages of 5 and 20 years, whereas type I can be seen at any age (see Table 3–2). An interesting but uncommon associated clinical finding with type II is partial lipodystrophy. The C3 component of complement may be depressed in type I and is commonly depressed in type II. The level in type II can be extremely low, and when the level is <10% of normal, the diagnosis is almost assured. The natural history in MPGN can vary dramatically. Spontaneous partial remission after an ANS presentation occurs in approximately one third of patients (*i.e.*, a return to a normal creatinine value although some proteinuria usually remains). The long-term prognosis is guarded in both types, with 10-year renal survival approx-

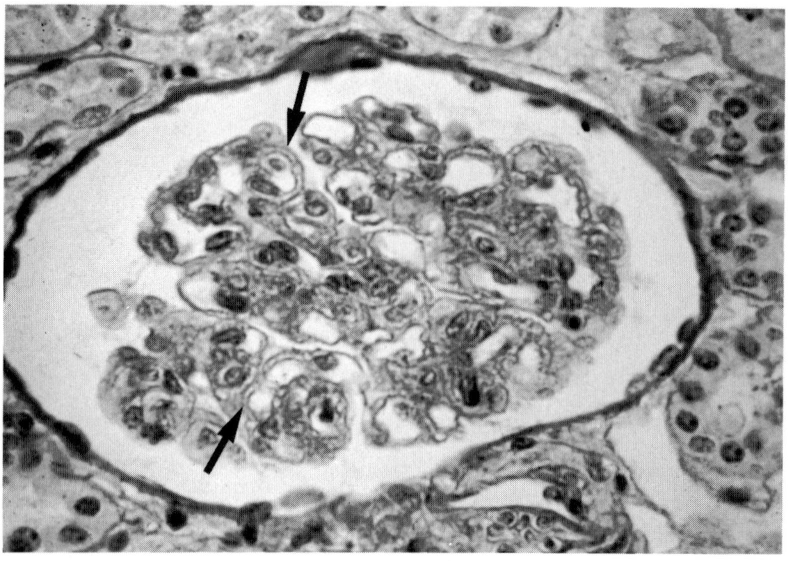

Figure 3–5. Membranoproliferative glomerulonephritis. A glomerulus shows lobulation secondary to the mesangial cell proliferation and matrix expansion. This expansion produces the apparent thickening of the peripheral capillary loops and the classic tram track appearance (arrows) in some areas, often visualized best on periodic acid–Schiff staining.

imately 40 to 50%. The prevalence of this type of GN has been decreasing during the past several years in most countries. The reason for this change is unknown. Treatment modalities have been hard to assess because of the variable natural history. Combined cytotoxic agents plus anticoagulant therapy, although initially thought to be helpful, have not proved to be of benefit. Long-term low-dose alternate-day steroids may modify the prognosis in children, but their use has not been proved in randomized clinical trials. The antiplatelet agent dipyridamole (225 mg daily) combined with acetylsalicylic acid (975 mg daily) has been demonstrated to preserve GFR better than placebo therapy, although no improvement in proteinuria was shown.

IgA/IgG Nephropathy (Berger's Syndrome)

Pathology. This histologic type is characterized by a variable degree of mesangial proliferation and increased mesangial matrix on light microscopy (Fig. 3–6). Diagnosis is confirmed by the presence of mesangial IgA in all glomeruli on immunofluorescence microscopy. IgG (65%) and/or IgM (20%) may accompany the IgA deposits. Electron microscopy confirms deposits in the mesangium with occasional extension into the subendothelial location. Anaphylactoid purpura (Henoch-Schönlein purpura) also has IgA mesangial deposition. This entity may be a systemic form of IgA nephropathy. The presence of fibrin in Bowman's space originally was believed to be confirmatory of anaphylactoid purpura, but it has now been described in many of the more active cases of pure IgA nephropathy.

Clinical Presentation and Treatment. The presentation is variable but classically includes recurrent macroscopic hematuria, minimal proteinuria, and well-preserved GFR. The gross hematuria can be quite severe, associated with loin pain and enlargement of the kidneys, and may be misdiagnosed as pyelonephritis. An ANS presentation occurs in only 10 to 20% of IgA cases, and a nephrotic presentation is also quite uncommon (*i.e.*, 10 to 15%). A history of an upper respiratory tract infection within 3 to 4 days of the gross hematuria, the absence of previous bladder infections, and the presence of RBC casts after careful examination of the urine usually are helpful in making the correct diagnosis. Phase microscopy of the urine may show poikilocytosis of the RBCs, confirming their glomerular origin. Although the majority of IgA patients do very well, it is now recognized that up to 50% will have a slow progression to end-stage renal failure over 10 to 20 years. Patients who present with severe hypertension, the nephritic syndrome, or nephrotic-range proteinuria or whose renal biopsies show interstitial fibrosis and glomerular obsolescence have a much worse prognosis. Serum IgA may be increased (50% of patients), but its level carries no prognostic significance. Similarly, although the finding of IgA and C3 deposits in the dermal capillaries may be of diagnostic importance, they have no relevance to outcome.

Various therapeutic agents have been tried, but the variability in the history of the disease, improper patient selection, and inadequate

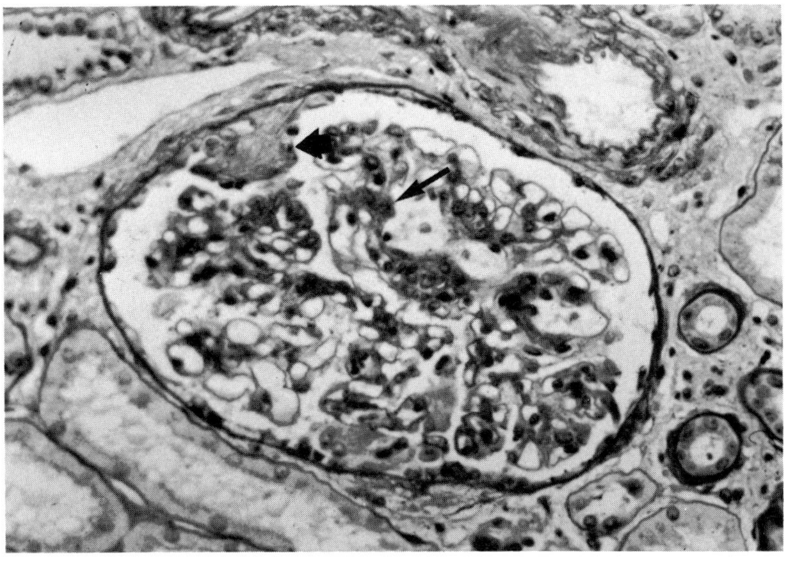

Figure 3–6. IgG/IgA nephropathy. The background mesangial proliferation and mesangial expansion give a prominence to the axial structure of the glomerulus (long arrow). The segmental (short arrow) crescents are more commonly present when the clinical presentation is with the acute nephritic syndrome associated with the IgA nephropathy.

sample size have made intervention studies with drugs such as steroids, cytotoxic agents, and phenytoin difficult to interpret. The latter is known to lower serum IgA levels, hence the rationale for its use.

An interesting feature may be the association of minimal change disease with IgA nephropathy. If a patient presents with heavy proteinuria, a normal GFR and blood pressure, and on biopsy only foot process fusion and mesangial IgA deposits are seen, a short course of prednisone (1 to 2 mg/kg for a maximum of 8 weeks) is warranted.

CASE SUMMARY 1

A 64-year-old man with known coronary artery disease presented with a history of a severe sore throat 2 weeks before admission. He experienced increasing shortness of breath, minimal swelling of his ankles, and some periorbital edema during the 4 days before presentation in the emergency room. On clinical examination, he was hypertensive (180/100 mm Hg), his jugular venous pressure was increased, he had crepitations in the bases of both lungs, and he showed 1+ peripheral edema. Examination of the urine showed 4+ proteinuria, trace glycosuria, and an active urine sediment with RBCs and RBC casts. His serum creatinine level was 150 μmol/L, his urea level was 13.5 mmol/L, and his electrolytes were normal. In the hospital, the patient was treated with diuretics and antihypertensive agents, but the creatinine continued to rise. Although it was thought that these findings most likely represented diffuse proliferative GN, the possibility of a crescentic histology could not be ruled out. A renal biopsy specimen therefore was obtained. It showed diffuse endocapillary proliferation on light microscopy, with large peripheral capillary deposits of IgG and C3 on immunofluorescence microscopy and subepithelial humps on electron microscopy. Symptomatic management was continued. The creatinine peaked at 350 μmol/L at day 10 and slowly declined into the normal range by 6 weeks. Diuretics and antihypertensive medication were tapered to zero over the same period.

CASE SUMMARY 2

A 42-year-old Asian woman had a history of an upper respiratory tract infection 4 days before her presentation in the emergency room with gross hematuria. She had minor complaints of back pain but no dysuria or frequency. She had had a similar occurrence 2 years earlier, at which time a urine culture was sterile and subsequent cystoscopy was normal.

On physical examination, she had borderline hypertension (130/90 mm Hg) and trace peripheral edema. Urinalysis showed RBCs with poikilocytosis and occasional RBC casts. Further laboratory examination revealed a protein excretion rate of 0.5 g/day and a normal creatinine clearance of 1.9 ml · $sec^{-1}/1.73\ m^2$. Her serum IgA level was elevated.

In discussion with the patient, it was suggested that she most likely had IgA nephropathy and that at this level of function nothing further needed to be done but continued careful observation. The patient wanted to be certain of her diagnosis for future planning of her career and a family. It was therefore decided to perform a renal biopsy, which showed mesangial cell proliferation and matrix expansion on light microscopy, occasional small segmental crescents and mesangial IgA, and a lesser amount of IgG deposit on immunofluorescence microscopy. There were no interstitial or tubular changes.

The diagnosis of IgA nephropathy was confirmed, and the patient was told that careful, regular monitoring was appropriate to watch for early signs of progressive renal disease or hypertension. A modest restriction in protein to 0.9 g/kg was suggested to the patient, with the explanation that it might reduce the workload of the kidneys and thus help preserve renal function.

SECONDARY FORMS OF ACUTE NEPHRITIS

The histologic patterns seen in secondary forms of acute nephritis are often indistinguishable from the primary types; therefore, pathology may not be helpful in determining the cause of the problem. The histologic changes, for instance, in diffuse proliferative lupus nephritis may look the same as in a patient with poststreptococcal GN.

> A specific diagnosis is usually made on the basis of the history, physical examination, and laboratory findings, not pathology.

The search for a cause is warranted in virtually all cases of ANS, because therapy and prognosis are so dependent on knowing both the pathology and etiology. Specific histologic findings are occasionally helpful, and these features are part of the outline in Table 3–3.

Presentation and Treatment

Diffuse Proliferative and Crescentic Lupus Nephritis

Disseminated lupus erythematosus (DLE) afflicts in 1 in 2000 females, with the peak age incidence between 15 and 45 years of age. There is a 5:1 female predominance. The pathology in the kidneys can vary from minimal involvement to circumferential crescents in 100% of the glomeruli. Approximately 20% of the time, the lesion is a diffuse proliferative type with or without crescents. Patients thus afflicted frequently present with ANS. Systemic manifestations may include the classic butterfly skin rash, arthritis or arthralgia, serositis, or neurologic features such as cerebritis. Laboratory abnormalities, which would support the diagnosis, include a positive antinuclear factor, suppression of both C3 and C4 complement components, elevation of anti-DNA antibodies, leukopenia, and thrombocytopenia. Management of these patients should initially be with steroids alone. High doses of prednisone, in the form of either oral therapy starting at 1 to 2 mg/kg for 1 to 3 months, or short courses of bolus methylprednisolone (5 to 10 mg/kg, given on alternate days during a 6- to 10-day period), followed by a lower dose of daily prednisone (0.5 to 1 mg/kg), are sufficient to induce a remission in more than 75% of lupus patients who present with ANS. Alternative forms of acute therapy include bolus cyclophosphamide (0.5 to 1 g/m^2, given at 4- to 6-week intervals). Some researchers have suggested that this therapy retards the development of scarring within the kidney and may be less toxic than high-dose steroids. The addition of plasmapheresis appears to be of little benefit. Total lymphoid irradiation has been tried in resistant cases but must be considered experimental at this time. A major consideration if disease activity persists is the risk:benefit ratio when using any of these potent and potentially dangerous therapies. Regardless of the response, careful monitoring for infection must be maintained because infection is now the leading cause of death in patients with lupus. Maintenance therapy is usually prednisone ($\leq$0.3 mg/kg) on alternate days. Azathioprine (2 to 3 mg/kg) or cyclophosphamide (1.0 mg/kg) is usually added if the disease flares on prednisone alone, especially if the minimum dose reached before relapse was $\geq$20 mg/day.

Polyarteritis Nodosa

Patients with classic polyarteritis nodosa present in their 60s with hypertension and evidence of vascular involvement as demonstrated by liver or bowel ischemia or infarction and/or neurovascular involvement with peripheral neuropathy or mononeuritis multiplex. This

Table 3–3. RENAL PATHOLOGY IN THE COMMON SECONDARY (SYSTEMIC) DISEASES THAT MAY PRESENT WITH ACUTE NEPHRITIC SYNDROME

Disease	Light Microscopy	Immunofluorescence	Electron Microscopy
Lupus nephritis Class 4 (diffuse)	Diffuse proliferation in ≥ 50% of glomeruli, variable size crescents ± segmental necrosis, wire loops ± hematoxylin bodies	Peripheral and mesangial deposits usually full house (i.e., IgG, A, M and complement components)	Subendothelial, mesangial, and occasionally subepithelial deposits
Polyarteritis nodosa	Focal segmental necrosis ± diffuse proliferation, occasional perivascular inflammatory infiltrate	Negative	No deposits
Wegener's granulomatosis	Focal segmental necrotizing glomerulonephritis, occasionally extensive necrosis with surrounding granulomatous reaction within the interstitium	Negative	No deposits
Anaphylactoid purpura (Henoch-Schönlein purpura)	Mesangial cell proliferation and increased mesangial matrix (segmental or diffuse). Presence of crescents 20–30%	IgA ± IgG ± IgM ± complement in the mesangium, fibrin-related products in the crescents	Mesangial ± subendothelial deposits
Mixed essential cryoglobulinemia	Endocapillary proliferation, monocytic cell infiltrate, intraluminal thrombi, and "double-contoured" glomerular basement membrane	IgG, IgM, and C3 deposits in peripheral capillary loops, often very "lumpy" in appearance	Regular amorphous deposits ± deposits with a fibrillar or crystalloid structure
Goodpasture's syndrome	Endocapillary proliferation plus compressed tuft by large circumferential crescents in 50 to 100% of glomeruli	Linear deposition of IgG ± complement along the capillary loops	No deposits but breaks in the basement membrane of the capillary loops ± breaks in the membrane of Bowman's capsule

variant more commonly presents with proteinuria and minor elevation of serum creatinine levels, but an acute nephritic presentation may occur. Microscopic polyarteritis variants (including the Churg-Strauss type, which usually implies a major pulmonary component often with a history of asthma and findings of pulmonary infiltrates and eosinophila) are more commonly found in young and middle-aged persons and in men more than in women. The pathology involves the small arterioles, capillaries, and venules. Other associated features may include skin petechiae or purpura, arthralgias, myalgias, and abdominal pain. Constitutional symptoms such as weight loss and fever may be prominent, and drugs such as penicillin, sulfa, and allopurinol are known to precipitate the disorder. The renal involvement is more extensive and the acute nephritic presentation more common than in the classic type. Autoantibodies directed against the cytoplasmic elements of the neutrophils (ANCA) detected by indirect immunofluorescence or enzyme-linked immunosorbent assay (ELISA) have been found in more than 70% of active cases of polyarteritis nodosa. Their presence is helpful in the diagnosis of the disease, although their pathogenetic and prognostic value is still being assessed. Biopsy of tissue other than renal, such as testis, seral nerve, or muscle, may confirm the vasculitis. This disorder is usually steroid responsive at doses of prednisone of 1 to 2 mg/kg initially, followed by a slow taper. Cytotoxic agents such as cyclophosphamide or azathioprine are commonly used in a dose similar to that given for lupus nephritis. Although not proved in control trials, they probably are of additional benefit or at least allow a lower daily dose of prednisone. This disease is lifelong, and relapses do occur; therefore, long-term monitoring is essential.

Anaphylactoid Purpura (Henoch-Schönlein Purpura)

This disorder was mentioned briefly under primary IgA nephropathy. Although the pathology may be identical, its systemic features, which may include skin, joint, gastrointestinal, and pulmonary components, make it distinct. The skin rash is usually purpuric and found on the dependent portions of the lower and upper extremities. The arthritis is usually mild and transient. Gastrointestinal involvement can be mild or severe and includes abdominal pain with melena and even bowel intussusception, especially in young children. Hemoptysis can also occur but is uncommon. The renal involvement is variable and includes isolated hematuria, proteinuria, the nephrotic syndrome, and in 5 to 20% of cases ANS with oliguria, hypertension, and even gross hematuria. The extrarenal manifestations of this disorder respond to corticosteroids, usually prednisone in a dose of 0.5 to 1.5 mg/kg over 4 to 6 weeks, but this therapy should be reserved for severe disease only. It is possible that with an acute nephritic presentation (often with crescents on biopsy), steroids are of renal benefit. A short course of either bolus methylprednisolone (0.5 to 1 g IV × 3) or oral prednisone (1 to 2 mg/kg), as in idiopathic crescentic GN, should be tried. The renal efficacy of this therapy has not been proved.

Wegener's Granulomatosis

Wegener's granulomatosis is a necrotizing, granulomatous vasculitis of uncertain etiology. It involves principally the respiratory and genitourinary systems. Upper respiratory tract involvement can be diverse and includes otitis media, sinusitis, epistaxis, conjunctivitis, and even gingivitis. Lung involvement may present as cough, hemoptysis, or increasing shortness of breath. Arthralgia, mild arthritis, fever, and weight loss can be other nonspecific symptoms. Rarely, the skin is involved with an ulcerative type of lesion. These symptoms may precede, appear at the same time, or be delayed compared to the genitourinary involvement. Renal disease is encountered in 80 to 90% of cases and is usually mild, with an abnormal urine sediment or modest proteinuria, but a rapidly progressive deterioration in renal function associated with extensive crescent formation and segmental necrosis may occur. Rarely, ureteric involvement with granuloma may produce obstruction, which can mimic the rapidly progressive glomerulonephritis form of Wegener's.

Antibodies to neutrophil cytoplasmic antigens are found in >90% of active cases. They produce a fine granular cytoplasmic staining on immunofluorescence. Whether there is a specific antibody for Wegener's granulomatosis that is not present in the other vasculitic syndromes is being debated. Other laboratory findings such as leukocytosis, eosinophilia, and thrombocytosis may occur but are nondiagnostic. Characteristic pulmonary findings on x-ray films are bilateral nodular infiltrates, which may cavitate. Sinusitis, even in asymptomatic patients, plus renal involvement almost clinches the diagnosis. Affected tissue from the respiratory tract shows typical necrotizing granulomatous lesions, which may include necrosis of small arteries and veins as well as a dense inflammatory infiltrate. The lesion is much more variable in the renal parenchyma, but a segmental and focal proliferative or necrotizing GN with or without crescents is generally seen. Immunofluorescence is generally negative, although scattered peripheral deposits of IgG, IgM, and C3 may occasionally be found. A combination of cyclophosphamide and prednisone therapy is recommended. Prednisone is initiated at 1 mg/kg in divided doses for 2 to 4 weeks. In acute fulminant cases, intravenous methylprednisolone (250 to 500 mg/day given on alternate days × 3 to 5 doses) may replace the initial oral prednisone. Cyclophosphamide is begun at 2 mg/kg/day and adjusted to maintain a neutrophil count between 1 and 1.5 $\times 10^9$/L. Pulse cyclophosphamide may be substituted for the oral regimen (*i.e.*, 0.5 to 1 g/m^2 every 4 to 8 weeks for up to 6 months). Optimum response seems to require prolonged therapy (*i.e.*, at least 6 to 12 months following subsidence of clinical disease activity). This type of combined therapy is associated with an 80 to 85% induced remission rate. However, up to 50% of these patients may suffer a relapse over a period of years; therefore, constant vigilance is required.

Mixed Cryoglobulinemia

The presence of cryoglobulins in the serum may be idiopathic or associated with an infectious, autoimmune, lymphoproliferative, or hepatic disease. The mixed type may present with ANS. A cryoglobulin consists of 2 or more immunoglobulin classes, one of which is a monoclonal paraprotein, usually IgM. Systemic features include purpura, fever, arthralgia, and features of vasculitis. Complement components, both C3 and C4, may be depressed or normal. The course of the renal disease is variable. Although as many as one third present with an acute nephritic or nephrotic/nephritic picture, less than 10% progress to renal failure. Deposits classically are found in the subendothelial location of the glomerular capillary loops and may be associated with an intense monocytic infiltrate. Perivascular cellular infiltrates may also be seen. When a high plasma level of cryoglobulins (cryocrit) is found, the addition of up to 20 courses of 4-L plasma exchanges over 30 days in addition to cyclophosphamide therapy (1 to 2 mg/kg) and oral or pulse prednisone (see vasculitis, above) are required. The natural history is extremely variable; therefore, efficacy studies using combined therapy are not available. Although long-term treatment may be required, an attempt should be made to achieve the lowest possible drug dosage because patients with this disorder are prone to serious life-threatening infections, and this risk is obviously heightened by concomitant immunosuppressive treatment.

Goodpasture's Syndrome

Goodpasture's syndrome occurs predominantly in young men and is secondary to the formation of an antibody that cross-reacts with both lung and glomerular basement membrane. Patients present with hemoptysis (which may be massive), dyspnea, and progressive anemia. An alveolar pattern to the infiltrate is seen on chest x-ray film. Renal involvement is indicated by an active urine sediment, modest proteinuria, and a rapidly rising creatinine level. Severe effects in one system (*e.g.*, lung) may occasionally be associated with a minor effect in the other (*e.g.*, kidney), but both organs frequently are significantly involved by the time therapy is instituted. The linear deposition of IgG with or without C3 on the glomerular basement membrane (and on the lung basement membrane) plus the presence of circulating antibody directed against glomerular basement membrane confirms the diagnosis. Although the serum antibody is ideally detected by a specific radioimmunoassay, a rapid diagnosis can be made in most severe cases in a routine pathology laboratory using a normal kidney target and an indirect immunofluorescence technique. Daily 4-L plasma exchanges to reduce the circulating antibody level combined with pulse methylprednisolone (250 mg/day × 5) and the addition of the cytotoxic agent cyclophosphamide (1 to 2 mg/kg) should be initiated as soon as the diagnosis is established. The duration of plasmapheresis is variable, but rarely is it necessary beyond 20 days. Cyclophosphamide is usually discontinued 8 to 10 weeks after the disease has subsided, and prednisone is slowly tapered to zero over 4 to 6 months. Relapses do occur in up to 25% of patients. Known aggravating factors include hydrocarbon exposure and smoking. These should be identified and eliminated. Although the overall response rate has been dramatically improved by this therapy, renal recovery is low in patients who have a creatinine level of >700 μmol/L, who are oliguric, or who have a high degree of glomerular obsolescence on biopsy at presentation. Risks of this aggressive therapy in patients with these markers must be carefully weighed, especially in the older age-group. Plasmapheresis may be required regardless of the renal status, because massive pulmonary hemorrhage often does not respond to immunosuppressive therapy alone.

CASE SUMMARY 3

A previously healthy 18-year-old male presents with a 2-day history of intermittent mild hemoptysis and some periorbital edema. He reported being a heavy smoker despite his occupation as a gas station attendant. He became acutely dyspneic the night before admission and in the emergency room had an episode of massive hemoptysis. On examination, he was acutely ill and had a respiratory rate of 36/minute and blood pressure of 110/80 mm Hg. He had bilateral crepitations throughout both lung fields. The costovertebral angle was not tender and he had only minor peripheral edema. The urine sediment showed numerous RBC casts, 30 to 50 RBCs per high-power field, and only a trace of protein. His serum creatinine level was 200 μmol/L, his urea level was 15 mmol/L, and his blood gases showed a modest respiratory acidosis and a pO_2 of 60 mm Hg.

Goodpasture's syndrome was strongly suspected, and using an indirect immunofluorescence technique, his serum showed intense linear staining along the target glomerular basement membrane. Intravenous pulse methylprednisolone (250 mg) and plasma exchange were begun immediately. Oral cyclophosphamide (2 mg/kg) was begun on day 4. Although his pulmonary hemorrhage had improved by that time, his creatinine level had risen to 450 μmol/L. A renal biopsy confirmed the diagnosis of Goodpasture's syndrome and the presence of large cellular crescents in 70% of the glomeruli. Therapy was continued with alternate-day pulse steroids and plasma exchange, and by day 14 his creatinine level started to decline. Plasma exchange was discontinued at day 20, when the antibody was no longer detected in the serum. The patient was switched from intravenous methylprednisolone to oral prednisone (1 mg/kg) at day 20. The cyclophosphamide was continued at 1 mg/kg, because his absolute neutrophil count remained $>1.0 \times 10^9$/L. His creatinine plateaued at 150 μmol/L at 1 month. His chest x-ray film was clear. Cyclophosphamide was discontinued after 6 months, and the prednisone tapered to zero by 8 months. The patient has stopped smoking, has changed his occupation, and is doing well after 2 years.

Suggested Readings

Ballo JE: Renal Vasculitis. Kidney Int 27:954, 1985.

Cattran DC, Cardella CJ, Roscoe JM, et al: Results of a controlled drug trial in membranoproliferative glomerulonephritis. Kidney Int 27:436, 1985.

Couser W: Rapidly progressive glomerulonephritis, pathogenetic mechanisms, and therapy. Am J Kidney Dis 11:449, 1988.

D'Amico G, Minetti L, Ponticelli C, et al: Prognostic indicators in idiopathic IgA mesangial nephropathy. Q J Med 228:363, 1986.

Donadio JV, Holley KE, Ferguson RH, et al: Treatment of diffuse proliferative lupus nephritis with prednisone and combined prednisone and cyclophosphamide. N Engl J Med 299:1151, 1978.

Hind CRK, Lockwood CM, Peters DK, et al: Prognosis after immunosuppression in patients with crescentic nephritis requiring dialysis. Lancet 1:263, 1983.

McCune WJ, Golbus J, Zeldes W, et al: Clinical and immunological effects of monthly administration of intravenous cyclophosphamide in severe lupus erythematosus. N Engl J Med 318:1423, 1988.

Nolle B, Specks O, Ludemann J, et al: Anticytoplasmic autoantibodies: Their immunodiagnostic value in Wegener's granulomatosis. Ann Intern Med 111:28, 1989.

Rodriquez-Iturbe B: Epidemic poststreptococcal glomerulonephritis. Kidney Int 25:129, 1984.

Roth DA, Wilz DR, Theil GB: Schönlein Henoch syndrome in Adults. Q J Med 55:145, 1985.

CHAPTER **4**

SODIUM AND POTASSIUM DISTURBANCES IN RENAL PATIENTS

Biff F. Palmer, Robert D. Toto, and Robert J. Alpern

Disorders of serum sodium and potassium are commonly encountered in clinical medicine. Acting with thirst and antidiuretic hormone (ADH), the kidneys are able to maintain the body's tonicity within well-defined limits despite being challenged with the extremes of intake of salt and water. In conjunction with factors that modulate the internal balance of potassium, the kidneys also defend the serum potassium within a narrow range when faced with similar environmental stresses. Because of the kidneys' pivotal role in these homeostatic systems, patients with renal dysfunction are particularly prone to disorders of sodium and potassium. In this chapter, mechanisms responsible for the maintenance of serum sodium and potassium concentrations are discussed, an approach to clinical disorders presented, and a rational discussion of treatment given.

REGULATION OF PLASMA SODIUM CONCENTRATION

Compartmentalization of Total Body Water

In an average man, total body water (TBW) is equal to 60% of body weight; this figure is 50% in women because of extra body fat, which is water free. Of the TBW, approximately two thirds is located intracellularly, whereas one third is located extracellularly. Of the extracellular fluid (ECF) volume, only one fourth is located within the intravascular space. In a 70-kg man with a TBW of 42 L, 28 L are located intracellularly, whereas only 14 L are located in the ECF and only 3.5 L are located in the extracellular intravascular compartment.

Osmolality and Tonicity

Osmolality is defined as the number of particles per kilogram of solution. Although plasma osmolality can be measured with an osmometer, a test that is clinically available, it can also be estimated using the following equation:

$$\text{Osmolality} = 2 \times [\text{Na}] + \frac{[\text{glucose}]}{18} + \frac{[\text{BUN}]}{2.8}$$

The concentration of sodium is multiplied by 2 because each sodium ion in the ECF is accompanied by an anion that also contributes to osmolality. This equation is very useful clinically in the calculation of the osmolal gap, which is the difference between the calculated osmolality and the measured osmolality. In general, a measured plasma osmolality more than 10 mOsm/L greater than the calculated osmolality indicates accumulation of an osmole not routinely measured. Such substances include ethanol, methanol, ethylene glycol, and acetone.

Whereas osmolality refers to all particles, tonicity refers only to those particles that cannot penetrate cell membranes and thus can lead to changes in cell volume. Such particles are considered *effective osmoles*. Isotonic solutions produce no water movement across cells. Hypertonic solutions cause cell shrinkage, whereas hypotonic solutions result in cell swelling. Clinically, tonicity is more important than osmolality because osmometers are able to measure only osmolality and cannot differentiate *effective* from *noneffective* osmoles. Patients with renal failure and with blood urea nitrogen (BUN) concentrations >100 mg/dl have high measured plasma osmolality, whereas plasma tonicity is normal. Urea passes freely across cell membranes and causes no change in cellular hydration. The body's homeostatic mechanisms ignore increases in osmolality due to ineffective solutes such as urea and make no attempt to lower osmolality. Under most clinical conditions, the plasma ECF tonicity is determined by the concentration of sodium salts and glucose and can be calculated using the previous equation, omitting the contribution of BUN.

Regulation of Tonicity

The body closely guards plasma osmolality within a narrow range through the interrelated actions of the renal concentrating and diluting mechanisms, secretion of ADH, and thirst. After glomerular filtration, salt and water are removed from the proximal tubules in an isosmotic fashion. Once filtrate reaches the diluting segments (ascending loop of Henle and early distal nephron), salt is removed from the tubular fluid but water is unable to be reabsorbed because this segment is impermeable to water. Thus, electrolyte-free water is generated. The tubular fluid then passes into the collecting duct, where permeability to water is determined by the level of ADH. In the absence of ADH, the collecting duct is water impermeable, and the dilute fluid formed in the diluting segment is excreted in the urine. In the presence of ADH, the collecting duct becomes water permeable, and because the medullary interstitium is hypertonic, water is reabsorbed and the urine can be concentrated up to 1200 to 1600 mOsm/L. **Therefore the requirements for maximal renal water excretion are (1) normal delivery of filtrate to the diluting segment of the nephron, (2) normal NaCl absorption in the diluting segment, and (3) suppression of ADH.**

The sensing mechanism for ADH secretion in response to osmolality is believed to be an osmometer in the hypothalamus. Increased concentration of effective osmoles in the ECF leads to shrinkage of the osmometer cells, thus sending a signal to the ADH-secreting cells of the hypothalamus to secrete ADH. Once plasma osmolality *increases* by approximately 10 mOsm/L above a preset threshold, mechanisms are invoked to stimulate thirst. *Thirst and access to water are the primary defenses against hypertonicity.*

Another important determinant of free-water excretion is decreased effective arterial blood volume. In response to decreases in effective arterial volume, (1) ADH is released, (2) thirst is stimulated, and (3) glomerular filtration rate (GFR) decreases and proximal salt and water absorption increase, both of which limit delivery to the diluting segment. These factors lead to renal water retention and expansion of the ECF volume. Because water is freely permeable across cell membranes, only one third of the retained water will remain in the ECF space, whereas two thirds will be sequestered in the intracellular space.

CLINICAL DISORDERS ASSOCIATED WITH HYPONATREMIA

The approach to hyponatremia in patients with either normal or impaired renal function begins with a consideration of serum osmolality to determine whether the low serum sodium level is associated with a hypotonic state. Hypotonic hyponatremia is further subdivided according to the volume status of the patient into hypovolemic, isovolemic, and hypervolemic forms (Fig. 4–1).

Isotonic and Hypertonic Hyponatremia

Before embarking on a workup of a low serum sodium level, one must determine if the hyponatremia is real. Circulating plasma is composed of 93% water and 7% solid (protein and lipid). In states of hyperproteinemia or hyperlipidemia, the solid phase of plasma is expanded, and the aqueous phase, to which sodium is confined, shrinks. The sodium concentration as measured in total plasma decreases despite the constancy of its concentration in plasma water. Measurements of osmolality are unaffected. Clues to the diagnosis of "pseudohyponatremia" include the measurement of a normal serum osmolality or the appearance of turbid plasma secondary to hyperlipidemia.

Hyponatremia can also occur because of fluid shifts from the intracellular to extracellular compartment as a result of the presence of nonsodium effective osmoles in the ECF space. These effective osmoles create an osmotic gradient for water movement from the intracellular space to the extracellular space, with resultant dilution of the serum sodium. These disorders result in the redistribution of water from one compartment to the other and can be associated with an isotonic or hypertonic state. Clinical exam-

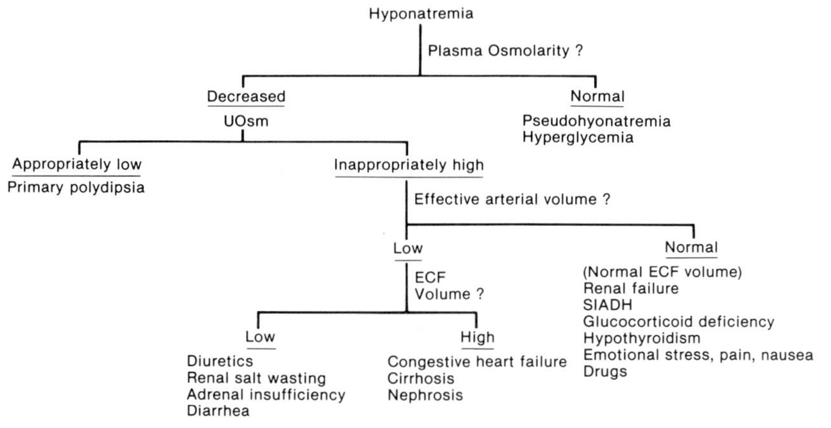

Figure 4–1. Approach to patients with hyponatremia.

ples include hyperglycemia, as seen in uncontrolled diabetes, or rarely hypertonic infusion of mannitol, used in the treatment of cerebral edema. **For every 100-mg/dl rise in glucose or mannitol, the serum sodium concentration quickly declines by 1.6 mEq/L.** As water intake increases and osmolality is returned to normal, serum sodium concentration decreases 2.8 mEq/L for every 100-mg/dl rise in glucose. A high measured osmolality resulting from ineffective osmoles such as urea does not cause a redistribution of water.

Hypotonic Hyponatremia

Hypotonic hyponatremia occurs when water intake is in excess of the kidneys' ability to excrete water. Because a normal kidney can excrete 20 to 30 L of water per day, the presence of hypotonic hyponatremia usually implies a defect in free-water excretion. The one exception is the unusual patient with primary polydipsia who drinks >20 to 30 L/day. In all other cases, the diagnostic approach is based on asking why urinary dilution is impaired. Patients with primary polydipsia can be identified by the presence of an appropriately dilute urine; all other patients will have inappropriately concentrated urine.

Total body sodium *content* is not reflected by the serum sodium concentration. It can be low, normal, or high in hyponatremic states and is best assessed by clinical evaluation of the ECF volume. Dividing the hypotonic states according to sodium content (or volume status) is useful, as each state is associated with a particular range of disorders, thus necessitating different therapeutic approaches.

Hypovolemic Hyponatremia

Loss of salt, whether from the gastrointestinal tract, skin, or kidneys, culminates in a series of hormonal and hemodynamic factors that signal renal water retention. As discussed earlier, the decreased effective arterial blood volume leads to decreased delivery of salt and water to the diluting segments of the kidneys, increased ADH levels, and thirst. Clinically, patients demonstrate the typical findings of a shrunken ECF volume: tachycardia, postural change in blood pressure and pulse, oliguria, and azotemia. In the absence of renal or adrenal disease and diuretic use, the urine sodium concentration will be low, reflecting the avid sodium reabsorption. Renal causes of volume depletion and hyponatremia are discussed below.

Diuretics. Diuretics are a common cause of hypovolemic hyponatremia. The hyponatremia in this setting is often accompanied by hypokalemic metabolic alkalosis. In addition to decreasing effective arterial blood volume, diuretics such as furosemide, ethacrynic acid, and thiazides decrease free-water excretion by directly inhibiting sodium reabsorption in the thick ascending limb and early distal tubule. Urinary sodium is high. Because loop diuretics inhibit generation of a hypertonic medullary interstitium, leading to inhibition of ADH-mediated water reabsorption, hyponatremia is much less common than with thiazide diuretics (when urinary concentration is unaffected).

Salt-Losing Nephropathy. Certain interstitial renal diseases can result in salt-losing nephropathy with resultant hypovolemic hyponatremia. In these diseases, sodium loss in the urine is significantly increased despite a contracted effective arterial volume. Examples include medullary cystic disease, analgesic nephropathy, partial urinary tract obstruction, and chronic interstitial nephritis. These patients may need to ingest supplemental NaCl to avoid depletion of ECF volume and secondary hyponatremia.

Mineralocorticoid Deficiency. Patients with Addison's disease develop a decreased effective arterial blood volume as a result of renal salt wastage secondary to lack of mineralocorticoid activity. These patients are hyperkalemic.

Hypervolemic Hyponatremia

The edematous states of congestive heart failure, cirrhosis, and in some cases nephrotic syndrome share a shrunken effective arterial blood volume that sets into motion the same pathophysiologic effects as noted with a contracted ECF volume. Thus, delivery of filtrate to the diluting segment is decreased, ADH levels are elevated despite the hypo-osmolar state, and thirst is increased. Urine sodium concentration is low, reflecting the low effective arterial volume. These patients are recognized clinically by the presence of edema.

Isovolemic Hyponatremia

Isovolemic hyponatremia is noted by the absence of edema and signs of a contracted ECF volume. Because effective arterial volume is not contracted, urine sodium is not low (*i.e.*, >20 mEq/L).

Renal Failure. In the setting of total suppression of ADH and normal renal function, the kidneys can excrete large quantities of water. For example, assuming that 20% of the normal GFR of 120 ml/min can be excreted as free water, one can calculate that a normal individual has the capacity to excrete 30 L of water per day. In the setting of renal failure, this capacity to excrete free water is truncated by limited delivery of filtrate to the diluting segment. A patient who has a GFR of 5 ml/min and excretes 20% of the filtered load of water will excrete only 1.4 to 1.5 L/day. **Thus, patients with chronic renal failure can develop hyponatremia by drinking more water than they deliver filtrate distally.**

Syndrome of Inappropriate ADH Secretion. In the setting of euvolemia, a concentrated urine and high ADH levels are inappropriate. The most common cause of this condition is the syndrome of inappropriate ADH secretion (SIADH). SIADH is generally associated with diseases of the central nervous system (CNS), usually those that affect the base of the brain, pulmonary diseases, and neoplasms (Table 4–1). These conditions lead to secretion of ADH that is inappropriate from the standpoint of both plasma osmolality and effective arterial volume. A number of other factors cause hypo-osmolality associated with euvolemia and can mimic SIADH.

Glucocorticoid Deficiency. With isolated glucocorticoid deficiency (normal mineralocorticoid activity), isovolemic hyponatremia can occur. This situation is seen in states of secondary hypoadrenalism resulting from decreased secretion of ACTH from the pituitary gland. These patients do not have salt wasting and possess an intact ECF volume. Persistent ADH secretion and decreased delivery to the diluting segment are responsible for the hyponatremia. Serum potassium level is normal.

Hypothyroidism. Lack of circulating thyroid hormone can result in hyponatremia. A decrease in GFR and increased circulating ADH account for the hyponatremia. Thyroid replacement will correct the abnormalities.

Emotional Stress, Pain, Nausea. These factors can result in the nonosmotic release of ADH. If water ingestion occurs at a time of nausea, pain, or acute psychosis, hyponatremia may ensue.

Drugs. Various drugs have been associated with either increased ADH release or augmented response of the kidneys to ambient

Table 4–1. DISORDERS ASSOCIATED WITH THE SYNDROME OF INAPPROPRIATE SECRETION OF ANTIDIURETIC HORMONE

Tumors	Pulmonary Diseases	CNS Disorders
Oat cell carcinoma	Tuberculosis	Brain tumor
Bronchogenic carcinoma	Lung abscesses	Encephalitis
Adenocarcinoma of pancreas	Viral and bacterial pneumonia	Subarachnoid hemorrhage
Hodgkin's disease		Acute intermittent porphyria
Thymoma		Head injury

ADH levels. These drugs are listed in Table 4–2.

TREATMENT OF HYPONATREMIA

The principal danger of hyponatremia or hypernatremia relates to effects on CNS function due to changes in brain size. Hyponatremia initially leads to cell swelling driven by the higher intracellular osmolality. The net result is equilibration of intracellular and extracellular osmolality at the expense of increased brain volume. Cells in general, and brain cells in particular, respond by decreasing the number of intracellular osmoles, secondarily causing water to move out and a return to normal cell size. If ECF osmolality decreases slowly, there will be no measurable cell swelling. This pathophysiologic sequence correlates well with clinical observations. If hyponatremia is slow in onset, neurologic symptoms and permanent brain damage are unusual, even if the decreases in sodium concentration and ECF osmolality are large. Conversely, if hyponatremia is rapid in onset, cerebral edema and significant CNS symptoms and signs can occur with lesser changes in serum sodium concentration (Table 4–3).

When treating a patient with hyponatremia, the sodium concentration should be raised at the rate at which it decreased. In a patient whose serum sodium concentration has declined slowly, neurologic symptoms are generally minimal, brain size is normal, and the number of intracellular osmoles is decreased. **Sudden return of ECF osmolality to normal values leads to cell shrinkage, neurologic symptoms, and possibly permanent brain damage.** Specifically, rapid correction has been associated with central pontine myelinolysis. Thus, it is recommended that serum sodium be corrected slowly in these patients. In a patient whose serum sodium concentration has decreased rapidly, neurologic symptoms are frequently present, as is cerebral edema. In this setting there has not been sufficient time to remove osmoles from the brain, and rapid return to normal ECF osmolality merely returns brain size to normal.

Table 4–2. DRUGS ASSOCIATED WITH HYPONATREMIA

ADH-Like Action	Stimulate ADH Release	Sensitize Kidney to ADH
Oxytocin	Chlorpropamide	Chlorpropamide
Deamino-D-arginine	Clofibrate	Cyclophosphamide
Vasopressin	Cyclophosphamide	Indomethacin
	Vincristine	Aminophylline
	Carbamazepine	
	Amitriptyline	
	Thiothixene	
	Nicotine	
	Morphine	

ADH, antidiuretic hormone.

Table 4–3. SYMPTOMS AND SIGNS OF HYPONATREMIA

Symptoms	Signs
Lethargy	Depressed sensorium
Muscle cramps	Hypothermia
Disorientation	Depressed deep tendon
Nausea	Reflexes
Agitation	Cheyne-Stokes respiration
	Seizures

Therapy of hyponatremia depends on several factors including the underlying cause, the rapidity of development, and the severity of symptoms and signs present. The initial approach in all cases is fluid restriction so that the degree of hyponatremia will not progress. The treatment of hypotonic hyponatremia is given in Table 4–4.

Rapid Correction of Hyponatremia

In patients who have acute hyponatremia and are demonstrating CNS signs or symptoms, rapid correction is indicated. Rapid correction of hyponatremia involves intravenous administration of hypertonic saline (usually 3% NaCl). Generally, an infusion rate is used that will **raise serum sodium concentration at a rate of 1 mEq/L/hr. Present evidence suggests that correction at a more rapid rate may be dangerous.** To calculate the amount of sodium required, one should use a volume of distribution of TBW. Although sodium is confined to the ECF space, in disorders of osmolality one is replacing an osmolar deficit present throughout the TBW.

$$(\text{Desired Na} - \text{actual Na}) \times \text{TBW} = \text{amount of Na required}$$

CASE SUMMARY 1

A 70-kg man with a history of chronic renal insufficiency presents with a serum sodium

Table 4–4. TREATMENT OF HYPONATREMIA

Correction	Low ECF Volume	Edema	Euvolemia
Acute			
Slow	Normal saline	Fluid restriction	Fluid restriction
Rapid 1 mEq/L/hr	Hypertonic saline	Hypertonic saline + furosemide	Hypertonic saline + furosemide
Chronic	Remove cause	Remove cause ? Demeclocycline	Remove cause Discontinue drug Hormone replacement Treat the cause of the syndrome of inappropriate ADH secretion Demeclocycline

ADH, antidiuretic hormone; ECF, extracellular fluid.

level of 110 mEq/L, has symptoms of stupor, and demonstrates seizure activity. In order to raise his serum sodium level to 130 mEq/L, one can calculate the amount of 3% saline needed.

$$\text{TBW} = 70 \text{ kg} \times 60\% = 42 \text{ L}$$
$$(130 \text{ mEq/L} - 110 \text{ mEq/L}) \times 42 \text{ L} = 840 \text{ mEq Na}$$

As each liter of 3% saline contains 513 mEq of sodium, one would administer 1.6 L of 3% NaCl over 20 hours in order to raise the serum sodium level by 1 mEq/L/hr.

Use of hypertonic saline alone may be associated with volume expansion that would be dangerous in the elderly or in patients with compromised cardiac function. Patients with impaired renal function are particularly prone to volume overload with such sodium loads. In this instance, a furosemide diuresis can be used. Hypertonic saline is infused at a rate equal to the urinary loss of sodium, chloride, and potassium that is induced by furosemide. For example, assume that furosemide administered at a dose of 1 mg/kg resulted in a urine output of 1000 ml/hr with a sodium concentration of 70 mEq/L. One can calculate that 136 ml of 3% NaCl will replace the excreted sodium and a net negative water balance of 864 ml has been achieved.

In order to calculate the total net negative fluid balance necessary to achieve the desired sodium concentration, one can use the following formulas:

$$\text{Body weight} \times 60\% = \text{TBW}$$
$$\text{or } 70 \text{ kg} \times 60\% = 42 \text{ L}$$
$$\text{TBW} - \frac{\text{Acutal Na [ ]}}{\text{Desired Na [ ]}} \times \text{TBW} = \text{amount of excess water}$$
$$\text{or } 42 - \frac{110}{130} \times 42 = 6.5 \text{ L}$$

When a serum sodium concentration of 130 mEq/L is obtained, one can simply place the patient on fluid restriction. In this manner, neurologic sequelae resulting from rapid correction of the serum sodium level can be avoided.

These formulas are to be used only as guidelines, and frequent monitoring of patients and serum sodium levels needs to be done during these rapid changes in fluid balance. With advanced renal failure, dialysis will be required to correct the hyponatremic state rapidly. Interestingly, patients treated with dialysis for hyponatremia frequently correct their hyponatremia very rapidly; however, this is generally well tolerated.

CLINICAL DISORDERS ASSOCIATED WITH HYPERNATREMIA

Although hyponatremia can occur in the setting of low, normal, or high osmolality, all instances of hypernatremia are associated with hypertonicity. Hypernatremia is indicative of a high sodium *concentration* but can occur with low, normal, or high total body sodium *content*. As a result, the hypertonic states can best be subdivided according to the ECF volume. A flow diagram outlining the approach to hypernatremia is depicted in Figure 4–2.

One of the most important points in understanding disorders of hypertonicity is to realize that **the primary defense against hypernatremia is thirst.** Thus, patients who have an intact thirst mechanism and who have free access to water do not become hypertonic and hypernatremic. If either the thirst mechanism is not intact (a specific lesion of the thirst center or a generalized decrease in mental status) or the patient does not have access to water, he or she is at risk for the development of hypernatremia.

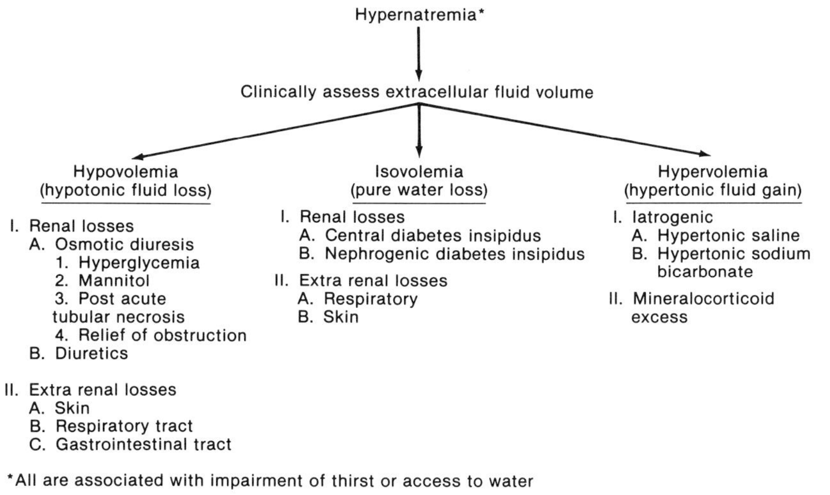

Figure 4–2. Approach to patients with hypernatremia.

The likelihood of a patient's developing hypernatremia is greater if he or she has, in addition, accelerated water loss or increased sodium intake.

Patients with chronic renal failure are predisposed to the development of hypernatremia, as the ability to concentrate the urine maximally is lost early in the development of renal insufficiency. The filtration of osmotically active particles into a smaller number of surviving nephrons results in a constant osmotic diuresis, diminishing the capacity to regulate sodium and water reabsorption. Damaged kidneys are also less responsive to circulating ADH. As renal failure progresses, the filtered load of water diminishes and the propensity toward excessive water loss is mitigated.

Hypovolemic Hypernatremia

Hypernatremia in the setting of a shrunken ECF volume indicates a loss of both sodium and water, but water to a greater extent. This loss of hypotonic fluid can occur through the gastrointestinal tract (diarrhea and vomiting), the skin (burns, fever, sweating), or the kidneys (osmotic diuresis, diuretics). Clinically, patients demonstrate signs of both dehydration and volume depletion.

Renal Losses

An osmotic diuresis typically results in losses of hypotonic fluid. Hyperglycemia in a patient with uncontrolled diabetes will produce such a diuresis. Acutely, hyperglycemia causes water to shift to the extracellular space from the intracellular compartment, resulting in a lowering of the serum sodium level in the setting of a high measured serum osmolality (hypertonic hyponatremia). Later, as hyperglycemia persists, hypotonic fluid lost in the urine will return sodium concentration to normal or above normal. **A normal or elevated serum sodium level in the presence of hyperglycemia is indicative of substantial fluid losses. Urea loads that occur after acute tubular necrosis and during the relief of urinary obstruction and infusion of mannitol can produce substantial urinary losses of hypotonic fluid.**

Hypervolemic Hypernatremia

In hypervolemic hypernatremia, there has been a gain of both sodium and water, but the gain in sodium has been greater. These situations often have iatrogenic causes, such as the administration of sodium bicarbonate to patients with metabolic acidosis or administration of hypertonic saline. Primary aldosteronism leads to expansion of the ECF space through its sodium-retaining effects, and serum sodium concentrations of 145 to 148 mEq/L are often found. In this setting, expansion of the effective arterial volume may suppress thirst.

Isovolemic Hypernatremia

Pure water loss, whether from mucocutaneous routes or from the kidneys, causes isovolemic hypernatremia. Because two thirds of pure water loss is sustained from within cells, patients will not become clinically volume depleted unless the water deficit becomes substantial.

Renal Water Losses. In the absence of an osmotic diuresis, polyuric hypernatremia, involving inappropriate water loss by the kidneys, is referred to as diabetes insipidus. Central diabetes insipidus refers to conditions in which ADH secretion from the posterior pituitary is

Table 4–5. CAUSES OF CENTRAL AND NEPHROGENIC DIABETES INSIPIDUS

Central Diabetes Insipidus	Nephrogenic Diabetes Insipidus
Posttraumatic	Familial (X-linked recessive)
Neurosurgery (hypophysectomy)	Amyloid
Tumors	Polycystic disease
1. Pituitary tumors	Sickle cell disease, trait
2. Craniopharyngioma	Postobstructive
3. Metastatic tumor (breast)	Hypercalcemia
Granulomatous disease	Hypokalemia
1. Sarcoid	Drugs
2. Histiocytosis X	Lithium
Meningitis, encephalitis	Demeclocycline
Drugs (nicotine, ethanol)	Methoxyflurane
Idiopathic	

inhibited despite the presence of hypertonicity. If ADH levels are appropriate for the existing hypertonicity but the urine is inappropriately dilute, the patient has ADH resistance or nephrogenic diabetes insipidus. The causes of central and nephrogenic diabetes insipidus are listed in Table 4–5.

Although renal water loss can lead to hypernatremia in patients with impaired thirst or access to water, most patients with diabetes insipidus have neither of these defects, and typically a patient presents with polyuria, polydipsia, and a normal serum sodium concentration. A useful approach to patients with polyuria is given in Figure 4–3. Once an osmotic diuresis is excluded as the cause of polyuria, the water deprivation test can be useful. It should be stressed that this test is not to be performed in the setting of existing hypernatremia. It is unnecessary, and further water restriction can lead to dangerous elevations of serum sodium concentration.

Water Deprivation Test. Primary polydipsia and central and nephrogenic diabetes insipidus can be distinguished by comparing the response of urinary osmolality to water deprivation and subsequent ADH administration. The water deprivation test is performed by water restriction until a patient is hypernatremic (serum sodium ≥145). ADH is then administered as 5 units of aqueous vasopressin subcutaneously, and urinary osmolality is monitored. In patients with central diabetes insipidus, the urine is not appropriately concentrated in response to water deprivation. Exogenous ADH administration will then result in dramatic reductions in urine volume and simultaneous increases in urine osmolality. In nephrogenic diabetes insipidus, circulating ADH levels are high but urine osmolality remains low and unresponsive to parenteral administration of ADH.

Patients who compulsively drink water also present with polyuria and polydipsia. With water deprivation, it is difficult to achieve hypernatremia, as these patients' urine can be concentrated. Exogenous ADH administration causes no additional response.

TREATMENT OF HYPERNATREMIA

Increases in ECF osmolality initially cause cell shrinkage within the brain. Signs and symp-

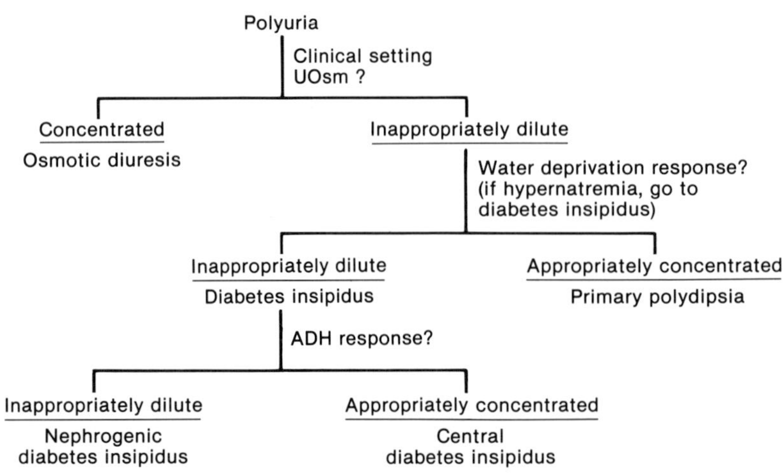

Figure 4–3. Approach to patients with polyuria.

toms include lethargy, weakness, fasciculations, seizures, and coma. This reduction in brain size may also cause rupture of cerebral veins with intracerebral and subarachnoid hemorrhage. The cells respond by the generation of intracellular osmoles, which pull water back into the cells, returning brain size to normal. These new intracellular osmoles include ions transported into cells, as well as other more poorly defined osmoles, referred to as idiogenic osmoles.

If extracellular osmolality is returned rapidly to normal during the therapy of hypernatremia, the extra intracellular osmoles will pull water into the brain cells, resulting in cerebral edema. Thus, in general, hypernatremia should be corrected slowly by water administration at a rate that leads to half correction in 24 hours.

Calculation of Water Deficit

One can calculate the water deficit using a volume of distribution of TBW, assuming that total body cations remain constant.

$$TBW_{present} \times [Na]_{present} = TBW_{normal} \times [Na]_{normal}$$

The differences between the two TBWs is the amount of water required to correct the serum sodium concentration.

CASE SUMMARY 2

A 70-year-old man with known chronic renal insufficiency is brought to the emergency room in a stuporous state. The patient has a serum sodium level of 170 mEq/L. The water deficit in this 75-kg man would be as follows:

$$\begin{aligned} 75\text{ kg} \times 0.60 &= 45\text{ L (TBW)} \\ 45\text{ L} \times 170\text{ mEq/L} &= TBW_{normal} \times 140\text{ mEq/L} \\ TBW_{normal} &= 54.6\text{ L} \\ 54.6\text{ L} - 45\text{ L} &= 9.6\text{ L water deficit} \end{aligned}$$

Correction of the water deficit would require 9.6 L of positive water balance. In order to avoid the development of cerebral edema, chronic hypernatremia in particular should be corrected slowly. The water deficit should be replaced at a rate that leads to half correction in 24 hours. The above calculation should be considered only a rough estimate. As with the treatment of hyponatremia, frequent monitoring of patients and serum sodium level is essential.

REGULATION OF SERUM POTASSIUM

Total body potassium is approximately 50 mEq/kg, such that 3500 mEq of potassium would be found in a 70-kg person. Of this, 98% is contained in the intracellular water and 2% in the ECF.

Internal Potassium Balance

The regulation of potassium distribution between the intracellular and extracellular space is referred to as internal potassium balance. Although the kidneys are ultimately responsible for maintenance of total body potassium, factors that modulate internal balance are important in the disposal of acute potassium loads. Factors affecting internal potassium homeostasis are as follows:

pH-Dependent Potassium Shifts. Metabolic acidosis promotes potassium exit from cells dependent on the type of acid present. Mineral acidosis (NH_4Cl or HCl) promotes the greatest efflux of potassium from cells, whereas organic acidosis (*i.e.*, lactic, beta-hydroxybutyric, or methylmalonic acid) results in no significant efflux of potassium. Acute respiratory acidosis results in only a small shift of potassium out of cells. Metabolic and respiratory alkalosis tend to lower the serum potassium level by promoting entry into cells.

Insulin. Insulin, perhaps by stimulating the sodium-potassium adenosine triphosphatase (ATPase), promotes the cellular uptake of potassium independent of its stimulation of glucose uptake. Increases in plasma potassium levels stimulate insulin release from the pancreas, which in turn enhances cellular uptake, restoring normal serum potassium levels. Thus, a functioning feedback loop exists for potassium and insulin.

Catecholamines. Beta-adrenergic agonists acting on $beta_2$ receptors stimulate the cellular uptake of potassium through a cyclic AMP-dependent activation of the sodium-potassium pump. Increased potassium intake leads to increases in catecholamine secretion that cause enhanced potassium uptake in muscle through $beta_2$ stimulation. The administration of beta-adrenergic agents such as epinephrine, salbutamol, and terbutaline all will result in hypokalemia. In the setting of beta blockade, a greater rise in serum potassium occurs after potassium loads and exercise. However, beta blockade has no effect on baseline potassium values. Alpha agonists inhibit potassium uptake by cells and alpha antagonists stimulate potassium uptake by cells.

Hypertonicity. Increases in ECF tonicity lead to a shift of fluid from the intracellular to the ECF compartment. The resultant cellular shrinkage concentrates intracellular potassium, providing a driving force for potassium efflux.

External Potassium Balance

Renal Potassium Excretion

All causes of chronic elevations or depressions in serum potassium levels can be related to disordered renal potassium handling. Potassium is freely filtered by the glomerulus but is extensively reabsorbed by the proximal tubules and loops of Henle so that approximately 10% of the filtered load reaches the distal nephrons. The distal nephrons secrete potassium into the tubular fluid, which will be excreted. Under most physiologic and pathologic conditions, potassium delivery to the distal nephrons remains small and does not vary, but rather the rate of secretion by the distal nephrons varies. Thus, the rate of potassium secretion in the distal nephrons will determine the rate of potassium excretion. The physiologic determinants of renal potassium excretion are as follows.

Mineralocorticoids. Aldosterone is a major determinant of potassium secretion. Aldosterone-induced stimulation of sodium reabsorption in the collecting tubules makes the luminal potential more negative, thus stimulating potassium secretion. In addition, mineralocorticoids directly stimulate potassium secretion in the distal nephrons.

Distal Delivery. Increased distal delivery of sodium stimulates distal sodium absorption, making the luminal potential more negative and thus increasing potassium secretion. In addition, increased luminal flow rate lowers luminal potassium concentration, secondarily stimulating potassium secretion.

The dependence of potassium secretion on distal delivery and aldosterone levels helps to make potassium excretion independent of volume status. When patients are volume overloaded, distal delivery is increased but aldosterone is suppressed. When patients are volume depleted, aldosterone is increased (secondary hyperaldosteronism) but distal delivery is decreased. In both of these states, potassium homeostasis is maintained.

Nonreabsorbable Anions. Because nonreabsorbable anions are not reabsorbed in the proximal tubules, they increase distal delivery of sodium and volume and secondarily increase potassium secretion by this mechanism. In addition, nonreabsorbable anions enhance potassium secretion by increasing the lumen-negative voltage in the cortical collecting tubules. Examples of poorly reabsorbable (or nonreabsorbable) anions are sulfate, phosphate, carbenicillin, and, under certain conditions, bicarbonate.

Potassium Intake. Chronic elevations in potassium intake lead to an adaptive process in the kidneys, associated with an increased activity of the basolateral membrane sodium-potassium ATPase of the collecting tubules, thus increasing cell potassium and ultimately increasing the rate of potassium excretion.

Low potassium intake leads to a decreased rate of potassium excretion. In the collecting tubules, there is not only a decreased rate of potassium secretion, but actually potassium reabsorption. The kidneys do not defend against hypokalemia as well as against hyperkalemia. On a zero-potassium diet, renal excretion of potassium will not decline below 5 mEq/day. A potassium-free diet combined with minimal stool losses of about 10 mEq/day requires intake of at least 15 mEq/day of potassium to stay in balance.

Extrarenal Potassium Excretion

Under normal circumstances, approximately 90% of an ingested potassium load is excreted in the urine, and 10% of the ingested load is excreted in the stool (5 to 15 mEq/day). Sweat with a mean potassium concentration of 9 mEq/L accounts for a small amount of potassium excretion (<5 mEq/day). In states of decreased renal function, the amount of potassium excreted in stool can increase to >20 mEq/day. Gastrointestinal and sweat potassium secretion is influenced by circulating aldosterone.

CLINICAL DISORDERS ASSOCIATED WITH HYPOKALEMIA

In the absence of physical and historical evidence of gastrointestinal or renal potassium losses, either a redistribution of potassium at the cellular level or laboratory error will account for a low serum potassium. The only spurious cause of hypokalemia is noted in leukemia patients with leukocyte counts of 100 to 250,000 mm^3; the leukocytes extract potassium from the serum.

Redistribution with Normal Total Body Potassium

The effect of alkalemia and, specifically, an increased bicarbonate concentration promoting potassium entry into cells has been discussed. Insulin excess, whether exogenous administration in a diabetic patient or endogenous secretion as in a normal person given a high-glucose load, will lower the serum potassium. Beta agonists used in the treatment of bronchospasm or in treating premature labor will effect similar potassium shifts. In a patient who has recently suffered a myocardial infarction, hypokalemia may result as a sequela of high circulating epinephrine levels and might predispose to arrhythmias in this clinical setting. Other clinical disorders resulting in an intracellular sequestration of potassium are treatment of megaloblastic anemia with vitamin B_{12}, hypothermia, and barium poisoning. Hypokalemic periodic paralysis is inherited in an autosomal dominant pattern and is characterized by episodic hypokalemia resulting in muscle weakness. A similar but noninherited syndrome has been encountered in thyrotoxic patients, often of Japanese descent.

Hypokalemia with Decreased Total Body Potassium

In the absence of a cellular redistribution, a low serum potassium level can result from inadequate dietary intake, extrarenal losses as from the gastrointestinal tract or skin, or renal losses. There are overlaps among these groups. The urinary potassium concentration serves as a useful guide in discerning between these possibilities. A urine potassium concentration of <20 mEq/L is suggestive of extrarenal losses, whereas a urine concentration of >20 mEq/L suggests renal potassium losses.

Inadequate Dietary Intake

Inadequate dietary intake of potassium is an unusual cause of hypokalemia. However, individuals who go extended lengths of time without potassium ingestion develop hypokalemia. Clinical situations associated with extremely potassium-deficient diets include anorexia nervosa, crash diets, alcoholism, and intestinal malabsorption. Increased renal potassium excretion owing to magnesium deficiency (which is often present in these clinical situations) may contribute to the observed hypokalemia.

Extrarenal Potassium Losses

Because sweat has a low concentration of potassium, sweating is an unusual cause of potassium depletion. However, during physical training, sweat losses can become substantial and potassium depletion may result.

Gastrointestinal syndromes are the most common clinical disorders of extrarenal potassium losses. Diarrhea leads to fecal potassium wastage and is associated with a normal anion gap acidosis. Although usually associated with a low urinary potassium concentration, the acidosis *per se* can lead to some degree of renal potassium wasting through increased distal delivery of sodium. In addition, the acidosis will result in potassium redistribution out of cells, leading to a degree of hypokalemia that is not as severe as the degree of potassium depletion.

Renal Potassium Losses

The effects of mineralocorticoids and distal delivery of sodium counterbalance each other; therefore, under normal circumstances, potassium excretion is independent of volume status. Decreases in volume status increase aldosterone secretion while they decrease distal delivery. Increases in volume status suppress aldosterone but increase distal delivery. Disruption of this balance explains many of the renal forms of hypokalemia. The causes of hypokalemia, grouped according to the physiologic determinants of renal potassium excretion, are listed in Table 4–6.

Primary Mineralocorticoid Excess. In conditions classified as primary mineralocorticoid excess, increases in mineralocorticoid activity cannot be attributed to decreased ECF volume or hyperkalemia. An increase in mineralocorticoids in the absence of volume contraction leads to a high incidence of hypertension, but edema is unusual. A so-called escape occurs before sufficient salt is retained for edema formation. In these conditions, normal or increased ECF volume leads to normal or increased distal delivery in the presence of high mineralocorticoid levels, and thus renal potassium wasting.

Decreased Salt Absorption Proximal to the Collecting Tubules. Inhibition of salt absorption

Table 4–6. RENAL CAUSES OF HYPOKALEMIA

Primary mineralocorticoid excess
1. Primary hyperaldosteronism
   a. Conn's syndrome
   b. Bilateral adrenal hyperplasia
2. ↑ Renin → ↑ aldosterone
   a. Renin-secreting tumor
   b. Renovascular hypertension
   c. Accelerated hypertension
3. ↑ Nonaldosterone mineralocorticoid
   a. Cushing's syndrome
   b. Licorice ingestion

Decreased salt absorption proximal to the collecting tubule
1. Diuretics
2. Osmotic diuretics
3. Bartter's syndrome
4. Magnesium deficiency
5. Distal delivery of nonreabsorbable anion
   a. Penicillins
   b. Ketoacidosis
   c. Metabolic alkalosis
   d. Proximal renal tubular acidosis
   e. Acetazolamide

Acid-base changes*
1. Metabolic alkalosis
2. Chronic metabolic acidosis

*Distal delivery of sodium is also important in these disorders.

proximal to the collecting tubules will increase distal delivery and lead to small degrees of volume depletion that secondarily elevate aldosterone levels. The combination of increased aldosterone levels and increased distal delivery leads to increased renal potassium wasting and hypokalemia. This group of disorders is different from the previous group, in that elevated aldosterone levels are appropriate for the mildly decreased ECF volume.

The most common cause of renal potassium wasting is diuretic ingestion. As is obvious from the previous discussion, any diuretic that acts proximal to the cortical collecting tubules increases renal potassium excretion. This includes diuretics that act in the proximal tubule such as acetazolamide, diuretics that act in the loop of Henle such as furosemide and ethacrynic acid, and diuretics that work in the early distal tubule such as the thiazides. Osmotic diuresis also leads to potassium wasting by this mechanism. Osmotic diuresis occurs in poorly controlled diabetes mellitus when serum glucose increases to higher levels than the proximal tubule can absorb. In addition, osmotic diuretics are used therapeutically in some conditions.

Bartter's syndrome is a rare condition in which there appears to be a primary defect in salt absorption in the loops of Henle. This leads to chronic increases in distal delivery and a chronic state of mild volume contraction. Patients are hypokalemic, with very high renin and aldosterone levels.

In certain conditions, sodium is delivered distally with a nonreabsorbable anion, increasing the lumen negative potential difference and leading to potassium wasting. All penicillins are nonreabsorbable anions, but only a few are given in sufficient quantities to lead to significant potassium wasting. Carbenicillin is an example of one of these. Ketoacids act as nonreabsorbable anions in patients with ketoacidosis due to diabetes, alcoholism, or starvation. Bicarbonate can function as a nonreabsorbable anion if delivered to the distal nephron in greater amounts than can be reabsorbed proximally. This occurs in active vomiting, in proximal renal tubular acidosis, and with acetazolamide administration.

Acid-Base Changes. All chronic acid-base disorders can lead to some degree of renal potassium wasting. However, metabolic alkalosis, both acute and chronic, clearly leads to the most marked degree of hypokalemia. This is because of increased collecting tubular cell potassium concentration, distal delivery of bicarbonate (behaving as a nonreabsorbable anion), and redistribution of potassium into cells. Metabolic acidosis may also lead to mild degrees of potassium depletion (due to decreased proximal salt absorption), but redistribution of potassium out of cells frequently prevents hypokalemia.

CLINICAL FEATURES OF HYPOKALEMIA

The most important clinical manifestations of hypokalemia occur in the neuromuscular system. Low serum levels lead to cell hyperpolarization, which impedes impulse conduction and muscle contraction. A flaccid paralysis typically develops in the hands and feet and moves proximally, eventually including the trunk and respiratory muscles. Death may occur from respiratory insufficiency.

Myopathy may also occur. In its most severe form, it can lead to frank rhabdomyolysis (muscle cell lysis) and renal failure. Potassium deficiency is believed to contribute to rhabdomyolysis occurring secondary to strenuous exercise. Hypokalemia can also lead to CNS changes with confusion and affective disorders and to smooth muscle dysfunction including paralytic ileus.

Cardiac complications of hypokalemia may also be important. The typical electrocardiogram (ECG) change is ST depression, T-wave flattening, and an increase in the amplitude of the U wave. This change, often misread as a widened QT, is nonspecific, often absent, and of little clinical use. It is well known that patients on cardiac glycosides have an increased incidence of premature ventricular contractions and supraventricular and ventricular tachyarrhythmias when hypokalemic. There is now concern that hypokalemia may predispose to these arrhythmias in patients not on these drugs.

Hypokalemia also causes a renal concentrating defect due to both a decrease in the medullary gradient and resistance of the cortical collecting tubule to ADH. Polyuria and polydipsia ensue. Hypokalemia can cause sodium retention and in some circumstances can contribute to metabolic alkalosis. Prolonged hypokalemia can also lead to tubulointerstitial nephritis and renal failure. Because insulin release is regulated partially by serum potassium, hypokalemia can lead to glucose intolerance.

TREATMENT OF HYPOKALEMIA

In treating patients with hypokalemia, it is useful but often difficult to ascertain the degree of the potassium deficit. **Serum potassium determinations can at times be misleading, as a normal or even increased potassium level can occur with significant total body potassium depletion.** In the absence of significant potassium shifts, a decline in the serum potassium from 4 to 3 mEq/L generally is associated with a deficit of 300 to 400 mEq intracellular potassium per 70 kg of body weight. A serum potassium concentration of 2 mEq/L reflects a deficit of approximately 600 mEq. Despite these guidelines, one should monitor the serum potassium level frequently during replacement therapy.

Potassium can be given orally or intravenously as the KCl salt. Potassium bicarbonate or citrate can be given if there is concomitant metabolic acidosis. The safest way to administer KCl is orally. KCl can be given in doses of 100 to 150 mEq/day. Liquid KCl tastes bitter and, like the tablet, can be irritating to the gastric mucosa. The microencapsulated or wax-matrix forms of KCl are better tolerated.

Intravenous administration of potassium may be necessary if a patient cannot take oral medications or if the potassium deficit is large and is resulting in cardiac arrhythmias, respiratory paralysis, or rhabdomyolysis. Intravenous KCl should be given at a maximum rate of 20 mEq/hr and maximum concentration of 40 mEq/L. Higher concentrations result in phlebitis. Replacement of KCl in dextrose-containing solutions can actually lower the serum level further secondary to insulin release. Thus, saline solutions are preferred. On rare occasions, higher concentrations of potassium may have to be given; frequent measurement of serum potassium and continuous ECG monitoring are essential in this case to prevent iatrogenic hyperkalemia.

Additional therapy of chronic hypokalemia involves the use of potassium-sparing diuretics such as amiloride, spironolactone, or triamterene. These agents are useful in situations of primary or secondary hyperaldosteronism. **Distal blockers must be used with caution in aged patients, in patients with renal insufficiency or diabetes, or in patients with other disorders that impair renal potassium excretion.**

CASE SUMMARY 3

A 26-year-old man with acquired immunodeficiency syndrome (AIDS) is being treated with amphotericin B for cryptococcal meningitis. He complains of weakness. Laboratory examination reveals the following (in mEq/L): sodium 134, potassium 2.0, chloride 104, CO_2 16. Arterial blood gas determinations showed pH 7.20 and pCO_2 40 mm Hg. His serum creatinine level is 2.4 mg/dl. An intravenous infusion of bicarbonate is started, and in 2 hours the patient complains of worsening weakness in his upper and lower extremities. Repeat arterial blood gas determinations showed pH 7.0 with pCO_2 increased to 60 mm Hg.

Amphotericin B is a nephrotoxic drug that can be associated with the development of distal renal tubular acidosis. Administration of bicarbonate without first correcting the potassium deficit precipitated symptomatic hypokalemia by shifting potassium into cells. **In patients with hypokalemic acidosis, one should always correct the serum potassium before correcting acidosis.**

CLINICAL DISORDERS ASSOCIATED WITH HYPERKALEMIA

As in the hypokalemic disorders, high serum potassium levels can occur in the setting of normal or altered body stores of potassium. The body has a marked ability to protect against hyperkalemia by means of regulatory mechanisms that excrete excess potassium quickly and mechanisms that redistribute excess potassium into cells until it is excreted. All causes of hyperkalemia therefore involve abnormalities in these mechanisms. The causes of hyperkalemia are listed in Table 4–7.

Pseudohyperkalemia

In approaching a patient with a high measured serum potassium concentration, it is important to remember that not all of these patients have true hyperkalemia. Because cell potassium concentrations are large and plasma potassium concentrations are small, small leaks of potassium out of blood cells can have large effects on measured serum potassium levels. Normally, when blood is allowed to clot before centrifugation, enough potassium is released from platelets to raise serum potassium by approximately 0.5 mEq/L. This variation is accounted for in the limits of normal. However, excessive errors can occur in the presence of marked thrombocytosis, marked leukocytosis, or hemolysis when obtaining blood samples. These conditions are referred to as *pseudohyperkalemia*.

Redistribution

Cellular redistribution is a more important cause of hyperkalemia than hypokalemia. As little as a 2% shift of intracellular potassium to the ECF results in a serum potassium level of 8 mEq/L. The effect of acidosis on cellular potassium redistribution has been discussed. Mineral acidosis by virtue of the relative impermeability of the chloride anion results in potassium shifts to the ECF. In contrast, organic acidosis does not cause hyperkalemia.

Table 4–7. CAUSES OF HYPERKALEMIA

Pseudohyperkalemia
Cellular redistribution
Acidosis
Cell shrinkage
Deficiency of insulin
Beta blockers
Hyperkalemic periodic paralysis
Cell injury
Excess intake (very rare)
Decreased renal excretion
Decreased distal delivery of sodium (oliguric renal failure)
Mineralocorticoid deficiency
Defect of cortical collecting tubule

Sudden increases in osmolality cause potassium to move out of cells. This shift is most often noted in diabetic patients. In fact, it is the hypertonic state as well as insulin deficiency that accounts for the relative hyperkalemia encountered in patients who have diabetic ketoacidosis and are potassium depleted. **Thus, potassium shifts out of cells are due to hyperosmolarity and insulin deficiency in ketoacidosis and due to cell ischemia in lactic acidosis.**

Beta-adrenergic blocking agents can interfere with the disposal of acute potassium loads. Other drugs that can result in hyperkalemia include the depolarizing muscle relaxant succinylcholine and severe digitalis poisoning. Hyperkalemic periodic paralysis is a rare autosomal dominant disorder characterized by repeated bouts of paralysis associated with hyperkalemia.

As 98% of the body's potassium is located within cells, cell death can result in substantial endogenous loads of potassium. Muscle breakdown from crush injury or rhabdomyolysis can be associated with a substantial increase in serum potassium concentration. Cell death as seen in tumor lysis syndromes can also be a source of substantial potassium loads. These syndromes are often associated with compromised renal function.

Although redistribution of potassium can result in hyperkalemia, the rise in potassium is generally mild and nonsustained. Prolonged and severe hyperkalemia implies the presence of concomitant decreases in renal potassium excretion.

Excessive Potassium Loads

In the presence of normal renal and adrenal function, it is difficult to ingest sufficient potassium to become hyperkalemic. It is even more difficult to do this on a chronic basis because of potassium adaptation. Rapid intravenous administration or intentional massive oral doses may exceed the excretory capacity of the kidneys, especially in the setting of severe sodium restriction.

Decreased Renal Excretion

Decreased renal excretion of potassium can be due to one or more of three abnormalities: decreased distal delivery of sodium, mineralocorticoid deficiency, and abnormal cortical collecting tubule function.

Decreased Distal Delivery of Sodium

As discussed previously, most filtered potassium is reabsorbed before the distal tubule. Potassium excretion is then determined by the rate at which potassium is secreted in the distal nephron. Acute decreases in GFR as occur in acute renal failure would therefore not be expected to have a marked effect on potassium excretion. Acute decreases in GFR may, however, lead to marked decreases in distal delivery of salt and water, which may secondarily decrease distal potassium secretion. Thus, when acute renal failure is oliguric, hyperkalemia is a frequent problem; when acute renal failure is nonoliguric, distal delivery is usually sufficient and hyperkalemia is unusual.

Chronic renal failure is more complicated than acute renal failure. In addition to the decreased GFR and secondary decrease in distal delivery, there is nephron dropout and less collecting tubule to secrete potassium. However, this is counterbalanced by a potassium adaptation, in which the remaining nephrons develop an increased ability to excrete potassium. This adaptation can be prevented by decreasing dietary potassium in proportion to the decrease in renal function. In addition, these patients possess two other defenses against hyperkalemia. First, in response to a potassium load they will redistribute the potassium into cells faster than normal individuals. Second, they have a markedly increased rate of potassium excretion in their stool. Thus, although patients with chronic renal failure do not excrete a potassium load as fast as normal persons, hyperkalemia is unusual until chronic renal failure has progressed to a GFR < 5 ml/min, frequently associated with an inability to excrete dietary NaCl. Hyperkalemia with a GFR of >10 ml/min should raise the question of decreased mineralocorticoid activity or a specific lesion of the cortical collecting tubule.

Decreased Mineralocorticoid Activity

Aldosterone deficiency can occur alone or in combination with decreased cortisol levels. Addison's disease is a deficiency of aldosterone and cortisol due to destruction of the adrenal glands. Certain enzyme defects can result in either isolated deficiency of aldosterone or adrenogenital syndromes associated with decreased mineralocorticoid activity. Heparin administration is associated with decreased adrenal secretion of aldosterone.

Angiotensin-converting enzyme inhibitors lead to hyperkalemia by decreasing levels of angiotensin II, a critical mediator of aldosterone secretion. Renin levels are high and aldosterone levels are low in all of these conditions.

The syndrome of hyporeninemic hypoaldosteronism accounts for most unexplained hyperkalemia in patients in whom the GFR and potassium intake would not be expected to result in hyperkalemia. Diabetic nephropathy and interstitial renal disease are the most common clinical entities associated with this syndrome. Other causes of renal disease associated with hyporeninemic hypoaldosteronism include analgesic nephropathy, urinary tract obstruction, sickle cell disease, systemic lupus erythematosus, and amyloidosis. Nonsteroidal antiinflammatory drugs are associated with decreased renin secretion. Additionally, these agents can cause hyperkalemia by decreasing GFR and reducing distal delivery of sodium. Cyclosporine administration is associated with the development of hyperkalemia in renal transplant patients. Although cyclosporine has a direct effect on the renal tubule, many patients taking this drug have low renin and aldosterone levels. These patients also may have a primary tubular defect at the level of the tubule independent of cyclosporine. $Beta_1$-receptor blockade also results in a hyporeninemic state.

Distal Tubular Defect

Certain interstitial renal diseases can affect the distal nephron specifically and lead to hyperkalemia in the presence of mild decreases in GFR and normal aldosterone levels. Many of these diseases are the same ones that can cause hyporeninemic hypoaldosteronism, and the impaired renin release and defect in tubular secretion frequently coexist. Examples include renal transplant, lupus erythematosus, amyloidosis, urinary obstruction, and sickle cell disease.

Potassium-sparing diuretics impair the ability of the cortical collecting tubule to secrete potassium. Amiloride and triamterene inhibit sodium reabsorption, thus abolishing the lumen negative potential and therefore inhibiting potassium secretion. Spironolactone competes with aldosterone and thus blocks the mineralocorticoid effect. Although these diuretics are useful in patients with a hypokalemic tendency, they weaken an important defense mechanism against hyperkalemia. They should therefore be avoided by patients with other defects that predispose to hyperkalemia (*i.e.*, diabetes mellitus, chronic renal insufficiency).

CLINICAL FEATURES OF HYPERKALEMIA

All of the clinically important manifestations of hyperkalemia occur in excitable tissue. As the potential across cell membranes is in part determined by the ratio of intracellular to extracellular potassium, hyperkalemia leads to depolarization of the resting membrane. Conduction velocity is markedly slowed as a result of this resetting of the threshold potential.

The heart is sensitive to this depolarizing effect, and changes are observable in the ECG. The progressive changes of hyperkalemia are as follows:

1. Peaking of T waves
2. ST segment depression
3. Widening of the PR interval
4. Widening of the QRS interval
5. Loss of the P wave
6. Sine wave pattern

The appearance of a sine wave pattern is a harbinger of impending ventricular fibrillation and asystole. The correlation of ECG changes with the serum potassium depends on the rapidity of onset of the hyperkalemia. Generally, with acute onset of hyperkalemia, ECG changes appear at a serum potassium level of 6 to 7 mEq/L. However, with chronic hyperkalemia, the ECG may remain normal up to a concentration of 8 to 9 mEq/L. The treatment of hyperkalemia is based more on the ECG than on the absolute serum value. All patients should have their serum potassium levels corrected, but patients with ECG changes should be treated emergently. **The presence of hypocalcemia, hyponatremia, and acidemia worsens the cardiac manifestations of hyperkalemia.**

Neuromuscular manifestations may also be noted with hyperkalemia. Paresthesias and fasciculations in the arms and legs are initially seen. As the serum potassium level continues to rise, an ascending paralysis with eventual flaccid quadriplegia supervenes. Trunk, head, and respiratory muscles classically are spared, but rarely respiratory failure can occur.

Acute Treatment of Hyperkalemia

The goals of therapy of acute hyperkalemia fall into three categories: first, to counteract the depolarizing effect on the myocardium; second, to shift potassium into cells; and third, to effect a net loss of potassium from the body.

Treatment with No Change in Potassium Balance

Calcium. The immediate treatment of life-threatening hyperkalemia is the administration of calcium, usually in the form of calcium gluconate (10% intravenously) or calcium chloride (10 ml). Calcium reduces the threshold potential (makes it less negative) and reduces the propensity for cardiac arrhythmias. The presence of late ECG changes such as an increasing PR interval or a widening QRS complex warrants treatment with calcium.

Treatment with Resultant Potassium Movement into Cells

Glucose and Insulin Therapy. Fifty percent dextrose in water, 50 ml, can be given as an intravenous bolus with 10 to 20 units of regular insulin or given as a continuous infusion over 1 to 2 hours. Administration of glucose and insulin shifts potassium into cells. Acute administration of glucose without insulin can potentially worsen hyperkalemia in diabetic patients by raising extracellular osmolality and causing potassium to shift into the extracellular space. If patients have a normal capacity for insulin secretion, however, glucose infusion lowers serum potassium by shifting potassium into cells. The effect of insulin and glucose can last for several hours.

Sodium Bicarbonate. Sodium bicarbonate administration (100 mmol [mEq] intravenously) through expansion of the ECF space results in dilution of the serum potassium level. Additionally, however, potassium is shifted into cells. The effects of sodium bicarbonate are short lived, usually lasting <1 hour. Complications of sodium bicarbonate therapy include volume overload, hypernatremia, and the precipitation of hypocalcemic tetany.

Beta$_2$ Agonists. Although not yet widely used, inhalation of beta$_2$ agonists such as fenoterol and albuterol or parenteral use of salbutamol can effect significant potassium shifts into cells. A recent study demonstrated that a dose of 10 to 20 mg of albuterol administered in a nebulized saline solution produced significant decreases in serum potassium levels without adverse effects in dialysis patients.

Treatment with Decreases in Total Body Potassium

The effects of calcium, bicarbonate, glucose and insulin, and $beta_2$ agonist therapy only temporarily correct the problem if excessive potassium stores have resulted in hyperkalemia. Therefore, measures to reduce total body potassium must soon be initiated. Although a decrease in the serum potassium level from 4 to 3 mEq/L is associated with a 300 to 400 mEq total body potassium deficit, only a 100 to 200 mEq excess of potassium is required to raise the plasma potassium concentration from 4 to 5 mEq/L.

Sodium Polystyrene Sulfonate (Kayexalate)

- 30 to 50 g resin orally, dissolved in 50 to 100 ml 20% sorbitol repeated every 2 to 4 hours.
- 50 to 60 g resin in 200 ml tap water administered rectally and retained 45 to 60 minutes. Repeat every 2 to 4 hours.

This resin acts as a sodium-potassium exchange resin and is usually given orally with sorbitol to promote rapid transfer through the gastrointestinal tract. One must monitor patients closely for evidence of volume overload, as significant sodium absorption can eventuate. When the resin is administered as an enema, potassium removal begins within 30 to 60 minutes, and 0.5 mEq of potassium is bound for every gram of resin. When the resin is given orally, 1 mEq of potassium is bound for every gram of resin, and onset begins in 3 to 4 hours.

Dialysis. Patients with serum potassium levels that are rapidly rising (rhabdomyolysis), or with significant hyperkalemia associated with renal failure, frequently require hemodialysis. As a patient is being readied for this procedure, the previously described treatments should be initiated. Hemodialysis can remove approximately 25 to 30 mEq of potassium per hour. Peritoneal dialysis is less efficient in removing potassium.

Treatment of Chronic Hyperkalemia

When faced with such a patient, a clinician should order measurement of a serum aldosterone level to help direct therapy. If a low value is obtained, 9α-fludrocortisone at doses of 0.1 to 0.3 mg daily is given. If aldosterone levels are normal, treatment with a diuretic such as furosemide or a thiazide to increase distal delivery of sodium is effective. However, aldosterone measurements are not rapidly obtainable, and a more practical approach can be used. One first assesses the volume status. Patients with a contracted ECF volume are best treated with fludrocortisone. If they are volume expanded or hypertensive, therapy with a diuretic is indicated. Patients should be counseled about low-potassium diets. Finally, some patients may have to be maintained on chronic Kayexalate therapy, with the dose and frequency titrated to the desired potassium level.

CASE SUMMARY 4

A 24-year-old white man with a 10-year history of insulin-dependent diabetes mellitus is referred for evaluation of hyperkalemia. The patient's only medications include split-dose insulin therapy and 600 mg of ibuprofen, which he takes for occasional joint pain. Laboratory examination reveals the following (in mEq/L): sodium 140, potassium 6.2, chloride 106, CO_2 22. The serum creatinine level is 2.5 mg/dl. Blood pressure is 150/105 mm Hg. A 24-hour urine collection reveals a creatinine clearance of 35 ml/min. An ECG is performed; results are normal.

Normally, the kidneys' ability to excrete potassium is maintained until the GFR falls below 10 ml/min. Hyperkalemia in the setting of a GFR >20 ml/min implies a defect in mineralocorticoid activity or a lesion within the cortical collecting duct. Diabetic patients have a high incidence of hyporeninemic hypoaldosteronism resulting from disease of the juxtaglomerular apparatus. Additionally, diabetic patients' use of a nonsteroidal antiinflammatory drug would predispose them to a hyporeninemic state. Therapy in the setting of a normal ECG would include discontinuation of ibuprofen, administration of Kayexalate, and dietary restriction of potassium. These patients are often hypertensive; therefore, a diuretic such as furosemide or a thiazide might be helpful in treating both the hypertension and hyperkalemia.

Suggested Readings

Anderson RJ: Hospital-associated hyponatremia. Kidney Int 29:1237–1247, 1986.

DeFronzo RA, Bia M: Extrarenal potassium homeostasis. *In* Seldin DW, Giebisch G (eds): The Kidney Physiology and Pathophysiology. New York, Raven Press, 1985, pp 1179–1206.

Linas SL, Berl T: Clinical diagnosis of abnormal potassium balance. *In* Seldin DW, Giebisch G (eds): The Regulation of Potassium Balance. New York, Raven Press, 1989, pp 177–205.

Mitch WE, Wilcox CS: Disorders of body fluids, sodium, and potassium in chronic renal failure. Am J Med 1982; 72:536–550.

Narins RG, Jones ER, Storm MC, et al: Diagnostic strategies in disorders of fluid, electrolyte, and acid-base homeostasis. Am J Med 72:536–550, 1982.

Robertson GL: Abnormalities of thirst regulation. Kidney Int 25:460–469, 1984.

Saxton CR, Seldin DW: Clinical interpretation of laboratory values. *In* Kokko JP, Tannen RL (eds). Fluids and Electrolytes. Philadelphia, WB Saunders, 1986, pp 3–62.

CHAPTER 5

ACID-BASE DISTURBANCES IN AZOTEMIC PATIENTS

David Z. Levine, Kevin D. Burns, and Marc B. Goldstein

This chapter provides an approach to the diagnosis and therapy of acid-base disturbances in azotemic patients. Acid-base physiology will not be reviewed in detail. Interested readers are referred to the reviews by Cohen and Kassirer and Narins and Emmett.

Rather, this discussion is restricted to particular derangements in patients with various types of renal disease. We first present a diagnostic approach to acid-base disorders, then focus mainly on the various causes of metabolic acidosis in renal patients. In addition, we describe an approach to patients with renal tubular acidosis (RTA) syndromes and comment briefly on metabolic alkalosis and respiratory acid-base disturbances.

DIAGNOSIS OF ACID-BASE DISTURBANCES IN RENAL PATIENTS

Many disorders of acid-base balance are initially detected from an evaluation of the arterial blood gas or serum electrolyte data in asymptomatic renal patients. The history often provides clues to the cause of the disturbance. However, renal patients may also present to the emergency room with a life-threatening acid-base disturbance and display certain physical signs that may suggest the diagnosis. For example, in severe metabolic acidosis, patients exhibit Kussmaul's respirations (tachypnea and increased tidal volume) and perhaps frank signs of congestive heart failure.* Bradycardia and hypotension may also be present. Severe alkalemia, on the other hand, may induce neuromuscular irritability (positive Trousseau's and Chvostek's signs), mental confusion, and cardiac arrhythmias.

*Severe acidemia causes sustained venoconstriction (increasing central blood volume), decreased myocardial contractility, and bradycardia with predisposition to ventricular arrhythmias. These effects all predispose to congestive heart failure.

> Suspect *severe* metabolic acidosis in renal patients presenting with Kussmaul's breathing, bradycardia, or hypotension.

An Approach to Evaluation of Blood Gas and Electrolyte Values

What is the Relationship Between pH and [H⁺]?

The $[H^+]$ of the extracellular fluid (ECF) is usually reported as its negative log, the pH. Because the negative log transformation results in data that are difficult to manipulate mentally and also obscures the magnitude of the change in $[H^+]$ in either direction, we encourage readers to think in terms of the $[H^+]$ rather than the pH. There are a number of "bedside" methods to convert the pH to $[H^+]$.

Fagen has pointed out that an *increase* in pH of 0.1 is equal to $0.8 \times [H^+]$, knowing that pH $7.00 = [H^+]$ of 100 nEq/L. This therefore yields the following relationship:

pH	$[H^+]$ (nEq/L)
7.00	100
7.10	80
7.20	64
7.30	51
7.40	41
7.50	32
7.60	24

The values in between can be obtained by interpolation—for example, pH 7.15 = $[H^+]$ of 64 + 0.5 (80 − 64) = 72 nEq/L. Similarly, the values for pH less than 7.00 ($[H^+]$ = 100 nEq/L) are obtained by multiplying the $[H^+]$ by 1.25—for example, pH 6.90 = $[H^+]$ of (100 × 1.25) = 125 nEq/L, pH 6.80 = $[H^+]$ of (125 × 1.25) = 156 nEq/L.

Another method of conversion (see Kassirer and Bleich) recognizes the fact that in the pH range often encountered clinically (7.28 to 7.45), there is a near linear relationship between pH and $[H^+]$, with a change of 0.01 pH units leading to a 1 nEq/L change in $[H^+]$ in the opposite direction. Beginning with a normal pH of 7.40 equivalent to a $[H^+]$ of 40 nEq/L, other values become as follows:

pH	$[H^+]$ (nEq/L)
7.46	34
7.44	36
7.40	40
7.36	44
7.33	47

Are the Reported Values Internally Consistent?

The Henderson equation gives the relationship between the $[H^+]$, pCO_2 and $[HCO_3^-]$ and can be used to verify the accuracy of the reported blood gas values.

$$[H^+] = K \times pCO_2/[HCO_3^-]$$

The value of the constant, K, is 23.9. This simple equation allows one to check for laboratory errors and to calculate the $[HCO_3^-]$ when provided with the pCO_2 and pH.

Many laboratories report the total carbon dioxide concentration ($[tCO_2]$), which represents $[HCO_3^-]$ plus dissolved CO_2 and carbonic acid (H_2CO_3). Because the latter two values are small in the absence of severe hypercapnia, $[tCO_2]$ usually is close to the value for $[HCO_3^-]$. However, the $[HCO_3^-]$ calculated from the pH and pCO_2 is in mEq/L plasma water, whereas the $[tCO_2]$ determined with other electrolytes is in mEq/L total plasma volume. Therefore, any process that reduces the water portion of the plasma (*e.g.*, hyperlipidemia) will result in a $[tCO_2]$ that is *lower* than the $[HCO_3^-]$ (cf. factitious hyponatremia).

Another useful way to check for internal consistency is to rearrange the Henderson equation and to use the value 25 for K, as follows:

$$pCO_2 = \frac{[H^+]\,[HCO_3^-]}{25}$$

As the value of K is 25, the relation between the pCO_2 and HCO_3^- is the relation between the $[H^+]$ and 25.

Note that for pH 7.00, $[H^+]$ = 100 nEq/L.

$$\text{Therefore, } pCO_2 = \frac{100 \times [HCO_3^-]}{25}$$

(100:25 = 4)

or approximately 4 times the $[HCO_3^-]$ at this pH.

Similarly, other *approximate* relations are as follows:

When pH = 6.90 ($[H^+]$ = 125 nEq/L), pCO_2 is 5 times the $[HCO_3^-]$.
When pH = 7.20 ($[H^+]$ = 64 nEq/L), pCO_2 is 2 1/2 times the $[HCO_3^-]$.
When pH = 7.30 ($[H^+]$ = 51 nEq/L), pCO_2 is twice the $[HCO_3^-]$.
When pH = 7.60 ($[H^+]$ = 24 nEq/L), pCO_2 equals $[HCO_3^-]$.

Using either this technique or the Henderson equation, it should be immediately apparent that one of the parameters is incorrect, when provided with the following laboratory results:

pH = 7.30 $[H^+]$ = 51 nEq/L
$[HCO_3^-]$ = 6 mEq/L pCO_2 = 32 mm Hg

The pCO_2 should be twice the $[HCO_3^-]$ in this case. The test should be repeated.

Therapy can be initiated in patients with a life-threatening disorder while the results are being checked, using clinical judgment to decide which of the three parameters is the most likely discrepant value.

What Is the Primary Acid-Base Disturbance?

If the reported values are consistent, the principal acid-base disturbances can be readily determined.

If the $[H^+]$ is increased, the patient has an acidemia, for which there are two possible explanations:

1. **Metabolic acidosis:** a primary reduction in $[HCO_3^-]$ and increase in $[H^+]$.
2. **Respiratory acidosis:** a primary increase in both $paCO_2$ and $[H^+]$.

If the $[H^+]$ is decreased, the patient has an alkalemia, for which there are also two possible explanations:

1. **Metabolic alkalosis:** a primary increase in $[HCO_3^-]$ and decrease in $[H^+]$.
2. **Respiratory alkalosis:** a primary decrease in both $paCO_2$ and $[H^+]$.

Is There an Appropriate Compensatory Response?

In each of these disorders, there is a physiologic compensatory change that minimizes the derangement in $[H^+]$. This compensation need not return the blood $[H^+]$ to normal. In fact, only in chronic respiratory alkalosis does the $[H^+]$ return to the normal range with the compensatory response.

The data on expected degrees of compensation are derived from normal subjects. Patients with renal disease may not compensate to the same extent, especially in respiratory disorders, in which the expected changes in renal H^+ secretion may not occur.

Compensatory responses for each primary disorder are as follows:

Metabolic acidosis: For every 1 mEq/L reduction in $[HCO_3^-]$ from 25 mEq/L, expect a 1 mm Hg reduction in $paCO_2$.

Metabolic alkalosis: For every 1 mEq/L increase in $[HCO_3^-]$ from 25 mEq/L, expect a 0.6 mm Hg increase in $paCO_2$.

Acute respiratory acidosis: For every 1 mm Hg increase in $paCO_2$, expect a 0.77 nEq/L increase in $[H^+]$. Or, for every 10 mm Hg increase in $paCO_2$, expect a 1 mEq/L increase in $[HCO_3^-]$.

Chronic respiratory acidosis: For every 1 mm Hg increase in $paCO_2$, expect a 0.33 nEq/L increase in $[H^+]$. Or, for every 10 mm Hg increase in $paCO_2$, expect a 3 mEq/L increase in $[HCO_3^-]$.

Acute respiratory alkalosis: For every 1 mm Hg reduction in $paCO_2$ from 40 mm Hg, expect a 0.74 nEq/L decrease in $[H^+]$. Or, for every 10 mm Hg reduction in $paCO_2$, expect a 2 mEq/L decrease in $[HCO_3^-]$.

Chronic respiratory alkalosis: For every 1 mm Hg reduction in $paCO_2$, expect a 0.17 nEq/L decrease in $[H^+]$. Or, for every 10 mm Hg reduction in $paCO_2$, expect a 5 mEq/L decrease in $[HCO_3^-]$.

Is a Mixed Acid-Base Disturbance Present?

A mixed acid-base disturbance is diagnosed when two or more acid-base disturbances coexist. Often, this is evident clinically only when the expected compensatory responses outlined earlier are not present for a given set of acid-base parameters. For example, if a patient has acute respiratory acidosis ($paCO_2$ = 60 mm Hg), we would expect the $[H^+]$ to be 55 nEq/L. The calculation follows:

In acute respiratory acidosis, we expect a 0.77 nEq/L rise in $[H^+]$ for each 1 mm Hg increase in $paCO_2$. Normal $paCO_2$ is 40; therefore, the increase in $[H^+]$ is $0.77 \times 20 = 15.4$. Because the normal $[H^+]$ is 40 nEq/L, the expected $[H^+]$ is $40 + 15.4 = 55$ nEq/L.

We can calculate the patient's expected $[HCO_3^-]$ from the Henderson equation, and it is $25 \times 60/55 = 27$ mEq/L. If this patient's actual blood gas values were pH 7.10, $[H^+]$ = 80 nEq/L, pCO_2 = 60 mm Hg, the $[HCO_3^-]$ is $25 \times 60/80 = 19$ mEq/L.

The patient's $[HCO_3^-]$ is much lower than expected, with an acute increase in $paCO_2$ to 60 mm Hg. Therefore, he also has metabolic acidosis in addition to the acute respiratory acidosis.

Mixed acid-base disturbances can also be identified by calculating the anion gap.

$$\text{Anion gap} = [Na^+] - ([HCO_3^-] + [Cl^-])$$

The normal plasma anion gap is 12 ± 2 mEq/L and is due to the negatively charged proteins, phosphate, sulfate, and other organic anions.

An increase in the anion gap by greater than 5 mEq/L usually indicates the presence of metabolic acidosis. Examples are lactic acidosis, ketoacidosis, the acidosis of end-stage renal disease, and metabolic acidosis due to intoxications. In these instances, the increase in the anion gap is roughly equal to the decrease in $[HCO_3^-]$. Otherwise, a mixed disturbance is present. That is, if the plasma anion gap has risen *less* than the decrease in $[HCO_3^-]$, a second process is lowering the $[HCO_3^-]$, either a normal anion gap type of metabolic acidosis or respiratory alkalosis.

If the increase in plasma anion gap greatly exceeds the decline in $[HCO_3^-]$, a second process has raised the $[HCO_3^-]$. There is either coexistent metabolic alkalosis or chronic respiratory acidosis.

METABOLIC ACIDOSIS IN RENAL PATIENTS

Mechanism

In normal persons, about 40 to 80 mmol H^+ are produced daily by hepatic metabolism of the dietary protein load. To maintain plasma $[HCO_3^-]$ at a constant level, H^+ must be excreted.*

The kidneys excrete the daily acid load in the form of ammonium (NH_4^+) and titratable acid (TA), mainly acid phosphate, with little HCO_3^- normally appearing in the urine. Free H^+, reflected by the urine pH, represents a trivial amount of acid.

The process of net acid excretion is impaired in renal failure, leading to metabolic acidosis. Renal net acid excretion, the sum of NH_4^+ plus TA minus bicarbonate, is reduced as a result of an impairment in the ability either to generate NH_4^+ in proximal tubular cells (thereby generating new bicarbonate) or to deliver NH_4^+ to the final urine. There may also be increased delivery of HCO_3^- out of the proximal nephron in renal failure, leading to a relatively alkalotic distal tubular fluid, which further impairs NH_4^+ trapping. Despite this, the urine pH in chronic renal failure is often less than 5.5, indicating that NH_4^+ availability is more impaired than is H^+ secretion. The consequence of this impaired ability to excrete acid is that dietary and endogenous acid production progressively titrate the plasma $[HCO_3^-]$ downward until a new steady state is reached. The fact that a new steady state is reached despite impaired renal HCO_3^- regeneration indicates that either H^+ production is reduced (decreased proton intake) or else some other source of acid buffering is mobi-

*The H^+ load is initially buffered by ECF HCO_3^- and intracellular buffers, but ultimately it must be eliminated in the urine if plasma $[HCO_3^-]$ is to be maintained.

Table 5–1. EXAMPLES OF METABOLIC ACIDOSIS IN AZOTEMIC PATIENTS

Patient	Plasma Acid-Base Values	Clinical Context	Diagnosis and Therapy
Chronic renal disease	$[HCO_3^-]$ = 20.8 mEq/L pH = 7.34 pCO_2 = 39.8 mm Hg	Long-standing disease. Anion gap slightly elevated. Serum creatinine = 4 mg/dl. Asymptomatic.	Mild metabolic acidosis of chronic renal disease. Alkali not usually administered. Effect of mild acidosis on bone is unclear. A mild degree of respiratory acidosis is present.
Chronic renal disease	$[HCO_3^-]$ = 13.2 mEq/L pH = 7.30 pCO_2 = 27.6 mm Hg	Well-known chronic patient. Anion gap elevated. Serum K = 6.2 mEq/L, creatinine = 6.6 mg/dl. Patient is dyspneic.	Consistent with acidosis of advanced renal failure with appropriate respiratory compensation. Therapy with $NaHCO_3$ or other alkali indicated; dyspnea and hyperkalemia should improve. Dialysis should be considered.
Postoperative oliguria	$[HCO_3^-]$ = 13.0 mEq/L pH = 7.14 pCO_2 = 40 mm Hg	24 hours before, patient had normal renal function and acid-base status. Now creatinine = 2 mg/dl, K = 6.4 mEq/L, anion gap = 28 mEq/L, BP = 95/60 mm Hg.	Metabolic acidosis complicated by superimposed respiratory acidosis (? pneumonia, ? oversedation). Metabolic acidosis cannot be attributed only to renal insufficiency as change in $[HCO_3^-]$ is too rapid. Hypotension and anion gap suggest lactic acidosis.
Dialysis patient	$[HCO_3^-]$ = 11.2 mEq/L pH = 7.27 pCO_2 = 25.2 mm Hg	Patient missed train, 4 days without dialysis. K = 6.8 mEq/L. Anion gap increased. Creatinine = 14.6 mg/dl.	Fall in $[HCO_3^-]$ consistent with 4 days anuria and "baseline" $[HCO_3^-]$ of about 20 mEq/L. Dialysis (preferably with HCO_3^-) is only treatment needed.
Nursing home patient	$[HCO_3^-]$ = 4.9 mEq/L pH = 7.00 pCO_2 = 36 mm Hg	69-yr-old woman said to have "intestinal flu." Creatinine = 4 mg/dl. BUN = 117 mg/dl. Obvious ECF volume contraction. Anion gap is normal. K = 4.0 mEq/L.	Acid-base values inconsistent (*i.e.*, pCO_2 = 20.4 mm Hg, if we assume pH and $[HCO_3^-]$ are correct). $NaHCO_3$ given to restore ECF volume and correct acidosis. Respiratory acidosis is present assuming HCO_3^- and pCO_2 are correct. Consider diarrhea as cause of normal anion gap metabolic acidosis. Exclude acidification defect (urine pH and NH_4^+). Absence of hyperkalemia in non–anion gap acidosis indicates K depletion requiring supplementary K.
Dialysis patient	$[HCO_3^-]$ = 9.2 mEq/L pH = 7.20 pCO_2 = 24.2	Cardiac patient is hypotensive on dialysis with mild ultrafiltration. Anion gap = 40 mEq/L. BP falls suddenly with nausea, hyperventilation. Large surface area dialyzer used for first time.	Lactic acidosis, of course, could be present as a result of too vigorous ultrafiltration or poor peripheral perfusion. However, "acetate acidosis" due to inability to metabolize acetate to bicarbonate may explain findings. Prove by showing high acetate levels and reversal of symptoms with $[HCO_3^-]$ dialysis.

lized. Negative calcium balance has been reported in renal patients, suggesting that acid is buffered by bone apatite, with protons displacing calcium ions.

The Anion Gap in Renal Failure

Although varying degrees of metabolic acidosis can be found in patients with differing degrees of renal dysfunction, as a *general* rule, the anion gap widens progressively with diminution in glomerular filtration rate (GFR). Certainly, when GFR is less than 20 ml/min, one can expect an increased anion gap.

The increase in unmeasured anions has been postulated to result from retention of unfiltered phosphate, sulfate, and other organic anions.

However, an anion gap greater than 30 mEq/L in a patient with renal failure should provoke a search for *another* cause of wide anion gap metabolic acidosis.

A decrease in the anion gap in renal failure may occur in states of hypoalbuminemia or in patients with multiple myeloma (paraproteins may carry a net positive charge).

> Calculation of the anion gap in a patient with renal failure may reveal another acid-base diagnosis: If the anion gap is greater than 30 mEq/L, the presence of another condition associated with high anion gap metabolic acidosis is suggested. If the anion gap is less than 10 mEq/L, hypoalbuminemia or multiple myeloma should be considered.

Clinical Presentations

(See Table 5–1 For Case Histories)

In acute anuric states or in functionally anephric dialysis patients, the plasma $[HCO_3^-]$ will decline at a fixed rate, determined by the rate of H^+ generation and the volume of the HCO_3^- space.

Consider a 70-kg patient with a single kidney who becomes completely anuric from renal artery thrombosis. At what rate will the plasma $[HCO_3^-]$ fall?

If one assumes a normal H^+ generation of 70 mmol/day, and the acid distribution (or HCO_3^- space) is 50% of body weight, then 70 mmol H^+/35 L = 2 mEq/L/day.

Acute renal failure may be accompanied by certain clinical disorders that may induce a more profound metabolic acidosis than that expected from uremia alone ($[HCO_3^-]$ <10 to 12 mEq/L). These are outlined in Table 5–2.

Table 5–2. SEVERE METABOLIC ACIDOSIS IN ACUTE RENAL FAILURE

Causes	Clinical Context
"Excess" H^+ production	Hypercatabolic states, burns, rhabdomyolysis
Lactic acidosis	Sepsis, hypovolemic shock
Diabetic ketoacidosis	Diabetics also experience renal failure
Ethylene glycol intoxication	Acute renal failure with anion gap >30 mEq/L, osmolal gap >15 mOsm, oxalate crystals in urine.

The patient with chronic renal failure and a stable serum creatinine level at 3 mg/dl (264 µmol/L) can be expected to have mild metabolic acidosis with plasma $[HCO_3^-]$ usually above 14 mEq/L. Certain renal diseases such as chronic pyelonephritis and analgesic nephropathy are associated with more severe metabolic acidosis because of a decrease in H^+ secretion and/or decreased NH_3 availability as a result of the damaged renal medulla.

In patients with chronic renal failure, certain medications may result in worsening metabolic acidosis. These medications are tabulated in Table 5–3. These possibilities should be kept in mind when a patient with renal insufficiency presents with plasma $[HCO_3^-]$ less than 10 mEq/L.

Therapy

In acute renal failure, treatment of metabolic acidosis is indicated when the plasma $[HCO_3^-]$ is very low (<10 to 12 mEq/L) and when a patient is fatigued or dyspneic from respiratory compensation.

Serious acidosis must be treated aggressively, because small changes in plasma $[HCO_3^-]$ or $paCO_2$ can have dramatic effects on acid-base status in these patients, as illustrated by the examples in Table 5–4.

Initial therapy should aim to remove patients from immediate danger by raising the plasma $[HCO_3^-]$ to greater than 10 mEq/L. The amount of $NaHCO_3$ required is determined by assuming that the volume of distribution of bicarbonate is at least 50% of the body weight.* Each ampule of $NaHCO_3$ contains 50 mEq

*With increasing acidemia, the volume of distribution of bicarbonate progressively increases.

Table 5–3. MEDICATIONS CAPABLE OF INDUCING SEVERE METABOLIC ACIDOSIS IN RENAL PATIENTS

Type	Indication	Clinical Context*
K^+-sparing diuretics	Hypertension, edematous disorders	Elderly patients, normal anion gap, hyperkalemia
Acetazolamide	Glaucoma	Elderly patients, normal anion gap
Angiotensin-converting enzyme inhibitors	Hypertension, congestive heart failure	Normal anion gap, hyperkalemia
Cholestyramine	Hyperlipidemia	Normal anion gap
Phenformin/metformin	Diabetes mellitus	Lactic acidosis, elevated anion gap

*The metabolic acidosis induced by these medications is a separate process, superimposed on the metabolic acidosis caused by renal insufficiency, which may be stable or may also become more severe as residual renal function is lost.

HCO_3^-. Therefore, an 80-kg patient with a plasma $[HCO_3^-]$ of 5 mEq/L would require at least 4 ampules (50 mEq/ampule) of $NaHCO_3$ to raise the plasma $[HCO_3^-]$ to 10 mEq/L, assuming no ongoing H^+ generation.

> In severe metabolic acidosis associated with renal insufficiency, initially raise the plasma $[HCO_3^-]$ to 10 mEq/L. Thereafter, progressively raise the plasma $[HCO_3^-]$ in accordance with the patient's ability to tolerate the sodium load.

The risks of acute administration of $NaHCO_3$ must be mentioned. Hypokalemia can be induced because of a shift of potassium into cells, and this can cause muscle weakness, leading to respiratory acidosis and worsening acidemia, especially in patients with RTA who tend to have hypocalemia. $NaHCO_3$ therapy may be hazardous in fluid-overloaded patients because of the sodium load. Such patients, if unresponsive to diuretics, may require early dialysis. Other temporizing measures to control acidemia are nasogastric suction, which can remove significant amounts of hydrochloric acid, and mechanical ventilation (especially important to decrease $paCO_2$ in patients with pulmonary edema and acute renal failure). Decreased serum ionized calcium can result from alkali therapy, leading to tetany.

In patients with chronic renal failure, therapeutic principles are similar. There is evidence in children that bone growth may resume with correction of acidemia. In adults, the benefits of alkali therapy for mild acidemia are less clear, although we have the clinical impression that a patient's sense of well-being is improved with correction of acidemia. The degree to which the acidemia is corrected in any given patient will depend on that patient's tolerance of the sodium load. Clearly, either congestive heart failure or worsening of hypertension may limit the amount of $NaHCO_3$ administered to any particular patient.

Treatment can be initiated with $NaHCO_3$ tablets. The usual dose is 600 mg four times a day (q.i.d.) (28.8 mEq HCO_3^-/day), but 1200 mg q.i.d. will often be necessary for complete correction of the acidemia. The use of Shohl's solution (sodium citrate-citric acid mixture) may provide relief for patients with abdominal bloating or belching; however, citrate may promote aluminum absorption, predisposing to toxicity. In hypocalcemic patients with volume overload, $CaCO_3$ supplements will provide a calcium and alkali source without causing excess ECF volume expansion.

METABOLIC ACIDOSIS IN DIALYSIS PATIENTS

Hemodialysis

From an acid-base standpoint, the goal of hemodialysis is to correct uremic acidosis and to provide enough base to buffer the H^+ gen-

Table 5–4. IMPACT OF SMALL CHANGES IN $[HCO_3^-]$ OR pCO_2 ON THE ACID-BASE STATUS OF PATIENTS WITH PLASMA $[HCO_3^-]$ OF 7 mEq/L

	pH	$[H^+]$ (nm)	pCO_2 (mm Hg)	$[HCO_3^-]$ (mEq/L)
A. Stable metabolic acidosis	7.12	75	22	7
B. Small reduction in hyperventilation	6.99	120	30*	7
C. Small decrease in plasma $[HCO_3^-]$	7.02	96	20	5*

*Note that the slight increase in pCO_2 in example B, or the small decrease in $[HCO_3^-]$ in example C, converts a modest acidemia into a severe one.

erated in the interdialytic interval. Hemodialysis patients often have a predialysis plasma [HCO_3^-] in the range of 16 to 20 mEq/L, the pH averaging 7.34. However, with the use of HCO_3^- dialysate and $CaCO_3$ as a phosphate binder, the predialysis plasma [HCO_3^-] may be in the normal range. The rise of plasma [HCO_3^-] after dialysis and its gradual decline in the interdialytic interval reflect the replenishment of alkali stores during dialysis and their depletion between treatments.

Acetate is a readily metabolizable source of alkali that has been used as a dialysate buffer since the early 1960s. It gained favor because of its stability and, unlike bicarbonate, did not lead to precipitation of calcium and magnesium in the bath.

In acetate hemodialysis, the plasma [HCO_3^-] decreases in the first half-hour of dialysis as a result of passive losses into the HCO_3^--free bath. Metabolism of acetate and generation of HCO_3^- must be brisk enough to offset these losses. In most patients, this is not a significant problem. In some patients, however, acetate metabolism may be impaired, and worsening metabolic acidosis may occur, associated with rising blood acetate concentration (and increased anion gap) during dialysis. This has also been described with high-efficiency hemodialysis, in which higher blood flows and larger surface area dialyzers are used. HCO_3^- losses across the dialyzer may exceed the metabolic conversion rate of acetate to HCO_3^- in this situation.

Reports of hypotension, unsuccessful ultrafiltration, and cardiac problems during acetate dialysis have led to increasing use of HCO_3^- as the dialysate buffer. The usual dialysate HCO_3^- concentration is 35 to 38 mEq/L. Uremic acidosis is corrected in a direct, physiologic manner, with blood pH rising throughout dialysis.

Peritoneal Dialysis

Lactate is used as a source of HCO_3^- in peritoneal dialysate. Its usual concentration is 35 mEq/L. This allows plasma [HCO_3^-] to be maintained at 20 to 22 mEq/L in most patients on continuous ambulatory peritoneal dialysis. With higher dialysate lactate concentrations (40 mEq/L), alkalemia may occur.

THE SYNDROMES OF RENAL TUBULAR ACIDOSIS

RTA comprises a group of conditions in which the renal ability to maintain acid-base balance is impaired. These patients present with a normal anion gap type of metabolic acidosis. They have hyperchloremia ([Cl^-] >110 mEq/L) unless hyponatremia is present. The basic defect leading to the renal acidosis may be located in the proximal or distal nephron, hence the separation into proximal and distal RTA. Both varieties are characterized by impaired renal NH_4^+ excretion.

One should suspect the presence of RTA in patients with normal anion gap metabolic acidosis and the absence of an increase in renal NH_4^+ excretion. Under normal circumstances, the renal response to chronic acidemia is to increase the urine NH_4^+ excretion 10-fold, from 40 to 400 mEq/day. The urine NH_4^+ concentration can be estimated from an evaluation of the urine [Na^+], [K^+], [Cl^-], urea, glucose, and osmolality. Because NH_4^+ is a cation, its excretion is usually in association with Cl^-, and the urine [Cl^-] markedly exceeds the [Na^+] + [K^+]. The excretion of NH_4^+ in conjunction with an unmeasured anion (*e.g.*, ketoacid anion) can be identified by the detection of a substantial (>40 mOsm) osmolal gap (measured osmolality >> calculated osmolality). The osmolality is calculated from the osmotic contribution of Na, K, Cl, urea, and glucose.

Proximal Renal Tubular Acidosis

Proximal RTA is due to a defect in proximal tubular H^+ secretion resulting in a failure to reabsorb filtered HCO_3^- with an acidemia due to bicarbonaturia. The H^+ secretory defect may be isolated or may be associated with other transport defects (urate, phosphate, glucose, amino acids), resulting in Fanconi's syndrome.

The diagnostic feature of proximal RTA is alkaline urine and a reduced plasma [HCO_3^-]. It is possible for these patients to excrete acid urine if some process (*e.g.*, diarrhea) lowers the plasma [HCO_3^-] below the new renal threshold, in which case the diagnosis is established by the administration of HCO_3^- and the detection of an alkaline urine while the plasma [HCO_3^-] remains below normal. Patients with proximal RTA also have reduced renal NH_4^+ excretion. Although the basis for this is not clear, a unifying concept to explain both impaired H^+ secretion and impaired NH_4^+ production in the proximal nephron would be alkalization of the proximal tubular cell.

Distal Renal Tubular Acidosis

Distal RTA is associated with impaired renal NH_4^+ excretion, which is the basis of the acidemia. There are two reasons for impaired NH_4^+ excretion:

1. Impaired distal nephron H^+ secretion
2. Impaired availability of NH_3 to the distal nephron

The urine pH can give insights into which mechanism is operative. Impaired H^+ secretion is generally associated with urine pH >5.3 whereas NH_3 defects are associated with urine pH <5.0. Combined defects may have an intermediate urine pH.

Further insights into the pathogenesis of distal RTA can be gained from the plasma [K^+]. If hypokalemia is present, an H^+ secretory defect is more likely, whereas if hyperkalemia is present, some process interfering with the generation or maintenance of the lumen negative potential difference is thought to be the basis of the problem. These would include the following:

1. Impaired distal sodium delivery
2. Mineralocorticoid deficiency
3. Impaired response to mineralocorticoid
4. Chloride shunt disorder

The steps involved in distal nephron H^+ secretion are as follows:

1. H^+ ATPase secretes H^+ into the distal lumen. This H^+ secretion is promoted by mineralocorticoid and inhibited by a lumen positive potential difference.

2. The minimization of a lumen positive potential difference requires the following:

A. Distal delivery of sodium

B. Reabsorption of sodium requires: mineralocorticoid secretion, normal receptor and postreceptor responses to mineralocorticoid

C. Anion impermeability

Isolated H^+ pump disorders will be associated with hypokalemia, as the lumen negative potential is normally generated and K^+ flows down its electrochemical gradient into the distal nephron lumen.

Any process reducing the biologic response to mineralocorticoid (see 2A and B, above) will be associated with hyperkalemia, as the lumen negative potential difference favoring K^+ addition to the luminal fluid is absent.

Abnormal anion reabsorption in this nephron segment (chloride shunt disorders) will also be associated with hyperkalemia due to dissipation of the lumen negative potential difference. These patients also have hypertension due to ECF volume expansion secondary to the sodium reabsorption with chloride rather than with potassium secretion (potassium excretion is equivalent to loss of sodium from the ECF; as potassium leaves the intracellular fluid for excretion, sodium enters the intracellular fluid).

In patients with hyperkalemia, ammoniagenesis may be inhibited, resulting in a lower urine pH (<5.0) if some H^+ secretion is preserved.

The clinical approach to patients with a normal anion gap metabolic acidosis should proceed as follows: Evaluate the urine [NH_4^+] from the urine electrolytes and osmolal gap.

1. If the urine [NH_4^+] is adequate (urine [Na^+] + [K^+] << urine [Cl^-]), look for a nonrenal cause of the acidemia (gastrointestinal HCO_3^- loss, acetazolamide, occult wide anion gap acidosis [*e.g.*, hypoalbuminemia masking the wide anion gap], posthypocapnia, or acid ingestion).

2. If the urine [NH_4^+] is low (urine [Na^+] + [K^-] > urine [Cl^-] and there is no osmolal gap, evaluate for RTA as detailed below.

Evaluation of Patients Suspected of Having Renal Tubular Acidosis

1. Obtain urine pH while patient is acidemic.

- If it is alkaline (>7), the patient has proximal RTA.
- If <5, the patient probably has a defect in NH_3 availability. Confirm by proceeding with the steps listed below.

2. Administer $NaHCO_3^+$ and correct hypokalemia if present.

- If urine pH was *not* initially alkaline, administer HCO_3^- until urine pH is >7.4. Assess plasma [HCO_3^-]; if it still is low, the patient has proximal RTA.
- If plasma [HCO_3^-] returns to normal before the urine becomes alkaline, proximal RTA is ruled out.

3. Once urine pH is >7.4, assess urine pCO_2.

- If the urine pCO_2 is <50 mm Hg, the patient has a H^+ pump defect.
- If the urine pCO_2 is >70 mm Hg, the H^+ pump is normal.
  - If the initial urine pH was <5.0, the patient's RTA is due to an ammoniagenesis disorder.
  - If the initial urine pH was >5.3, the patient's RTA is due to back diffusion of H^+ from the lumen (amphotericin B).

Renal Tubular Acidosis in Renal Transplant Patients

Hyperchloremic metabolic acidosis, due to RTA, is the most common acid-base disturbance in patients undergoing renal transplantation. In the first few months after transplantation, proximal RTA can occur in association with resolving secondary hyperparathyroidism. In addition, Fanconi's syndrome has also been described in the early posttransplant period. These defects usually resolve within a few months.

In long-standing renal allografts, the development of distal RTA has been linked to episodes of acute and chronic rejection. A defect in distal tubule H^+ secretion has been postulated to occur in these patients. Aldosterone deficiency and hyperkalemia have also been reported.

The antirejection drug cyclosporine induces distal RTA in up to 20% of renal transplant recipients. There is some evidence to suggest that the drug causes hyporeninemic hypoaldosteronism with impaired tubular response to aldosterone. There are also data compatible with the presence of a chloride shunt disorder in some of these patients. Careful monitoring of the dose of cyclosporine and control of hyperkalemia are the mainstays of therapy.

METABOLIC ALKALOSIS IN RENAL PATIENTS

Metabolic alkalosis can progress rapidly to frank alkalemia in patients with established renal disease. This is because any process that *initiates* metabolic alkalosis will be perpetuated by the inability of the poorly functioning kidneys to excrete excess HCO_3^- in the urine. This is especially important when the GFR is severely reduced (<20 ml/min).

Patients with end-stage renal disease often experience nausea and vomiting as the major symptoms heralding the necessity for dialysis. In this setting, loss of acid caused by vomiting will first tend to correct the preexisting metabolic acidosis of renal failure, and then progress to alkalemia. An increase in blood pH >7.60 is potentially life-threatening and must be corrected promptly.

Another common example of rapidly progressing metabolic alkalosis occurs in patients who undergo nasogastric suction without sodium chloride replacement. ECF volume depletion and decreased GFR reduce the body's ability to excrete HCO_3^-, causing sustained metabolic alkalosis.

Management. The management of renal patients with metabolic alkalosis will depend on the severity of the alkalosis and the degree of depression of GFR. Severe alkalemia can cause cardiac arrhythmias, soft-tissue calcification, and neuromuscular irritability. Patients with severe alkalemia may require intravenous administration of a source of acid such as dilute HCl, arginine HCl, or ammonium chloride, over several hours. Alternatively, patients can be dialyzed with a high Cl^-/low HCO_3^- dialysate to correct the disturbance.

Patients who have mild renal insufficiency (whether due to prerenal azotemia or established renal disease) and who also have metabolic alkalosis will respond to cautious administration of sodium chloride or indeed potassium chloride, bearing in mind the hazards of potassium supplements in renal patients. If gastric acid loss is the cause of the alkalosis, use of antiemetics, H_2 blockers, and discontinuation of nasogastric suction (if permissible) will also diminish hydrochloric acid loss.

RESPIRATORY ACID-BASE DISTURBANCES IN RENAL PATIENTS

Although the ventilatory response to metabolic acidosis appears to be normal in patients with varying degrees of renal insufficiency, it is not clear whether appropriate changes occur in plasma $[HCO_3^-]$ when renal patients have superimposed respiratory disturbances. For example, can a kidney with a GFR of 30 ml/min generate sufficient HCO_3^- to prevent severe acidemia in a patient with severe chronic hypercapnia? There are no data available to answer this question, although one might expect to see coexistent metabolic acidosis in patients who have renal failure and respiratory acidosis. This combination is particularly hazardous, as it can lead to profound acidemia.

Respiratory alkalosis occurs commonly in renal patients. This is especially true in hemodialysis patients, because arterial CO_2 can diffuse across the dialyzer and cause alkalemia.

Renal patients not uncommonly develop triple acid-base disturbances, in which metabolic acidosis and metabolic alkalosis accompany respiratory acidosis or alkalosis.

Suggested Readings

Cohen JJ, Kassirer JP: Acid-base metabolism. *In* Maxwell MH, Kleeman CR (eds): Clinical Disorders of Fluid and Electrolyte Metabolism, 3rd ed. New York, McGraw-Hill, 1980.

Fagen TJ: Estimation of hydrogen ion concentration. N Engl J Med 288:915, 1973.

Kassirer JP, Bleich HL: Rapid estimation of plasma carbon dioxide from pH and total carbon dioxide content. N Engl J Med 272:1067, 1965.

Narins RG, Emmett M: Simple and mixed acid-based disorders: A practical approach. Medicine 59:161, 1980.

CHAPTER 6

OBSTRUCTIVE UROPATHY

Saulo Klahr

Obstructive uropathy is of great importance to clinicians because it is a common entity that is treatable and often reversible. Patients with obstructive uropathy may exhibit a diversity of clinical syndromes, but very often they present with symptoms and signs of acute or chronic renal failure. The diagnosis of obstructive uropathy should be considered in various settings but particularly in patients presenting with acute renal failure. **In most instances, the renal failure due to obstructive uropathy is reversible, and surgical procedures or instrumentation may completely reverse the clinical picture.**

DEFINITIONS

The structural or functional changes in the urinary tract that impede the normal flow of urine are known as obstructive uropathy. Obstructive nephropathy is produced as a consequence of impaired flow of urine or tubular fluid. Hydronephrosis is the dilatation of the urinary tract that sometimes may occur in the absence of a defined anatomic obstruction.

INCIDENCE

Obstructive uropathy is common. It occurs at all ages. Hydronephrosis has been found on postmortem examination of 3.5 to 3.8% of adults, with equal distribution between males and females. Hydronephrosis, mostly due to congenital anomalies of the urinary tract, is found at autopsy in about 2% of children. More than 2 million men and women in the United States have kidney stones. Four of every five patients with stones are men, usually between the ages of 20 and 40 years. After the age of 60, obstructive uropathy occurs more frequently in men than in women as a result of the increased incidence of benign prostatic hypertrophy and carcinoma of the prostate. In middle-aged women, complete obstructive uropathy may be due to pelvic cancer and retroperitoneal fibrosis. It has been calculated that 166 patients per 100,000 population were hospitalized in the United States in the year 1985 with a presumptive diagnosis of obstructive uropathy. Obstructive uropathy was the fourth leading diagnosis on discharge among patients with kidney and urologic disorders, with a rate of 242 patients per 100,000 discharged. In 1985, in the United States, 387 patient visits per 100,000 population visits were attributed to obstructive uropathy.

CAUSES

The specific causes of obstructive uropathy are numerous (Table 6–1) but a simple classification is based on both clinical and anatomic features. Clinical features include the age and sex of the patient. Obstruction of the urinary tract in individuals younger than 15 years of age is usually due to congenital anomalies, and the lesions are more frequently located at the level of the posterior urethra or ureteropelvic junction. In women, cervical cancer causes obstruction near the ureterovesical junction. Pregnancy is another common cause of urinary tract obstruction. In elderly men, benign prostatic hypertrophy and carcinoma of the prostate are common causes of lower urinary tract obstruction.

Obstruction may occur at the level of the upper urinary tract—that is, above the uretero-

This work was supported by U.S.P.H.S. NIDDK grants DK-09976, DK-07126, and DK-40321.

The author would like to thank Ms. Pat Verplancke for her help in the preparation of this chapter.

Table 6–1. CAUSES OF URINARY TRACT OBSTRUCTION

Upper Urinary Tract	Lower Urinary Tract
Intrinsic causes 1. Intraluminal a. Intratubular deposition of crystals (uric acid) b. Ureter: urolithiasis, blood clots, renal papillae, fungus ball 2. Intramural a. Ureteropelvic junction or ureterovesical junction dysfunction b. Ureteral valve, ureteral polyp, ureteral stricture *Extrinsic causes* 1. Vascular lesions a. Aneurysm: abdominal aorta, iliac vessels b. Aberrant vessels: ureteropelvic junction c. Venous: retrocaval ureter, puerperal ovarian vein thrombophlebitis d. Fibrosis following vascular reconstructive surgery 2. Originating in the reproductive system a. Uterus: pregnancy, prolapse, tumors, endometriosis b. Ovary: abscess, tumors, ovarian remnants c. Gartner's duct cyst, tubo-ovarian abscess 3. Lesions of the gastrointestinal tract: Crohn's disease, diverticulitis, appendiceal abscess, tumors, pancreatic tumors, abscess, cysts 4. Diseases of the retroperitoneum a. Retroperitoneal fibrosis (idiopathic, radiation) b. Inflammatory: tuberculosis, sarcoidosis c. Hematomas d. Primary retroperitoneal tumors (lymphoma, sarcoid, etc.) e. Tumor metastatic to the retroperitoneum (cervix, bladder, colon, prostate, etc.) f. Lymphocele g. Pelvic lipomatosis	1. Phimosis, meatal stenosis, paraphimosis 2. Urethra: strictures, stones, diverticulum, posterior or anterior urethral valves, periurethral abscess, urethral surgery 3. Prostate: benign prostatic hyperplasia, prostatic calculi, abscess, prostatic carcinoma 4. Bladder a. Neurogenic bladder: spinal cord defect or trauma, diabetes, multiple sclerosis, cerebrovascular accidents, Parkinson's disease b. Bladder neck dysfunction c. Bladder calculus d. Bladder cancer 5. Trauma a. Straddle injury b. Pelvic fracture

vesical junction or at the level of the lower urinary tract: bladder, urethra, and bladder neck. The obstruction may be intrinsic (intraluminal or intramural) or extrinsic. Intraluminal obstruction may be due to renal stones, blood clots, or sloughed renal papillary tissue and tends to occur more frequently in the ureteropelvic or ureterovesical junctions. However, it may occur at other levels as well. Within the kidneys, obstruction of the tubular lumen may occur as a result of deposition of crystals, particularly sulfonamides, uric acid, and acyclovir. Intramural obstruction may be due to structural or functional abnormalities of the wall of the urinary tract. Functional obstruction may be due to the presence of aperistaltic segments at the level of the ureter or impaired peristaltic activity such as a neurogenic bladder. Structural anomalies include inflammation of the wall of the genitourinary tract, such as is encountered in certain infections (tuberculosis), or abnormal growth of the cells of the urinary wall, such as benign or malignant tumors.

The extrinsic causes of obstructive uropathy are best classified according to the system of origin of the obstructing lesion. Most extrinsic lesions causing obstruction originate in the reproductive system. These include pregnancy, pelvic malignancies (particularly carcinoma of the cervix), and ovarian pathology, as well as abnormalities of the uterus, such as prolapse or endometriosis. Extrinsic obstruction may be due to vascular abnormalities, including aneurysms of the aorta or iliac vessels or the presence of aberrant vessels. Other lesions that may obstruct the ureter originate in the gastrointestinal tract or in the retroperitoneal space, including Crohn's disease, colorectal cancer, retroperitoneal fibrosis, or metastases of tumors to the retroperitoneum. The latter two disorders may cause slowly progressive obstruction with few clinical manifestations. Most of the causes previously cited produce obstruction of the upper urinary tract. The causes of lower urinary tract obstruction include lesions of the urethra, the prostate, and the bladder. Urethral strictures are usually secondary to chronic instrumentation or gonococcal infections. Malignant and benign tumors of the bladder are infrequent causes of obstruction. **In men, prostatic hypertrophy is the most common cause of obstruction of the lower urinary tract. In fact, about 80% of men over 60 years of age may have benign prostatic hypertrophy and some evidence of bladder dysfunction.** Neurogenic vesical dysfunction (neurogenic bladder) can result from upper neuron damage and produce involuntary micturition (spastic bladder dys-

Table 6–2. CLASSIFICATION OF URINARY TRACT OBSTRUCTION

Location
Upper urinary tract (above ureterovesical junction)
Lower urinary tract (below ureterovesical junction)
Duration
Acute (hours)
Subacute (days)
Chronic (weeks or months)
Degree
Complete or total (high-grade obstruction)
Incomplete or partial (low-grade obstruction)

function) or lower spinal tract injury and give rise to a flaccid atonic bladder. In both settings, significant residual urine may develop, resulting in ureterovesical reflux, ureteral dilatation, and increased pressure in the upper urinary tract. Drugs such as tranquilizers (diazepam), anticholinergics, antihistamines, and alpha-adrenergic stimulators can cause bladder dysfunction and urinary retention.

CLINICAL MANIFESTATIONS

The clinical manifestations of urinary tract obstruction vary depending on the location, duration, and degree of the obstruction (Table 6–2). The clinical manifestations of upper and lower urinary tract obstruction differ. Patients with total obstruction may present with acute renal failure and anuria. Partial obstruction may cause polyuria or fluctuating urine output alternating from oliguria to polyuria. Pain is more common in acute than in chronic obstruction. **Obstructive uropathy may occur without symptoms or with overt clinical manifestations and laboratory findings highly suggestive of obstruction.**

Major clinical syndromes of obstruction are summarized in Table 6–3. The symptoms suggestive of obstruction include urinary tract infection (usually refractory to treatment), abdominal flank pain, or a tender palpable kidney. Pain is a frequent symptom in obstructive uropathy, particularly in patients with ureteral calculi. Acute ureteral obstruction may be manifested by a steady crescendo flank pain radiating to the labia, the testicles, or the groin. The acute attack may last less than half an hour or as long as a day. Pain radiating into the flank during micturition is said to be pathognomonic of ureterovesical reflux. On the other hand, patients with chronic, slowly progressive obstruction such as those with retroperitoneal fibrosis may not report a history of pain at all. Anuria occurs with complete bilateral obstruction or with unilateral obstruction in a patient with a solitary kidney. Polyuria and sodium wasting and defects in acidification and potassium excretion may occur in patients with partial ureteral obstruction. **A pattern of changing urine output, particularly alternating periods of oliguria and polyuria, strongly suggests the presence of obstructive uropathy.**

Lower urinary tract obstruction may be manifested by difficulties in micturition, including a decrease in the force and caliber of the urinary stream, intermittency, postvoid dribbling, hesitancy, and nocturia. Urgency, frequency, and urinary incontinence can be due to incomplete emptying of the bladder. Obstruction may develop in patients with established chronic renal disease and can cause an acceleration in the rate of progression of the renal insufficiency. Occasionally, end-stage renal failure may be due to chronic obstructive uropathy that has had an asymptomatic course. Gross hematuria can occur, particularly in patients who develop

Table 6–3. CLINICAL PRESENTATIONS OF OBSTRUCTIVE UROPATHY

Presentation	Cause
Acute renal failure	Complete bilateral obstruction (or complete obstruction of a solitary kidney)
Chronic renal failure	Severe partial bilateral obstruction
Flank pain and/or enlarged tender kidney	Unilateral obstruction: partial or complete
Polyuria, polydipsia, sodium wasting and/or renal tubular acidosis	Chronic partial obstruction or postobstructive diuresis
Bladder symptoms: hesitancy, incontinence, decreased caliber of urine stream	Obstruction of lower urinary tract (bladder neck, bladder pathology)
Repeated or refractory urinary tract infections	Any obstructive lesion, but most commonly lower urinary tract
Hypertension	Increased extracellular fluid volume (bilateral obstruction); increased renin-angiotensin (unilateral obstruction)
Polycythemia	Increased renal production of erythropoietin (presumably due to renal ischemia during obstruction)

obstruction as a consequence of stones. Hypertension can be coincidental or can occur as a consequence of obstruction. It can be due to expansion of the extracellular fluid or to the increased secretion of renin-angiotensin. In elderly individuals, hyperkalemic hyperchloremic metabolic acidosis may occasionally be seen as a consequence of obstructive uropathy. Polycythemia has been described and presumably is due to increased secretion of erythropoietin by the obstructed kidney. In neonates and infants, obstructive uropathy may not be suspected until failure to thrive, voiding difficulties, fever, hematuria, or symptoms of renal failure appear. Oligohydramnios at the time of delivery should raise the suspicion of obstructive uropathy. Patients with obstruction occasionally may present with acute pyelonephritis, high fever, costovertebral angle pain, and tenderness. Bacteremia may occasionally be the presenting picture. In males, the presence of urinary tract infection should suggest possible obstruction, and an intravenous pyelogram (IVP) may be required. This is not the case in females, in whom urinary tract infection is common in the absence of obstruction.

DIFFERENTIAL DIAGNOSIS

The differential diagnosis varies depending on the clinical presentation and clinical symptoms. Patients presenting with anuria and acute renal failure should be evaluated for other potential causes of acute renal failure such as ischemia, administration of nephrotoxins, and so on. Patients with partial obstruction and polyuria may mimic the entity of nephrogenic diabetes insipidus. Patients with obstruction presenting with hyperchloremic hyperkalemic metabolic acidosis should be distinguished from patients who have the same syndrome on the basis of low levels of renin and aldosterone secretion. Renal colic due to stones may mimic flank pain due to gastrointestinal pathology. In children, the manifestations of obstructive uropathy can include gastrointestinal symptoms such as nausea, vomiting, and abdominal pain.

DIAGNOSIS

Although in some instances the diagnosis of obstruction is obvious, in other cases it is difficult to establish. When obstructive uropathy is strongly suspected, appropriate tests should be obtained. **Because obstruction may result in irreversible renal damage, the sooner the diagnosis is made and the sooner appropriate therapy is instituted, the better the prognosis will be.**

History and Physical Examination

Detailed history with emphasis on some of the clinical manifestations previously described is of great importance. On physical examination, a palpable tender kidney may be found. In patients with partial obstruction, volume depletion may occur, and the signs of intravascular volume depletion may be evident, including hypotension, tachycardia, and so on. In patients with complete obstruction, on the other hand, signs of fluid overload may be present at admission. It is always important to look for the presence of a distended bladder by careful percussion of the suprapubic area. **Rectal examination is essential in elderly men to rule out the presence of a markedly enlarged prostate. A pelvic examination in women is necessary to rule out pelvic malignancy.**

Laboratory Evaluation

The laboratory evaluation may or may not be helpful. The urine sediment may be normal in many instances except in those individuals who have urinary tract infection and/or stones, in which case hematuria, white blood cells, and bacteria may be seen in the urine sediment. Proteinuria is usually absent. Other laboratory determinations that should be obtained include measurements of urea nitrogen, creatinine levels, and electrolytes in serum. The latter may reveal hypernatremia in patients with partial obstruction due to severe water losses, the presence of hyperchloremic hyperkalemic acidosis, or the presence of acidosis due to a renal tubular defect in hydrogen secretion. A urine culture should be obtained to determine whether there is infection of the urinary tract. Obstructive uropathy impairs the ability to concentrate the urine, and most patients with obstruction cannot excrete maximally concentrated urine. However, patients with acute or chronic renal failure, but without obstruction may also have a concentrating defect.

Radiologic Studies

Several radiologic techniques can be used to diagnose suspected upper urinary tract obstruction. These techniques include plain abdominal x-ray films, sonography, computed tomography, excretory urography, retrograde pyelography, isotopic renography, pressure flow studies, and voiding cystography.

Sonography is a noninvasive test that should be the initial screening procedure used in the diagnosis of obstruction (Fig. 6–1*A*). The main finding detected by sonography is dilatation of the urinary tract, which is seen in 90% of instances, even in the absence of excretory function. In a few instances, sonography may give false-positive results suggesting obstruction, because anatomic variations of the pyelocalyceal system may be interpreted as dilatation of the urinary tract. In patients with acute obstruction, on the other hand, dilatation of the urinary tract may not occur and sonography may be unrevealing. Sonography may also provide false-negative results in patients with obstruction and severe dehydration or in those with a "frozen" pelvis, due to malignancy. Radiologic evaluation may be initiated by obtaining a plain film of the abdomen or renal tomograms without the administration of dye. Using these procedures, the clinician can assess renal and bladder morphology and differences in size between the two kidneys or can determine the presence of a large bladder suggestive of outlet obstruction. Ureteral calculi may be also visualized on the plain film of the abdomen (the kidney-ureter-bladder [KUB] workup).

Computed tomography provides excellent resolution and is a very accurate technique to detect dilatation of the pelvis and collecting system (Fig. 6–1*B*). This technique is particularly valuable for identification and localization of an obstructing lesion, especially those lesions located in the retroperitoneal space. Computed tomography can be done without or with the injection of contrast material.

IVP is used to investigate suspected upper urinary tract obstruction (Fig. 6–2). The excretion of dye may be delayed in patients with a low glomerular filtration rate (GFR) because of a decrease in the filtered load of the contrast medium. In such patients, the examination should be extended until the collecting system and the site of obstruction are identified. This may require obtaining delayed films sometimes as long as 24 hours after the injection of the radiocontrast. An IVP is not helpful in patients with severely compromised renal function (creatinine greater than 5 mg/dl) because visualization of the urinary tract is poor in these individuals.

Retrograde pyelography requires the retrograde injection of radiocontrast and is used to visualize the ureter and collecting system when an IVP cannot be done or is not justified because of a history of allergic reactions to contrast material or other contraindications. This procedure can identify both the site and the cause of the obstruction (Fig. 6–3). It is helpful to include a postdrainage film, which is usually obtained 10 minutes after the retrograde injection of the radiocontrast. If the dye is not retained in the collecting system, obstruction is unlikely. Urinary tract infections may be a consequence of retrograde pyelography. If ob-

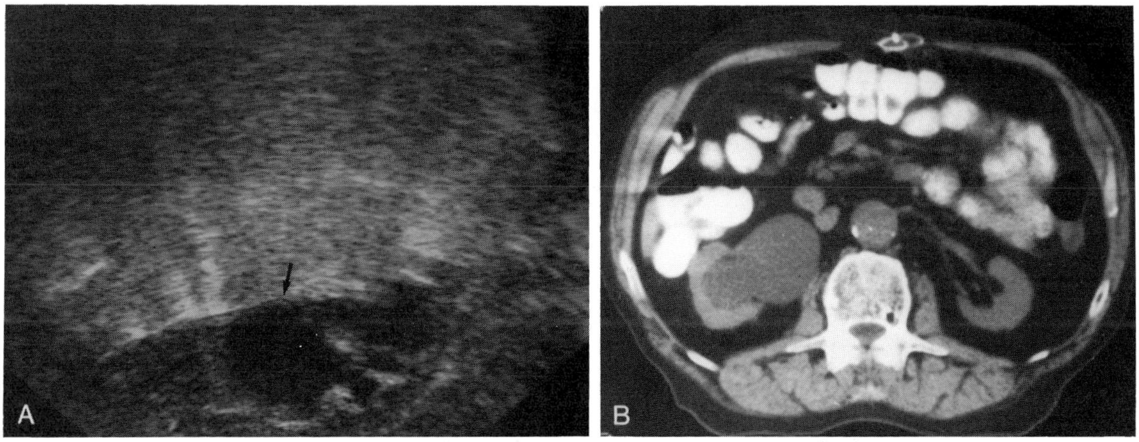

Figure 6–1. *(A)* Ultrasonogram, longitudinal section, illustrating chronic urinary tract obstruction secondary to a large recurrent cancer of the bladder. The different echogenicity is indicated by the arrow. *(B)* A computed tomogram obtained in the same patient revealed, in the absence of injection of contrast material, chronic hydronephrosis. The attenuation value of the widened pyelocalyceal system equals that of water. There is also thinning of the renal parenchyma, which is a characteristic of long-standing severe hydronephrosis. (Reproduced with permission from Massry SG, Glassock RJ: Textbook of Nephrology, 2nd ed. Baltimore, Williams & Wilkins, 1989.)

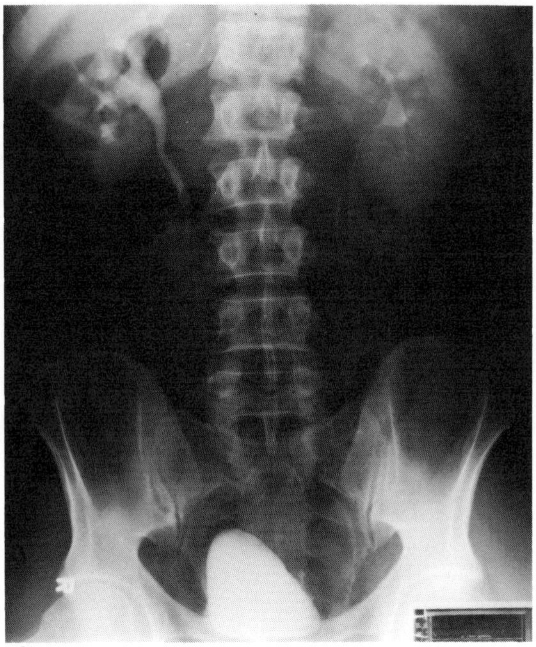

Figure 6–2. Intravenous pyelogram (IVP) of a patient admitted with the chief complaint of renal colic. A flat film of the abdomen (KUB) revealed the presence of a radiopaque density suggestive of a ureteral stone. The IVP reveals dilatation of the upper right ureter, the pelvis, and calyceal system of the right kidney (notice the difference between the renal pelvis and calyces of the right and left kidneys). There was an abrupt change in the diameter of the right ureter below the site where the stone had been impacted. At this site, the dye stopped and the stone is now seen as a radiolucent area. (Reproduced with permission from Massry SG, Glassock, RJ: Textbook of Nephrology, 2nd Ed. Baltimore, Williams & Wilkins, 1989.)

struction is present, the risk of producing infection that is difficult to control with conventional therapy is great. **Hence, if obstruction is diagnosed during retrograde pyelography, it is imperative to provide adequate drainage to avoid the development of infection in an obstructed urinary tract.**

Isotopic renography consisting of the intravenous injection of a radionuclide and gamma camera studies can be used to diagnose upper urinary tract obstruction. This test can be combined with intravenous furosemide administered 20 to 30 minutes after injection of the isotope. Conceptually, the diuretic should cause a rapid washout of the isotope in a dilated nonobstructed system. Persistence of the isotope suggests that the system is not only dilated but also obstructed. Although the isotopic renogram is relatively noninvasive and can be performed in most hospitals and clinics, it is seldom the definitive test in establishing the diagnosis of obstruction. Decreased renal func-

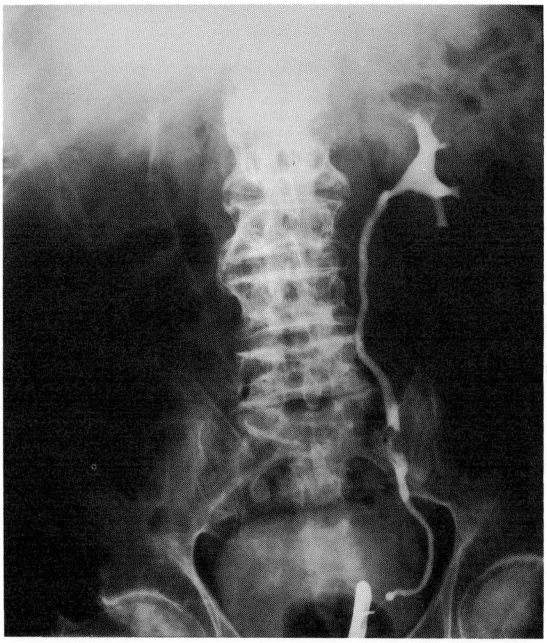

Figure 6–3. Retrograde pyelogram in a patient who was admitted with the chief complaints of hematuria and dull flank pain. A computed tomogram revealed mild dilatation of the pelvis and calyces of the left kidney. The same computed tomogram, at the level of the pelvis, revealed a soft-tissue density located on the left side. When a retrograde pyelogram of the left ureter and pelvis was performed, an irregular mass was detected in the ureter at the level of the pelvis. At surgery, this was found to represent a transitional cell carcinoma of the ureter. (Reproduced with permission from Massry SG, Glassock, RJ: Textbook of Nephrology, 2nd ed. Baltimore, Williams & Wilkins, 1989.)

tion significantly limits the usefulness of this technique because the diuretic response to furosemide may be absent, making interpretation of the test difficult.

Obstruction of the upper urinary tract occasionally is difficult to diagnose using the techniques previously described. Pressure flow studies may be needed to establish the diagnosis. Fluid is perfused in the collecting system at a rate of 10 ml/min, and the differential pressures between the bladder and the collecting system are determined. A differential pressure greater than 20 cm H_2O indicates obstruction, and a pressure between 15 and 20 cm H_2O is equivocal in diagnosing obstruction. An evaluation of the rise in pelvic pressure during perfusion diuresis also provides useful information.

Diagnosis of Lower Urinary Tract Obstruction

Obstruction of the lower urinary tract may be evaluated by the use of cystoscopy, radiologic tests, and urodynamic tests. Cystoscopy allows visualization of the entire urethra and the bladder during the same procedure. However, the procedure requires anesthesia in children and young adults. The anterior urethra can be assessed by retrograde urethrogram, which is performed by occluding the urethral meatus using a syringe or a catheter and injecting contrast medium. In most cases, the external urethral sphincter generates enough resistance to permit distention of the anterior urethra and demonstrate obstructive lesions. However, a retrograde urethrogram is not adequate to evaluate the posterior urethra. This anatomic area is best examined by an excretory or retrograde cystogram. The two tests combined provide a complete study of the urethra.

Urodynamic tests with measurements of the urine flow rate per unit of time are useful to evaluate bladder outlet obstruction. Measurement of the urine flow rate is a noninvasive test that examines the interplay between the expulsive force of the detrusor muscle and urethral resistance. Maximum flow rate is useful in assessing bladder outlet obstruction. Because micturition requires the coordinated effects of expulsive force and urethral resistance, a decrease in bladder tone or an increase in resistance (*e.g.*, due to prostatic hypertrophy) may produce symptoms of bladder outlet obstruction.

Cystometrography can be used to observe the force of the detrusor muscle. The procedure quantitates the pressure-volume relationship of the bladder. Dyssynergia of the bladder sphincter is reflected in the inability of the external sphincter to relax the contraction of the detrusor muscle and is encountered in patients with neurologic disorders. This type of resistance is better analyzed by electromyography and urethral pressure profiles.

TREATMENT

The treatment of urinary tract obstruction has both medical and surgical components. **Emergency medical treatment may be required when gram-negative septicemia is present in patients with complete or partial obstruction.**

Gram-negative septicemia due to pyelonephritis should be treated aggressively. Appropriate urine and blood cultures should be obtained, and appropriate antibiotics should be administered immediately without waiting for the results of the cultures. When the culture results are available, appropriate modifications in antibiotic therapy can be made if the organism or its sensitivity to antibiotics is different from that initially presumed to be present. Acute renal failure may be a life-threatening event, particularly if hyperkalemia and severe acid-base imbalance are present. Dialysis may be required. In some instances, acute relief of the obstruction by a nephrostomy or the placement of a stent in the ureter may allow for enough return of renal function to stabilize the situation. The presence of partial obstruction with electrolyte depletion may require the administration of appropriate fluids. The presence of hypernatremia in children with partial obstruction may require the administration of water in excess of sodium to decrease the concentration of sodium in serum. In patients with fluid overload due to complete obstruction, administration of fluid should be avoided to avoid causing congestive heart failure and pulmonary edema. The treatment of urinary tract obstruction also includes other considerations such as the need for surgery or instrumentation. **Complete bilateral ureteral obstruction presenting as acute renal failure requires rapid intervention.**

The site of obstruction frequently determines the approach. If the obstruction is distal to the bladder, introduction of a urethral catheter may suffice. Suprapubic cystostomy sometimes may be necessary. If, on the other hand, the obstruction is located in the upper urinary tract, placement of nephrostomy tubes or passage of a retrograde ureteral catheter may be required. Tubes should be placed in both obstructed renal calyces because the potential for functional recovery of either kidney is not easily predicted. Surgical intervention can be delayed for a few weeks or even months in patients with low-grade acute obstruction or partial chronic obstruction. However, prompt relief of partial obstruction is indicated when (1) there are multiple repeated episodes of urinary tract infection, (2) a patient has significant symptoms (flank pain, dysuria, voiding dysfunction), (3) there is urinary retention, and (4) there is evidence of recurrent or progressive renal damage.

Management of Upper Urinary Tract Obstruction

Stones are the most frequent cause of ureteral obstruction. Their treatment includes relief of pain, elimination of obstruction, and treatment of infection. Pain can be relieved by intramuscular injection of a narcotic analgesic. Stones less than 5 mm in diameter usually do not require surgical intervention or instrumentation because about 90% of these calculi pass spontaneously. If the stones are 5 to 7 mm in diameter, however, only about half will pass. Stones larger than 7 mm in diameter usually are not passed spontaneously. Increased fluid intake to achieve urine volumes of at least 1.5 to 2 L/day may help mobilize the stone. **Surgery or instrumentation for calyceal/ureteral stones is indicated when there is persistent colic, urinary tract infection, complete obstruction, a calculus greater than 7 mm in diameter or a smaller calculus that has not moved despite a prudential time and increased fluid intake.**

New procedures such as endourology and the application of extracorporeal shock-wave lithotripsy have allowed for the management of ureteral stones without the need for open surgery. Calculi located distal to the pelvic brim can be approached from below. They can be removed from the ureter using various loops or baskets, and this procedure is successful in about 70% of patients. If it fails, dilatation of the ureter or ultrasonic disintegration of the stone can be accomplished using the ureteral renoscope. Thus, the need for open surgery for distal ureteral calculus is rare. Broad-spectrum antibiotics are useful when infections complicate renal calculi. Choice of antibiotic depends on appropriate urine cultures and sensitivities. It should be remembered, however, that relief of obstruction is indispensable for successful antimicrobial therapy.

Nephrostomy is the insertion of a tube through the kidney into the renal pelvis to provide urine drainage. The procedure can be done under fluoroscopy using local anesthesia. Complications of nephrostomy include perirenal hemorrhage and acute obstruction due to clots. Dislodgment of the nephrostomy tube should be considered an emergency, and the tube should be replaced immediately. Long-term complications of nephrostomy tubes include calculus formation, infection, and pyelonephritis that may lead to renal insufficiency.

Treatment of Lower Urinary Tract Obstruction

Urethral and bladder neck obstruction requires surgery in patients who have recurring infections and are ambulatory, particularly when reflux, renal parenchymal damage, total urinary retention, repeated bleeding, or other severe symptoms are present. Obstruction secondary to benign prostatic hyperplasia does not always progress. Therefore, a patient with minimal symptoms, no infection, and a normal upper urinary tract may be safely monitored until he and his physicians agree that surgery is desirable.

When obstruction is due to abnormal bladder function, dynamic studies are essential to determine therapy. The main goals of therapy should be (1) to establish the bladder as a urine storage organ without causing renal parenchymal injury and (2) to provide a mechanism for bladder emptying that is acceptable to a patient. Patients can be divided in two groups: those with atonic bladder secondary to lower motor neuron injury and those with unstable bladder function due to upper motor neuron disease. A neurogenic bladder in patients with diabetes mellitus is usually due to lower motor neuron disease. If patients void at regular intervals, they sometimes achieve adequate emptying of the bladder. These patients occasionally respond to cholinergic agents. Recent reviews on the use of bethanechol chloride (Urecholine), 50 mg orally, have seriously questioned its long-term use. In such patients, overdistention of the bladder may impair emptying. Thus, bladder outlet obstruction may be a major problem. Alpha-adrenergic blockers relax urethral sphincter tone but have only limited success because of their side effects. **The best treatment for patients with significant residual urine and recurrent bouts of urosepsis is the establishment of clean intermittent catheterization at regular intervals.**

The goal should be to catheterize four to five times per day such that the amount of urine drained from the bladder is not in excess of 400 ml. This technique is successful but requires that patients accept treatment and be carefully trained.

In patients with hypertonic bladder function, the major goal is to improve the storage function of the bladder. The use of anticholinergic agents such as oxybutynin (Ditropan), 5 mg every 4 to 6 hours, may be indicated. Chronic clean intermittent catheterization occasionally is necessary. In a patient with a neurogenic bladder, a chronic indwelling catheter should be avoided if possible. **In the presence of lower urinary tract obstruction, surgical diversions are indicated if (1) deterioration of renal function occurs despite conservative measures, (2) there is intractable incontinence, (3) there is a small contracted bladder, and (4) there are multiple bladder fistulae.** An ileal conduit is the operation of choice for permanent diversion. The ureters are anastomosed to a small isolated ileal sac with a stoma through the skin. This procedure decreases the time of contact of the urine with the intestinal mucosa and does not lead to the metabolic acidosis commonly encountered in patients whose ureters drain into the sigmoid colon. However, stomal obstruction or an antiperistaltic or very long loop may increase the time that the bowel mucosa is exposed to the urine, leading to metabolic acidosis of comparable degree to that in patients with ureteral diversion to the sigmoid colon.

Treatment of Postobstructive Diuresis

Postobstructive diuresis refers to the marked natriuresis and diuresis that follow relief of obstructive uropathy. This diuresis is characterized by the excretion of large amounts of sodium, potassium, magnesium, and other solutes. Although of self-limited duration, the losses of salt and water may result in hypokalemia, hyponatremia or hypernatremia, hypomagnesemia, and/or marked contraction of the extracellular fluid volume with peripheral vascular collapse.

In many patients, however, a brief diuresis after relief of obstruction may represent a normal response to expansion of the extracellular fluid volume that occurred during the period of obstruction. This postobstructive diuresis is physiologic and does not compromise a patient's volume status. Postobstructive diuresis in this setting can be prolonged by overzealous administration of salt and water after relief of obstruction. Fluid replacement is justified only when excessive losses of sodium and water are inappropriate for the volume status of a patient and are presumably due to an intrinsic tubular defect for sodium and water reabsorption. Fluid replacement is guided in large part by the volume and composition of the urine. Intravenous fluid replacement should be provided when tachycardia and orthostatic hypotension are present. **To distinguish between inappropriate diuresis and appropriate excretion of fluid retained or excess fluid administered, it may sometimes be necessary to decrease fluid replacement to levels less than those of urine output and observe patients carefully for signs of volume depletion.**

Weighing patients daily and making laboratory determinations of the electrolyte composition of the plasma are necessary to adjust fluid replacement. Urine losses of salt and water are usually replaced with half normal saline to which sodium bicarbonate and potassium chloride are added. Magnesium can be replaced by adding magnesium sulfate (supplied as 2-ml ampules containing 8 mEq of magnesium) to the NaCl solution. In some instances, phosphate replacement may be necessary. Either 42% sodium phosphate (15-ml ampules containing 45 mmol of phosphate and 60 mEq of sodium) or 46% potassium phosphate (15-ml ampules containing 45 mmol of phosphate and 66 mEq of potassium) may be added to 5% dextrose or half normal saline.

Treatment of Other Complications of Obstructive Uropathy

Severe hypertension is sometimes observed concomitantly with obstructive uropathy. Relief of obstruction, particularly bilateral, may lower the blood pressure. In this case, the hypertension was probably due to expansion of the extracellular fluid volume. Patients with unilateral obstruction may require antihypertensive therapy to decrease blood pressure levels. Because in some of these patients the hypertension is more likely the result of an increased release of renin and angiotensin, drug therapy may be required. In patients with end-stage renal disease due to obstructive uropathy, renal transplantation may be performed. However, appropriate drainage into an ileal conduit may be necessary. In these patients, the original kidneys may have to be removed, particularly if repeated infections have occurred in the past. In this way, a potential site of infection is eliminated before patients are given immunosuppressive therapy required in renal transplantation.

Suggested Readings

Klahr S, Bander SJ: Obstructive nephropathy. *In* Massry SG, Glassock RJ (eds): Textbook of Nephrology, 2nd ed., Vol II. Baltimore, Williams & Wilkins, 1989, pp 889–909.

Klahr S, Buerkert J, Morrison A: Urinary tract obstruction. *In* Brenner BM, Rector FC Jr (eds): The Kidney, 3rd ed. Philadelphia, WB Saunders, 1986, pp 1443–1490.

Klahr S, Clayman RV, Bahnson RR: Management of obstructive uropathy. *In* Bayless TM, Brain MC, Cherniack RM (eds): Current Therapy in Internal Medicine, 2nd ed. Toronto, BC Decker, 1987, pp 1066–1071.

Klahr S, Harris K, Purkerson ML: Effects of obstructive uropathy on renal functions. Pediatr Nephrol 2:34–42, 1988.

CHAPTER 7

DIABETIC NEPHROPATHY

Richard J. Glassock and Sharon G. Adler

DEFINITIONS AND TERMINOLOGY

Diabetic nephropathy is an all-encompassing term used to identify disorders of kidney structure and function that arise secondary to diabetes mellitus, either of the insulin-dependent (type 1) or non–insulin-dependent (type 2) variety. As such, this definition includes disorders that affect the glomeruli, tubules, interstitium, and intrarenal vasculature. The term *kidney disease of diabetes mellitus* is often used interchangeably with diabetic nephropathy. *Diabetic glomerulopathy* is a more specific term that refers to the disorders of glomerular structure and function that arise as a consequence of long-standing diabetes mellitus.

Two principal morphologic variants of diabetic glomerulopathy are recognized: (1) diffuse diabetic intercapillary glomerulosclerosis and (2) nodular diabetic glomerulosclerosis (the Kimmelstiel-Wilson lesion) (Fig. 7–1). Although morphologically distinct, these two forms of diabetic glomerulopathy are viewed as a part of a continuum of diabetes-induced abnormalities of the glomerular capillaries and associated supporting structures.

In addition to its associated disorders of renal structure and function, diabetes mellitus may also be implicated in extrarenal diseases involving the genitourinary tract. These disorders, which have important clinical consequences, include unilateral or bilateral extrarenal arterial vaso-occlusive disease (atherosclerosis), ascending urinary tract infection, ureteric obstruction secondary to sloughed papillae or localized mycelial fungal growths, bladder dysfunction secondary to autonomic neuropathy, and vulvovaginal infections. In addition, functional disorders, in part related to extrarenal abnormalities, may influence renal function in important ways. Examples might include congestive heart failure, renal tubular acidosis, abnormalities of adrenal steroidogenesis secondary to insulin deficiency, and diarrhea and/or nausea and vomiting secondary to visceral autonomic insufficiency (*e.g.*, diabetic gastroparesis). Thus, it is important to recognize that diabetes mellitus may be attended by a wide variety of kidney and urinary tract disorders. The fluid and electrolyte abnormalities that accompany diabetes, such as diabetic ketoacidosis and hyperosmolar coma, are beyond the scope of this brief discussion. The principal focus of this chapter is on the progressive renal disease that is the direct consequence of the abnormal milieu engendered by diabetes mellitus *per se*. Because diffuse diabetic glomerulosclerosis and nodular diabetic glomerulosclerosis are found to be the underlying causes of progressive renal failure in most patients with long-standing diabetes mellitus (either type 1 or type 2), the clinical features, natural history, and management of diabetic glomerulopathy are discussed.

DIABETIC GLOMERULOPATHY: CLINICAL DESCRIPTION

Diabetic glomerulopathy evolves over many years (often decades) (Fig. 7–2). The clinical manifestations of the disorder depend on the stage of evolution in which it is detected. It is believed that diabetic glomerulopathy evolves through these stages in a similar fashion in both type 1 and type 2 diabetes mellitus, although longitudinal studies of the progress of diabetic glomerulopathy have largely been conducted in type 1 (insulin-dependent) diabetes mellitus. Diabetic glomerulopathy evolves gradually in four fundamental stages. The initial stage begins with the onset of clinically recognized abnormalities in glucose homeostasis or sometimes before overt hyperglycemia. This initial stage is

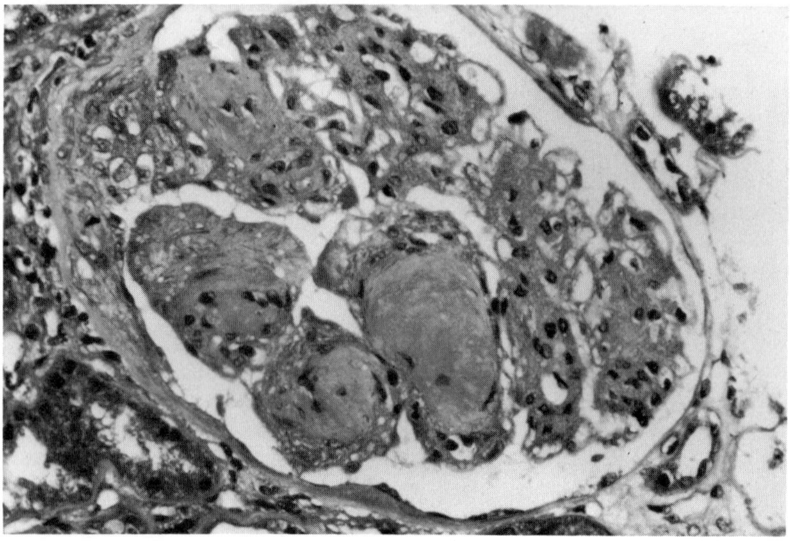

Figure 7–1. Nodular diabetic glomerulosclerosis—Kimmelstiel-Wilson lesion (PAS, × 500).

characterized by a substantial increase in glomerular filtration rate (sometimes as much as 40 to 50% greater than normal), increased renal plasma flow, and increased renal length and volume. A transient increase in albumin excretion, above the normal range (greater than 15 micrograms per minute) but below that which is readily detectable by standard qualitative tests, is also often present. This transient "microalbuminuria" quickly disappears on institution of insulin therapy and partial correction of hyperglycemia. This initial proteinuria may also be associated with a rise in β_2-microglobulin excretion, suggesting that it may at least in part be of tubular origin. However, with partial correction of hyperglycemia, the increase in glomerular filtration rate does not return to normal and renal size remains increased. Renal biopsies at this stage will demonstrate an increase in mesangial volume and perhaps some mild thickening of the capillary basement membranes.

Among patients who have type 1 diabetes mellitus and maintain excellent glycemic control (hemoglobin A_{1c} values <8%), no further progression beyond this stage may be noted. In fact, approximately 30 to 40% of all patients with type 1 diabetes mellitus *never* develop any overt signs of diabetic glomerulopathy. In addition to having excellent glycemic control, these patients seem to lack a family history of hypertension and themselves remain normotensive. However, the majority of patients with type 1 diabetes mellitus and an unknown but probably similar fraction of patients with type 2 diabetes mellitus eventually progress to the second stage, designated as incipient or early diabetic glomerulopathy. The usual time period between the onset of abnormal glucose homeostasis and the onset of incipient glomerulopathy is 7 to 10 years. If incipient glomerulopathy has not developed within 15 years of the onset of abnormal glucose homeostasis, it is increasingly unlikely that it will develop thereafter.

The second stage of diabetic glomerulopathy, called incipient glomerulopathy, is heralded by the onset of *persistently* abnormal urinary excretion rates of albumin, usually >30 μg/min. This excretion rate is well below the limit of detection of the usual qualitative tests for albumin excretion. Detection of this microalbuminuria depends on more sensitive colorimetric, radioimmune, or immunoenzymatic assays. On occasion, persistent microalbuminuria may be preceded by intermittent episodes of microalbuminuria exacerbated by intercurrent illness and/or exercise. Microalbuminuria is unassociated with an increase in excretion rate of β_2-microglobulin, indicating its glomerular origin.

At the onset of this stage, the glomerular filtration rate remains elevated, the kidneys continue to be enlarged, and a slight increase in blood pressure (mean arterial pressure) is observed. This rise in arterial pressure is usually 5 to 10 mm Hg, and many patients may remain

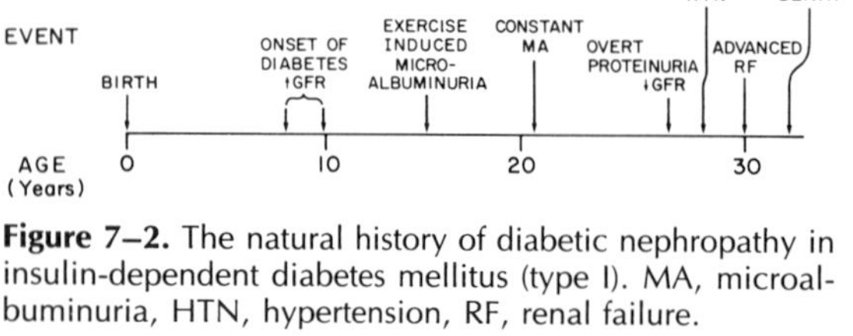

Figure 7–2. The natural history of diabetic nephropathy in insulin-dependent diabetes mellitus (type I). MA, microalbuminuria, HTN, hypertension, RF, renal failure.

within the so-called normotensive range (*e.g.*, <140/90 mm Hg). Background retinopathy may begin to demonstrate a transition to proliferative retinopathy during this stage. In the absence of dramatic improvement in glycemic control or antihypertensive therapy, urinary albumin excretion rates continue to increase slowly during the next several years, and at the end of 5 to 10 years most patients will have progressed to overt proteinuria (albumin excretion rates >200 μg/min and urinary total protein excretion rates of >500 mg/day). As the urinary albumin excretion rate rises, blood pressure rises further and in most patients reaches frank hypertensive ranges. Glomerular filtration rate simultaneously declines from supranormal levels into the range of normal values for nondiabetic subjects of comparable size, age, and sex. During the stage of incipient glomerulopathy, the rate of increase of albumin excretion can be influenced by glycemic control and by reduction of arterial pressure by antihypertensive agents. The rate of rise of albumin excretion and the relationship between albumin excretion rate and blood pressure are better defined for type 1 than for type 2 diabetes mellitus.

Excellent glycemic control combined with rigorous control of blood pressure may arrest the disease at the stage of incipient glomerulopathy; however, many patients will continue to progress to the next stage of overt glomerulopathy. The time that elapses between the onset of incipient nephropathy and the onset of overt nephropathy averages 7 to 10 years. More rapid progression may occur in those patients who develop more severe hypertension, particularly when combined with very poorly regulated glycemia.

The onset of the stage of overt glomerulopathy is heralded by the development of qualitatively detectable abnormal proteinuria, usually in excess of 500 mg/day (or >200 μg/min of albumin excretion). At the onset of this stage, most if not all patients have unequivocal hypertension, which at times may be severe. The glomerular filtration rate will have decreased to normal or slightly subnormal values. The rate of decline of the glomerular filtration rate is variable from patient to patient but overall averages about 0.8 to 1.1 ml/min/month. In this regard, it is important to emphasize that creatinine is a very poor marker for glomerular filtration in the presence of proteinuria and renal disease. **Because of increasing tubular secretion of creatinine, the creatinine clearance *overestimates* the true glomerular filtration rate (sometimes by a factor of 2 or more), and a substantial decline in glomerular filtration rate can occur even with a normal serum creatinine concentration. The kidneys remain enlarged.**

Renal biopsies at this stage reveal further expansion of the mesangial zones by the accumulation of an acellular matrix and distinct thickening of the glomerular capillary walls. Some biopsy specimens reveal a distinct intercapillary nodular glomerulosclerosis at this stage. Excellent glycemic control at this time seems to have little effect on the future rate of progression; however, vigorous antihypertensive therapy may reduce the magnitude of proteinuria and slow the subsequent rate of decline of glomerular filtration rate.

Most patients progress to frank nephrotic syndrome with urinary protein excretion rates of >3.5 g/day and accompanying hypoalbuminemia, hypercholesterolemia, and edema. Proliferative retinopathy appears and progresses. Blood pressure continues to rise and may require multiple antihypertensive agents for management. The glomerular filtration rate continues to decrease, and by definition, when this decline is accompanied by a distinct rise in serum creatinine and blood urea nitrogen above normal levels, a patient has entered the final stage of azotemic glomerulopathy. The time elapsed from the onset of overt glomerulopathy to azotemic glomerulopathy averages 3 to 5 years. The rate of progression can be significantly influenced by vigorous antihypertensive therapy.

The onset of the phase of azotemic glomerulopathy is heralded by a distinct and abnormal elevation in serum creatinine and/or blood urea nitrogen. The glomerular filtration rate has decreased to 30 to 50% of normal nondiabetic values corrected for age, sex, and body size. Patients at this stage have heavy proteinuria, hypertension, edema, and often hypoalbuminemia. In addition, they may also be suffering from extrarenal manifestations such as ischemic heart disease, congestive heart failure, peripheral vascular insufficiency and neuropathy, severe proliferative retinopathy, cerebral vascular accidents, or occlusive renal vascular disease. The kidneys remain large, although late in the stage of azotemic glomerulopathy they may gradually experience a reduction in size.

Renal biopsies reveal advanced glomerulosclerosis, often with a nodular transformation. In addition, substantial degrees of vascular and tubulointerstitial disease are found. Excellent glycemic control at this stage has little effect on the rate of progression. Rigorous blood pressure control may significantly slow the decline of glomerular filtration rate, however, but even with normalization of blood pressure, patients slowly and predictably progress to end-stage renal disease (ESRD). The rate of progression, as measured by the rate of decline in glomerular filtration rate, may accelerate in the last few months before ESRD develops. Severe nephrotic syndrome with marked hypoalbuminemia and difficult-to-manage edema may accompany the early phases of azotemic glomerulopathy. Proliferative retinopathy may rapidly progress, leading to blindness. Peripheral and autonomic neuropathy and peripheral and coronary artery disease may further complicate the picture. The time elapsed from the onset of azotemic glomerulopathy to ESRD averages 2 to 5 years but in patients with very poorly controlled blood pressure may be even shorter.

OTHER RENAL DISEASES IN PATIENTS WITH DIABETES MELLITUS

Although diabetic glomerulopathy is the most common renal parenchymal disorder encountered among patients with diabetes mellitus, it is important for clinicians to recognize that several other renal disorders may occur in diabetic patients and may contribute significantly to renal morbidity and mortality. A detailed description of these disorders is beyond the scope of this discussion, but brief mention and description of several of these entities is appropriate.

Renal Arterial Occlusive Disease

Patients with diabetes mellitus are subject to a dramatically increased risk of large-vessel atherosclerotic disease. Such atherosclerosis may affect one or both renal arteries. Unilateral renal arterial stenosis, secondary to atherosclerosis, may dramatically aggravate the underlying tendency to hypertension. Afflicted individuals may present with sudden worsening of hypertension, difficult-to-control hypertension, grade 3 or 4 hypertensive retinopathy, lateralizing abdominal bruits, disparity in renal size, and hyperreninemia. A high index of suspicion is required in order to make the diagnosis. Captopril scintigraphy may be a useful screening test; however, percutaneous transfemoral renal arteriograms or intraarterial digital subtraction angiography is required to substantiate the diagnosis. However, in the setting of incipient, overt, or azotemic glomerulopathy, the administration of radiocontrast agents may induce acute renal failure (see below).

Bilateral renal arterial atherosclerotic occlusive disease represents an important although uncommon, cause of progressive renal failure in patients with diabetes mellitus. Such patients have hypertension out of proportion to the degree of manifestations of diabetic glomerulopathy, chiefly proteinuria. They also may present with renal failure in the absence of proliferative diabetic retinopathy. Abdominal bruits will frequently be present. A disparity of renal size may be observed as a result of the unequal severity of the occlusive process. Again, a high index of suspicion is required for the diagnosis. **Bilateral renal arterial occlusive disease should always be suspected when acute renal failure or a substantial decline in glomerular filtration rate follows the administration of angiotensin-converting enzyme inhibitors or an acute lowering of systemic arterial pressure with any antihypertensive agent**. The only definitive way of detecting this disorder is radiographic imaging of the renal arteries using contrast media.

Acute Renal Failure Secondary to Contrast Media or Nonsteroidal Antiinflammatory Agents

Patients with diabetes mellitus, particularly those with early, overt, or azotemic glomerulopathy, are at increased risk of developing acute renal failure (acute tubular necrosis) following contrast media injection, such as with an intravenous pyelogram or a renal arteriogram. The renal failure is often mild and reversible and is chiefly of a nonoliguric variety. The risk of acute renal failure may be decreased by diminishing the total dose of contrast media, volume expansion before contrast media injection, or by the use of an osmotic diuretic (mannitol) in conjunction with the contrast media injection.

Nonsteroidal antiinflammatory agents may also induce a functional form of acute renal failure in patients with diabetes mellitus, particularly those with concomitant congestive heart failure due to coronary artery disease. In such patients, glomerular filtration rate rapidly declines on administration of the drug and usually quickly returns to baseline when the drug is discontinued. On rare occasions, tubulointerstitial nephritis may complicate the use of these drugs.

Renal Medullary and/or Papillary Necrosis

Patients with diabetes mellitus are at increased risk of developing medullary and/or papillary necrosis in association with partial lower urinary tract obstruction or with acute ascending bacterial pyelonephritis. Necrotic papillae may be passed into the urine, and acute renal failure may develop.

Urinary Tract Infection

The incidence and prevalence of urinary tract infection may be slightly increased in patients with diabetes mellitus, particularly females. Relapses of infection following treatment are common, especially in the presence of abnormal bladder emptying or impaired renal function. On rare occasions, such urinary tract infections may be complicated by the development of granulomatous pyelonephritis. This disorder principally affects one or the other kidney and results in an enlarged, poorly functioning or nonfunctioning kidney. It is often mistaken for a renal malignancy. Rarely, fungal infection of the urinary tract may lead to ureteric obstruction from mycelial phase growth of the organism (fungus ball). Diabetic patients are also at increased risk for developing the uncommon entity known as emphysematous pyelonephritis, in which gram-negative gas-forming bacterial organisms rapidly induce necrosis of the kidney.

Renal Tubular Acidosis

Patients with diabetes mellitus, particularly those with incipient or early overt glomerulopathy, may develop a form of renal tubular acidosis known as type 4 (hyperkalemic) renal tubular acidosis. These patients also have low plasma renin levels. Aldosterone secretion rates are abnormally low in relationship to the concomitant hyperkalemia. The pathogenesis of this syndrome is quite diverse. In some patients, a primary defect in renin secretion may be at fault; in others, an abnormality of aldosterone production may be the underlying cause. This complication seldom requires any direct therapy, although the hyperkalemia and acidosis may sometimes result in morbidity. Hyperkalemia is particularly hazardous in patients with coronary artery disease and disorders of atrioventricular conduction.

Nondiabetic Glomerular Disease

Because diabetes mellitus is a relatively common disorder, it is not surprising that a significant proportion of patients with diabetes presenting with overt renal disease are found to have non–diabetes-related lesions on careful investigation. These are most common in patients with type 2 diabetes mellitus presenting with proteinuria and/or hematuria but are also found among patients with type 1 diabetes mellitus presenting with proteinuria and/or hematuria 5 years or less from the onset of insulin dependency. **Clues to the presence of a nondiabetic lesion underlying a disorder of renal function in a diabetic patient include rapid onset, absence of proliferative glomerulopathy, "active" urinary sediment (dysmorphic hematuria and red blood cell [RBC] casts), absence of hypertension, small kidneys, tubular proteinuria, eosinophiluria, and normal hemoglobin A_{1c} values.** The presence of either hematuria or tubular proteinuria may not be a reliable or discriminatory observation. However, it should be emphasized that some patients with diabetic glomerulopathy may present with hematuria RBC casts in addition to glomerular proteinuria. The origin of the RBCs in the urine of patients with diabetic glomerulopathy is unknown but could relate either to concomitant hemorrhagic cystitis, papillary necrosis, or a ruptured glomerular microaneurysm. Dysmorphic hematuria is noted only when RBCs derive from a renal origin.

Clinicians should retain a high index of suspicion for nondiabetic glomerular disease in patients who have type 2 diabetes mellitus and present with renal failure and proteinuria and also in patients who have type 1 diabetes mellitus and present with proteinuria and/or renal failure 5 years or less from the onset of insulin dependency. The nondiabetic renal lesions that occur in patients with diabetes mellitus are heterogeneous, but there appears to be an increased prevalance of idiopathic membranous glomerulonephritis, minimal change disease, and poststreptococcal glomerulonephritis. Amyloidosis, for unknown reasons, is quite uncommon. Renal biopsies sometimes may be required for definitive separation of diabetic glomerulopathy from nondiabetic glomerular disease. In otherwise typical cases of diabetic glomerulopathy, a clinical diagnosis is sufficient and renal biopsies are ordinarily not performed.

MANAGEMENT OF DIABETIC GLOMERULOPATHY

A detailed discussion of the management of hyperglycemia, ketoacidosis, nonketotic hyperosmolar coma, and other fluid and electrolyte problems that occur in patients with diabetes mellitus is beyond the scope of this chapter. Nevertheless, it is extremely important to emphasize that many of the renal complications of diabetes mellitus can be avoided or substantially decreased by rigorous attention to the management of the diabetic state *per se*. For example, strict control of blood glucose to maintain the hemoglobin A_{1c} levels below 8% seems to diminish substantially the risk of subsequent development of diabetic glomerulopathy. It may also reduce the risk of the attendant extrarenal complications, particularly large-vessel atherosclerosis, by returning lipid levels toward normal. The extent to which strict control of blood glucose at nearly euglycemic levels will reduce the complications of diabetes will not be definitely known until the results of a large prospective trial (The Diabetes Control and Complications Trial) are released sometime in 1994. Ultimately, successful whole or segmental pancreas or islet cell transplantation may avoid all of the late complications of diabetes mellitus, including renal disease. Additionally, early treatment of newly diagnosed type 1 diabetes mellitus with immunosuppressive agents (*e.g.*, cyclosporine) may ultimately prevent irreversible damage to beta cells and lead to a cure for diabetes mellitus. For now, clinicians (and patients) need to recognize the importance of metabolic control in the prevention of later complications, particularly those affecting the kidneys and blood vessels. Whether rigorous metabolic control will also beneficially affect the course of retinopathy is unknown.

Because only about 60% of patients with diabetes mellitus will ultimately develop diabetic glomerulopathy, it would be helpful to be able to identify those patients at risk at the onset of their disease. At present, such risk stratification at the onset of disease is not possible; however, patients with diabetes mellitus who have a strong family history of hypertension seem to have a significantly increased risk of later developing glomerulopathy. Perhaps in the future, genetic analysis (*e.g.*, HLA genotype) may uncover a genetic basis for susceptibility for diabetic glomerulopathy. For now, clinicians must rely on careful follow-up observation to detect the earliest manifestations of diabetic glomerulopathy.

Serial measurements of urinary albumin excretion appear to be the best method for early detection of incipient glomerulopathy. For such measurements to be interpreted reliably, they need to be carried out under carefully controlled conditions of activity, glycemic and blood pressure control, protein and water intake, and medications. Studies performed during urinary tract infection are of no value. Decisions should be based on measurements repeated on several occasions. Twenty-four-hour urine collections or overnight urine collections seem to be most reliable. Accurate and quantitative measurement of albumin in urine samples is essential. This can be accomplished by radioimmunoassay, enzyme-linked immunoabsorbent assays, or specialized colorimetric techniques. Screening may be accomplished by the use of special, highly sensitive dye-impregnated paper strips. **Persistent albumin excretion of >30 μg/min can be regarded as evidence of early or incipient glomerulopathy and identifies the patients who, in the absence of intervention, have an 85% or greater likelihood of evolving to overt glomerulopathy in the next 5 to 10 years.**

The exact relationship between the development of microalbuminuria and overt glomerulopathy is best established in type 1 diabetes mellitus and is less well understood in type 2. Periodic screening for microalbuminuria should be initiated after 5 years of insulin dependency in type 1 diabetes mellitus and at the time of diagnosis of type 2. In patients with type 2, the presence of microalbuminuria seems to correlate best with morbidity and mortality from macrovascular disease than it does with progressive diabetic glomerulosclerosis. Exercise-induced microalbuminuria in diabetic patients seems not to have great prognostic value.

Greatly elevated glomerular filtration rates, especially in conjunction with high hemoglobin A_{1c} values, may also be used to stratify patients into a high-risk category. Patients with persistent microalbuminuria should be managed with an intensive regimen of insulin to secure optimal glycemic control without an unacceptable occurrence of hypoglycemic episodes. Careful attention to concomitant lipid disorders is also important.

Blood pressure should be monitored carefully and frequently. Although such treatment is controversial, many researchers believe that antihypertensive agents, particularly angiotensin-converting enzyme (ACE) inhibitors, should be prescribed to diabetic patients (particularly those with type 1 diabetes mellitus) at the onset of persistent microalbuminuria irrespective of the actual blood pressure level. Because most patients with microalbuminuria will have experienced a significant rise in blood pressure, compared with values obtained in the premicroalbuminuric stage, an argument could be made that hypertension actually exists even though the absolute values decrease below the conventional definition of abnormal blood pressure (*i.e.*, 140/90). It should be emphasized that the renal circulation in diabetes mellitus is in a vasodilated state (primarily at the afferent arteriole); therefore, systemic arterial pressure is being transmitted to a greater extent to the glomerular capillaries in diabetic individuals then in nondiabetic persons. Certain agents, particularly ACE inhibitors, may reduce this capillary hypertension (by relaxing efferent arterioles) even in the absence of an effect on the prevailing systemic arterial pressure. If glomerular capillary hypertension is involved in the pathogenesis of progressive glomerulopathy, such a therapeutic approach will likely be beneficial. This proposition is now being tested in prospective randomized controlled trials. Early studies seem to indicate that rigorous metabolic control, combined with lowering of the capillary and/or systemic mean arterial pressure, decreases microalbuminuria or retards its progression to overt proteinuria and thus may delay or prevent the evolution to overt glomerulopathy. Whether this scenario will also apply to type 2 diabetes mellitus is unknown.

Dietary protein restriction may have effects similar to those of ACE inhibitors but seems to reduce capillary hypertension by increasing afferent arteriolar resistance. Thus, the effects of ACE inhibitors and protein restriction may be additive. Unfortunately, because many patients with type 2 diabetes mellitus present with overt glomerulopathy, the opportunity for intervention at an earlier stage is not available.

The management of patients with overt glomerulopathy (Table 7–1) is focused primarily on rigorous control of blood pressure. Almost all patients with overt glomerulopathy will have some evaluation of mean arterial pressure. Rigorous metabolic control of hyperglycemia is less important in overall management. The method of lowering blood pressure in patients with overt glomerulopathy may be less important than the magnitude of the decline in blood pressure. Thus, ACE inhibitors, beta blockers, calcium channel antagonists, vasodilators, and sympatholytic drugs all may be of equal effectiveness when comparisons are made at equivalent levels of blood pressure lowering. Nonetheless, on theoretical grounds and based on some experimental evidence, ACE inhibitors

Table 7–1. MANAGEMENT OF DIABETIC GLOMERULOPATHY

Stage	Management
Initial	Optimal glycemic control (Hemoglobin A_{1c} values <8%) Prudent diet* Monitor blood pressure and albumin excretion
Incipient glomerulopathy	"Tight" glycemic control Optimal blood pressure control (MAP ≤95 mm Hg) Prudent diet* Reduce hyperlipidemia (?)
Overt glomerulopathy	Avoid severe hyperglycemia and/or metabolic acidosis Rigorous blood pressure control (MAP 90 to 100 mm Hg) Modest protein restriction (?) Reduce hyperlipidemia (?)
Azotemic glomerulopathy	Avoid severe hyperlgycemia and/or metabolic acidosis Rigorous blood pressure control (MAP 90 to 100 mm Hg) Modest protein restriction (0.6 mg/kg/day) Reduce hyperlipidemia
End-stage glomerulopathy	Renal transplantation Pancreas transplantation Dialysis

*Prudent diet: 21 to 26 kcal/kg body weight (at ideal body weight for sex and age); 20% protein (vegetable > meat), not to exceed 1.0 g/kg/day; 50% carbohydrate (unrefined > refined); 25% fat (polyunsaturated > saturated); fiber, 40–50 g/day (cereal derived); cholesterol, lowest attainable; sodium chloride not to exceed 4 to 6 g/day.

MAP, mean arterial pressure: diastolic pressure plus ⅓ of pulse pressure (systolic minus diastolic pressure)

and beta blockers may be preferred to calcium channel antagonists and vasodilators because the latter agents generally do not cause a diminution in the magnitude of proteinuria.

On rare occasions, the use of ACE inhibitors may be associated with an aggravation of type 4 hyperkalemic renal tubular acidosis. Quite commonly but not universally, urinary protein excretion rate falls significantly (by 50% or more) after treatment with ACE inhibitors. No decrease or only slight decline in urinary protein excretion rates is observed when other antihypertensive agents are used.

The goal of blood pressure lowering should be to maintain mean arterial pressure between 90 and 95 mm Hg. Somewhat higher values might be accepted in patients with serious underlying cerebral or coronary arterial occlusive disease, because there is evidence that too great a reduction in mean arterial pressure in these patients may be associated with a rising prevalence of cerebral vascular accidents or myocardial infarction.

The effectiveness of antihypertensive therapy may be judged by serial measurements of glomerular filtration rate and urinary protein excretion rate. A beneficial effect should be associated with a substantial decline in the rate of deterioration of glomerular filtration rate and by a reduction in urinary protein excretion. Limited studies have shown that protein restriction to values around 0.5 to 0.6 g/kg/day will reduce the magnitude of proteinuria and stabilize the glomerular filtration rate. Because blood pressure control was also improved, it is difficult to be sure whether the limitation of protein intake or the salutary effect on blood pressure was responsible for the observed retardation of the progression of renal disease. Controlled trials are in progress to answer this important question. **For the time being, modest protein restriction, limitation of cholesterol intake, high soluble-fiber intake, and a high ratio of polyunsaturated to saturated fat in the diet would seem to be reasonable for diabetic patients in general.**

RENAL REPLACEMENT THERAPY IN END-STAGE DIABETIC NEPHROPATHY

Diabetic nephropathy progresses to ESRD in approximately 40 to 50% of insulin-dependent and 30 to 60% of non–insulin-dependent patients with diabetes mellitus. The wide range in the latter group is largely due to differences in the populations studied, the higher percentage noted in certain groups such as Native Americans. The prevalence of comorbid conditions, most notably hypertension, also influences the likelihood of the development of renal failure. Representation of diabetics in ESRD programs reflects not only the prevalence of end-stage diabetic nephropathy in a given population, but also reveals the commitment of resource allocation of given societies to the treatment of ESRD in general and to diabetic patients within that group in particular. In the United States, diabetic nephropathy has become the most common primary renal diagnosis cited for patients with ESRD (33%), followed closely by hypertensive nephrosclerosis (30%). In the diabetic group, 40% of the patients are insulin dependent, 57% non-insulin dependent, and 3% unspecified. In contrast, the frequency of diabetic patients receiving renal replacement therapy in the United Kingdom was 11.1% in 1984. The differences between the United States and United Kingdom dialysis populations reflect differences in social priorities as well as differences in patient population base.

It should be appreciated, however, that not every diabetic patient approaching ESRD should necessarily undergo renal replacement therapy. In a minority of individuals with severe, untreatable, unrelenting diabetic complications (*e.g.*, peripheral vascular disease with multiple amputations, debilitating cerebrovascular accidents, confining and untreatable cardiovascular ischemia, refractory congestive heart failure, uncontrollable fecal incontinence, severe gastroparesis, or autonomic or peripheral neuropathy), prolongation of life with dialysis or transplantation may be an inappropriate choice. Ideally, frank and informative sessions with patients and their families well in advance of the need for a decision should help to provide the perspective necessary to make an appropriate decision. For the majority of patients, however, renal replacement therapy sustains life and provides an acceptable quality of life.

Although survival for diabetic patients treated for ESRD has been improving, these individuals do not fare as well as their ESRD counterparts without diabetes. Taken together, actuarial survival of diabetic patients with ESRD treated with dialysis may be as low as 50% at 2 years, irrespective of the type of renal replacement therapy offered. In general, the older a patient with diabetes is at the time of initiation of renal replacement therapy, the worse the prognosis. Two-year survival of diabetic patients who are older than 65 years and are on renal replacement therapy (other than renal transplantation) may be as low as 25%.

Patients with diabetes tend to require renal replacement therapy when they have higher levels of residual renal function than nondiabetic persons with ESRD. This is because of the additive effects of diabetes superimposed on uremia. Diabetic patients are more likely to experience intractable hyperkalemia (and acidosis) due to insulin deficiency, hyporeninemia, and hypoaldosteronism. Nausea, vomiting, and resultant malnutrition due to gastroparesis may be difficult to distinguish from that of uremia alone, although diabetic vomiting is more likely to be nocturnal whereas uremic vomiting tends to occur closer to mealtimes. Poor glycemic control can induce myopathy and simulate the fatigue and general malaise of uremia. Peripheral and autonomic neuropathy is common to both. Finally, the prevalence of left ventricular dysfunction in diabetic patients may limit the patients' tolerance for volume overexpansion, especially with superimposed uremia.

Hemodialysis

In the United States, approximately 80% of diabetic patients receiving renal replacement therapy are treated by in-center hemodialysis, compared with only 47% of these patients in the United Kingdom. In-center hemodialysis is a viable option for patients with impaired vision, who may otherwise have difficulty with self-care (approximately 25% of diabetic patients with ESRD are blind). Initial concerns about heparinization and increased ocular pressure during dialysis worsening diabetic retinopathy appear now to be unfounded. However, placement of vascular access sites in diabetic patients with marked peripheral vascular disease continues to be a challenge. Arteriovenous fistulas with adequate flow rates are more difficult to create with the narrowed atheromatous arteries frequently encountered in diabetic patients, and these access sites are slow in maturing. Arteriovenous grafts, although shorter lived, may be the access site of choice. However, both fistulas and grafts may induce steal syndromes causing ischemia in hands, legs, and feet. Rarely, the presence of a fistula or graft may induce high-output congestive heart failure in a patient previously in tenuous balance. Permanent indwelling subclavian vein Silastic catheters may occasionally be required if hemodialysis is the option of choice when fistulas and grafts meet with failure.

Additional difficulties in performing hemodialysis in diabetic patients include the problems arising from impaired autonomic responses during periods of rapid ultrafiltration, resulting in hypotension. Bicarbonate rather than acetate hemodialysis baths may help minimize the frequency of hypotension. Addition of glucose (200 mg/dl) to the bath prevents hypoglycemia during dialysis. Although continued maintenance of euglycemia and treatment of hypertension in the ESRD period should minimize progressive extrarenal disease and prolong survival in diabetic patients, cerebral, coronary, and peripheral vascular disease continue to take their toll in these patients earlier than in their nondiabetic counterparts with ESRD.

Continuous Ambulatory Peritoneal Dialysis

For a number of reasons, continuous ambulatory peritoneal dialysis (CAPD) offers theoretical advantages over hemodialysis as a treatment modality for ESRD in diabetic patients. No vascular access site is required. Dialysis can proceed without heparin, and rapid changes in fluid balance that induce cardiovascular stress do not occur. Insulin can be added to the peritoneal fluid, where it enters the portal circulation, a more physiologic route of entry than the subcutaneous route. Simplified transfer systems have been developed, allowing for the training of patients without vision. Thus, CAPD offers diabetic patients the same advantages of self-reliance and freedom from a hemodialysis center that it offers nondiabetic persons, with additional benefits of specific importance to diabetes sufferers. However, despite its theoretical advantages, the CAPD technique failure rate is higher in diabetic than nondiabetic individuals. This is largely because of higher peritonitis rates in diabetic patients, especially in those with impaired vision, and difficulties these patients have in the self-maintenance of fluid balance, alternately inducing hypotension or complications of fluid overload. In patients with many episodes of peritonitis, loss of peritoneal vascular surface area limits the success of the technique. Glucose absorption from the CAPD solutions may exacerbate hyperlipidemia, especially hypertriglyceridemia, a concern in patients with prevalent atherosclerotic disease. It is possible that amino acid or polyglucose-containing CAPD solutions may lessen this problem to some extent. Finally, as in nondiabetic persons, the burden of three to four daily exchanges often results in emotional burnout and loss of enthusiasm for the technique. In the United States, a minority of diabetic patients undergo CAPD, whereas in the United Kingdom, this is the treatment modality of 51% of diabetic patients treated for ESRD.

Renal Transplantation

There is general agreement that in selected diabetic patients, early renal transplantation offers the best hope for achieving a near normal life-style. In eligible patients, transplantation should ideally be performed when the endogenous creatinine clearance is approximately 10 to 15 ml/min (corresponding to a glomerular filtration rate of 5 to 7 ml/min) and before malnutrition, severe vascular disease, or irreversible autonomic or peripheral neuropathy is present. Candidates should be assessed for the presence of significant coronary artery stenosis, and angioplasty or bypass should be performed before elective renal transplantation when indicated. In one study, left main or three-vessel disease or severe left ventricular failure was associated with a 62% mortality rate after renal transplantation. In contrast, carefully selected, pretreated diabetic patients undergoing renal transplantation can have an excellent prognosis. At the University of Minnesota, 2-year graft survival in 360 diabetic recipients was 83% between 1979 and 1984 and is now even higher with more frequent and experienced use of cyclosporine.

In the past, transplants from living related donors were the modality of choice, but with increased graft survival with the use of cyclosporine, the timing rather than the source of the graft seems most critical. Undeniably, even carefully selected diabetic patients present greater problems than nondiabetic persons in the operative and postoperative periods. Graft anastomosis may be more difficult because of the presence of recipient atherosclerotic plaque lesions. The use of high-dose steroids for the treatment of acute rejection may make glycemic control difficult. Long-term steroid use may accelerate cataract formation and atherogenesis, and some have argued that progressive severe peripheral vascular disease requiring amputation may be even more common in transplanted diabetic patients than in those undergoing maintenance dialysis. The presence of a neurogenic bladder may predispose an immunosuppressed diabetic renal transplant recipient to frequent urinary tract infections or even pyelonephritis.

Finally, progression of the vascular, retinal, and neuropathic disorders of diabetes continues unabated after transplantation. For this reason, there has been some interest in the transplantation of the pancreas in diabetic patients. Data from the International Pancreas Transplant Registry show that between 1983 and 1986, 82% of the 707 patients receiving a pancreas transplant also had either a prior or a concurrent renal transplant. Fifty-four percent of these patients did not require insulin 1 year later, and 85% were still alive at 1 year. Theoretically, a successful pancreas transplant might slow or reverse diabetic retinopathy, nephropathy, vasculopathy, and neuropathy. In practice, even successful pancreas transplants may not prevent the progression of retinopathy. However, in a small number of patients, decrements in glomerular mesangial volume have been reported compared with measurements before pancreas transplant, and preliminary evidence suggests that a successful pancreas transplant may improve autonomic neuropathy. In summary, in selected patients, early renal transplant, possibly with simultaneous pancreas transplantation, is the renal replacement therapy of choice for diabetic patients.

CASE SUMMARY 1

R.P. is a 15-year-old girl who developed insulin-dependent diabetes mellitus at age 8. She has been noncompliant with her medical regimen and has been hospitalized repeatedly for episodes of ketoacidosis. She now presents with a severe episode of candida vulvovaginitis. She takes 18 units of NPH insulin in the morning and 10 units of regular insulin in the evening.

Physical examination reveals a thin female with a blood pressure of 136/90 mm Hg, pulse of 90 beats per minute, and temperature of 37°C (98.6°F). The optic fundi reveal only grade 1 background diabetic retinopathy. Other than for severe vulvovaginitis, results of the examination are normal.

Laboratory studies reveal hemoglobin of 13.6 g/dl, and a white blood cell (WBC) count of 6800 mm^3. Serum creatinine level is 0.5 mg/dl, serum electrolytes are normal, and nonfasting blood glucose level is 240 mg/dl. The urinalysis reveals 4+ glucose, many WBCs, no RBCs, and no protein.

In addition to treating this patient's vulvovaginitis, what additional studies should be performed?

Several timed urine specimens should be studied for albumin excretion once her vulvovaginitis has been cleared with appropriate antimicrobial agents. If urinary albumin excretion is consistently greater than 30 μg/min, R.P. should be managed vigorously in order to achieve optimal glycemic control, including the possible use of constant subcutaneous insulin infusion methods. Consideration should also be given to lowering her blood pressure with small doses of an ACE inhibitor. Her albumin excretion rate should be monitored carefully, as she is at risk for the subsequent development of overt diabetic glomerulopathy.

CASE SUMMARY 2

A.G. is a 46-year-old American Indian woman who presents with severe hypertension. She has had non–insulin-dependent diabetes mellitus for 7 years and has been treated with diet and oral hypoglycemic agents. Her blood pressure was under excellent control with oral clonidine until 1 month ago, when it became much more severe and refractory to therapy. One week ago she developed visual acuity loss.

Physical examination reveals a moderately obese-appearing chronically ill woman. Her blood pressure is 190/120 mm Hg, pulse 86, and temperature 37°C (98.6°F). The optic fundi reveal grade 4 hypertensive retinopathy and background diabetic retinopathy with hemorrhages, exudates, and papilledema. Her heart is enlarged, and an atrial gallop can be heard. Her chest is clear. Her abdomen reveals a bruit in the left epigastric region and bruits over both femoral arteries. Pitting pretibial edema is 1+. Laboratory studies reveal hemoglobin of 10.8 g/dl, and a WBC count of 7800 mm^3. Serum electrolyte determinations reveal mild hyponatremia and hyperkalemia. Her serum creatinine level is 1.5 mg/dl, and a random blood glucose level is 180 mg/dl. Urinalysis reveals 1+ protein, 2+ glucose, and no cellular elements. An electrocardiogram shows left ventricular hypertrophy, atrial hypertrophy, and strain.

In addition to control of blood pressure with intravenous sodium nitroprusside, what additional investigations are now warranted?

Studies to evaluate the presence of a unilateral renal arterial stenosis should be undertaken, including radionuclide studies of renal blood flow and a renal arteriogram. The rapid onset of severe, drug-refractory hypertension in a middle-aged woman with long-standing non–insulin-dependent diabetes mellitus should raise the strong suspicion of an atherosclerotic renal arterial lesion, especially in the presence of the lateralizing abdominal bruit.

CASE SUMMARY 3

F.W. is a 46-year-old man with long-standing insulin-dependent diabetes mellitus. Approximately 4 years ago he developed severe proteinuria, edema, and hypertension. He was placed on an antihypertensive regimen consisting of diuretics and vasodilators, and despite a modest decline in his blood pressure, heavy proteinuria persisted and renal insufficiency gradually developed. One month ago, he began to develop symptoms of nausea and vomiting, particularly in the morning. A serum creatinine level was found to be 6.0 mg/dl; his serum electrolytes demonstrated mild hyperkalemia and metabolic acidosis. Visual acuity has recently been decreasing, and proliferative retinopathy has been noted by his ophthalmologist. F.W. complains of occasional numbness and tingling in his lower extremities at night.

Physical examination reveals a blood pressure of 170/105 mm Hg, a pulse of 72 beats per minute, and a temperature of 37°C (98.6°F). F.W. is a pale, chronically ill man who appears somewhat older than his stated age. His optic fundi reveal advanced proliferative diabetic retinopathy. His heart is enlarged and he has an atrial gallop. His extremities reveal 2+ pitting pretibial edema. Ankle and knee jerks are absent bilaterally. Laboratory studies reveal a hemoglobin of 8.6 g/dl, hematocrit of 26%, and WBC count of 9000 mm^3. Serum electrolyte levels reveal modest hyperkalemia, metabolic acidosis, and hyponatremia. Serum creatinine level is 7.1 mg/dl; random blood glucose level is 190 mg/dl. Electrocardiogram reveals left ventricular hypertrophy.

What would be the best approach to long-term therapy for this man?

F.W. should be considered a candidate for renal transplantation, either from a living related or a cadaveric donor. He may require hemodialysis or continuous ambulatory peritoneal dialysis to stabilize his uremic state; however, because of advanced proliferative retinopathy and neuropathy, he would be more likely to benefit from renal transplantation. In advance of transplantation, he may require an evaluation for asymptomatic ischemic heart disease, because long-standing diabetes mellitus, hypertension, and lipid disorders may have predisposed him to developing coronary artery disease.

Suggested Readings

Brenner BM, Stein JH (eds): The Kidney in Diabetes Mellitus. Vol. 20. Contemporary Issues in Nephrology. New York, Churchill Livingstone, 1989, pp 1—234.

Friedman EA, L'Esperance FA (eds): Diabetic Renal-Retinal Syndrome, Vol 2. Prevention and Management. New York, Grune & Stratton, 1982.

Friedman EA, L'Esperance FA (eds): Diabetic Renal-Retinal Syndrome, Vol 3. Therapy. New York, Grune & Stratton, 1986.

Mogensen CE, Jensen HA (eds): Hypertension and Diabetic Complications. Diabetic Nephropathy 4:1–59, 1985.

Mogensen CE, Mauer SM, Kjellstrand CM: Diabetic nephropathy. *In* Schrier RW, Gottschalk CW (eds): Diseases of the Kidney, 4th ed. Boston, Little, Brown & Co., 1988, pp 2395–2438.

CHAPTER 8

RENAL DISEASE AND HYPERTENSION IN PREGNANCY

Jason G. Umans and Marshall D. Lindheimer

This chapter discusses renal disorders and high blood pressure in pregnant women, first reviewing the anatomic and physiologic changes in gestation and their clinical relevance to detecting and managing disease. The section on the kidneys is devoted to acute renal failure and chronic parenchymal diseases including allograft recipients. Only the features of urinary tract infection unique to pregnancy are addressed. Because more than three fourths of the hypertensive disorders of gestation are due to preeclampsia and essential hypertension, the section on high blood pressure is primarily devoted to these two entities.

STRUCTURAL AND FUNCTIONAL CHANGES IN NORMAL PREGNANCY

Normal pregnancy is accompanied by both structural and functional changes in the kidneys, urinary tract, and systemic vasculature. Familiarity with these changes is the key to interpreting both clinical and laboratory data from pregnant patients who may have renal disease or hypertension.

Urinary Tract

During pregnancy, kidneys increase in size and the intrarenal collecting system and ureters become significantly dilated. The latter change is present by the end of the first trimester and may persist through the third postpartum month. However, despite the presence of sometimes marked ureteral dilatation, it is unclear whether there is increased vesicoureteral reflux during pregnancy. It remains unresolved whether these changes are secondary to humoral (*e.g.*, estrogen, progesterone, or prostaglandins) or mechanical (*i.e.*, the enlarged uterus) factors. Although ultrasonographic studies show dilation before significant uterine enlargement, most studies still favor the mechanical hypothesis. For instance, ureteral pressure in standing or supine women in their third trimester increases only above the level of the pelvic brim. It decreases rapidly when the extrinsic pressure of the enlarged uterus is removed when a woman assumes a lateral decubitus or knee-chest position or after cesarean delivery of the fetus. Radiographic studies have shown that ureteral dilatation terminates at the pelvic brim, suggesting that mechanical obstruction is due to the pressing of the uterus on the ureter as it crosses the iliac artery. This set of circumstances leads to the so-called iliac sign on pyelography. Because the urinary tract is physiologically dilated, as shown by the renal ultrasonogram in Figure 8–1, frank urinary tract obstruction may be difficult to diagnose during gestation. A distention syndrome may occur in late pregnancy; it is characterized by abdominal pain, marked hydronephrosis, and a variable increase in serum creatinine level and is managed by placement of ureteral stents.

Urinary stasis in the dilated tract may lead to errors in collection of timed urine samples and may increase the frequency with which urinary tract infection progresses to pyelonephritis in a gravida. Collection errors may be minimized by hydrating patients and placing them in lateral recumbency before the beginning and completion of a timed urine collection.

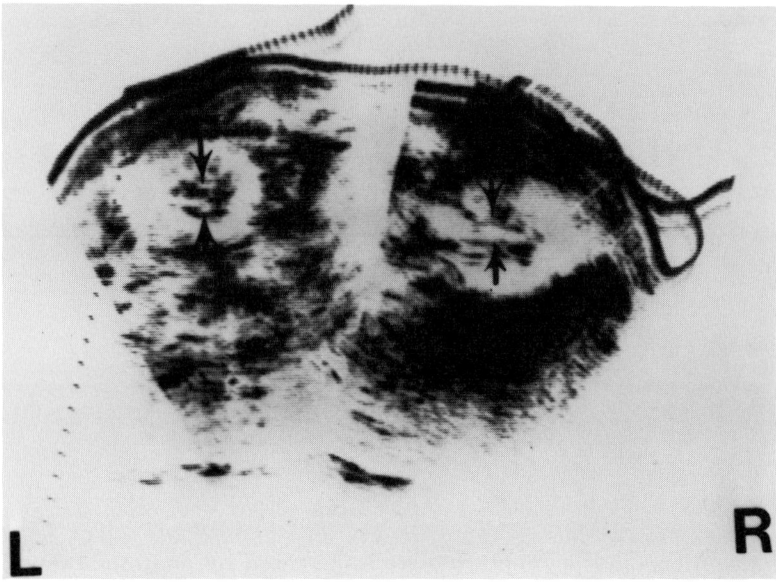

Figure 8–1. Renal ultrasonography demonstrating dilated intrarenal collecting system in a normal gravida *without* obstructive uropathy.

Renal Hemodynamics and Solute Handling

Increases in glomerular filtration rate (GFR) and renal plasma flow (RPF) occur early in gestation, become maximal at about 150% of preconception values by the end of the first trimester, and persist until near term. After gestational week 36, GFR (as assessed by 24-hour creatinine clearance) may decrease by 20% and even, rarely, to nonpregnant levels. Because creatinine production remains constant during gestation, its increased clearance (GFR) predicts a lower normal range for serum creatinine in pregnancy. Norms for creatinine and urea nitrogen decrease from means of 0.7 and 12 mg/dl (62 μmol/L and 4.3 mmol/L) in a nonpregnant woman to 0.5 and 9 mg/dl (44 μmol/L and 3.3 mmol/L), respectively, in a gravida. Thus, levels of urea nitrogen and creatinine that would usually appear normal may reflect renal disease in a pregnant patient.

Increased GFR may also contribute to the increased proteinuria, glycosuria, and aminoaciduria that normally accompany gestation. The upper limit for normal proteinuria should be doubled to 300 to 500 mg/24 hr in a gravida. The increased filtered loads of glucose and amino acids, along with decreases in their tubular reabsorption, explain the increases in their urinary excretion during normal gestation. Increased GFR and decreased tubular reabsorption also lead to decrements of plasma urate in normal pregnancy to levels below 5 mg/dl (297 μmol/L).

Acid-Base Regulation

Pregnant women normally hyperventilate to a pCO_2 of about 30 mm Hg and compensate for this respiratory alkalosis by decreasing their serum bicarbonate level to a mean value of 20 to 22 mEq/L, resulting in a mean arterial pH of 7.44. Although the decreased renal bicarbonate threshold may result in more alkaline urine during gestation, the kidneys' ability to augment excretion of titratable acid and ammonium following an acid load is unimpaired. Despite this, the lower steady-state bicarbonate in a gravida puts her at a theoretical disadvantage in coping with sudden severe metabolic acidosis, as might result from sepsis, acute renal failure, or diabetic ketoacidosis.

Volume Homeostasis and Osmoregulation

The usual maternal weight gain during gestation is 12.5 kg, half or more of which is due to volume expansion, with an increase of about 6 to 8 L in total body water, 4 to 6 L of this in the extracellular compartment, and a 50% increase in plasma volume. This volume expansion is accompanied by cumulative retention of about 900 mEq sodium. The increase in intravascular volume occurs most rapidly during the second trimester, whereas the increases in the interstitial compartment are greatest in the third trimester. This physiologic hypervolemia is sensed as normal by a gravida; therefore, salt depletion or volume contraction, from the new gravid set-point back toward nongravid values, provokes all of the homeostatic mechanisms designed to defend circulating volume and blood pressure. Because volume expansion and the resultant hemodilution are signs of normal physiologic adaptation in pregnancy, diuretic therapy and salt restriction have little place in routine obstetric management.

For reasons that are incompletely understood, all elements of the renin-angiotensin-aldosterone system (prorenin, active renin, plasma renin activity, angiotensin II, and aldosterone) are increased in normal pregnancy. A gravida's vascular responsiveness to angiotensin II is quite blunted, however, and the elevated levels of mineralocorticoid do not lead to hypertension, hypokalemia, or excess salt retention.

Plasma osmolality begins to decline immediately after conception, reaching a nadir 8 to 10 mOsm/kg below the nonpregnant level by gestational week 10. This hypotonic state, which is associated with predictable hyponatremia, is maintained until about 2 weeks postpartum. This change in tonicity is due to decrements in the osmotic thresholds for both thirst and vasopressin (antidiuretic hormone [ADH] or arginine vasopressin [AVP]) release. As in the case of volume regulation, a gravida senses the new (hypotonic) set-point as normal and thus appropriately concentrates and dilutes her urine around a plasma osmolality 10 mOsm/kg lower than in the nonpregnant state.

The other important change in osmoregulation is due to a substantial increase in the metabolic clearance rate of circulating AVP. This is in part a result of an increase in a circulating vasopressinase of placental origin. This increase in vasopressin clearance may be responsible for several syndromes manifested by transient diabetes insipidus of pregnancy, one due to the combined effects of a subclinical lesion of central diabetes insipidus and the increased clearance of the endogenously produced hormone and a second directly due to excessive quantities of circulating vasopressinase. These syndromes remit after delivery, and the second form can only be treated with 1-desamino-8-D-AVP (DDAVP), a vasopressin analogue resistant to enzymatic degradation.

Blood Pressure Regulation

Mean arterial pressure decreases early in pregnancy so that second-trimester diastolic blood pressure is often 10 to 15 mm Hg below postpartum levels. Blood pressure normally increases during the third trimester, approaching nonpregnant levels at term. Because cardiac output may increase 30 to 50% in early gestation, the decrease in blood pressure denotes an even larger decrement in peripheral vascular resistance. The cause of this early and persistent systemic vasodilation remains obscure. Of note, blood pressures that would appear normal in a nonpregnant patient may be abnormally elevated in a gravida, and likewise, the usual early gestational fall in diastolic pressure may mask antecedent hypertension.

Table 8–1 summarizes many of these anatomic and physiologic alterations in gestation, noting their clinical relevance and implicating some of these changes in several syndromes peculiar to gestation.

RENAL DISEASE PRESENTING IN PREGNANCY

This section addresses the presentation and management of urinary tract infection and renal failure in gravidas without prior known renal disease.

Infection

The incidence of asymptomatic bacteriuria is 4 to 7% in pregnancy, similar to that in sexuallly active nonpregnant women. This similarity is surprising in light of the factors that would appear to favor urinary tract infection in a gravida (*e.g.*, ureteral dilation, urinary stasis, and increased urinary nutrient content). The significant difference is that in pregnancy, 40% of patients with asymptomatic bacteriuria will progress to overtly symptomatic urinary tract infection or pyelonephritis. Thus, early screening and treatment of bacteriuria are important in a gravida. A woman with sterile urine at her first antenatal visit will not likely develop bacteriuria during her pregnancy. **A confirmed positive urine culture requires determination of antibiotic sensitivities, treatment for 2 weeks, and subsequent surveillance urine cultures throughout gestation. Antibiotic selection depends on both bacterial sensitivities and published Food and Drug Administration (FDA) guidelines regarding potential risk to the fetus.** Short-acting sulfonamides and first-generation cephalosporins are used commonly.

Pyelonephritis, which may occur in as many

Table 8–1. GESTATIONAL ALTERATIONS IN RENAL STRUCTURE AND FUNCTION

Alteration	Manifestation	Clinical Relevance
Increased renal size	Renal length approximately 1 cm greater on roentgenograms.	Postpartum decreases in renal size should not be mistaken for parenchymal loss.
Dilatation of renal pelves, calyces, and ureters	Resembles hydronephrosis on intravenous pyelography or renal ultrasonography (usually more marked on right).	Do not mistake for obstruction; defer elective pyelography to at least 3 months postpartum; retained urine may lead to errors in timed collections; may be responsible for "distention syndrome"; upper tract infections are more virulent.
Increased renal hemodynamics	Glomerular filtration rate and effective renal plasma flow both increase 30–50%.	Serum creatinine and urea nitrogen values decrease, with normal Cr <0.8 mg/dl; urinary protein, glucose, and amino acid excretion all increase; serum urate falls to <5 mg/dl.
Changes in acid-base regulation	Compensated primary respiratory alkalosis with decreased renal bicarbonate threshold.	Arterial pCO_2 decreases 10 mm Hg, and serum bicarbonate falls by 4–5 mEq/L. An asthmatic with a pCO_2 of 40 or less may already manifest CO_2 retention.
Water metabolism	Osmoregulation of vasopressin release is altered, and metabolic clearance rate of vasopressin is increased.	Plasma osmolality decreases 10 mOsm/L (serum sodium by 5 mEq/L). Increased vasopressin clearance may cause certain transient diabetes insipidus-like syndromes.
Volume homeostasis	Intravascular volume increases 40% early in pregnancy. Interstitial volume increases >2 L after midgestation.	Volume changes must be considered in the rare gravidas maintained on dialysis.
Blood pressure regulation	Arterial pressure normally decreases 10 mm Hg by second trimester.	Patients with antecedent mild essential hypertension may be undiagnosed in early pregnancy and misdiagnosed as preeclamptic when pressure rises near term.

as 2% of pregnancies, has been associated with prematurity, intrauterine growth retardation, fetal demise, and an increased incidence of maternal sepsis. Thus, treatment of upper urinary tract infection should be rapid and aggressive, requiring parenteral antibiotics in an inpatient setting. Pregnant patients with pyelonephritis usually defervesce quickly but are likely to suffer a relapse or become reinfected later in gestation. Avoiding such an outcome requires appropriate oral antibiotic therapy for 3 to 4 weeks, followed by either frequent surveillance urine cultures or continued antibiotic prophylaxis until term.

Renal and perinephric abcesses are infrequent complications of infection during gestation. They must, however, be included in the differential diagnosis of resistant postpartum fever. Culture of voided urine is futile in the immediate puerperium, when the incidence of positive cultures approaches 20% and suprapubic aspiration is preferred.

Patients with bacteriuria during pregnancy have a higher than normal incidence of predisposing occult urinary tract pathology, and some believe they may therefore benefit from postpartum radiographic evaluation.

Acute Renal Failure

Acute renal failure (ARF) once occurred with a bimodal distribution during pregnancy. Those cases at 12 to 18 weeks of gestation were due to septic abortion, whereas those near term were related most commonly to preeclampsia, placental abruption, or volume depletion. The earlier peak, which formerly accounted for the overwhelming majority of cases, has been all but eradicated in industrialized countries by liberalized abortion laws. Thus ARF severe enough to require dialytic therapy, which once had an incidence as high as 1 in 2000, now occurs rarely (*i.e.*, less than 1 in 20,000 gestations). The etiologic and pathologic lesion in virtually all cases of ARF is acute tubular necrosis, although a minority present with patchy or sometimes complete bilateral renal cortical necrosis. Cortical necrosis is a rare lesion in the nonpregnant state. It occurs somewhat more frequently during gestation and is usually associated with placental abruption and concealed uterine hemorrhage at 32 to 34 weeks. Of note, women with the patchy variety may initially show considerable return of function, but chronic renal failure often ensues.

A gravida is uniquely sensitive to sepsis as a cause of ARF. Also, although her blood volume is increased, she is at least as sensitive to volume loss as a nonpregnant woman, a factor of special importance because a gravida may suffer large blood losses due to clinically inapparent intrauterine hemorrhage.

Two unusual causes of ARF are unique to pregnancy: acute fatty liver of pregnancy and idiopathic postpartum renal failure. The former is characterized by severe hepatic dysfunction late in pregnancy or immediately postpartum, may result in renal failure secondary to either intravascular coagulation or hemodynamic instability, and carries a significant risk of mortality due to hepatic failure. Earlier data suggested a maternal mortality of 75%, whereas the current figure of less than 10% likely reflects more accurate diagnosis of mild disease. The differential diagnosis includes fulminant hepatitis or hepatic necrosis, and immediate delivery may be beneficial.

Idiopathic postpartum renal failure (postpartum hemolytic-uremic syndrome), an even more uncommon disorder, usually presents as severe hypertension and uremia in the puerperium following an uncomplicated pregnancy. Some presentations may be less obvious, with nearly normal blood pressure and oliguria. These women occasionally have extrarenal manifestations including cardiac and central nervous system dysfunction and evidence of microangiopathic hemolytic anemia. The cause of this disease is obscure, with some suggested possibilities including a viral infection, an abnormal immunologic response, deficiencies in antithrombin III or vasodilator prostaglandins, effects of retained placental fragments, and drug effects due to ergot alkaloids, oxytocin, or oral contraceptives prescribed postpartum. Renal pathology may resemble that seen in the hemolytic-uremic syndrome, in scleroderma kidney, or in malignant nephrosclerosis. There is an increased incidence of bleeding after renal biopsy in these patients. Treatment is aimed at blood pressure control and dialytic support through ARF. Some researchers have suggested benefit from early use of heparin, exchange transfusion, or infusion of blood products including antithrombin III concentrates, although supporting data for these interventions are not yet adequate. The possible role of retained placenta suggests dilatation and curettage for women presenting soon after delivery. In spite of therapy, the disease usually progresses to severe renal insufficiency and historically has had a high mortality.

Dialysis During Pregnancy

Management of acute or chronic renal failure is similar to that in nongravid patients and may include either peritoneal dialysis or hemodialysis. A gravid uterus is not a contraindication to placement of a new peritoneal catheter, which should be made under direct vision and high in the abdomen. Because urea and presumed uremic toxins may readily traverse the placenta, early aggressive prophylactic or intensified (daily) dialysis should be empirically instituted to attempt to maintain blood urea nitrogen less than 50 mg/dl (18 mmol/L).

Suggested alterations in the hemodialysis prescription during pregnancy are outlined in Table 8–2. Although experience is limited, chronic ambulatory peritoneal dialysis may offer a success rate in excess of the 20 to 25% expected in pregnant patients with chronic renal failure maintained on hemodialysis. This preference may be due to the maintenance of a more constant intrauterine milieu and the avoidance of rapid intradialytic fluid shifts and hypotension.

PREGNANCY WITH PREEXISTING RENAL DISEASE

Renal parenchymal disease was formerly considered a contraindication to pregnancy. A number of recently published studies dating from 1980, although largely retrospective and uncontrolled, suggest prognoses better than previously thought. They both suggest specific guidelines for management of certain renal diseases in a gravida and permit a few generalizations.

Women with renal disease but well-preserved GFR and no hypertension (or easily controlled blood pressure) will likely have a successful pregnancy. In fact, many such patients manifest increases in GFR during gestation, a favorable prognostic sign. Women with glomerular disease often demonstrate nephrotic-range proteinuria, which is usually not a sign of progressive disease. Further, although certain renal diseases may first become clinically apparent or worsen during gestation, their natural course and long-term prognosis seem not to be affected by pregnancy. Although this generalization is true of most disorders, prognosis is different in women with collagen vascular disease, and several entities provoke controversy in the literature, as discussed later.

In patients with moderately decreased GFR

Table 8–2. MODIFICATIONS OF HEMODIALYSIS PRESCRIPTION DURING PREGNANCY

Modification	Rationale
Intensified or daily dialysis to keep BUN <50 mg/dl, with increased dialysis required in the last trimester.	The fetus is exposed to uremic toxins of maternal origin, and fetal outcome is poor when dialysis merely avoids maternal uremic symptoms. The fetus produces >0.5 g of urea daily at term, and maternal BUN rises during the last trimester.
Monitor predialysis potassium and increase dialysate potassium concentration to 3–3.5 mEq/L as needed.	Daily dialysis may result in hypokalemia.
Lower dialysate alkali so as to maintain serum bicarbonate between 18 and 22 mEq/L. Use bicarbonate rather than acetate dialysis.	Attempt to mimic the normal compensated respiratory alkalosis of pregnancy. Daily dialysis may result in delivery of alkali in excess of daily acid production. There are no data on acetate metabolism in a gravida.
Lower dialysate sodium concentration to 134 mEq/L.	Attempt to mimic the normal hypo-osmolality of pregnancy.
Avoidance of large fluid shifts by daily dialysis and use of isolated ultrafiltration for large intradialytic weight gains. Treatment of intradialytic hypotension by liberal use of saline infusions.	Episodic hypotension or rapid fluid shifts may result in fetal distress and premature labor.
Use minimal heparin, given by constant infusion.	Although heparin does not cross the placenta, its use is associated with fetal loss.
Increase estimated dry weight by 0.5–1 kg/month during the first 6 months and by 0.25–0.5 kg/week during the last trimester, while following blood pressure and physical exam closely.	Attempt to mimic physiologic volume expansion of pregnancy.

(serum creatinine >1.5 mg/dl, 132 μmol/L) or those with difficult-to-control moderate or severe hypertension, the prognosis is more guarded. Approximately one third will suffer accelerated renal functional deterioration or hectic blood pressure swings during the pregnancy.

Severe renal dysfunction (serum creatinine >3 mg/dl, 265 μmol/L) often causes infertility. In the instances when such patients conceive, the likelihood of a successful pregnancy is less than 50%, and significant maternal morbidity is likely.

GENERAL GUIDELINES FOR EVALUATION AND MANAGEMENT

All pregnant women with renal disease should be managed by a team including both a high-risk fetal-maternal specialist and a nephrologist. In addition to all usual screening tests, initial laboratory evaluation should include the following: an assessment of GFR by creatinine clearance; careful urinalysis, screening of urine culture, and 24-hour urine collection for total protein excretion; measurement of serum electrolytes, urea nitrogen, albumin, cholesterol, urate, glutamic-oxaloacetic transaminase, glutamic-pyruvic transaminase, lactate dehydrogenase; and prothrombin time, partial thromboplastin time, and platelet count. This data base may, in part, serve as a baseline for detecting superimposed preeclampsia, as discussed later.

Follow-up should include biweekly visits until gestational week 32 and weekly visits thereafter. All renal parameters should be assessed at least every 4 to 6 weeks. Fetal assessment, including electronic monitoring, should commence by gestational week 32.

GLOMERULAR DISEASES

The course of most glomerular diseases in pregnancy is determined by the level of renal function and blood pressure before conception. Significant disagreement exists regarding the course of IgA nephropathy in pregnancy, with some investigators finding no adverse effect on the course of disease and others reporting worsened proteinuria, renal function, hypertension, and renal lesions on biopsy. It appears, however, that there is a greater tendency toward hypertension in these patients.

Likewise, controversy surrounds the effect of gestation on the course of focal glomerulosclerosis and mesangioproliferative glomerulonephritis. One small series suggested an excess of severe hypertension, proteinuria, renal functional loss, and fetal loss, whereas two other small series failed to observe an accelerated loss of renal function with gestation.

SYSTEMIC LUPUS ERYTHEMATOSUS AND OTHER COLLAGEN VASCULAR DISEASES

The effects of pregnancy on the activity and progression of both renal and extrarenal manifestations of systemic lupus erythematosus (SLE) are not uniformly predictable. This is not surprising in light of the lack of prognostic accuracy in nonpregnant patients with this disease. Although outcome is poorer than in most other glomerular disorders, most patients with preserved renal function fare well. Prognosis is most favorable when a patient is normotensive and the disease has been quiescent for at least 6 months. There is a marked increase in spontaneous abortion in those patients with anticardiolipin antibodies.

Because of the unpredictable course of disease during pregnancy, renal function should be evaluated at least monthly, and clinical and laboratory markers of disease activity should be followed closely. It is important to realize that proteinuria may increase significantly without any change in disease activity and that superimposed preeclampsia may be difficult to differentiate from an exacerbation of lupus glomerulonephritis.

Pharmacologic management during gestation commonly includes steroids, nonsteroidal antiinflammatory drugs, and azathioprine (Imuran). Nonsteroidal agents should not be used near term to avoid possible effects on the fetal ductus arteriosus. We try to avoid chloroquine (FDA class C) and do not prescribe cyclophosphamide (FDA class D). The role of aspirin or antiplatelet therapy for patients with anticardiolipin antibodies is still unclear. Because fetal exposure to a specific maternal autoantibody, anti-Ro (SS-A), is associated with congenital fetal heart block, susceptible fetuses should have heart rate traces carefully monitored after midgestation.

In contrast to the usually favorable outcome in patients with lupus, prognosis is poorer in patients with either scleroderma or polyarteritis nodosa. Anecdotal reports of severe maternal morbidity and mortality during gestation in these patients suggest that pregnancy not be undertaken and that early unanticipated pregnancies be terminated.

NEPHROTIC SYNDROME

Preexisting nephrotic syndrome with well-preserved renal function is not a contraindication to pregnancy, although there is a higher incidence of intrauterine growth retardation. Normal increases in GFR and renal venous pressure may exacerbate proteinuria and simulate worsened underlying disease. **Although serum albumin decreases and edema usually worsens during pregnancy, diuretic use should be minimized if possible because it may result in severe intravascular volume depletion and impaired uteroplacental perfusion.** Likewise, the hypercoagulable state associated with normal pregnancy may exacerbate that due to the nephrotic syndrome, resulting in more frequent thromboembolic episodes during gestation. These patients do not receive routine prophylactic anticoagulation, although if anticoagulation is required, heparin should be used because it does not readily cross the placenta. The hyperlipidemia associated with the nephrotic syndrome is rarely treated during gestation, and there is little experience with use of hypolipidemic drugs in gravidas. Finally, these patients are at increased risk for infection and should have repeated screening for asymptomatic bacteriuria.

In the past, many investigators recommended high-protein diets in an attempt to maintain serum albumin levels in patients with the nephrotic syndrome. More recently, it has been suggested that low dietary protein intake may paradoxically lessen proteinuria, improve albumin kinetics, and minimize glomerular hyperfiltration. **However, because of the unknown effects of dietary protein limitation on a developing fetus, we cannot yet advocate this intervention in gravidas.**

Most of the other glomerular lesions associated with the nephrotic syndrome have been described in pregnant patients, yet preeclampsia remains the most common cause of nephrotic proteinuria presenting during pregnancy. The importance of a specific diagnosis before instituting therapy in these patients is therefore emphasized.

DIABETIC NEPHROPATHY

Although many pregnant insulin-dependent diabetics may already have occult nephropathy and are more likely to become preeclamptic, they will rarely suffer renal complications or deterioration during gestation. They are at greater risk for urinary tract infection, and recent studies imply that microalbuminuria may predict hypertension as well as other complications. Patients with overt nephropathy but well-preserved renal function usually have successful pregnancies, although they are likely to have either new or worsening hypertension, significant increases in proteinuria, and reversible decrements in renal function. The presence of hypertension along with nephropathy denotes a poorer prognosis.

TUBULOINTERSTITIAL DISEASES

Polycystic kidney disease often remains undetected during pregnancy, as hypertension or functional deterioration is often not manifest until after the childbearing years. Patients with the disease have an increased risk of preeclampsia.

Chronic pyelonephritis is more prone to exacerbation during pregnancy. Both frequent surveillance urine cultures and high fluid intake are prudent interventions. Reflux nephropathy is one of the most common renal diseases occurring in young women. Although some investigators believe that pregnancy has a negative impact on the course of the disease, it is more likely that poor outcome is manifest in the subset of patients with hypertension and moderate renal insufficiency before conception. These patients require frequent surveillance urine cultures and aggressive treatment of urinary tract infection throughout gestation.

Noninfectious interstitial nephritis has a prognosis similar to that of glomerular disease in pregnancy—that is, good outcome if GFR is well preserved and hypertension is absent. Again, these patients are prone to renal failure when salt restricted or volume depleted. Renal tuberculosis does not seem to be affected by pregnancy.

NEPHROLITHIASIS

Urinary calcium excretion may increase twofold during gestation, most likely as a result of increased calcitriol-dependent intestinal calcium absorption. The resultant increased urinary supersaturation with respect to calcium salts as well as urinary stasis would seem to favor enhanced stone formation in a gravida. However, the incidence of symptomatic nephrolithiasis is less than 0.5%, not different from that in nonpregnant women. Known stone-forming patients are not at increased risk for recurrence during gestation. The lack of an expected gestational increase in stone formation may be due to many factors, including enhanced urinary excretion of citrate, magnesium, and crystal growth inhibitory glycoproteins.

Clinical presentation of stone passage is similar to that in nongravid patients, usually including pain, often with nausea and emesis. Complications may include urinary tract infection and premature labor. Diagnostic evaluation differs in a gravida in that radiographic procedures are avoided if possible. Ultrasonography may be helpful; however, its sensitivity may be impaired because most symptomatic stones in pregnancy are located in the ureters and because the ureters are physiologically dilated even in the absence of obstruction. In the case of antibiotic-refractory pyelonephritis, declining renal function, or symptoms unresponsive to conservative therapy for presumed stone disease, a limited excretory urogram may be key to appropriate diagnosis and management.

Conservative therapy with bed rest, hydration, and analgesics will result in spontaneous passage of more than 50% of symptomatic stones. If possible, it is prudent to delay urologic intervention until after delivery. However, pregnancy should not be a deterrent to necessary surgery, which should use a team approach including intraoperative fetal monitoring. Except for analysis of recovered stones, metabolic evaluation of patients should be delayed until at least 3 months after delivery and lactation. Treatment of hypercalciuria with thiazide diuretics or of hyperuricosuria with xanthine oxidase inhibitors is best avoided during pregnancy. Reasonable therapy in a gravida includes adequate hydration to maintain a daily urine output of 2.5 L and, in the case of uric acid stone disease, oral alkali intake to maintain a urine pH of 6.0.

RENAL TRANSPLANT RECIPIENTS

There has now been considerable experience with successful pregnancies in renal transplant recipients. A substantial risk of both fetal and maternal complications remains, including rejection, renal deterioration (approximately 10% of patients), or hypertension (approximately 30% of patients) in pregnancies that continue beyond the first trimester. Preterm delivery and intrauterine growth retardation are likewise increased. Nevertheless, 90% of these pregnancies will have a successful outcome. These patients are at special risk for infectious complications as a result of their chronic immunosuppression. The presence of a renal allograft poses no unique contraindications to spontaneous vaginal delivery. Guidelines for transplant recipients who desire a pregnancy are outlined in Table 8–3.

The occurrence of third-trimester proteinuria (>2 g/day in 40% of these patients), hypertension (in approximately 30%), and drug-induced laboratory abnormalities all make the diagnosis of preeclampsia even more problematic in these patients. Likewise, considering the risks that aggressive antirejection therapy poses to the fetus, clinical suspicion of acute rejection is more likely to require renal biopsy for definitive diagnosis.

Management of these patients requires a team approach with attention to blood pressure control, serial assessment of renal function, monitoring for allograft rejection, aggressive diagnosis and treatment of infection, and surveillance of fetal well-being. Antenatal visits should be biweekly up to 32 weeks and weekly thereafter. Potential fetal complications requiring active pediatric intervention may include adrenocortical insufficiency and severe neonatal infection.

HYPERTENSION IN PREGNANCY

Hypertension complicates almost 10% of all pregnancies, with a higher incidence in nulliparas and women carrying multiple fetuses. It remains a major cause of morbidity and mortality for both mother and child and is often difficult to diagnose by clinical criteria alone.

Classification of Hypertension in Pregnancy

It is useful to classify hypertension occurring during pregnancy as preeclampsia, chronic hypertension, chronic hypertension with superimposed preeclampsia, or transient hypertension of (late) pregnancy.

Table 8–3. GUIDELINES FOR RENAL ALLOGRAFT RECIPIENTS CONTEMPLATING PREGNANCY

Good general health for at least 2 years after transplantation.
Stable renal function with serum creatinine of 2 mg/dl or less.
No significant proteinuria.
Normal blood pressure or easily managed hypertension.
No evidence of graft rejection.
Stable antirejection therapy at maintenance doses of prednisone: 15 mg/day or less; azathioprine: 2 mg/kg/day or less; cyclosporin A: safe doses not yet clearly established, but less than 5 mg/kg/day.
No evidence of collecting system obstruction or dilatation.
Stature compatible with good obstetric outcome.

Preeclampsia

Diagnosis and Clinical Evaluation. Preeclampsia is a disorder unique to pregnancy. It is most frequent in nulliparas and is characterized by hypertension and proteinuria, often accompanied by edema and sometimes by a coagulopathy. It usually occurs after gestational week 20, most frequently near term.

Hypertension in the third trimester is defined as either a sustained blood pressure of 140/85 mm Hg or an increase of 30 mm systolic and 15 mm diastolic over readings in early gestation. Signs favoring the diagnosis of preeclampsia may include the sudden appearance of proteinuria, the rapid accumulation of edema, and the appearance or progression of one or more of the following: hemoconcentration, hypoalbuminemia, liver function or coagulation abnormalities, and elevated serum urate (realizing that in pregnancy values greater than 4.5 mg/dl may be abnormal). The diagnostic utility of elevated serum iron levels, low antithrombin III levels, and hypocalciuria are subjects of ongoing investigation.

Pathophysiology. The pathophysiology of hypertension in preeclampsia is still obscure, although alterations in the systemic vasculature appear to favor vasospasm and contribute to blood pressure lability by rendering arteries more sensitive to the effects of endogenous vasopressors. Although normal pregnant women are relatively refractory to the vasopressor effect of infused angiotensin II, women who are destined to become preeclamptic may begin to lose this refractoriness weeks before manifesting any disease. As might be expected in hypertension due to a primary increase in systemic vascular resistance, invasive hemodynamic studies have shown untreated preeclamptic patients to have lower cardiac output, lower ventricular filling pressures, and markedly elevated systemic vascular resistance as compared with normotensive gravidas at term. Uteroplacental perfusion is often compromised, leading to an association with intrauterine growth retardation. Renal hemodynamics decrease approximately 25% in patients with preeclampsia.

There may also be alterations in prostaglandin metabolism in patients with preeclampsia, favoring vasoconstrictor over vasodilatory metabolites. This latter thesis has led to a number of recent and ongoing clinical trials of aspirin in the prophylaxis of preeclampsia in high-risk pregnancies. Limitations in the size and design of the published studies do not yet allow us to recommend low-dose aspirin as routine chemoprophylaxis against preeclampsia.

Complications. Two life-threatening complications of preeclampsia must be recognized promptly. The first is characterized by fulminant microangiopathic hemolytic anemia, hepatic dysfunction, and coagulopathy. **This syndrome, termed HELLP (Hemolysis, Elevated Liver enzymes, Low Platelet count), is an emergency requiring prompt termination of pregnancy.** The second complication is progression of preeclampsia to a convulsive phase termed *eclampsia.* **Incipient or manifest eclampsia likewise requires immediate termination of pregnancy, and this recognition has led to a decreased incidence of the disorder**. These syndromes are sometimes so severe as to necessitate intensive care monitoring including pulmonary artery catheterization.

Pathology. Renal biopsy discloses a pattern of glomerular pathology unique to preeclampsia. The glomeruli typically are enlarged and relatively bloodless as a result of endothelial cell hypertrophy rather than proliferative changes. Electron microscopy demonstrates hypertrophy and vacuolization of lysosomes in endothelial and sometimes mesangial cells. This lesion has been called *glomerular capillary endotheliosis* and is shown in Figure 8–2. Other findings may include subendothelial and mesangial dense deposits and interposition of mesangial cell cytoplasm or matrix along the basement membrane. The relationship of immunohistochemical abnormalities or lesions of focal and segmental glomerular sclerosis to preeclampsia is unclear and is the subject of some debate. The renal lesions typical of preeclampsia appear to be reversible with time.

Renal biopsy studies suggest that the clinical diagnosis of preeclampsia may be incorrect in 25% of nulliparas and more than half of multiparous patients. However, it is rare for results of antepartum renal biopsy to modify management of such patients. Therefore, although renal biopsy carries no greater risk in pregnant patients when there is attention to blood pressure control and coagulation status, it is indicated only rarely. Antepartum renal biopsy, however, may be useful in the following situations: sudden unexplained renal functional deterioration before 32 weeks of gestation, symptomatic and difficult-to-manage nephrotic syndrome occurring before 32 weeks of gestation, and *de novo* presentation with an active urinary sediment, proteinuria, and renal dysfunction during pregnancy.

Treatment. All patients in whom preeclampsia is suspected should be hospitalized. Fetal maturity is assessed, and if the patient is near term and the fetus mature, induction is the therapy of choice. Temporizing measures appropriate earlier in gestation include bed rest and antihypertensive medications to keep diastolic blood pressure at or below 100 mm Hg. **Early termination is indicated in the setting of uncontrollable blood pressure, renal functional deterioration, hepatic dysfunction, coagulopathy, or fetal compromise**. Hyperreflexia and impending eclamptic convulsions are usually treated with parenteral magnesium sulfate, with therapy monitored by serum levels and assessment of deep tendon reflexes. Magnesium sulfate administration, the domain of fetal-maternal specialists, usually commences with a slow intravenous loading dose of 4 g of magnesium

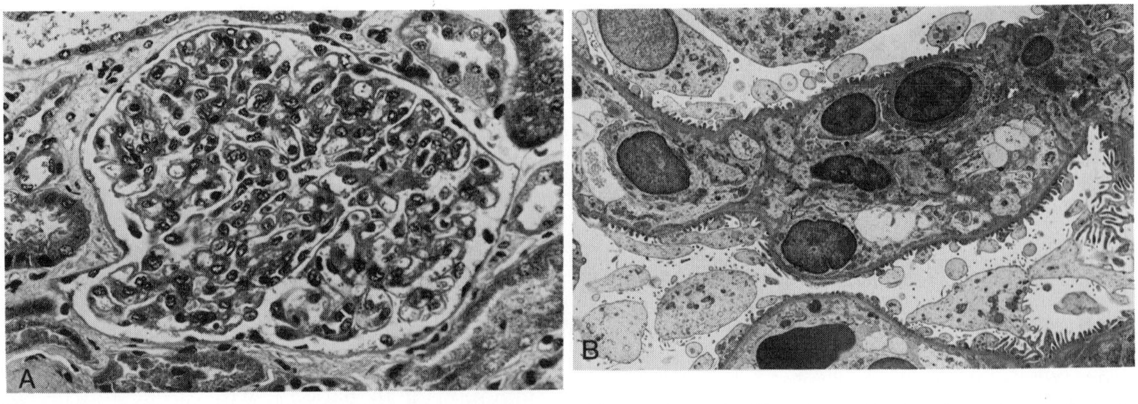

Figure 8–2. *(A)* Light micrograph of a glomerulus of a patient with preeclampsia. The glomerulus is enlarged and relatively bloodless, with the capillary lumina obstructed by swollen endothelial cells. *(B)* Electron micrograph from a glomerulus of a patient with preeclampsia. The capillary lumen is obstructed by hypertrophied endothelial cells. Note that epithelial foot processes are relatively well preserved.

Table 8–4. DRUGS USED IN TREATMENT OF SEVERE PERIPARTUM HYPERTENSION

Hydralazine	Drug of choice, administered parenterally. Initial dose is 5 mg, followed by 5–10 mg every 20–30 minutes. Tachycardia and headache are common side effects, and neonatal thrombocytopenia has been reported.
Diazoxide	Currently recommended second-line drug for use when hydralazine proves inadequate. Titrate dose with repeated 30-mg boluses, rather than the larger doses used in nonpregnant patients. May result in arrested labor and neonatal hyperglycemia.
Labetalol	Given parenterally as repeated boluses, may replace diazoxide as second-line drug.
Nifedipine	Given orally or sublingually. Favorable results reported in limited trials. Magnesium may potentiate the effect of calcium channel entry blockers and result in severe hypotension.

sulfate heptahydrate, followed by a maintenance infusion of 2 to 3 g/hr as needed to maintain serum levels between 6 and 8 mEq/L. Decreased renal function may result in magnesium accumulation to toxic levels (*i.e.*, >10 mEq/L), requiring dose adjustment. Overdosage may result in respiratory arrest and may be treated by administration of intravenous calcium gluconate.

Severe peripartum hypertension can usually be controlled with intravenous hydralazine, although some centers successfully use parenteral diazoxide, labetalol, clonidine, or oral nifedipine. Nitroprusside should be avoided because of fetal toxicity. The ongoing debate about the desired level of blood pressure reduction reflects our continued uncertainty concerning the degree to which uteroplacental blood flow is autoregulated. We currently recommend target diastolic levels of 90 to 105 mm Hg. Specific recommendations are outlined in Table 8–4.

Chronic Hypertension

Diagnosis. Most of these patients suffer from essential hypertension, which may first become manifest during pregnancy. Although only a very small subset of these patients have secondary hypertension, the unusually morbid course of pheochromocytoma in pregnancy makes screening of urinary catecholamines or metabolites prudent if any clinical suspicion is aroused. Patients with chronic hypertension are more likely to develop superimposed preeclampsia. The diagnosis of chronic hypertension depends primarily on a history of documented hypertension before conception or very early in pregnancy and secondarily on physical evidence of arteriolar or end-organ damage (*e.g.*, as detected by funduscopic examination).

Complications. Most women with essential hypertension have uncomplicated pregnancies. However, complications of chronic hypertension in pregnancy may include superimposed preeclampsia, acute renal failure, placental abruption, intrauterine growth retardation, and midtrimester fetal demise. The occurrence of these complications appears to exhibit covariance with maternal age and the duration of hypertension. Thus, women at greatest risk are those who are older than 30 years or who have evidence of end-organ damage.

Antihypertensive Therapy. Treatment of

Table 8–5. ANTIHYPERTENSIVE DRUGS IN PREGNANCY

Centrally acting α_2 agonists	Alpha-methyldopa is proven safe and effective by large randomized trials with long-term follow-up. Possible side effect is neonatal tremor. Usual dosage is 250–500 mg every 8 hours, up to a maximum of 2 g/day. Clonidine is embryotoxic in some animals.
β receptor antagonists	Atenolol and metoprolol are most extensively tested and appear both safe and effective. Adverse effects suggested by human and animal studies may include infants that are small for gestational dates, fetal and neonatal bradycardia, hypoglycemia, and impaired fetal tolerance of hypoxia.
Combined β and α_1 blockers	Labetalol is as effective as methyldopa. A possible contribution to retroplacental hemorrhage is under investigation.
Calcium entry blockers	Nifedipine appears effective, and safety of chronic use is under investigation.
Direct arteriolar vasodilators	Hydralazine is used frequently in combination with methyldopa. Usual dosage is 25–50 mg every 6 hours. There is only trivial experience with minoxidil.
Diuretics	Most authorities do not use these drugs for blood pressure control in pregnancy.
Angiotensin-converting enzyme inhibitors	These drugs are contraindicated in pregnancy, as they have been associated with neonatal renal failure and caused fetal death in several animal studies.

mild hypertension in pregnancy is a subject of ongoing debate. Most clinicians would withhold drug therapy until diastolic blood pressures are 90 mm Hg in the second trimester and 100 mm Hg near term. Younger patients, however, may require earlier intervention. There are few reliable and well-designed trials assessing safety and efficacy of antihypertensive medications in pregnancy. Current recommendations are outlined in Table 8–5.

Superimposed Preeclampsia

Some women with chronic hypertension may develop proteinuria and an exacerbation of their hypertensive disease in late pregnancy. These findings may be accompanied by more labile hypertension, renal dysfunction, oliguria, and evidence of disseminated intravascular coagulation. Fetal outcome is poorer in superimposed preeclampsia than in preeclampsia occurring in a previously normotensive woman. Maternal morbidity is likewise greater, and superimposed preeclampsia accounts for most cases of cerebral hemorrhage in pregnancy. **This combination of disorders signals a medical emergency and also carries a high risk of recurrence in any future pregnancies.**

Transient Hypertension

This category includes women who probably represent a diversity of underlying diagnoses. They typically present in the third trimester with nonproteinuric hypertension that normalizes by 10 days postpartum. It is prudent to treat nulliparas with this presentation as if they were preeclamptic. Most patients, including the multiparous ones, are likely destined to have essential hypertension later in life.

Selected Readings

Brown MA: Sodium and plasma volume regulation in normal and hypertensive pregnancy: A review of physiology and clinical implications. Clin Exp Hypertens [B]7:265, 1988.

Cunningham FC: Urinary tract infections complicating pregnancy. Clin Obstet Gynecol 1:891, 1987.

Davison JM: Pregnancy in renal allograft recipients: Prognosis and management. Clin Obstet Gynecol 1:1027, 1987.

Ferris TF: Renal diseases. *In* Burrow GN, Ferris TF (eds): Medical Complications During Pregnancy, 3rd ed. Philadelphia, WB Saunders, 1988, pp 277–302.

First MR, Pollak VE: Pregnancy and renal disease. *In* Schrier RW, Gottschalk CW (eds): Diseases of the Kidney, 4th ed. Boston, Little, Brown & Co, 1988, pp 2533–2559.

Hou S: Peritoneal dialysis and hemodialysis in pregnancy. Clin Obstet Gynecol 1:1009, 1987.

Lindheimer MD: Diagnosis and management of hypertension complicating pregnancy. Am J Kidney Dis (Suppl 1)13:17, 1989.

Lindheimer MD, Davison JM: Renal biopsy in pregnancy. To b--- or not to b---. Br J Obstet Gynecol 94:932, 1987.

Lindheimer MD, Katz AI: Preeclampsia: Pathophysiology, diagnosis and management, Annu Rev Med 40:233, 1989.

Lindheimer MD, Katz AI: The kidney and hypertension in pregnancy. *In* Brenner BM, Rector FC Jr (eds): The Kidney, 4th ed. Philadelphia, WB Saunders, 1990.

Lindheimer MD, Katz AI, Ganeval D, et al: Acute renal failure in pregnancy. *In* Brenner BM, Lazarus JM (eds): Acute Renal Failure, 2nd ed. New York, Churchill Livingstone, 1988, pp 597–620.

CHAPTER 9

PEDIATRIC NEPHROLOGY

Norman M. Wolfish and Alfred Fish

MATURATION OF RENAL FUNCTION

At birth, renal function is related to gestational age rather than birth weight, length, or surface area. Thus, the glomerular filtration rate (GFR) of a prematurely born infant is much lower than that of a small-for-date neonate of equivalent weight. Postnatally, the kidneys must assume the secretory functions formerly performed by the placenta. Birth thus initiates a functional maturation regardless of gestational age or maturity.

GFR is low in newborns then slowly increases throughout infancy and, when corrected for surface area, reaches adult values by 12 to 18 months of age (Table 9–1). Other factors such as the interplay of renin-aldosterone, prostaglandins, antidiuretic hormone (ADH), catecholamines, and the sympathetic nervous system influence the developmental progress of kidney function. GFR is low as a result of a combination of various factors: high renal vascular resistance, low renal fraction of cardiac output, decreased intraglomerular filtration pressure due to anatomic immaturity, low glomerular perfusion and hydraulic permeability, and reduced effective blood volume.

Because neonates and infants are anabolic, their protein metabolism is efficient and their urea production low. Thus, the serum and urine content of urea is lower than adult values. Because serum creatinine level reflects muscle mass, this value is less in infants than in older children; neonatal levels, however, reflect maternal serum levels, decreasing during the first week of life (see Table 9–1).

GFR (in ml/min/1.73 m^2) may estimated by the following formula:

$$\frac{0.55 \times \text{length (cm)}}{\text{serum creatinine (mg/dl)}} \text{ or } \frac{0.33 \times \text{length (cm)}}{\text{serum creatinine (mmol/L)}}$$

Tubular function is *proportional* to GFR, thus preserving glomerulotubular balance. Although absolute rates for reabsorption (T_{max}) of amino acids, glucose, phosphate, and bicarbonate are lower in infants than in adults, the *ratio* per unit of GFR is similar to that in adults.

Serum bicarbonate is lower in infants and young children (20 to 21 mmol/L) than in adults (24 to 27 mmol/L), partly because of a low renal threshold for bicarbonate, demonstrating a functional immaturity of the proximal tubule. Distal tubular acidification is intact, and infants are capable of acidifying the urine to pH 4.8. Although urinary ammonia production and excretion lag behind that of an older child in response to an acid load, the higher serum phosphate level may act as a systemic buffer and obviates the need for large increases in ammonia secretion.

Maximum urinary concentrating capacity in neonates is less than in infants and children (Table 9–2). Infants have short loops of Henle and a high rate of medullary blood flow, both of which contribute to this limitation, as does

Table 9–1. NORMAL VALUES

Age	BUN		Creatinine		GFR
	mg/dl	*mmol/L*	*mg/dl*	*mmol/L*	*ml/min/1.73m²*
Neonates (1–4 weeks)	3–10	1.07–3.57	0.6–1.0	53.0–88.4	38–48
Infants (4 weeks–2 years)	5–10	1.78–3.57	0.25–0.4	22.1–48.6	58–103
Children (2–10 years)	5–15	1.78–5.35	0.23–0.7	22.1–61.9	110–135
Adolescents	5–17	3.57–6.07	0.53–1.22	46.9–107.9	110–135

Table 9–2. MAXIMUM URINE CONCENTRATION

Age	mOsm/kg	Specific Gravity
Neonate	600–800	1.018–1.021
2 months	700–1200	1.021–1.024
2–12 months	800–1400	1.024–1.032

the relative insensitivity of the distal tubule to ADH and reduced urinary excretion of osmotically active substances, specifically urea (see above).

The serum phosphate level is higher in infants (4.5 to 6 mg/dl or 1.1 to 1.6 mmol/L) and slowly decreases throughout childhood to reach adult values before puberty. Immediately after birth there is a relative hypoparathyroidism due to a limited secretory capacity of the neonatal parathyroid gland. This hypoparathyroidism, coupled with a low GFR, a reduced tubular responsiveness to parathormone, and an infant's relative high dietary phosphate intake, is partially responsible for maintaining the elevated level of serum phosphorus. Because calcium has a reciprocal relationship to phosphate, levels tend to be low in neonates. The interplay of relative hypoparathyroidism, tendency to acidosis, activity of renal alpha$_1$-hydroxylase, and availability of 1,25 dihydroxyvitamin D_3 all tend to favor a low serum calcium level.

NEPHROLOGIC PROBLEMS IN NEONATES

At least 90% of premature and 93% of full-term infants void in the first 24 hours of life. Failure to pass urine after the first 30 hours of life is usually associated with abnormalities of perfusion-filtration (*i.e.*, urine formation) or obstruction (Table 9–3).

A presumptive diagnosis of acute renal failure (ARF) is made in a neonate if urine output is less than 1 ml/kg/hr, serum creatinine level is greater than 1.0 mg/dl (90 mmol/L), and blood urea nitrogen level (BUN) is greater than 20 mg/dl (7.5 mmol/L) (*i.e.*, similar to maternal serum values). ARF is most often secondary to perinatal asphyxia or shock, in which both renal blood flow (RBF) and GFR are reduced, causing oliguria or anuria. The reduction in function is proportional to the severity of the asphyxia but is usually completely reversible if extensive parenchymal injury has not occurred. The eventual prognosis for normal renal function in these circumstances is excellent.

Clinical clues to the diagnosis of renal failure include respiratory distress, cardiac failure, pallor, poor feeding, low-set ears, and auricular anomalies. A palpable bladder suggests lower tract obstruction, whereas enlarged kidneys may be associated with hydronephrosis, cysts, renal vein thrombosis, or tumor. Hematuria (gross or microscopic), proteinuria, and red blood cell (RBC) casts are often observed. Seizures may be due to hyponatremia, hypocalcemia, disseminated intravascular coagulation, or hypertension (blood pressure greater than 90/65 mm Hg in term infants and 80/45 in preterm infants).

> Presumptive diagnosis of ARF in a neonate is made when neonatal BUN and serum creatinine levels are greater than maternal values.

Since the most common cause of ARF is hypovolemia, a fluid challenge of 20 ml/kg of

Table 9–3. CAUSES OF ACUTE RENAL FAILURE IN THE NEWBORN PERIOD

Prerenal
Hypotension–hypovolemia
  Septic shock
  Maternal antepartum hemorrhage
  Twin-to-twin transfusion
  Cardiac surgery
Congestive heart failure
Hypoxia-asphyxia
Dehydration

Renal
Congenital anomalies
  Infantile polycystic kidneys
  Cystic dysplasia
  Hypoplasia
  Bilateral agenesis
Acute tubular necrosis
  Asphyxia
  Dehydration
  Shock
  Nephrotoxins
Vascular
  Renal vein or arterial thrombosis
  Cortical necrosis
  Disseminated intravascular coagulopathy
Inflammatory
  Pyelonephritis
  Toxoplasmosis
Syphilis

Postrenal (obstruction)
Posterior urethral valves
Urethral diverticulum
Neurogenic bladder
Ureterocele
Ureteropelvic or ureterovesical obstruction and hydronephrosis
Tumors—nephroblastoma, mesoblastic nephroma

saline or 10% dextrose in H_2O over 1 to 2 hours may be indicated. If an infant still fails to pass urine, furosemide (Lasix) (2 mg/kg IV) can be used. Diagnosis of continuing oliguria-anuria may require ultrasonography, differential radionuclide evaluation, or the cautious use of intravenous urography (radiographic dyes may induce acute tubular necrosis [ATN] in neonates) or cystography.

Differentiation of prerenal from renal failure may be assisted by calculating the fractional excretion of sodium (FE_{Na}). In prerenal failure, it is usually less than 3 to 5% in term infants and slightly higher in premature infants. Fluid requirements in neonates are restricted to balancing insensible, renal, and nonrenal losses with intake. For neonates, average daily water needs (in ml/kg/day) are as follows: insensible 60, fecal 20, plus urinary losses. Insensible water loss is increased under radiant heaters or with fever and is decreased with respirator therapy.

HEMATURIA IN CHILDREN

Hematuria is not an uncommon urinary finding in children, its reported prevalence varying from 0.7 to 2.5% of the school-age population. Hematuria most often is microscopic and may represent no more than a variant of normal. Gross hematuria is readily observable and more alarming, although the causes in children may be less serious than in adult patients. An important clue to the site of bleeding is RBC morphology. Glomerular bleeding or bleeding that originates in the upper nephron results in RBCs that pass through the nephron, undergoing morphologic changes ranging from burr cell appearance to gross alterations in size and shape having a *dysmorphic* appearance. Because bleeding from the calyces and distal urinary system directly adds RBCs to the urine, the RBCs do not undergo morphologic alterations and are *isomorphic* in appearance. The prognosis of asymptomatic hematuria is controversial but appears to depend on the quantity of RBCs in the urine and the presence of proteinuria.

Dysmorphic RBCs thus usually indicate glomerular injury or inflammation. Diagnostic investigation with radiologic or cystographic evaluation is rarely informative. Renal ultrasonography may be helpful in *certain* renal parenchymal disorders (poststreptococcal glomerulonephritis, acute glomerulonephritis [AGN] membranoproliferative glomerulonephritis [MPGN], or other chronic renal diseases) in which kidney size is *increased*, and there is generalized *increased* echodensity (the latter is usually compared with liver, which normally has greater echodensity or echotexture than kidney). However, patients with isomorphic urinary RBCs likely have a nonglomerular origin of hematuria such as stone, tumor, or structural causes and might benefit by visualizing the renal urinary system. Table 9–4 lists the more common causes of hematuria in children and underscores the relative infrequent requirement for radiologic or urologic procedures.

> Dysmorphic RBCs usually indicate glomerular bleeding.
>
> Isomorphic RBCs are usually of a nonglomerular origin.

Isolated microscopic hematuria in children tends to be benign, whereas careful evaluation of gross hematuria frequently results in an identifiable cause, thus investigation is likely to be productive. IgA nephropathy is one of the more common causes of gross or microscopic hema-

Table 9–4. COMMON CAUSES OF HEMATURIA IN CHILDREN

Glomerular
Benign recurrent or persistent
Sporadic, physiologic (fever, exercise, etc.)
Familial
Glomerulonephritis
Postinfectious
Membranoproliferative
Rapidly progressive (crescentic)
Lupus nephritis
Hemolytic uremic syndrome
Henoch-Schönlein (anaphylactoid purpura) nephritis
Hereditary (Alport's) nephritis
IgA nephropathy (Berger's)
Nephrotoxins
Extraglomerular
Trauma
Cystic diseases—polycystic, multicystic, microcystic
Neoplasm—Wilms' tumor
Sickle cell disease or trait
Pyelonephritis
Hydronephrosis
Interstitial nephritis
Renal hemangiomas
Idiopathic hypercalciuria
Nephrolithiasis
Nonrenal
Urinary tract infection
Calculi
Foreign body
Meatal ulceration
Left renal vein compression

turia. A definitive diagnosis can only be made by immunofluorescent observation of mesangial IgA deposits on renal biopsy, because serum levels of IgA may frequently be normal. Although progression to renal insufficiency is unusual in children, prognosis is guarded because 5 to 15% of adults may develop renal deterioration. Idiopathic hypercalciuria without nephrolithiasis is another cause of hematuria; acceptable levels of urinary calcium excretion are less than 4 mg/kg/24 hr (0.1 mmol/kg/24 hr) or a urinary calcium:creatinine ratio less than 0.21 if measured in mg/dl (or 0.7 when measured in mmol/L).

The initial investigation of a child with persistent hematuria should include qualitative estimate of RBCs and casts by urinalysis, cellular morphology to assist in the localization of the bleeding, urine culture, a calcium:creatinine determination, and a 24-hour urine collection for protein, creatinine clearance, and calcium excretion. Blood is evaluated for creatinine, urea, immunoglobulins, complement, and antistreptococcal antibody titers, and for antinuclear antibodies and antiDNA antibodies. Radiography, sonography, radionuclide scans, cystography, cystoscopy, and biopsy may be warranted under specific circumstances. Renal biopsy is usually not indicated in mild asymptomatic microscopic hematuria in the absence of proteinuria and with normal renal function. Because the risk of chronic renal failure appears to increase with quantitative increasing hematuria, renal biopsy may be indicated if significant hematuria persists for longer than 1 year.

> Hematuria associated with proteinuria or reduced renal function has a worse prognosis than isolated hematuria.

PROTEINURIA IN CHILDREN

Isolated proteinuria (without hematuria) is not uncommon in children and may be detected in up to 1.5% of school-age children. The level at which proteinuria becomes *significant* varies with age and has been defined as 0.4 mg/kg/hr. Premature and newborn infants may have *transient* proteinuria for the first 1 to 2 weeks of life. Transient proteinuria also occurs with febrile illnesses, infectious and inflammatory disorders, and exercise, but it rapidly resolves. *Postural* or *orthostatic* proteinuria occurs in children and adolescents, especially during the rapid phase of growth. Protein excretion rarely exceeds 1 g/24 hr in these circumstances and varies from the recumbent to the erect position. *Persistent* or *fixed* proteinuria is detectable at all times, may slowly but progressively increase, and deserves a full nephrologic evaluation.

GLOMERULONEPHRITIS

Several forms of glomerulonephritis have been defined on the basis of the nature of the glomerular immunopathologic findings (Table 9–5) and the presence of hypocomplemetemia.

> The hallmark of glomerulonephritis is the presence of hematuria, proteinuria, and casts in the urine.

Forms of Glomerulonephritis

Postinfectious Glomerulonephritis. These patients characteristically present with gross hematuria and tea-colored urine. Edema due to fluid overload and oliguria, along with hypertension secondary to hypervolemia, is observed. Documentation of streptococcal infection (pharyngitis, pyoderma), elevated levels of antistreptococcal (ASO, anti-DNAase B) antibodies, and hypocomplementemia establish the diagnosis. This condition has an excellent prognosis. Kidney biopsy is not required. Careful management of fluid and electrolyte balance and control of elevated blood pressure ensure an uneventful recovery.

Systemic Lupus Erythematosus. When hypocomplementemia is present with glomerulonephritis, systemic lupus erythematosus (SLE) needs to be ruled out. This disorder is usually associated with fever, arthropathy, skin rash, and glomerulonephritis. The diagnosis of SLE nephropathy is established by kidney biopsy. A generally favorable prognosis in children is now achieved with aggressive use of steroid and immunosuppressive therapy.

Membranoproliferative Glomerulonephritis. Type I MPGN is usually a variably progressive form of glomerulonephritis that is characterized on kidney biopsy by mesangial cell interposition in peripheral glomerular capillary loops. A peripheral lobular distribution of C3 and IgG is found by immunofluorescence. Type II MPGN (also called *dense deposit disease*) is associated

Table 9–5. IMMUNE-MEDIATED GLOMERULONEPHRITIS

Condition	Etiology/Chronicity	Serum C3	Immunopathologic Change	Pathogenesis
Postinfectious	Streptococcal and other agents/acute	Low	Diffuse small subendothelial and subepithelial deposits	Immune complex
Systemic lupus erythematosus	Antinuclear (anti-DNA) antibodies/acute and chronic	Low	Subendothelial, mesangial, subepithelial deposits	Immune complex/ autoimmune
Membranoproliferative	Unknown/chronic	Low	Mesangial interposition and immune deposits	Immune complex
IgA nephropathy	Unknown/acute and chronic	Normal	IgA mesangial deposits	Immune complex
Goodpasture's syndrome	Anti-GBM antibodies to NC1 domain type IV collagen/acute	Normal	Linear IgG deposition along GBM	Anti-GBM nephritis/ autoimmune

GBM, glomerular basement membrane.

with double linear (tram-track) deposits of C3 and diffuse deposition of dense material in the glomerular basement membrane and mesangium on electron microscopy. Both conditions are associated with hypocomplementemia and have clinical features of glomerulonephritis with an active urine sediment, proteinuria, loss of renal function, and hypertension. Overall, the prognosis in both diseases is poor, type II MPGN being worse.

IgA Nephropathy

IgA nephropathy (Berger's disease) is a mild form of glomerulonephritis characterized by recurrent episodes of microscopic and/or gross hematuria. This condition, which is the most common form of glomerulonephritis in children, on presentation is usually associated with normal renal function, normal serum complement levels, normal blood pressure, and no proteinuria. The diagnosis can be established if the serum IgA is elevated, and kidney biopsy is usually not indicated. Tissue studies have revealed mild focal segmental glomerulonephritis with mesangial cell proliferation. Prominent IgA deposits characteristically are detected in the mesangium by immunofluorescent microscopy, and immune dense deposits are seen by electron microscopy. The course of this disorder is characterized by recurrent episodes of hematuria associated with upper respiratory tract infections, and it is usually nonprogressive in children. The onset of hypertension, reduced renal function, or proteinuria may herald the onset of progressive glomerular injury, and a kidney biopsy should be performed.

Goodpasture's Syndrome

Goodpasture's syndrome is a severe form of crescentic proliferative glomerulonephritis associated with pulmonary hemorrhage. This autoimmune condition is mediated by antibodies to the glomerular basement membrane. Goodpasture's antigen has been identified as the NC1 domain of type IV (basement membrane) collagen. Some patients have only glomerulonephritis without pulmonary involvement. Proteinuria, hematuria, and rapid loss of renal function are frequently encountered. Kidney biopsy reveals crescentic glomerulonephritis with diffuse cellular proliferation. By immunofluorescent microscopy, characteristic linear deposition of IgG and C3 along the glomerular basement membranes is seen. These patients frequently require dialysis, and therapy is also directed toward reduction and elimination of circulating autoantibodies to glomerular basement membrane by plasmapheresis and immunosuppression. The prognosis in this condition is guarded.

Hemolytic-Uremic Syndrome

Hemolytic-uremic syndrome (HUS) is a clinical syndrome characterized by progressive renal failure associated with hemolytic anemia and thrombocytopenia. This condition has become more prevalent and since 1983 has been associated with infectious diarrhea due to *Escherichia coli* 0157:H7 contamination of meat and milk. Although other pathogens have been implicated, recent epidemics of HUS have been clearly related to this organism, which can be identified in the stool. Patients have a prodrome of severe, often bloody diarrhea for 2 to 7 days before the onset of renal failure. It appears that the pathogenesis of HUS relates to the development of localized intravascular coagulation, with microthrombotic events affecting capillary beds throughout the body. When this occurs in the renal glomerular capillary network, GFR declines and renal failure develops. Progressive hemolytic anemia and thrombocytopenia are due to intravascular coagulation. This condition, which is closely related to thrombotic thrombocytopenic purpura, may also be associated with central nervous system involvement, seizures, and hemiparesis. The clinical picture in these patients is characterized by severe renal failure, hypokalemia, and acidosis. The diagnosis is established clinically, and kidney biopsy is not indicated. Treatment involves careful management of fluid and electrolyte balance and correction of hematologic parameters by transfusion of packed RBCs and platelets. Management of renal failure by peritoneal dialysis or hemodialysis is usually needed and may be required for periods up to 3 to 4 weeks until renal function returns. The overall prognosis in these patients is very good, with the majority having complete recovery and restoration of normal renal function, although 15 to 20% of children may develop hypertension 3 to 5 years after the onset of the disease. A small number of patients have varying degrees of patchy cortical necrosis, resulting in residual renal insufficiency and chronic renal failure.

NEPHROTIC SYNDROME IN CHILDHOOD

Children presenting with nephrotic syndrome in childhood have the typical features of this condition, including extensive edema and fluid retention, hypoproteinemia, proteinuria, and hypercholesterolemia.

> The majority of afflicted children between the ages of 18 months and 7 years have a steroid-responsive form of nephrotic syndrome.

The investigation of children with nephrotic syndrome is directed at determining whether minimal change nephrotic syndrome of childhood (nil lesion) is the likely diagnosis (Table 9–6). These patients have normal blood pressure and renal function, proteinuria without cells or cellular casts, normal C3 and C4 levels, and negative fluorescent antinuclear antibody studies. When these clinical parameters have been established, a trial of steroid therapy using prednisone is recommended. Disappearance of proteinuria and resolution of the nephrotic syndrome with steroid therapy additionally confirm the likely diagnosis of minimal change nephrotic syndrome of childhood. A trial of steroid therapy within 6 to 8 weeks in this manner is not recommended for those children with evidence of glomerulonephritis (*i.e.*, hematuria, azotemia, oliguria, or hypertension). A kidney biopsy is indicated in children with nephrotic syndrome when there is evidence of glomerulonephritis or in those children who do not respond to a trial of steroid therapy. This approach can be taken because prior therapy does not alter the biopsy findings and does not pose a clinically significant delay in establishing the actual diagnosis. The likelihood of minimal change nephrotic syndrome of childhood is less after the age of 8 years, and these patients usually undergo kidney biopsy so that a specific diagnosis can be established.

> The prognosis of nil lesion nephrotic syndrome of childhood is favorable, with most children outgrowing the condition during adolescence.

Therapy of nil lesion nephrotic syndrome involves the use of prednisone (2 mg/kg/day in three divided doses) until proteinuria is absent for 1 week, and then therapy is changed to 2 mg/kg every other day as a single morning dose. Diuretic therapy with furosemide may be used to control excessive edema and ascites during the overt nephrotic stage. Steroid toxicity, growth failure, hypertension, fluid retention, and infection are major risks complicating the course of treatment in these patients. Children having frequent relapses of this disorder may be candidates to receive cyclophosphamide.

Focal glomerular sclerosis is a related condition with a poorer prognosis. The nephrotic state is often resistant to steroid therapy, and the diagnosis is established by kidney biopsy. Hypertension and progressive renal failure are frequent accompaniments and lead to renal insufficiency. Recurrence of focal glomerular sclerosis has been observed in some patients who have had renal transplantation.

CONGENITAL MALFORMATIONS OF THE URINARY TRACT

For ease of classification (Table 9–7), congenital malformations of the kidneys can be thought

Table 9–6. NEPHROTIC SYNDROME OF CHILDHOOD

	Steroid Responsive	Steroid Resistant
Clinical		
Renal function	Normal	Normal or reduced
Blood pressure	Normal	Normal or elevated
Urinalysis	Occasional hematuria	Hematuria
	Hyaline casts	Cellular or granular casts
	Proteinuria	Proteinuria
Serology		
C3, C4	Normal	Normal or low
FANA	Negative	Negative or positive
Biopsy		
Light microscopy	Minimal change	Focal sclerosis or glomerulonephritis
Immunofluorescence	Negative	Positive
Electron microscopy	Foot process fusion	Immune deposits

FANA, fluorescent antinuclear antibodies.

of as abnormalities of renal parenchymal morphogenesis, structural abnormalities of the collecting system, or renal cysts. With the advent of prenatal ultrasonography, various congenital renal malformations are incidentally uncovered, some of which are isolated to the kidneys, others associated with several nonrenal structural defects, most commonly of the central nervous system. The most common prenatal renal obstructive lesions are hydronephrosis, often associated with ureteropelvic junction obstruction, and hydroureter due to ureterovesical junction obstruction. If bilateral hydronephrosis and hydroureter are present, posterior urethral valves should be considered. Other intrauterine structural anomalies frequently encountered include polycystic kidney disease, uni- or bilateral multicystic dysplasia, hypoplasia, aplasia, or agenesis. There may be associated maternal polyhydramnios, indicating poor fetal renal concentrating capacity. Oligohydramnios is a serious prognostic factor because it often suggests reduced fetal renal function and is associated with bilateral pulmonary hypoplasia and facial dysmorphism. Potter's syndrome is an association of severe bilateral renal hypoplasia, aplasia or agenesis, pulmonary hypoplasia, and a characteristic flattened facies due to oligohydramnios. It is most often incompatible with postnatal life because of the pulmonary hypoplasia.

Table 9–7. CONGENITAL RENAL MALFORMATIONS

Abnormalities of parenchymal morphogenesis
Amount
Agenesis
Aplasia
Hypoplasia
Differentiation
Dysplasia
Location
Ectopy
Abnormalities of the collecting system
Hydronephrosis
Hydroureter
Reflux
Renal cysts
Nonhereditary
Simple
Multicystic
Multilocular
Hereditary
Cortical
Medullary
Polycystic

Functional disturbances may accompany congenital malformations. Concentrating and acidification defects occur with alterations of medullary architecture (*e.g.*, hydronephrosis, cysts), whereas diminished GFR will accompany hypoplasia and dysplasia. Severe (especially bilateral) structural anomalies (*e.g.*, hydronephrosis or multicystic disease) have associated dysplastic elements that will result in combined glomerular and medullary functional deficits.

Aplasia, Hypoplasia, Dysplasia

Renal hypoplasia is usually unilateral and inconsequential, but it may be segmental and associated with hypertension or bilateral and accompanied by dysplasia and reduced GFR. Renal dysplasia may be unilateral or bilateral and is often associated with hypoplasia or multicystic disease. Dysplasia is frequently accompanied by reduced GFR and/or hypertension. When multicystic disease is present, polydipsia and polyuria will be predominant symptoms. A unilateral multicystic dysplastic kidney does not usually require removal if asymptomatic. About 25% involute spontaneously over several months to years, and there is no proven association with renal malignancies.

Hydronephrosis

Hydronephrosis is due to obstruction at either the ureteropelvic or ureterovesical junction or to obstruction from the posterior urethral valves in the urethra. Ureterovesical obstruction is associated with hydroureter of the affected side(s) and dilated renal pelvis with varying degrees of calyceal clubbing and parenchymal thinning. A test to decide whether surgical repair is indicated is the furosemide washout. If good clearance of the radioisotope during the excretory phase of the venogram is obtained, then correction is usually not required.

Reflux

Vesicoureteral reflux is a congenital ureteric anomaly with lateral displacement of the ureteral orifice in the bladder wall. Renal maldevelopment (dysplasia) and concomitant abnormalities in urinary concentration and GFR may be present in these infants.

Reflux is the most frequent abnormality associated with urinary tract infection (UTI) (up to 30%) and is demonstrable by cystography either during micturition only (high-pressure) or during bladder filling (low-pressure reflux). Grade 1 reflux ascends to the renal pelvis, grade 2 reflux fills the pelvis but has well-maintained calyceal cupping, grade 3 reflux is associated with calyceal clubbing and ureteropelvic dilatation, grade 4 reflux is accompanied by calyceal clubbing and evidence of pyelonephritis (loss of renal parenchyma), and grade 5 reflux superimposes elements of hydronephrosis, loss of renal parenchyma, and scarring. Prognosis is directly related to the degree of reflux. Grades 1 and 2 are associated with a high degree of spontaneous resolution (70 to 85%) over several years, providing the urine remains sterile. This may necessitate prolonged prophylactic antibiotic therapy (6 months of daily single-dose therapy). Grades 4 and 5 reflux have a low rate of spontaneous resolution (5 to 10%), even with meticulous urinary antisepsis, and usually require ureteral reimplantation. Grade 3 reflux is intermediate in response to antibiotic therapy and deserves several years of medical therapy before surgical repair is considered.

Posterior Urethral Valves

Posterior urethral valves are a congenital anomaly causing bladder outlet obstruction and bilateral hydroureter, hydronephrosis, and often renal dysplasia and renal failure. The bladder is distended and palpable, and the urinary stream is of poor quality. This is a common cause of renal failure in young male infants, but the diagnosis may not be made until UTI occurs.

Renal Cysts

Polycystic Kidney Disease. Cystic renal disease in children accounts for 10% of children in end-stage renal disease. The major cystic disorders (see Table 9–7) are autosomal dominant polycystic kidney disease (ADPKD), autosomal recessive polycystic kidney disease (ARPKD), multicystic dysplastic kidney, and juvenile nephronophthisis. ADPKD is best detected by ultrasonography and has been detected *in utero* as well as in early infancy. Although hypertension may be an associated complication, very few children will develop evidence of renal failure, and the onset of renal insufficiency is usually delayed until middle age. Screening family members with genetic markers for the ADPKD gene on chromosome 16 is 99% reliable and is advisable to identify other members at risk and assist in genetic counseling. In contrast, ARPKD is frequently recognized at birth or in early infancy, presenting as a palpable abdominal mass that is either kidney or liver. This disorder should be distinguished from the dominant form by radiology or ultrasonography and the severity of the disease at presentation, rapidity of progression, presence of hepatic or biliary involvement, careful family pedigree, and chromosome characterization. Most children with ARPKD have a poor prognosis, requiring renal transplantation in childhood until the third decade of life. However, patients with ADPKD may be expected to have adequate renal function.

Medullary Cystic Disease or Juvenile Nephronophthisis. Like polycystic kidney disease, medullary cystic disease exists as both an autosomal recessive and dominant form, and as in polycystic kidney disease the recessive form has an earlier onset and progresses more rapidly than the dominant form. Both are associated with multiple microcysts in the medulla, periglomerular fibrosis, polydipsia, polyuria, late-onset hypertension, and progressive renal insufficiency. The recessive form, juvenile nephronophthisis, is associated with growth failure and anemia and is the fourth most common cause of end-stage renal disease in children.

The two disorders do not differ from each other significantly other than by different age of onset and genetics.

Multicystic Kidney. Multicystic kidney usually occurs unilaterally and is frequently associated with ureteral stenosis or atresia and renal dysplasia. Various degrees of renal insufficiency occur if there is bilateral involvement. Bilateral disease should be suspected in any infant who has obvious unilateral disease and whose GFR does not mature appropriately.

URINARY TRACT INFECTION

UTI is one of the more common bacterial infections of childhood. The risk of a girl's developing symptomatic UTI during childhood is about 3%, but the risk is 0.1% for a boy. UTI is secondary to congenital malformation with obstruction of the urinary tract more often in boys than in girls. More than 50% of the patients with symptomatic infections will have more than one recurrence. About 20 to 30% have ureteral reflux, and 5 to 10% have associated structural defects. Of children with symptomatic infections, 5 to 10% will develop renal scarring during childhood, and about 1% will become hypertensive or uremic. However, the majority of children with recurrent UTI will have no demonstrable cause identified and may have a bladder that is unusually susceptible to bacterial infection (*Escherichia. coli*) related to bacterial virulence, adhesion, host blood groups, and other factors.

Clinical Presentation

Newborns with UTI usually present with signs of sepsis: fever, anorexia, vomiting, failure to thrive, and persisting jaundice. Older infants and children with upper UTI present with spiking fever, chills, or abdominal or loin pain, and frequently with lower UTI symptoms such as frequency, urgency, dysuria, incontinence, and occasionally hematuria. Hematuria is frequently associated with UTI and, if present, is usually accompanied by symptoms of dysuria or pyelonephritis.

Physical examination should include assessment of height percentile, blood pressure determination, a search for extrarenal congenital anomalies (ears, anus, vertebrae), kidney palpation, examination of the genitalia (specifically an ectopic meatus in boys, labial fusion in girls), and an evaluation of the urine stream on voiding.

> Only 30 to 40% of children with recurrent UTI have a demonstrable structural defect.

Indications for Radiologic Investigation (Renal Sonogram and Voiding Cystogram)

1. *Apparent first infection:* Radiologic investigation is indicated in all infants and toddlers (up to 3 years) with their first documented or symptomatic infection; in all boys with documented infection irrespective of age; when a renal mass is palpated, suggesting hydronephrosis; and when hypertension and/or uremia is present.
2. *Recurrent infections:* Radiologic investigation is indicated in children of all ages and both sexes, although the yield decreases with increasing age greater than 10 years.
3. *Recurrent asymptomatic bacteriuria:* Cystoscopic evaluation is usually not necessary unless major bladder abnormalities are present.

Treatment

The major antibiotics used in children with UTI are summarized in Table 9–8. The usual therapy for acute UTI lasts from 10 to 14 days. Prolonged therapy for reflux should continue for 6 months. Trimethroprim and sulfamethoxazole or nitrofurantoin are usually used for such prolonged therapy, using a single daily dose for prophylaxis. Some children with frequent recurrent UTI without congenital anomalies will also benefit from prophylactic treatment. Megatherapy (*i.e.*, one-dose therapy) does not appear

Table 9–8. ANTIBIOTIC THERAPY OF UTI IN CHILDREN

Drug	Daily Dosage	Intervals
Amoxicillin	35–50 mg/kg	q 8 hr
Sulfamethoxazole	50 mg/kg for 2 days, thereafter 25 mg/kg	q 12 hr
Sulfisoxazole	100–200 mg/kg	q 6 hr
Nitrofurantoin	3–5 mg/kg	q 6 hr
Trimethoprim	6 mg/kg	q 12 hr
Sulfamethoxazole	30 mg/kg	q 12 hr
Cephalexin	30 mg/kg	q 6 hr

to offer any major advantages over a 10-day to 2-week course and has the potential of inducing drug toxicity in a young child with immature detoxification mechanisms.

HYPERTENSION

Acute elevation of blood pressure in children is most commonly encountered in the postoperative period, especially in those patients undergoing urologic surgery. These problems usually relate to metabolic effects of anesthesia combined with fluid and electrolyte administration during surgery. In other circumstances, fluid overload, acute glomerulonephritis, chronic pyelonephritis, vasculitis, renal dysplasia, coarctation of the aorta, and renal artery stenosis may be the cause of acute hypertensive crises in children.

> Because acute hypertensive events may be associated with congestive heart failure, papilledema, and seizures, it is essential to lower the blood pressure quickly and safely.

In these circumstances, orally administered medications are usually not feasible, although we have found that oral doses of liquid nifedipine (0.25 to 0.5 mg/kg) can be effective ("bite and swallow" capsules). Several agents can be administered parenterally, being used sequentially until satisfactory lowering of blood pressure is achieved. Hydralazine (0.2 to 0.4 mg/kg IV) is useful and gives a rapid effect; because repeated administration after the second dose may result in flushing, tachycardia, headache, and nausea, another drug should be tried thereafter. Labetalol is an effective intravenous beta-adrenergic blocker and is given at 1 to 3 mg/kg/hr. Similarly, diazoxide (2 to 5 mg/kg given by rapid IV bolus) will effectively lower blood pressure with sustained effect over several hours. These agents can be administered repeatedly as needed and are safely used with close patient observation. Patients requiring sodium nitroprusside must have close blood pressure monitoring in an intensive care unit to adjust the rate of continuous drug administration. The dosage varies between 0.5 and 0.8 μg/kg/min IV. Retention of thiocyanate or cyanide and lactic acidosis are rarely a problem in patients with normal or moderately reduced renal function.

The long-term management of chronically hypertensive pediatric patients is related to the nature and etiology of the hypertensive state. Drugs used in the treatment of children with chronic hypertension are outlined in Table 9–9.

> It is essential to completely investigate a child with hypertension to establish a specific diagnosis. The younger the child, the less likely is essential hypertension.

Because of the atherogenic potential of long-term thiazide diuretics and beta-adrenergic blockers, we have moved away from their use in chronically hypertensive children. Nevertheless, thiazide therapy can be useful in children with renal disease when the creatinine clearance is greater than 50 ml/min/1.73 m^2. Loop diuretics (furosemide, bumetanide, metolazone) are used when renal function is further impaired. In situations where states of mineralocorticoid excess exist, the use of spironolactone or triamterene may be helpful.

Angiotensin-converting enzyme inhibitors have become popular in treating hypertensive children. Captopril (1 to 6 mg/kg/day in three

Table 9–9. CHRONIC ANTIHYPERTENSIVE THERAPY

Drug	Dose (mg/kg/day)	
	Starting	***Maximum***
Diuretics		
Hydrochlorthiazide	1	2–3
Furosemide	1	12
Bumetanide	0.02–0.05	0.3
Metolazone	0.1	3
Spironolactone	1	3
Triamterene	2	6
Converting enzyme inhibitors		
Captopril	1	6
Enalapril	0.15	0.6
Calcium channel blockers		
Nifedipine	0.25	3
Nicardipine	0.25	2
Adrenergic blocking agents		
Propranolol	1	8
Atenolol	1	8
Adrenergic agonist		
Clonidine	0.005	0.03
Vasodilator agents		
Hydralazine	0.75	7.5
Minoxidil	0.1–0.2	1

to four doses) and enalapril (0.1 to 0.6 mg/kg/day in one to two doses) are used. Frequent monitoring of total leukocyte counts is needed to detect bone marrow suppression. Calcium channel blocking agents are also used as first-line drugs. Nifedipine (0.25 to 3 mg/kg/day in three to four doses) and the long-acting agent nicardipine (0.25 to 2 mg/kg/day in two to three doses) are effective.

The alpha$_1$-adrenergic blocking agent prazosin and clonidine, a central alpha$_2$-adrenergic agonist, are second-line drugs used in the treatment of hypertension in children. In some situations, the addition of a beta-adrenergic blocking agent such as propranolol and the longer-acting drug atenolol can be used. In particularly resistant hypertensive states, the effective vasodilator minoxidil can be employed. This drug acts directly on systemic arterioles; hypertrichosis is an undesirable side effect limiting its long-term use.

ACUTE RENAL FAILURE

ARF is diagnosed when rapid reduction in GFR results in oliguria with urine volumes less than 0.5 ml/kg/hr in infants or less than 500 ml/1.73 m^2/day in older children. Some causes of ARF are outlined in Table 9–10.

Fractional excretion of sodium (FE_{Na}) is helpful in determining the nature of renal failure. FE_{Na} is calculated using the following formula:

Table 9–10. CAUSES OF ACUTE RENAL FAILURE

Prerenal
- Dehydration and hypovolemia
- Congestive heart failure

Renal
- Vascular
  - Renal vein thrombosis
  - Vasculitis
  - Hemolytic uremic syndrome
- Glomerular
  - Acute glomerulonephritis
  - Rapidly progressive glomerulonephritis
- Tubular
  - Acute tubular necrosis
  - Shock, cardiac surgery, toxic nephropathy
  - Urate nephropathy
  - Sepsis
- Interstitial
  - Acute interstitial nephritis
  - Acute pyelonephritis

Postrenal
- Obstruction
  - Congenital—posterior urethral valves
  - Acquired—tumor, lymphoma

$$\%\ FE_{Na} = \frac{urine_{Na}/serum_{Na}}{urine_{Cr}/serum_{Cr}} \times 100$$

Prerenal causes of renal failure are associated with low (<1%) FE_{Na} values. The importance of recognizing a prerenal cause of renal failure relates to directing treatment toward correction of hypovolemia or heart failure, resulting in resolution of oliguric renal failure.

The most common cause of acute renal failure in children is ATN with an FE_{Na} greater than 1 to 2%. This condition is usually reversible and is associated with necrosis of renal tubular epithelium. The pathogenesis and etiology relate to anoxia (shock, cardiac surgery, asphyxia, dehydration) and nephrotoxins (antibiotics, chemotherapeutic agents, accidental poisoning, rhabdomyolysis).

> Successful resolution of ARF in children depends on correction and elimination of factors leading to renal failure and meticulous management of fluid, electrolyte, and acid-base balance.

The following guidelines are given for the management of ARF in children:

Management of Acute Renal Failure

1. Volume replacement, if necessary (insensible losses plus urinary output).
2. Mannitol or furosemide: Mannitol is given IV at a dosage of 0.5 g/kg (2.5 ml/kg of 20% solution). Furosemide is given IV at 1 mg/kg. Bumetanide is more potent and less ototoxic. The dosage is 0.05 mg/kg.
3. Hyperkalemia becomes an emergency if electrocardiographic changes are observed or if serum potassium rises above 7 mEq/L. The following steps should be taken: Eliminate all sources of potassium intake. Infuse hypertonic (7.5%) sodium bicarbonate; 3.3 ml/kg (3 mEq/kg) will raise blood pH and lower serum potassium by causing an intracellular potassium shift. Alternatively, infuse 1 ml/kg of solution of 50% glucose containing 1 unit of insulin per 3 g glucose. Infuse calcium chloride, 10 mg/kg (0.1 ml/kg of 10% solution) to assist in lowering serum potassium levels. Administer Kayexalate (1 g/kg orally or by retention enema with 10 ml of 70% sorbitol) and repeat as necessary every

4 hours. This method takes several hours and is not the treatment of choice in life-threatening circumstances.

4. Peritoneal dialysis or hemodialysis is indicated if there is severe and persistent renal failure, intractable hyperkalemia, hypertension, or cardiac failure.

Techniques of Peritoneal Dialysis in Children

1. The amount of peritoneal fluid starts at 10 ml/kg and can be increased slowly to 35 to 45 ml/kg/cycle.

2. Hypertonic peritoneal dialysis solutions (4.25% glucose) are indicated in children with hypervolemia and cardiac failure or hyperkalemia. A solution containing 1.5% glucose should be used for maintenance.

3. Potassium is added to the solution as indicated.

4. Serum electrolytes should be monitored frequently and intravenous solutions adjusted accordingly.

5. Fluid balance is calculated from the intravenous infusion, the accumulated negative peritoneal balance, and urine output on a daily basis.

CHRONIC RENAL FAILURE

The causes of chronic renal failure (CRF) in children differ from those in adults (Table 9–11). Renal malformations and obstructive uropathy with infection are more prevalent in younger children, whereas chronic glomerulonephritis is an important etiologic factor in older children and adolescents. Overall prevalence in children varies from 3 to 6 per million population per year, whereas in adults it varies from 40 to 60 per million.

Table 9–11. CAUSES OF END-STAGE RENAL DISEASE IN CHILDREN UNDER AGE 15 YEARS (FROM CANADIAN RENAL FAILURE REGISTRY, 1981–1987)

Cause	Number	Percent
Chronic glomerulonephritis (including focal segmental glomerulonephritis, hemolytic-uremic syndrome, anaphylactoid purpura nephritis)	73	35
Renal malformations (including cystic hypoplastic, dysplastic disorders)	64	31
Obstructive Uropathies (including pyelonephritis and hydronephrosis)	53	25
Hereditary disorders (including Alport's syndrome, cystinosis	19	9
Total	209	100

Progressive renal insufficiency in childhood results in problems that are unique to children. As renal function declines, failure to thrive, reduced growth, delayed puberty, and metabolic bone disease become major problems. Management of these patients is directed toward controlling these abnormalities. High caloric intake with cautious reduction of protein intake to minimum recommended daily allowance levels is recommended. Calcium supplements and added vitamin D therapy are used. Progressive phosphorus retention is difficult to control even with the use of phosphate binders. Aluminum-containing phosphate binders are discouraged because of potential aluminum toxicity.

When the various therapeutic modalities become less effective, failure to thrive and a lesser quality of life become evident. At this point, replacement of renal function is required. Peritoneal dialysis or hemodialysis is a step to eventual kidney transplantation. Bilateral nephrectomy may be indicated in children with hypertension and a history of complicated urinary tract anomalies and infection. The overall results of transplantation in children of all ages, including young infants, continue to improve. Despite problems of toxicity from steroids and immunosuppression, survival is high, along with variable restoration of growth velocity. It is anticipated that with more effective approaches to immunosuppression, the results of kidney transplantation in children will continue to improve.

FLUID AND ELECTROLYTE THERAPY IN CHILDREN

Infants and children develop dehydration more readily than adults. The various causative factors include a greater surface (evaporative) area per unit weight, higher metabolic rate, greater proportion of total body water in the extracellular phase, and a lesser ability to concentrate the urine maximally.

Using the concept of *balance*, maintenance intravenous therapy must equal all body fluid losses minus the water gained through metabolism (Table 9–12). The volume and composition of normal fluid and electrolyte losses from the body are 1800 ml/m^2/day, with a net gain

Table 9–12. WATER BALANCE IN CHILDREN BASED ON BODY SURFACE AREA

In			Out		
Source	*ml/m²/day*	*Tonicity (mOsm/kg)*	*Source*	*ml/m²/day*	*Tonicity (mOsm/kg)*
Water of metabolism	300	0	Skin and lungs (insensible losses)	500–900	30–50
Usual dietary intake*	1500	100	Gastrointestinal	10–100	100
			Renal	300–800	300
Total	1800	0	Total	1800	100

*Represents usual maintenance requirements (*i.e.*, 1500 ml/m²/day of fluids with a tonicity of 100 mOsm/kg or one third isotonic).

of 300 ml/m²/day, making a net loss of 1500 ml/kg/m²/day of approximately 100 mOsm or one third isotonic fluid. This represents maintenance requirements of intravenous fluids. Because solute losses in most circumstances approximate this osmolal relationship and the body induces various compensatory mechanisms, the most common type of dehydration observed in children is isotonic. If *solute* losses are in excess of this relationship, then hypotonic dehydration may result. Conversely, if water losses exceed solute losses, the result will be hypertonic dehydration.

> Maintenance fluid requirements = 1500 ml/m²/day of one third isotonic fluid

Intravenous fluid requirements must take into account the following:

1. Previous losses (as assessed by the degree of dehydration [Table 9–13])
2. Maintenance fluid requirements (1500 ml/m²/day)
3. Ongoing losses (replaced by equal volume and tonicity)

In general, mild dehydration may require only oral hydration with hypotonic electrolyte solutions (50 to 75 mOsm/kg) if vomiting is not a problem. Moderate and severe dehydration require intravenous replacement, the more severe the volume depletion, the more rapid the replacement (Table 9–14). If isotonic dehydration is present, 0.25 to 0.33% saline in 5% dextrose in water is recommended (except in shock, when isotonic fluids are required).

Correction of hypotonic (hyponatremic) dehydration may be calculated by the following formula:

$$\text{Amount of sodium required} = [\text{sodium deficit}] \times [\text{volume of distribution}] = [135 - \text{serum Na}^+ \text{ observed}] \times [\text{body weight in kg} \times 0.6]$$

Half is added to initial replacement fluids, the remainder over 24 hours. Hyponatremia should not be corrected faster than 5 to 8 mEq/L/12 hr. A general guide to replacement follows:

Serum Sodium (mEq/L)	NaCl Concentration (in D_5W)
130–135	0.25–0.33%
125–130	0.5%
120–125	0.9% (isotonic)
<120	may use 3–5% saline judiciously

Correction of *hypertonic dehydration* depends on the degree of volume contraction. If it is mild to moderate, then very slow correction (*i.e.*, at maintenance rates, ignoring the degree of dehydration) over 2 to 3 days using hypotonic fluids (one sixth to one fourth isotonic) may be attempted. If volume depletion is moderately severe to severe, necessitating large volumes for fluid replacement, intracellular osmotic shifts may occur if hypotonic fluids are chosen and rapidly administered, with resulting cerebral edema and seizures. Thus, isotonic fluids should initially be used to correct only the volume depletion in the first 24 hours. Then fluids at maintenance rates and of gradually decreasing tonicity (isotonic decreasing slowly

Table 9–13. DEGREE OF DEHYDRATION AS PERCENTAGE OF WEIGHT LOSS

	Mild	Moderate	Severe	Shock
Infants	<5%	5–10%	10–15%	>15%
Children	<3%	3–8%	8–12%	>12%

Table 9–14. RATE OF REPLACEMENT THERAPY IN DEHYDRATION

	Moderate	Severe	Shock
½ of replacement	6–8 hours	4–6 hours	20 ml/kg ½ in ½ hour, remainder in 1–2 hours

to one third isotonic) may be given during the next 2 to 3 successive days to lower the serum sodium level gradually.

Metabolic acidosis, the most common acid-base disturbance accompanying dehydration in children, is corrected with sodium bicarbonate when the systemic bicarbonate level is less than 15 mmol/L, using the following formula:

Required bicarbonate = [base deficit] × [volume of distribution (*i.e.*, bicarbonate space)] or
= [desired bicarbonate* − measured bicarbonate] × [body weight kg × 0.5].

One half is given during a 2- to 4-hour period, the remainder over 18 to 24 hours. There is a danger of hypocalcemic tetany or seizures if long-standing acidosis is rapidly and completely corrected. Ongoing or severe acidosis such as salicylate intoxication may require continuous high-dose bicarbonate therapy. There is a danger of inducing hypertonicity, intracerebral hemorrhage, and convulsions, especially in younger children.

Addition of potassium to fluid replacement should not begin until there is evidence of adequate renal function. Usual potassium concentrations (as KCl) added to intravenous fluids vary from 10 to 50 mEq/L.

*Desired bicarbonate should not be greater than 10 mmol above the measured bicarbonate.

Selected Readings

Aoni EF, Lalmand TB, Didier F, et al: Multicystic dysplastic kidney: Natural history, in utero diagnosis, and postnatal follow-up. J Urol 138:1420, 1987.

Gruskin A (guest ed): Pediatric nephrology. Pediatr Clin North Am 34:3, 1987.

Holliday MA, Barrett TM, Vernier RL: Pediatric Nephrology, 2nd ed., Baltimore, Williams & Wilkins, 1987.

Tune BM, Mendoza SA, Brenner BM, et al: Pediatric Nephrology in Contemporary Issues in Nephrology, Vol 12. New York, Churchill Livingstone, 1984.

Vehaskari MD: Asymptomatic hematuria a cause for concern? Pediatr Nephrol 3:240, 1989.

Wolfish NM, McLaine PN, Martin D: Renal vein entrapment syndrome. Clin Nephrol 26:96, 1986.

CHAPTER 10

STONE DISEASE

Roger A. L. Sutton

INCIDENCE AND CLINICAL PRESENTATION

Renal stone disease is the most common upper urinary tract disorder, affecting more than 5% of the North American population at least once, men more commonly than women, and recurring at an average rate of about 10% per year. The most common clinical presentation is with renal colic, and most such episodes terminate with the spontaneous passage of gravel or a small stone. However, renal stones may present with renal pain, hematuria, or symptoms of associated infection. They also may be discovered incidentally on radiography or ultrasonography. Renal colic may resemble other medical conditions; the diagnosis is generally confirmed by the finding of hematuria and by the demonstration of the stone and/or hydronephrosis on a flat plate, excretory urogram, or renal ultrasonogram. Of the common stone types, only uric acid is radiolucent, but uric acid stones are detected by ultrasonography.

SURGICAL CONSIDERATIONS

This chapter emphasizes the diagnosis of the cause of stone formation and the prevention of recurrent stone formation. The surgical management of stone disease requires the involvement of a urologist. It has changed remarkably in the past decade, with advances in endoscopic (transurethral and percutaneous) lithotripsy, including ultrasonic, electrohydraulic, and laser techniques, and in 1980 with the introduction of extracorporeal shock-wave lithotripsy (ESWL). ESWL allows the successful noninvasive treatment of most small stones less than 1 to 2 cm in diameter.[1] Larger stones usually require debulking, for example by percutaneous lithotripsy. Second-generation (and later) extracorporeal shock-wave lithotripters no longer require immersing a patient in a water bath and cause less discomfort, thus requiring less anesthesia. Complications of ESWL include hematuria, renal colic, and occasionally ureteric obstruction by stone debris. Although hematuria is usual after ESWL, overt renal damage is uncommon, but the possibility that subsequent hypertension might result has not been excluded. Not every renal stone requires removal; the physician and patient may choose to leave small asymptomatic renal stones *in situ*.

PATHOGENESIS AND CLASSIFICATION

In order for stones to form in the urinary tract, the urine must be supersaturated with a stone constituent. Natural inhibitors of stone formation are present in normal urine—for example, inhibitors of calcium oxalate stone formation include citrate and the recently recognized glycoprotein inhibitor nephrocalcin. Other constituents may act as promoters—for example, uric acid promotes calcium oxalate stone formation. The mode of action of promoters and inhibitors is not fully understood and may operate at the level of initial formation or nucleation of crystals, crystal growth, or crystal aggregation. For example, there is recent evidence that citrate, in addition to complexing calcium, may be a powerful inhibitor of aggregation of calcium oxalate crystals and may in this way reduce the risk of crystal aggregates becoming arrested during flow down the urinary tract.

Chemical Composition

Renal stones may conveniently be classified by their chemical composition (Table 10–1).

> The opportunity to determine the composition of a stone should never be missed.

Stone analysis may be performed by several techniques, including wet chemical analysis (kits), infrared spectroscopy (which can be semiquantitative), and optical crystallography.

Causes of Stones

Various chemical types of kidney stones, classified according to their causes (Table 10–2), form the basis for investigative protocols for stone patients and for attempts at prevention of stone recurrence.

Table 10–2. CAUSES OF STONE FORMATION

Calcium stones (calcium oxalate and/or phosphate)
- Hypercalciuria
  - Idiopathic hypercalciuria (including hypercalciuria induced by high dietary sodium, calcium, and protein)
  - Primary hyperparathyroidism
  - Sarcoidosis
  - Vitamin D and/or calcium excess (including milk-alkali syndrome)
  - Renal tubular acidosis (RTA type 1)
- Hyperoxaluria
  - Enteric hyperoxaluria
  - Idiopathic hyperoxaluria (including hyperoxaluria related to high dietary oxalate, protein, ascorbic acid)
  - Hereditary hyperoxaluria (types 1, 2, and others)
- Hyperuricosuria
  - Dietary purine excess
- Hypocitraturia
  - Idiopathic
  - Renal tubular acidosis type 1 (complete or incomplete)
  - Acetazolamide ingestion
  - Diarrhea, exercise, high protein intake
- Medullary sponge kidney
- Low urine volume
- Idiopathic calcium stones—no detectable metabolic predisposition

Uric acid stones
- Persistent low urine pH
- Hyperuricosuria (primary and secondary)

Struvite stones
- Urinary tract infection with urease-producing organisms

Cystine stones
- Hereditary cystinuria

Others (see Table 10–1)

INVESTIGATION AND DIAGNOSIS OF THE CAUSE OF STONES

A careful history, together with appropriate laboratory investigations, identifies an underlying cause of stone formation in at least 80% of patients. Physical examination is rarely helpful.

History and Physical Examination

Previous stone episodes should be documented in order to assess the activity of the stone disease. Information should be obtained on previous stone analysis. A positive family history may be obtained in patients with idiopathic hypercalciuria, renal tubular acidosis, cystinuria, gout, and other disorders. A past history of bowel disease or resection or of urinary tract infections or surgery may be important.

Table 10–1. RENAL STONE COMPOSITION

Composition	Approximate % of Stones
Calcium oxalate	75
Calcium phosphate	25
Uric acid	10
Struvite	10
Cystine	1
Others: matrix, artifact, xanthine, ammonium urate, 2,8-dihydroxyadenine, triamterene, silicate	

A diet history is essential in stone patients. It will identify contributing factors such as ingestion of supplements of calcium or vitamin D or C, excess protein and purine intake, excess oxalate intake, or low fluid intake. The assistance of a dietitian is very helpful. Ingestion of acetazolamide (for glaucoma) predisposes to calcium phosphate stones; triamterene may occasionally contribute to stone formation. A past or current history of hypertension may be important in influencing the choice of prophylactic treatment for stones.

Laboratory Investigations

Table 10–3 lists a reasonable minimum laboratory workup for a patient in whom stones are of unknown composition or are known to contain calcium.

> Metabolic investigation (especially 24-hour urine analysis) is best deferred for 2 to 3 months after a stone episode or ESWL, because test results may be temporarily affected.

The information to be derived from these tests includes the following:

Flat Plate, Excretory Urogram and Renal Ultrasonography

Radiologically, calcium stones are denser than bone; cystine and struvite stones are of intermediate density; and uric acid stones are radiolucent. Staghorn calculi are most commonly composed of either struvite or cystine. A excretory urogram will identify anatomic abnormalities that may predispose to urinary tract infection and struvite stones and is essential for the diagnosis of medullary sponge kidney (tubular ectasia). Extensive nephrocalcinosis in association with calculi most commonly occurs in renal tubular acidosis, primary hyperparathyroidism, and medullary sponge kidney.

Urinalysis, Culture, and pH

Struvite ('coffin lid') and cystine (hexagonal) crystals are pathognomic of infection with urease-producing organisms and cystinuria, respectively. Infection with an organism that can be urease producing (Table 10–4), together with a highly alkaline urine (pH >7), strongly suggests that stones may be struvite. Urease-producing organisms may be present in urine cultures at low colony counts (<50,000) but should not be ignored. Stone material obtained at operation should be crushed and cultured. The biofilm matrix secreted by these bacteria may isolate colonies from the urinary environment and contribute to the difficulty in eradication. An early morning urine pH greater than 5.5 in the absence of infection is consistent with type 1 renal tubular acidosis (RTA). In the incomplete form, the patient does not have a systemic acidosis. An acid-loading (ammonium chloride) test is required to confirm the diagnosis. Patients with complete or incomplete type 1 RTA generally have low urinary citrate excretion. Urinary tract infection may also cause hypocitraturia. A persistent urine pH less than 5.5 is commonly present in uric acid stone formers and may be idiopathic or secondary to chronic diarrhea. The nitroprusside test is used to screen for cystinuria. Determinations of 24-hour urinary cystine excretion may be helpful in treating the disease.

Table 10–3. RENAL STONES: LABORATORY INVESTIGATION

Stone analysis
Radiology (flat plate, excretory urogram, ultrasonography)
Urinalysis, culture, urine pH
Qualitative cystine test (cyanide, nitroprusside)*
Blood chemistry
Serum calcium and albumin × 2
Inorganic phosphorus
Urea
Creatinine
Electrolytes
Uric acid
24-hour urine × 2, ambulatory, ingesting normal food and fluid intake
Volume
Creatinine
Calcium
Sodium
Oxalate
Uric acid
Citrate
(Urea)

*Not required if stone analysis has ruled out cystine stones.

Table 10–4. UREASE-PRODUCING ORGANISMS IMPLICATED IN STONE FORMATION

Proteus (all species)
Pseudomonas
Klebsiella
Providencia
Citrobacter diversus
Morganella morganii
Enterobacter cloacae
Ureaplasma urealyticum
Staphylococcus saprophyticus

Blood Chemistry

Hypercalcemia most frequently indicates underlying primary hyperparathyroidism in a stone former, although vitamin D intoxication and sarcoidosis are other possible causes. Hypercalcemia in primary hyperparathyroidism is often long-standing and may be borderline. Repeated values should be obtained, and with high or borderline values parathyroid hormone (PTH) determination is useful, particularly using the new "intact" PTH assays.

> Hypercalcemia with a high PTH level in an active stone former is generally a sufficient basis on which to recommend parathyroid exploratory surgery by an experienced parathyroid surgeon.

The electrolytes may show a hyperchloremic acidosis in type 1 RTA, in an acetazolamide-treated patient, and occasionally in primary hyperparathyroidism. It is associated with low urinary citrate excretion in type 1 RTA (complete or incomplete) and in acetazolamide-treated patients.

Hyperuricemia sometimes accompanies hyperuricosuria but is of little diagnostic value. Hypouricemia is a hallmark of hereditary xanthinuria.

24-hour Urinalysis

Twenty-four-hour urine collections should be made while patients are ingesting their normal diet. Table 10–5 summarizes normal ranges for 24-hour urine composition. Analysis of these urine specimens provides the following information:

Volume. Urine volume is frequently below average (1500 ml/day in adults) in stone patients, indicating a need to increase fluid intake.

Calcium. Hypercalciuria is defined in Table 10–5. The higher the calcium excretion, the greater the risk of stone recurrence. Causes of hypercalciuria include idiopathic hypercalciuria, primary hyperparathyroidism, excess ingestion of calcium or vitamin D, and sarcoidosis. Idiopathic hypercalciuria has been subdivided into so-called absorptive, renal, and other types, but the subdivisions are now believed to have little practical importance. Idiopathic hypercalciuria is exacerbated by high sodium or protein intakes.

Sodium. Urinary sodium level reflects salt intake and is helpful in determining if sodium restriction is indicated.

Oxalate. Oxalate levels may be markedly increased (more than 1.5-fold above the upper limit of normal) in enteric hyperoxaluria (associated with bowel bypass or resection, in which urinary citrate is also low) and in hereditary hyperoxalurias, and it may be mildly increased in patients with idiopathic calcium stone formation.

Table 10–5. NORMAL 24-HOUR URINE COMPOSITION

	Male	Female
Volume (ml)	1500 ml	
Calcium (mmol)	<7.5	<6.25
Oxalate (μmol)	<440	
Uric acid (mmol)	<4.8	<4.5
Citrate (mmol)	>1.0	
Cystine	<60 mg (0.25 mmol)	
Creatinine (mmol)	0.16 mmol/kg/day	

> Small increases in urinary oxalate output may be more important in calcium oxalate stone formation than proportionately similar increases in calcium excretion.

High dietary protein, oxalate, and ascorbic acid, as well as dietary calcium restriction, may contribute to this mild hyperoxaluria. Determination of urinary glycolate, a metabolic precursor of oxalate, at present available mainly in research laboratories, may be helpful in differentiating the various causes of hyperoxaluria. Urinary glycolate level is increased in type 1 hereditary hyperoxaluria and may be increased along with oxalate levels in response to a high protein intake.

Uric Acid. Hyperuricosuria may be exogenous, related to high dietary purine intake, or endogenous, as in gouty urate overproducers. Hyperuricosuria may contribute to both calcium oxalate and uric acid stones.

Citrate. Hypocitraturia may indicate type 1 RTA, acetazolamide ingestion, or other conditions associated with mild acidosis (diarrhea, strenuous exertion, or high protein intake). It may be caused by urinary tract infection. Hypocitraturia is also a frequent finding in idiopathic calcium stone formers.

Creatinine. Creatinine excretion depends on the muscle bulk of the patient and averages about 0.16 mmol/kg/day. Creatinine excretions varying by more than 10% may indicate incomplete 24-hour collections.

Urea. Twenty-four-hour urinary urea excretion may be used as an index of approximate protein intake using the following formula: protein (grams per day) $=$ 0.18 $\times$ mmol urea per day $+$ 14.

Cystine. Twenty-four-hour cystine excretion may be useful in guiding therapy of cystinuria.

MEDICAL PROPHYLAXIS OF STONES

Preventive treatment is available for most of the diagnostic categories of stone formers listed in Table 10–2. The problem for a physician often is to decide how aggressively to treat the disorder. Although stones are painful, they are not life-threatening, and there is therefore a natural reluctance to give therapy that could have long-term serious side effects. For example, although thiazide diuretics or allopurinol may help a substantial proportion of calcium oxalate stone formers, both of these agents have the potential to cause serious side effects. Thiazides may adversely affect lipids and increase the risk of atheroma, and allopurinol may cause severe liver toxicity.

> Stone disease requires very long term treatment, and the current emphasis is on altered diet and fluid intake first, followed by drugs only if necessary.

Aggressiveness of treatment will depend on the frequency of stones and on other factors such as a patient's own inclinations.

An approach to stone prevention in each of the major diagnostic categories is summarized in the paragraphs that follow.

Calcium Stones

Idiopathic Hypercalciuria. Dietary factors that may contribute to hypercalciuria should first be corrected. This approach requires the help of a dietitian. Moderation of the intake of calcium (<800 mg/day), vitamin D (no supplements), sodium (100 mEq/day), and protein (1 g/kg/day) is recommended. If hypercalciuria and stones persist, treatment with a thiazide diuretic may be considered. A dose of chlorthalidone (25 mg PO daily) or hydrochlorothiazide (25 to 50 mg PO daily) may be used. Higher doses appear to be no more effective for stone prevention. Failure to respond to a thiazide diuretic with a lowering of urinary calcium excretion may result from excessive salt intake. Recurrence of stones during thiazide therapy may relate to hypocitraturia secondary to potassium depletion or to maintenance of poor urine volume. Neutral phosphate or potassium citrate has been recommended and may be as effective as thiazide diuretics, but they have not undergone prospective randomized study.

Primary Hyperparathyroidism. The presence of active stone formation in primary hyperparathyroidism is generally regarded as an indication for parathyroid exploration by an experienced parathyroid surgeon.

Enteric Hyperoxaluria. Dietary oxalate restriction should be strictly observed and attempts made to increase urine volume. Sodium bicarbonate or potassium citrate may be used to correct accompanying hypocitraturia; decreased fat intake or cholestyramine may help, as may oral calcium or magnesium supplements. Treatment in enteric hyperoxaluria must be individualized and is often not completely effective. A bowel bypass may ultimately need to be revised to correct stone formation.

Hereditary Hyperoxaluria. Hereditary hyperoxaluria may be helped with oral pyridoxine supplements and neutral phosphate.

Idiopathic Mild Hyperoxaluria. Restriction of dietary protein and oxalate intake is indicated. High-oxalate foods include leafy vegetables (*e.g.*, rhubarb and spinach), chocolate, nuts, unprocessed teas, and some juices (*e.g.*, grapefruit). Dietary calcium restriction may cause mild hyperoxaluria by preventing binding of oxalate to calcium in the gut lumen and, if undertaken, should be accompanied by dietary oxalate restriction.

Hyperuricosuric Calcium Oxalate Stone Formers. Restrict dietary purine intake (meat, fish, and poultry). If this does not correct hyperuricosuria, allopurinol (100 to 300 mg/day) may be required.

Hypocitraturia. Supplementary alkalis, either potassium citrate or sodium bicarbonate (1 to 2 mmol/kg/day), will increase urinary citrate excretion. Potassium citrate may be preferable, because potassium supplements have less tendency than sodium to increase calcium excretion. Potassium citrate (20 to 25 mEq t.i.d.) may be given as K-Lyte or Urocit-K.[3]

Uric Acid Stone Formers. Persistent aciduria is generally a more important contributing cause of uric acid stones than is hyperuricosuria. Thus urinary alkalization, which need only maintain a pH of 6, should be achieved by providing patients with urinary pH paper strips (nitrazine), together with sodium bicarbonate tablets, and determining the dose required to ensure that urine pH is never less than 6.0. In case of special difficulty in increasing the urine pH to 6, which particularly may occur in the early morning, a single dose of acetazolamide (Diamox), 250 mg at bedtime, may be helpful. Continuous use of acetazolamide does not result in urinary alkalinization. In hyperuricosuric patients, allopurinol (100 to 300 mg/day) may be a useful adjunct. Uric acid stones should dissolve *in situ* with this therapy.

Struvite Stones. Struvite stones should be eradicated with ESWL and/or surgery, and then vigorous attempts must be made to control urinary tract infection with antibiotics. Unfortunately, these attempts often fail in patients with an abnormal urinary tract. The drug acetohydroxamic acid, a urease inhibitor excreted in the urine when given orally, can correct the high urine pH and ammonium content despite continuing infection with a urease-producing organism. The drug has some undesirable side effects, but it can be effective in preventing stone growth.[4]

Cystine Stones. A high urine volume secondary to increased fluid intake may occasionally be sufficient to cause stone dissolution. Alkalization may be helpful, but cystine solubility does not increase markedly until pH is greater than 7.5, a level that is difficult to achieve. Continuing cystine stone formation requires drug therapy, generally penicillamine.[3] The dose of penicillamine can be determined by measuring urinary cystine concentrations in its presence. This is cumbersome, and an alternative is to estimate the dose of penicillamine based on daily cystine output. Cystine solubility is approximately 250 mg/L of urine. If a patient excretes 900 mg of cystine per day and has a urine volume of 2 L, sufficient penicillamine is required to complex 400 mg of cystine. Because 250 mg of penicillamine reduces cystine by about 100 mg, this patient would require approximately 4 × 250 mg of penicillamine daily. There is a high incidence of side effects with penicillamine. An alternative agent, alpha-mercaptopropionyl glycine (MPG), may cause fewer side effects.

CASE SUMMARY 1

A 45-year old airline pilot presents with a history of spontaneous passage of three stones in the past 5 years, analyzed as calcium oxalate. X-ray films show an asymptomatic 1-cm-diameter radiopaque stone in the right kidney. Laboratory investigation shows normal results of blood chemistry tests, urinalysis, and culture. Two 24-hour urine specimens collected while the patient was ingesting his normal diet had volumes of 1500 and 1600 ml, calcium of 9.8 and 10.3 mmol, sodium of 180 and 210 mmol, uric acid of 6.1 and 6.3 mmol, oxalate of 350 and 390 μmol, and citrate of 2.9 and 3.5 mmol.

Thus, this patient has hypercalciuria associated with a high urinary sodium and uric acid output.

Diet survey indicated a normal calcium intake (800 mg/day), a high protein intake, and a predilection for salty food.

The patient was advised to increase his fluid intake (eight 8-ounce glasses of water per day) and to decrease sodium and protein intake. He was also referred to a urologist for consideration of ESWL, in view of his occupation.

He returned to the clinic 2 months later, following ESWL. Twenty-four-hour urinary uric acid and sodium excretion were now normal, but urinary calcium remained 9 mmol/24 hours. In view of persisting hypercalciuria and his occupation, treatment with chlorthalidone (25 mg PO daily) was recommended and resulted in correction of the hypercalciuria. He has not formed further renal calculi.

CASE SUMMARY 2

Mary K. is now 48 years old. She had two stones at age 40 and 47. The first passed spontaneously, and the second required ESWL. Stone analysis showed calcium oxalate and phosphate. Urine culture was sterile. Laboratory investigations showed serum levels of calcium to be 2.9 and 2.8 mmol, phosphate 0.8 mmol, creatinine 75 mmol, sodium 140 mmol, potassium 4.0 mmol, chloride 100 mmol, and CO_2 24 mmol. Twenty-four-hour urine volume was 2010 ml; urine content of calcium was 9.2 mmol, sodium 98 mmol, uric acid 3.0 mmol, oxalate 220 μmol, citrate 3 mmol, and creatinine 8.9 mmol.

This woman has hypercalcemia and hypercalciuria. She has no history of excessive calcium or vitamin D intake. Further investigation showed "intact" PTH, 15 pmol/L (normal $<$ 10). Ultrasonography of the neck showed an enlarged right lower parathyroid gland. Mary K. underwent successful removal of a right lower parathyroid adenoma. Follow-up 3 months later showed normocalcemia and normocalciuria.

CASE SUMMARY 3

Jacob S. is a 30-year-old man with a history of numerous episodes of renal colic with spontaneous stone passage in the past 5 years. Stones were analyzed as calcium phosphate. X-ray film showed extensive bilateral nephrocalcinosis. Early morning urine had a pH of 6.0 and was sterile on culture. Blood chemistry determinations showed calcium 2.1 mmol, phosphorus 0.9 mmol, sodium 136 mmol, potassium 2.5 mmol, chloride 110 mmol, CO_2 18 mmol, and creatinine 90 mmol. Twenty-four-hour urine volume was 2346 ml; urine content of sodium was 101 mmol, potassium 115 mmol, calcium 7.5 mmol, oxalate 300 mmol, citrate 0.1 mmol, creatinine 10.6 mmol, and uric acid 3.1 mmol. This man has a low plasma bicarbonate concentration, hyperchloremia, and hypokalemia. Blood gases showed a compensated metabolic acidosis. These findings are typical of type 1 RTA. Jacob S. also has calcium phosphate stones (which are more frequent than calcium oxalate in RTA), borderline hypercalciuria, and marked hypocitraturia.

Treatment was initiated with sodium bicarbonate 6 g/day (1 mmol/kg/day). Serum electrolytes normalized (potassium 4.0 mmol, bicarbonate 24 mmol), but urinary citrate remained low (0.8 mmol/day). An increase in the sodium bicarbonate level to 12 g/day was associated with normal serum electrolytes and correction of hypocitraturia (2.0 mmol/day). On this treatment, further stone formation has not occurred, but nephrocalcinosis persists.

CASE SUMMARY 4

This 28-year-old man has a long-standing history of Crohn's disease, for which extensive small-bowel resection has been performed. He has had three renal calculi in the past 6 months. He has chronic diarrhea requiring symptomatic treatment and is also receiving prednisone therapy. Stone analysis shows calcium oxalate. Blood chemistry evaluation shows normal concentrations of calcium, creatinine, and sodium; potassium is 3.0 mmol; total CO_2 is 20 mmol, and magnesium is 0.6 mmol. Twenty-four-hour urine volume is 750 ml; content of urine sodium is 50 mmol, potassium 55 mmol, calcium 2 mmol, magnesium 1.1 mmol, oxalate 1100 μmol, citrate 0.3 mmol, creatinine 9.5 mmol, and uric acid 3.0 mmol.

This man has a low urine volume, hyperoxaluria, hypocitraturia, and a low urinary output of sodium, potassium, calcium, and magnesium, presumably associated with malabsorption. Stone prophylaxis was recommended with an increase of fluid intake (to the limit of toleration), strict dietary oxalate restriction, and treatment with potassium citrate (25 mEq t.i.d.). One month later, 24-hour urine volume was 1500 ml; the content of urine sodium was 60 mmol; potassium was 100 mmol; calcium was 2.5 mmol; magnesium was 1.2 mmol; oxalate was 500 μmol; citrate was 2.5 mmol; creatinine was 9.0 mmol; and uric acid was 4.0 mmol.

On this treatment, the patient has shown no evidence of further stone formation during the following year. However, he has persistent mild hyperoxaluria with diarrhea and steatorrhoea.

CASE SUMMARY 5

This 55-year-old man has a long history of gout. He presents with hematuria and renal pain. Flat plate shows no stone. Ultrasonography shows a stone in the right renal pelvis. Intravenous pyelography shows a filling defect lying free in the right renal pelvis. Blood chemistry evaluation shows normal levels of calcium, phosphate, urea, creatinine, and electrolytes. Uric acid level is elevated. Twenty-four-hour urine collection shows normal levels of sodium, calcium, citrate, oxalate, creatinine, and uric acid.

The patient is presumed to have a uric acid stone, probably associated with persistent low urine pH. Serial urine pH through a 24-hour period showed that the pH was persistently 5.5 or less.

Treatment with sodium bicarbonate was recommended. The patient determined that 6 g of sodium bicarbonate taken in four divided doses was sufficient to keep his urine pH at or above 6 throughout the 24 hours. On this therapy, the presumed uric acid stone apparently dissolved, because it did not pass and was no longer demonstrable on ultrasonography after 2 months. He has remained stone free.

CASE SUMMARY 6

This 22-year-old woman passed one small stone 1 year previously. The stone was not analyzed. She presented with renal pain and on ultrasonography had a stone in the right kidney. On a flat plate, the stone was radiopaque. She was referred for ESWL. Blood chemistry determinations were normal. Urinalysis showed cystine crystals. Analysis of stone debris following lithotripsy showed cystine. Twenty-four-hour urinary cystine excretion was 1.1 g/day. Following treatment with lithotripsy, the patient was stone free. A high fluid intake was recommended, but she was unable to maintain a daily urine output greater than 2 L. Potassium citrate was given for urine alkalization. Ultrasonography after 6 months showed reappearance of a renal stone, and a repeat 24-hour urine collection again showed 1.1 g of cystine. Penicillamine therapy was recommended, increasing to a dose of 6 × 250 mg daily based on the estimation that 2 L of urine would hold 500 mg of cystine in solution, requiring complexing of the remaining 600 mg by penicillamine. Penicillamine was introduced gradually and with appropriate monitoring of the blood count and of the urine for protein, but no adverse side effects were noted. Three years later, the woman is stone free, on penicillamine, and under regular supervision in the stone clinic.

References

1. Finlayson B, and Thomas WC Jr: Extracorporeal shock wave lithotripsy. Ann Intern Med 101:387, 1984.
2. Lingeman JE, Woods JR, Toth PD: Blood pressure changes following extracorporeal shock wave lithotripsy and other forms of treatment for nephrolithiasis. JAMA 263:1789, 1990.
3. Pak CYC (ed): Renal Stone Disease. Pathogenesis, Prevention and Treatment. Boston, Marthinus Nijhoff Publishing, 1987.
4. Williams JJ, Rodman JS, Peterson CM: A randomized double-blind study of acetohydroxamic acid in struvite nephrolithiasis. N Engl J Med 311:760, 1984.

Selected Readings

Coe FL, Parks JH (eds): Nephrolithiasis: Pathogenesis and Treatment, 2nd ed. Chicago, Yearbook Medical Publishers, 1988.

Sutton RAL (guest ed): Symposium on Urolithiasis. Mineral and Electrolyte Metabolism 13:209–304, 1987.

CHAPTER 11

EDEMATOUS STATES AND HEPATORENAL SYNDROME

Mortimer Levy

EDEMA

The extracellular fluid (ECF) is normally partitioned so that about 25% of the total circulates within the vascular compartment as plasma and the remainder (75%) is found within the interstitial space and lymphatics. A tendency toward hypovolemia is defended against by the retention of urinary sodium and by readjusting the transvascular partitioning of ECF to permit less ultrafiltration from capillaries or augmented capillary reabsorption from the interstitial space, as well as mobilization of lymphatic fluid into the venous compartment. Hypervolemia is defended against by increasing the urinary excretion of salt and water and by increasing ultrafiltration of plasma so that more plasma saline is shunted into the interstitial space.

The physiologic factors normally regulating the transvascular partitioning of ECF are collectively called the Starling forces. These include capillary hydrostatic pressure, plasma colloid oncotic pressure, and free fluid interstitial hydrostatic pressure. Other contributing factors are oncotic pressure within the interstitial fluid, integrity of the capillary wall, hydraulic conductivity of the capillary endothelium, surface area of capillaries available for ultrafiltration, and the efficiency of regional lymphatic flow.

Edema may be defined as an excess of fluid within the interstitial or nonvascular space of a given organ that is detectable by visual or other clinical means. Edema may be subcutaneous within the lower extremities (which is what most physicians think of when they think of edema) but may also be localized to the periorbital, digital, or presacral areas or to the lungs or a serous cavity (*e.g.*, ascities within the peritoneal space). Edema appears when the volume of fluid leaving capillaries overwhelms the ability to return it to the vascular compartment. Edema may be localized to a given vascular territory or may have the potential for occurring in all vascular beds. Localized edema may result from the following conditions:

1. Excess arteriolar inflow (*e.g.*, immersing hands in warm water)
2. Venous hypertension (*e.g.*, venous obstruction)
3. Localized change in capillary permeability (*e.g.*, angioedema)
4. Localized lymphatic obstruction

In clinical practice, the most common cause of true localized edema is venous hypertension. However, **localized edema may appear as the first manifestation of generalized edema, largely because normal postural considerations cause relative venous hypertension of the lower extremities.**

Collections of true localized edema (*e.g.*, associated with thrombophlebitis) rarely if ever are associated with significant perturbations to circulating plasma volume or to neuroendocrine disturbances such as increased plasma levels of renin, aldosterone, or catecholamines or mobilization of the sympathetic nervous system. This is probably because the fluid losses in localized edema from the vascular compartment are usually modest and because interstitial fluid from uninvolved areas may be mobilized to replenish the vascular compartment and so correct any tendency toward hypovolemia.

Generalized Edema

Although localized causes of edema such as venous obstruction or lymphatic obstruction may cause extensive accumulation of extravascular fluid, the edema is generally confined to the involved vascular territories. In disease states associated with generalized edema, the potential for edema exists for all vascular territories, although edema will not be found in all areas of the body because of postural considerations (*i.e.*, ease of venous drainage for areas above the heart and difficulty of venous return for areas below the heart).

The more important generalized edema states are listed in Table 11–1.

Because edema is a syndrome and has multiple causes, the associated clinical features vary depending on the underlying disease. However, certain physiologic disturbances are common to all generalized edema states (Table 11–2).

In order for generalized edema to accumulate, three conditions must be fulfilled. First, there must be a sufficient disturbance at the level of the capillary bed to force large volumes of fluid out of the vascular compartment. Because the disease states causing edema tend to be chronic and the Starling forces must therefore undergo gradual perturbation, it seems clear that the disturbed Starling forces sufficient to force fluid out of the circulation must be an end-state phenomenon. Second, **for detectable edema to accumulate, urinary sodium retention must occur to continually replenish the vascular compartment.** This is because in generalized edema the tendency for fluid to leave the circulation is widespread over an extensive vascular territory. Were it not for continuous sodium retention and replenishment of the circulating plasma, volume contraction would soon bring edema formation to an end. This tendency for urinary sodium retention maintains normal or even expanded plasma volume in most of the edema states. Third, the interstitial compartment must be able to accept large volumes of edema. Under normal physiologic conditions there exist various "safety" factors that ensure that the interstitial space is kept "dry." Only when these factors are overwhelmed (*e.g.*, by limited drainage ability of regional lymphatics) will detectable volumes of fluid collect within the interstitial space as edema.

Table 11–1. SOME COMMON CAUSES OF GENERALIZED EDEMA

Diseases of the kidney
Acute and chronic renal failure
Acute glomerulonephritis
Nephrotic syndrome
Cirrhosis of the liver
Heart failure
Cyclical edema of women
Capillary-leak syndromes
Drugs (e.g., minoxidil, estrogens)

Table 11–2. PHYSIOLOGIC DISTURBANCES IN EDEMA STATES

Reduction in urinary sodium and water excretion
Plasma volume expansion (at least in preedema phase)
Bilateral ankle swelling (ascites with cirrhosis; periorbital and digital edema with nephrotic syndrome)
Nocturnal cough and dyspnea when supine
Weight gain
Nocturia
Exertional dyspnea
Pallor
Fatigue, lassitude

All of these conditions suggest that there is usually an extensive period of sodium retention before the formation of edema, because the Starling forces deteriorate over a period of time and the safety margin within the interstitial space presumably takes some time to become overwhelmed.

Incipient Edema

In most of the syndromes associated with generalized edema, the pathophysiologic disturbances occur slowly over at least several months. During this interval of time, sufficient salt and water may be retained to increase body weight, but may not yet appear as clinically obvious edema. Indeed, some 4 to 5 L of fluid may accumulate in the ECF before patients or their physicians might actually observe pitting edema. During this interval and depending on the magnitude of dietary salt intake, the following symptoms of incipient edema may be elicited with careful questioning: weight gain; exaggerated diurnal swings in weight; nocturia; cough and/or dyspnea in supine position; increasing fatigue and dyspnea on exertion; relative oliguria; subjective symptoms: "shoes too tight," "rings too tight"; and periorbital edema on awakening.

Therapy of Edema

Although specific therapy for the specific edema states will be discussed in detail later in this chapter, several general principles may be applied to the treatment protocols of *all* edema states. Such therapeutic options are discussed in the paragraphs that follow.

Dietary Manipulation

Because urinary retention of salt and water is characteristic of patients who are actively forming edema, attention must be closely paid to dietary intake. If the kidneys are capable of excreting only 40 to 50 mEq of sodium per day because of flagrant nephrotic syndrome or congestive heart failure (CHF), dietary intake in excess of this amount will simply be retained to add to the edema. In patients who have entered a phase of active edema formation, and particularly those who are proving refractory to therapy, it is not inappropriate to document daily urinary excretion of sodium and to adjust the diet accordingly. In practical terms, for ambulatory patients, it is very difficult to reduce sodium intake below 30 to 40 mEq/day. Less stringent curtailment, on the order of 50 to 60 mEq/day, is often sufficient to ameliorate the situation, however. Reduction of salt intake often permits patients to achieve sodium balance. Restriction of salt intake is particularly effective in dialysis-independent uremic patients. **Because in stable chronic renal failure urinary excretion of salt and water often remains fixed and at high values, dietary curtailment of salt and water intake often leads to rapid clearing of the edema, even without diuretics and particularly if a patient is given bed rest to help mobilize the edema.**

In planning dietary restriction of sodium, it is helpful to recall that 1 g of NaCl contains 17 mEq sodium whereas 1 g of sodium contains 43 mEq Na^+. By avoiding the salt shaker at meal time and by omitting salt from the preparation of foods and cooking water, as well as avoiding prepared and preserved foodstuffs that are notoriously high in salt, dietary sodium intake can easily be reduced to the order of 50 to 70 mEq/day.

For those patients who cannot tolerate a reduction in dietary salt but who feel they must have it, salt substitutes are available. These usually contain potassium salts, however, and great care must be taken before they are used in the presence of oliguric states or uremia and with concomitant use of potassium-sparing diuretics or angiotensin-converting enzyme (ACE) inhibitors.

Postural Considerations

When a human assumes the orthostatic position from the supine, some 700 to 800 ml of blood that has been below the diaphragm (when gravity has no effect on the circulation) is mobilized and returns to the central thorax. Bed rest, particularly with leg elevation, is an effective way of initiating diuresis and natriuresis (central activation of volume receptors) and thereby mobilizing edema. Indeed, there is some evidence that slight head-down posture is even more effective in refractory cases.

Ultrafiltration

The widespread availability of various procedures for the rapid removal of edema means that ultrafiltration from the vascular compartment can be achieved either rapidly for life-threatening pulmonary edema or more slowly for anasarca, which is not particularly life-threatening. Acute peritoneal dialysis with 2.5 or 4.25% glucose solutions using 30- to 40-minute dwell times is one technique available; another would be continuous arteriovenous hemofiltration using ultrapermeable cartridges. These techniques, particularly the latter, can easily remove 400 to 1500 ml/hr. Ultrafiltration using dialysis equipment is another option for rapid fluid removal.

Diuretics

Diuretics inhibit sodium reabsorption within the nephrons and increase the percentage of glomerular filtrate that is excreted as urine. The subsequent decrement in plasma volume and rise in colloid oncotic pressure then permit the mobilization of edema from the interstitial space into the vascular compartment, where it becomes available for renal excretion. The diuretic response has thus been translated into a mobilization response. Because any edema state imposes physiologic restrictions on the ease with which fluid may be returned to the vascular compartment, as a result of either the elevated venous pressures or reduced colloid oncotic pressures (or both in combination), overzealous diuresis poses the danger of producing hypovolemia. If this occurs, renal perfusion may then decline and the diuresis may come to an end. In addition to prerenal failure, relative hypotension (with further orthostatic decline) and biochemical features peculiar to hypovolemia may ensue (*e.g.*, hyponatremia, hyperuricemia, hypokalemia, or hyperkalemia if sufficient azotemia and oliguria supervene). The complications of overzealous diuresis are summarized in Table 11–3. The nonhemodynamic complications of diuretics are summarized in Table 11–4.

Features of the diuretics most commonly used today are summarized in Table 11–5.

Table 11–3. COMPLICATIONS ASSOCIATED WITH DIURETIC-INDUCED FLUID LOSSES

Azotemia
Hypotension with orthostatic exaggeration
Dizziness if hypotension with orthostatic exaggeration is sufficiently severe
Hypercalcemia
Hyperuricemia
Hyponatremia
Magnesium depletion
Hypokalemia and metabolic alkalosis (hyperkalemia and acidosis with potassium-sparing agents)
Weakness and easy fatigability

Another diuretic sometimes used is acetazolamide (Diamox). This agent, acting on the proximal tubule and producing a bicarbonate diuresis, is sometimes used in intoxications to alkalize the urine, or to treat hyperuricosuric states or even alkalemia. It has no place in the routine therapy of edema.

The potassium-sparing diuretics must be used cautiously in the elderly, particularly if they are obese or diabetic, because of the potential for provoking type 4 renal tubular acidosis (RTA) and for aggravating hyperkalemia. They should *not* be used with ACE inhibitors because of the property of these antihypertensive drugs to increase serum potassium levels (inhibition of aldosterone effect). Because they act at the most distal nephron sites, where perhaps only 1 to 2% of the available filtered sodium load is available for tubular reabsorption, they are, of necessity, weak diuretics. **Their major uses are in the conservation of potassium and for causing mild sodium loss when a gentle diuresis is necessary to preserve the physiologic status of a patient (*e.g.*, with cirrhosis of the liver).**

Principles of Diuretic Management

Except for life-threatening situations (*e.g.*, acute pulmonary edema), diuresis should be judicious and fluid loss should probably not exceed 1 kg/day lest the problems of hypovolemia (described earlier) become predominant. Diuresis should proceed at a pace that allows adequate mobilization from the extravascular compartment to keep up with diuretic-induced losses from the circulation.

Table 11–4. COMPLICATIONS OF DIURETICS UNRELATED TO FLUID LOSSES

Hyperglycemia
Hyperlipidemia
Acute pancreatitis (thiazide group)
Skin rashes
Acute interstitial nephritis (thiazide, furosemide, triamterene)
Intratubular crystallization (stones)—triamterene
Gastrointestinal upset
Ototoxicity (furosemide)

Patients should preferably maintain bed rest and continue dietary salt curtailment to maximize the beneficial effects of the diuretics.

Edema of the gastrointestinal mucosa is often present and may reduce absorption of oral medication from the gastrointestinal tract. If a patient is proving refractory to oral medication in the presence of extensive edema that could be affecting the gastrointestinal mucosa, it may be worthwhile to switch to intravenous administration.

When a patient is proving refractory to a single diuretic (usually loop active), it may be wise to add a diuretic thought to be active at other sites. Useful additions include metolazone and other thiazides. Metolazone is thought to act at the level of the proximal convoluted tubule, as well as the cortical diluting site. Moreover, unlike other thiazides, metolazone continues to be active even when the GFR is quite depressed (<35 ml/min). In this way, extra sodium is delivered to the loops of Henle, which may then be acted on by the loop-active diuretic. A thiazide added to a loop-active diuretic such as furosemide often augments the natriuresis.

Specific maneuvers in specific disease states will often potentiate the use of diuretics. These include (1) placing a pregnant woman in the third trimester in the left lateral position to improve renal hemodynamics; (2) reduction of afterload in patients suffering from CHF with ACE inhibitors or other vasodilators, which often improves renal perfusion and suboptimal diuresis; (3) infusion of ascites or albumin solutions to cirrhotic patients before initiating diuresis; and (4) keeping a woman with idiopathic cyclical edema at bed rest while initiating diuresis.

Once "dry weight" has been reached, one should consider stopping the diuretic, reducing the dose, or even administering the drug on alternate days to minimize diuretic side effects.

As noted earlier, great care should be used when giving potassium-sparing diuretics so that concomitant clinical circumstances do not produce life-threatening hyperkalemia.

Treatment of Underlying Disorder

In addition to manipulating dietary salt, diuretic regimens, and activity, it is worthwhile

Table 11–5. FEATURES OF COMMONLY USED DIURETICS

Common Brand Name	Generic Name	Usual Dosages	Remarks
Hydrodiuril	Hydrochlorothiazide	25–100 mg q.d.	Not recommended if GFR <35 ml/min. Oral dose active within 2 hr, beware of hypokalemia and hyponatremia.
Hygroton	Chlorthalidone	50–100 mg q.d. or alternating days	Long acting, >24 hr. Not recommended for routine use.
Lasix	Furosemide	20–80 mg q.d.	Rapid onset; <0.5 hr; potent; effective when GFR <35 ml/min. Effects last 6 hr.
Edecrin	Ethacrynic acid	50–150 mg q.d.	Similar for furosemide Longer acting (~8 hr).
Zaroxolyn	Metolazone	1–10 mg q.d.	Effective with GFR <35 ml/min. Potentiates action of loop-active diuretics. May cause profound diuresis and hypokalemia in susceptible patients.
Potassium-sparing agents			
1. Aldactone	Spironolactone	25–100 mg q.i.d.	Gradual onset (2–3 days). Not recommended when GFR <25 ml/min. Danger of hyperkalemia and acidosis.
2. Midamor	Amiloride	5–20 mg q.d.	Contraindicated when GFR <25 ml/min. May cause hyperkalemia. Effects may last 2–24 hr.
3. Dyrenium	Triamterene	100–300 mg q.d.	Contraindicated when GFR <25 ml/min. Long lasting, up to 16 hr. May cause hyperkalemia. Blood dyscrasias, triamterene stones, and interstitial nephritis may be a problem.
4. Dyazide	Triamterene/ hydrochlorothiazide mixture	50 mg 1 tab b.i.d. 25 mg	Commonly used in family practice when potassium sparing desired. Should not be used with K^+ supplements or other potassium-sparing agents. Avoid use when GFR <35 ml/min. Incidence of hyperkalemia rises with increasing age.

to direct specific therapy to treatment of each of the underlying disorders responsible for generalized edema. Thus in CHF, depending on clinical circumstances, the use of digoxin, antihypertensives, and ACE inhibitors for afterload reduction, together with antiarrhythmic agents, might be indicated as well as agents to augment coronary artery perfusion.

In nephrotic syndrome, adjustment of protein intake and the use of specific agents such as prednisone and cyclophosphamide may be indicated to treat the underlying glomerulopathy.

In cirrhosis of the liver, refractory ascites may respond to LeVeen valve shunting.

Many centers have begun to perform large-volume (about 4.0 L) paracentesis every second or third day, supplemented by intravenous albumin infusion to make up for the protein loss. This has proved to be an effective and safe way to control tense ascites.

There is also great advantage to converting tense ascites to soft ascites. By relieving excessive pressure on the abdominal vena cava, venous return and therefore cardiac output may be increased, and a previous refractory response may then prove amenable to the same diuretics.

It must be remembered in treating severe edema that major physiologic constraints (*e.g.*, venous hypertension) and/or a reduction in the serum albumin level will limit mobilization of interstitial fluid into the vascular compartment. **Therefore, any maneuver that tends to empty the vascular space (*e.g.*, diuretics or ultrafiltration) must be done sufficiently cautiously to prevent significant hypovolemia with subsequent hypotension and reduced renal perfusion.**

CASE SUMMARY 1

A 56-year-old obese man who had been an insulin-dependent diabetic for 22 years presented to hospital with severe dyspnea and extensive anasarca. He was found to have ascites, right pleural effusion, and 4+ edema of the lower extremities. Examination revealed a blood pressure of 210/118 mm Hg, pulse rate of 96/min, jugular venous distention, and rales in both lung bases. Urinary protein was 4+, and the sediment was "active." Blood urea nitrogen (BUN) was 30 mg/dl, serum creatinine level was 1.92 mg/dl, and serum albumin level was 3.0 g/dl.

Although the referring physician's initial impression was that the patient had nephrotic syndrome (secondary to diabetes), it was clear that more than a glomerulopathy was present. The elevated venous pressure and pulmonary edema in the presence of hypertension and a relatively well-preserved serum albumin level suggested that CHF rather than nephrotic syndrome was largely responsible for the edema. Subsequent therapy with antihypertensive drugs, diuretics, bed rest, and control of dietary salt intake was associated with rapid clearing of the edema. Although serum creatinine level initially rose to 2.2 mg/dl, it decreased to 1.65 mg/dl several weeks later. Unless specifically contraindicated, use of ACE inhibitors would be expected to reduce arterial pressures, improve cardiac output, and reduce urinary protein losses.

HEPATORENAL SYNDROME

Physicians have long recognized that there is an intimate relationship between severe hepatobiliary disease and acute renal failure (ARF). Unfortunately, these relationships have often been poorly defined, so that the term hepatorenal syndrome (HRS) has been inappropriately applied. We now recognize, for example, that the ARF frequently accompanying acute obstructive jaundice (particularly if a patient is subjected to surgery) most often takes the form of acute tubular necrosis (ATN) and is less commonly functional in nature. The cause of ATN in this setting is not clear but probably includes a combination of factors, such as volume contraction, sepsis, endotoxemia, and jaundice.

HRS does not develop in acute biliary disorders and usually occurs in a clinical setting of advanced alcoholic cirrhosis with ascites. It may also be present in severe acute viral hepatitis, in fulminating alcoholic hepatitis, in Budd-Chiari syndrome, and in some patients with hepatic cancer, as well as in other circumstances where there is acute and severe primary liver damage.

In a setting of severe liver disease, usually alcoholic cirrhosis of the liver, HRS may be defined as the onset of acute, progressive renal failure that shows two major features: (1) there is no apparent clinical cause for the renal failure, and (2) the biochemical features of the urine indicate the presence of functional prerenal failure. This latter aspect implies severe underperfusion of the nephron mass.

This definition excludes clinical events such as polyarteritis, leptospirosis, shock, or drug intoxication, in which both the liver and kidneys may be the target of some common insult, but implies that the ARF is due to marked renal underperfusion brought about by some singular cause of renal vasoconstriction that is presumably related to the advanced liver failure.

Pathophysiology

The term HRS is widely abused and is often applied incorrectly to cases of ARF occurring in the presence of liver disease. The basis for such imprecision lies in the clinical setting in which HRS most commonly occurs, alcoholic cirrhosis of the liver with ascites. Consider the major pathophysiologic features involved. As alcoholic cirrhosis progresses, partial obstruction to hepatic venous outflow develops, eventually causing portal venous hypertension. As liver function continues to deteriorate, hypoalbuminemia supervenes. Because of these and other factors, large amounts of hepatic and splanchnic lymph form and cannot be drained away to the venous system by the regional lymphatics and thoracic duct. The overflow collects in the peritoneal space as ascites. We thus have a situation in which large volumes of blood may be sequestered within the mesenteric venous circulation and large volumes of fluid may be sequestered as a third space within the peritoneal compartment. These events will lead to progressive arterial hypovolemia, which is invariably compounded by poor dietary intake of salt.

Once a patient is hypovolemic, the only reasonable source for vascular replenishment is the large ascitic depot. The disturbed Starling forces existent in the portal circulation (venous hypertension and low colloid osmotic pressure), however, do not favor reabsorption of ascites into the vascular compartment; indeed, continuing filtration of fluid is more likely to occur. Thus, by the very nature of the underlying disease, cirrhotic patients are prone to develop significant arterial hypovolemia. If, in this clinical setting, a prerenal type of ARF develops, it is grossly misleading to label this HRS, for there are clearly identifiable causes of the renal ischemia. **In other words, conferring a diagnosis of HRS on a cirrhotic patient suffering from arterial volume depletion is no more helpful than using the term *cardiorenal syndrome* to describe a patient who has severe CHF and progresses to ARF on a prerenal basis.** Strictly speaking, therefore, the diagnosis of HRS should be reserved for those circumstances in which renal underperfusion is not due to arterial hypovolemia but rather due to some unique cause of selective intrarenal vasoconstriction.

Selective Renal Vasoconstriction: Possible Causes

Several lines of evidence suggest that a primary increase in intrarenal vascular resistance is the major cause of HRS.

Tristani and Cohn infused large volumes of iso-oncotic dextran into cirrhotic patients with oliguric renal failure. One group, clearly hypovolemic, responded to the infusion with an increase in cardiac output, a decrease in systemic vascular resistance, and a rise in renal blood flow. A second group, with higher plasma volumes, failed to respond with a change in cardiac output (already normal), systemic vascular resistance, or renal blood flow. Therefore, there clearly is a group of cirrhotic patients with oliguric ARF in whom volume contraction is not the cause of renal ischemia, but rather is selective renal vasoconstriction. Even in a group of patients who did respond to acute volume expansion with a marked increment in cardiac output and renal perfusion, renal vasoconstriction often persisted, requiring the local intraarterial infusion of vasodilators to restore renal blood flow toward normal.

Epstein and colleagues have demonstrated that the renal blood flow in patients with HRS does not correlate with the level of cardiac output. Using radioactive xenon washout techniques, these investigators were able to demonstrate that comparable reductions of renal cortical blood flow were found in patients with either high or low cardiac output. This situation (*i.e.*, in HRS) is unlike that found in patients with another basic cause of arterial hypovolemia, congestive heart failure, in which cortical flow does correlate directly with cardiac output.

If cirrhotic patients with HRS are subjected to portal venous decompression by surgical means, renal perfusion often remains fixed despite large increments in cardiac output.

On removal of the diseased liver and transplantation of a healthy liver, the kidney commences forming urine. Alternatively, a kidney that is removed from a cirrhotic patient and transplanted into a new host will attain normal function.

Selective angiography of the kidneys in patients with HRS reveals intense diffuse vasoconstriction. If this procedure is repeated postmortem, the vasculature is seen to be quite normal.

If local vasoconstrictor influences are the primary determinant of renal ischemia in HRS, what factors might mediate the vasoconstrictor response?

Table 11–6 summarizes the suggested possible causes of selective renal vasoconstriction in HRS. A discussion of the merits of each of these possibilities is beyond the scope of this chapter, and interested readers should consult recent reviews on this topic. At present, the view held by most investigators is that renal perfusion in health (and disease) is maintained by modulating vasoconstrictor influences of catecholamines and angiotensin II with the vasodilating influence of intrarenal prostaglandins and other autocoids such as kinins. It has been suggested that if the intrarenal generation of vasodilator prostaglandins declines, unopposed vasoconstriction may cause HRS in a clinical setting of cirrhosis. Although there is some support for this view, this hypothesis is somewhat controversial and at the moment must be considered speculative. **No matter what the exact cause(s) of renal vasoconstriction, it is important to emphasize that HRS cannot be diagnosed unless it is reasonably clear that arterial hypovolemia has been ruled out as a likely cause of the renal ischemia.** Studies have emphasized the possible role of efferent renal sympathetic nerves and the augmented intrarenal generation of vasoconstrictor prostaglandins (thromboxanes).

Clinical Features

Table 11–7 summarizes the major clinical features usually observed in HRS. In North

Table 11–6. POSSIBLE CAUSES OF SELECTIVE RENAL VASOCONSTRICTION IN HEPATORENAL SYNDROME

Endotoxemia
Increased sympathetic activity and circulating catecholamines
Increased activity of the renin-angiotensin system
Hepatic encephalopathy
False neurotransmitters
Decreased intrarenal vasodilator prostaglandins or kinins
Increased intrarenal vasoconstrictor prostaglandins
Release of unidentified humoral agents from diseased liver

Table 11–7. HEPATORENAL SYNDROME: MAJOR CLINICAL FEATURES

Usually occurs only in hospitalized patients
No apparent clinical cause
Ascites usually present
No consistent relationship to jaundice
May be a temporal relationship to advent of hepatic encephalopathy
Marked oliguria is present
Relative hypotension may be present

America, HRS occurs in an overwhelming number of patients with alcoholic cirrhosis of the liver. It is rarely observed in ambulatory patients (except those with alcoholic hepatitis) and usually occurs once a cirrhotic patient has been admitted to the hospital. It must be emphasized, however, that because of profound and extensive muscle atrophy usually observed in these patients, the serum creatinine level does not accurately reflect GFR. It has been determined as well that creatinine clearance in these patients probably overestimates true GFR by approximately 20%. **Thus, ambulatory out-of-hospital patients with severe cirrhosis but without overt oliguria may already have a profound reduction in GFR despite apparently normal levels of serum creatinine.** The worsening of kidney function once admitted to hospital suggests that a reduction in salt intake and/or excessive diuresis by a managing physician may in reality be inducing relative arterial hypovolemia in a patient already partially volume contracted and with some degree of renal failure already present. Sequential observations in cirrhotic patients over many months and even years indicate that blood volume tends to decrease (from expanded levels), and this decrement is accompanied by the appearance of azotemia.

Oliguria as an isolated finding, without a progressive rise in serum levels of creatinine or BUN, does not imply ARF. There are many causes of oliguria in cirrhotic patients (poor dietary intake of salt, protein, and calories; inability of the liver to form urea; some degree of arterial hypovolemia; increased plasma levels of vasopressin and aldosterone), and low urinary output may be physiologic, considering a patient's condition. Only if the oliguria is accompanied by progressive azotemia or if there is a depressed value for creatinine clearance can a diagnosis of ARF be made.

It is difficult to know the true incidence of HRS in cirrhotic patients because the syndrome has been defined so many different ways and there may be so many different causes of renal failure. Probably 40 to 80% of all hospitalized cirrhotic patients have some degree of renal failure. True HRS is probably found in only 10 to 20% of those patients who present with ARF; the remainder probably have prerenal failure. A large teaching hospital (600 to 900 beds) will probably see no more than six to eight cases per year of true HRS, depending on the type of community the hospital serves.

Laboratory Features and Diagnosis

Table 11–8 summarizes the major laboratory features of HRS.

Because HRS is due to intense renal underperfusion, it comes as no surprise that the manifestations found in the urine are those of prerenal failure. Moreover, if a patient is very jaundiced, the sediment may be quite active, because this latter condition often causes the appearance of an active sediment with red blood cells, tubular cells, and granular casts in the absence of morphologic renal disease.

The diagnosis of HRS in a cirrhotic patient depends on the presence of at least two features: the ARF is prerenal in type, and significant arterial hypovolemia is not present. It may often not be possible to reach this conclusion until adequate intravenous fluid replacement has been administered. The biochemical features of the urine occasionally may be ambiguous, and it may not be possible to decide whether HRS or ATN is actually present.

The urine volume is usually quite depressed, and the urinary sodium concentration very low (usually <10 to 15 mEq/L) and sometimes may be 0 mEq/L. Despite the intense oliguria (100 to 600 ml/day), the serum creatinine may not reach high levels and may stabilize at 7 to 8

Table 11–8. HEPATORENAL SYNDROME: LABORATORY FEATURES

Urine:	Marked oliguria
	Low urinary sodium (usually <15 mEq/L)
	Elevated creatinine concentration and osmolality
	Renal failure index ($U_{Na}/U/P_{cr}$ <1.0)
	Slight proteinuria may be present
	Sediment is usually inactive, mild activity compatible with jaundice
	Urine is generally acid
Plasma:	Severe disturbance of usual liver function test results
	Marked hyponatremia may be present
	Hypokalemia may be present
	Rise in serum creatinine is usually progressive

mg/100 ml. Once renal failure is present and progressing, arterial blood pressure may decrease, and the serum sodium concentration may decline to very low levels (<125 mEq/L).

Several investigators have remarked on the relationship between spontaneously developing ARF in cirrhotic patients and the appearance of hepatic encephalopathy. Resolution of the renal failure has sometimes accompanied resolution of the hepatic coma or precoma. In some series, encephalopathy has been present in at least half the cases of HRS. Finally, a diagnosis of HRS implies that other causes of ARF (obstruction, severe urinary sepsis, nephrotoxic drugs, or an acute glomerulopathy) have been ruled out. Of course, HRS may, after some time (days or weeks), progress to ATN. Death from nonrenal factors may also occur when the serum creatinine is very low (2.5 to 4.0 mg/100 ml).

Therapy

Avoidance

The most desirable strategy to follow in dealing with patients who are hospitalized for severe alcoholic cirrhosis and ascites is a strategy of avoidance. Based on the features of the cirrhotic process outlined earlier in this chapter, it is clear that such patients are physiologic time bombs in whom vascular replenishment from the ascitic depot may not keep pace with the many opportunities for vascular emptying. Accordingly, one should avoid extensive, rapid diuresis; extensive removal of fluid by paracentesis (unless replaced by albumin infusions); rapid and extensive intravenous infusion (unless judged necessary), for fear of expanding and rupturing varices; giving any drug that might cause vomiting and/or significant diarrhea; or inappropriately reducing the dietary salt intake.

If tense ascites is present, it should be relieved in an attempt to increase venous return and cardiac output. Normally, the presence of ascites in the peritoneal space increases the intraperitoneal pressure according to the height of the fluid column. In tense ascites, however, because of elastic recoil of the abdominal musculature, the pressure increases beyond what would be expected from the height of the column of fluid, and compression of the vena cava may occur with a resultant decline in venous return.

All fluid losses (*e.g.*, bleeding, diarrhea) should be vigorously replaced. Diuresis should not be attempted unless the edema and ascites are either extensive or are causing some specific problem (*e.g.*, respiratory embarrassment or bulging of an umbilical hernia). Diuresis should not be initiated with the potent loop-active diuretics such as furosemide or even thiazides, but rather with the less potent diuretics such as spironolactone or triamterene, which act on the most distal segments of the nephron. These drugs produce a gentle, slow diuresis permitting adequate time for vascular replenishment.

Indeed, spironolactone is the initial diuretic of choice. It should be started in doses of 25 to 50 mg q.i.d. and then increased at weekly intervals by 25 mg q.i.d. The daily dose should not exceed 100 mg q.i.d. Only if this dosage is not producing the required response should a thiazide or furosemide be added. It must be remembered that cirrhotic patients probably can transfer no more than 900 ml/day across the peritoneal membranes. It is probably wise, therefore, to limit diuretic-induced weight loss to ½ to 1 pound/day, unless peripheral edema is present to help buffer the diuretic losses. Severe hyponatremia and ARF may be the result of overenthusiastic use of diuretics.

Other than hyperkalemia, the most troublesome complications of spironolactone are RTA and painful gynecomastia.

The underlying disorder should be vigorously treated before the advent of HRS.

Treatment of Cirrhosis

For cirrhosis of the liver, treatment would focus on the following areas:

Nutrition. Provide adequate calories and nutrients. If a patient can tolerate it, the daily protein intake should be 80 to 100 g. When there is danger of encephalopathy, the daily protein intake should be restricted to 40 g. About half of the calories should be given as carbohydrates. Vitamins should be provided. Salt should not be restricted unless there is clear evidence (24-hour urine collections) that salt retention is present. Many cirrhotic patients with ascites are able to handle a modest salt intake.

Electrolyte Abnormalities. Such abnormalities as hyponatremia and hypokalemia should be corrected by reducing free-water intake or by administering a potassium supplement.

Ammonia Levels. These should be kept low by providing gentle cleansing enemas if constipation is present, by giving neomycin (4 to 8 g/day) either by mouth or by a retention enema (2.0 g/200 ml isotonic saline given t.i.d.), or by giving lactulose (40 to 160 g daily).

Infections. Search for and treat infections vigorously. Cirrhotic patients are immunosuppressed and may spontaneously develop infections such as peritonitis. Remember that endotoxemia has been suggested as a cause of HRS.

Treatment of Other Underlying Diseases

For diseases other than cirrhosis, other modalities of therapy should be used (e.g., portacaval fistula for Budd-Chiari syndrome).

Avoid drugs that may compromise renal function *(e.g.,* cyclooxygenase inhibitors such as indomethacin). Current concepts indicate that under conditions that might exist in a cirrhotic patient, such as arterial hypovolemia, the renal vasoconstriction resulting from elevated plasma levels of catecholamines and angiotensin is modulated by the augmented intrarenal generation of prostaglandin E_2, a renal vasodilator. Interfering with prostaglandin production would allow unopposed renal vasoconstriction to exist. Indeed, a reversible form of ARF has been reported in cirrhotic patients following administration of indomethacin.

Treatment of Hepatorenal Syndrome

Once HRS has developed, institute the therapeutic strategies discussed in the paragraphs that follow.

First, ensure that there is no volume contraction, because HRS and prerenal failure are almost impossible to differentiate. If there is any question of vascular underfilling, patients should be given large volumes of fluid intravenously, either saline or, preferably, a colloid solution. The dangers of overexpansion are the rupture of esophageal varices or augmentation of ascites and edema formation. However, the infusion of colloid sufficient to raise central venous pressure to normal levels, combined with intravenous diuretics, is often rewarded with a brisk diuresis. One of the problems with intravenous infusion is that the abnormal Starling forces tend to force fluid into mesenteric venous channels or into the peritoneal space. Thus, infused fluid may not adequately reexpand the arterial blood volume.

The reinfusion of ascites combined with intravenous furosemide in an attempt to reverse oliguria offers only transient results and is largely a wasted effort.

The most important advance in the treatment of ARF in liver disease has been the availability of the LeVeen peritoneovenous valve. This valve, which serves to pump fluid continuously from the peritoneal space to the venous system, is capable of mobilizing large volumes of ascites within 2 to 3 days. It thus serves as an iatrogenic, synthetic thoracic duct. Not only does it mobilize ascites, it effectively prevents its reformation. Thus, large volumes of protein-rich saline are quickly returned to the vascular compartment—and stay there. Many patients respond to this maneuver (especially when combined with a diuretic) with a brisk natriuresis. The blood pressure and cardiac output rise, plasma levels of renin and aldosterone decline toward normal, and glomerular filtration rate and renal blood flow may rise dramatically.

The response to the LeVeen valve offers a diagnostic test on pragmatic grounds. A positive response implies that the patient was quite hypovolemic and that the basis of ARF was not HRS. Assuming that the shunt is functioning properly and that ATN has been ruled out, a lack of response suggests true HRS *(i.e.,* ARF because of selective intrarenal vasoconstriction in the absence of hypovolemia). **Experience with this device during the past 5 years suggests that many patients with ARF in the setting of cirrhosis and ascites may recover their renal function.** This circumstance in turn suggests that many of these patients may not have had true HRS, but rather hypovolemic prerenal failure. These shunts may be left in place for many months, and if patients stop drinking, there may be a remarkable improvement in both nutritional status and liver function. However, many centers have become disenchanted with the LeVeen valve because of the extensive array of complications that may occur.

A common error made in use of the LeVeen shunt is to wait too long *(i.e.,* until a patient is moribund) before its insertion. If ARF or HRS is advancing and is unresponsive to fluid challenges, good nutrition, diuretics, and other therapies, one should insert the valve early while the patient is well enough to profit from a possible restoration of renal function. Once inserted and functioning, the valve may be left in place as long as required or as long as no complications develop. The common complications are as follows:

1. Disseminated intravascular coagulation
2. Continuous leak of ascites from the abdominal incision
3. Thrombosis of the jugular vein

4. Infection of the shunt and peritonitis
5. Variceal hemorrhage
6. Pulmonary edema
7. Early cessation of shunt function (?clotting)

Heart failure, bleeding varices, peritonitis, and severe hepatic encephalopathy are the major contraindications to valve insertion.

Hemodialysis or peritoneal dialysis has no place in the treatment of HRS. Because the underlying problem is severe liver disease, use of these procedures (which are dangerous in cirrhotic patients) does not add to long-term survival. A possible exception to this statement is in the case of HRS that may accompany severe acute viral hepatitis; here, tiding a patient over while waiting for adequate liver regeneration may be indicated. Use of renal vasodilators or catecholamines to raise blood pressure offers only temporary improvement and is generally not indicated. Considering the high morbidity and mortality accompanying portal systemic shunting procedures, such procedures are to be discouraged.

The recovery rate from true HRS is poor, and the advent of this complication in cirrhosis usually means that death is near.

Hepatorenal Syndrome: A Summary Statement

HRS is a functional or prerenal type of ARF that occurs most commonly in a clinical setting of severe alcoholic cirrhosis of the liver. Because the very nature of the cirrhotic process mandates a tendency toward arterial hypovolemia, it is to be expected that prerenal failure may frequently be present. Indeed, there is clinical evidence that glomerular filtration rate declines in cirrhotic patients as blood volume begins to decrease from markedly expanded levels during the course of the disease. In a consideration of the causes of ARF, HRS cannot be diagnosed unless arterial hypovolemia can be ruled out with certainty. This is not usually possible; therefore, a trial of volume expansion is usually in order. Strictly speaking, HRS can be diagnosed only if it can be demonstrated that a patient is not responding to intravascular volume expansion (assuming that ATN is not present). This can most readily be accomplished using the LeVeen peritoneovenous valve, which mobilizes ascites, expands the plasma volume, and prevents ascites reformation. Because a diagnosis of HRS should be confined to those patients in whom there is isolated intrarenal vasoconstriction in the absence of arterial hypovolemia, a lack of response to a LeVeen valve would, for the moment, appear to be a simple and pragmatic method of differentiating between true HRS and prerenal failure.

The mechanism underlying an increase in intrarenal vascular resistance is unknown, but it may be due to an imbalance between the availability of intrarenal vasodilator prostaglandins and the vasoconstrictor effects of catecholamines and angiotensin or an excess of vasoconstrictor prostaglandins (thromboxanes). HRS augurs poorly for the health of the patient and may proceed to ATN.

Selected Readings

Better OS, Chaimovitz C: The hepatorenal syndrome. *In* Schrier RW, Gottschalk W (eds): Diseases of the Kidney, 4th ed. Boston, Little, Brown & Co, 1988, pp 1489–1500.

Dibona GF: Renal neural activity in hepatorenal syndrome. Kidney Int 25:841, 1984.

Epstein M: The hepatorenal syndrome. Hosp Pract 24:65, 1989.

Epstein M, Lifschitz M: Renal eicosanoids as determinants of renal function in liver disease. Hepatology 7:1359, 1987.

Gordon JA, Anderson RJ: Hepatorenal syndrome. Semin Nephrol 1:37, 1981.

Levy M: The edematous patient. *In* Schrier RW (ed): Manual of Nephrology, 2nd ed. Boston, Little, Brown & Co, 1985.

Levy M: Hepatorenal syndrome. *In* Seldin DW, Giebisch G (eds): The Kidney: Physiology and Pathophysiology, 2nd ed. New York, Raven Press, 1990.

Rose B: Clinical Physiology of Acid-Base and Electrolyte Disorders, 3rd ed. New York, McGraw-Hill, 1989.

Seldin DW, Alpern RJ: Pathophysiology of edema formation. *In* Seldin DW, Giebisch G (eds): The Kidney: Physiology and Pathophysiology, 2nd ed. New York, Raven Press, 1990.

Staub NC, Taylor AE: Edema. New York, Raven Press, 1984.

Tristani FE, Cohn GN: Systemic and renal hemodynamics in oliguric hepatic failure: effect of volume expansion. J Clin Invest 46:1891–1894, 1967.

CHAPTER 12

DRUG USE IN RENAL PATIENTS AND THE EXTRACORPOREAL TREATMENT OF POISONINGS

Suzanne K. Swan and William M. Bennett

The kidneys provide the primary route of elimination from the body for most therapeutic agents or their pharmacologically active metabolites. Many drugs, whether excreted by renal or nonrenal means, exert toxic effects in the setting of reduced renal function. Thus, the impact of renal dysfunction on the pharmacokinetic and pharmacodynamic properties of a given drug poses a complicated challenge for physicians prescribing for such patients. Patients with impaired renal function must be maintained within a narrow therapeutic range, avoiding toxicity at one end and subtherapeutic dosing at the other. In this chapter, basic pharmacologic principles will be reviewed and applied to the setting of renal failure. Dosage recommendations will appear in tabular form, with brief discussions centering on specific agents.

PHARMACOKINETICS

Drugs and their active metabolites undergoing renal excretion require dosage adjustments in the setting of renal insufficiency. Dosage modification cannot simply be based on decreased renal excretion because alterations in other pharmacokinetic factors also are involved with drug metabolism (Table 12–1).

Absorption rates of many drugs are altered in patients with renal failure. Uremia-induced vomiting, delayed gastric emptying, and sluggish gut motility secondary to neuropathic changes may contribute to diminished absorption. Aluminum-containing phosphate binders can complex with drugs such as tetracyclines to block absorption by forming insoluble compounds. Phosphate binders can retard gastrointestinal motility. Bowel wall edema, as encountered in nephrotic, cirrhotic, and congestive failure states, may slow drug absorption as well.

Table 12–1. PHARMACOKINETIC FACTORS ALTERED BY RENAL FAILURE

Absorption	Protein binding
Volume of distribution	Biotransformation

Volume of distribution and degree of protein binding for a given agent predict plasma and tissue levels. The volume of distribution is altered by azotemia but not in a predictable fashion. Most acidic drugs such as penicillins exist in their unbound or pharmacologically active form to a greater degree in patients with renal failure than in persons with normal renal function. Organic acids that accumulate in the uremic milieu are thought to displace acidic drugs from their binding sites or alter the binding proteins themselves. Consequently, a greater proportion of unbound or "free" drug is present in the plasma. This same mechanism also provides higher concentrations of substrate for drug-metabolizing enzymes in the liver. If drug metabolites are excreted by nonrenal means, elevated levels of unbound parent compound may be balanced by increased drug clearance rates secondary to hepatic metabolism. Drugs with decreased protein binding in uremia are listed in Table 12–2.

Biotransformation can be affected by impaired renal function. Most drugs are metabolized in the liver by oxidative pathways. Renal failure generally has little effect on these reactions. Exceptions to this involve more rapid oxidation of phenytoin, digitoxin, and propranolol. Quinidine, in contrast, is oxidized more slowly in the presence of renal failure. Other metabolic conversions (*e.g.*, acetylation, hydrolysis, reduction) are normal or modestly slowed in the setting of renal insufficiency. If a drug has active metabolites dependent on renal excretion, significant reductions in dosage are necessary to avoid markedly elevated plasma concentrations.

DOSAGE REGIMENS

A stepwise process can be used to establish drug dosage regimens for patients with renal failure. This approach will aid in achieving therapeutic drug levels while avoiding toxicity (Table 12–3).

1. Calculate Creatinine Clearance

Because blood urea nitrogen (BUN) and serum creatinine levels *per se* are insensitive measures of renal function, creatinine clearance (C_{cr}) is traditionally used to approximate glomerular filtration rate (GFR). The fact that lean body mass and age correlate with C_{cr} directly and inversely, respectively, allows the use of serum creatinine to estimate the C_{cr}.[1]

$$C_{cr} = \frac{(140 - \text{age})\ (\text{body weight in kg})}{72 \times \text{serum creatinine level}}$$

In women, multiply the result by 0.85. It is important to remember that this formula represents only an approximation of renal function. If a patient has acute renal failure, a C_{cr} of less than 10 ml/min should be assumed for purposes of drug dosage adjustment.

Table 12–2. SOME DRUGS IN WHICH PROTEIN BINDING IS DECREASED IN UREMIA

Acids	Bases
Barbiturates	Diazepam
Cephalosporins	Morphine
Clofibrate	Triamterene
Dicloxacillin	
Diazoxide	
Furosemide	
Penicillin G	
Phenytoin	
Salicylate	
Sulfonamides	
Valproate	
Warfarin	

Adapted from Bennett WM: *In* Schrier RW, Gottschalk CW (eds): Diseases of the Kidney, 4th ed. Boston, Little, Brown & Company, 1988, p 3442.

Table 12–3. ESTABLISHING DOSAGE REGIMENS

1. Assess renal function with creatinine clearance
2. Choose a loading dose
3. Choose a maintenance dose
4. Monitor drug levels

2. Choose a Loading Dose

For most drugs in the setting of normal renal function, a steady-state concentration is achieved after 3.3 drug half-lives. Because renal failure may prolong an agent's half-life, simply reducing drug dosages would be a therapeutic error because such a strategy would delay attainment of a steady-state concentration and therapeutic drug levels. Thus, a loading dose needs to be given for most drugs. This dose usually does not vary from the initial dose given to patients with normal renal function. An exception to this rule is digoxin, for which 50 to 75% of the usual loading dose should be given because of its reduced volume of distribution in renal failure. In patients with significant volume contraction superimposed on renal failure, it may be prudent to lower the standard loading doses of aminoglycosides by 25% to avoid ototoxicity.

3. Choose a Maintenance Dose

Once a loading dose is administered, a maintenance regimen in patients with renal failure may be determined by either one of two methods. First, the dosing interval can be lengthened by the following formula:

$$\text{Dosing interval} = \frac{\text{normal } C_{cr}}{\text{patient's } C_{cr}} \times \text{normal interval}$$

Alternatively, each individual dose can be reduced and given at standard intervals:

$$\text{Dose} = \frac{\text{patient's } C_{cr}}{\text{normal } C_{cr}} \times \text{normal dose}$$

The first or *varying interval* method can potentially lead to periods of subtherapeutic drug levels. Conversely, the latter or *varying dose* method allows for more constant drug levels but risks toxicity due to higher trough levels. Thus, the interval method is preferable for aminoglycosides whereas the dosage method is more applicable to anticonvulsants and antiarrhythmics.

4. Monitor Drug Levels

Simply varying the dose or dosing interval is usually not sufficient when adjusting drug regimens for renal failure. Monitoring drug levels when possible may be necessary to ensure therapeutic levels while avoiding toxicity. Drug assays may only measure protein-bound concentrations while significantly underestimating plasma levels of the active form of the drug. An example of this is illustrated by phenytoin. In renal failure, a greater proportion of this drug exists in the unbound or free state. Standard drug levels do not reflect this increase in physiologically active compound. However, associated with decreased protein binding, a faster rate of clearance may be achieved as a result of increased availability of unbound drug to undergo hepatic metabolism. As a result of these opposing factors, no dosage adjustment is generally needed. The therapeutic range, however, is reduced to 4 to 8 μg/ml from 10 to 20 μg/ml, reflecting the increased proportion of active drug present.[2]

For patients receiving hemodialysis, attention must be paid to dose scheduling and the necessity to give supplemental doses to replace lost body stores. Dialysis clearance of a drug depends primarily on its molecular weight and degree of protein binding. As protein binding increases, dialysis clearance decreases. Likewise, the smaller the compound (less than 500 daltons), the more drug will be removed during a dialysis treatment. In general, scheduled doses should be given after dialysis if possible. Additionally, if a significant portion of a drug is removed, supplemental doses should be given after each dialysis session.

Information compiled from numerous sources is presented in tabular form for dosage adjustments in patients with renal failure (Tables 12–4 through 12–6).[3] It must be emphasized that these are general recommendations and thus must be individualized for each patient after considering all the variables affecting a patient's handling of a drug. A few comments on specific drug categories and dosage adjustments for renal insufficiency follow.

Nonsteroidal Antiinflammatory Drugs. Because of their efficacy, over-the-counter accessibility, and numerous clinical indications, nonsteroidal antiinflammatory drugs (NSAIDs) are commanding more attention as nephrotoxic agents. Renal impairment secondary to NSAIDs can be broadly categorized into two types. The first and more common form involves pathophysiologic responses to renal prostaglandin inhibition. Vasoconstriction underlies this response, and the characteristic clinical features are outlined in Table 12–7. Patient risk factors that predispose to this form of drug-induced renal failure have been identified (Table 12–8).

The second and less recognized form of NSAID nephrotoxicity involves drug hypersensitivity resulting in interstitial nephritis and often nephrotic-range proteinuria. This form of renal failure typically has a protracted course; it is insidious in onset and slow in resolution. Long-term use of NSAIDs and the development of papillary necrosis are clearly linked. Although phenacetin-containing analgesics were viewed as etiologic agents in the past, many NSAIDs have been implicated in the development of papillary necrosis with prolonged use.[4]

Specific recommendations for dosage reduction of NSAIDs are not well defined. In patients at risk for developing acute renal failure, NSAID use should be avoided. Sulindac has been suggested to be a "nephroprotective" NSAID, but several cases of acute renal failure associated with its use have been reported.[4] If NSAID use is necessary, particularly on a chronic basis, close monitoring of C_{cr} as well as urinalysis should be performed at regularly scheduled intervals.

Diuretics. Patients with impaired renal function often require diuretic therapy to avoid volume overload. Loop diuretics, such as furosemide, bumetanide, and ethacrynic acid, exert their effect from the luminal side of the tubule. As a result of extensive protein binding, most diuretics cannot undergo glomerular filtration and must be secreted by organic anion pumps in the basolateral membrane into the tubular lumen. In azotemic states, organic acids compete with and displace diuretics from these transport channels. As a result, dosage increments are often necessary to achieve the desired diuretic response. An effective dose must initially be established, one that renders a natriuretic response. This is accomplished by doubling subsequent doses every 30 to 60 minutes until a ceiling dose is reached or diuresis occurs (Table 12–9). With the clinically available loop diuretics, ototoxicity is most likely to occur with ethacrynic acid but has also been reported with furosemide and bumetanide.

Aminoglycosides. Widespread use of aminoglycoside antibiotics for life-threatening infections continues. Because of a narrow therapeutic window and GFR-dependent excretion, close attention must be paid to dosage regimens, drug levels, changes in renal function, and concomitant nephrotoxic drug use. As ami-

Table 12–4. ANTIMICROBIAL AGENTS

Drug	Route of Excretion	Method of Adjustment	$C_{cr} > 50$	$C_{cr} = 10–50$	$C_{cr} < 10$	Dialysis
AMINOGLYCOSIDE ANTIBIOTICS						
Amikacin	R	D	60–90	30–70	20–30	Yes
		I	12	12–18	24	
Gentamicin	R	D	60–90	30–70	20–30	Yes
		I	8–12	12	24	
Tobramycin	R	D	60–90	30–70	20–30	Yes
		I	8–12	12	24	
Netilmicin	R	D	60–90	30–70	20–30	Yes
		I	8–12	12	24	
ANTIFUNGAL DRUGS						
Amphotericin B (nephrotoxic; produces hypokalemia, renal tubular acidosis)	NR	I	24	24	24–36	No
Flucytosine	R	D	50	30–50	20–30	Yes
Ketoconazole	H	D	Unch	Unch	Unch	No
ANTITUBERCULOUS DRUGS						
Ethambutol	R	I	24	24–36	48	Yes
Isoniazid	H	I	8	8	8–12	Yes
Rifampin	H	I	Unch	Unch	Unch	No
ANTIVIRAL AGENTS						
Acyclovir	R	I	8	24	48	Yes
Amantadine	R	I	12–24	48–72	168	No
CEPHALOSPORINS						
Cefamandole	R	I	6	6–8	12	Yes
Cefazolin	R	I	8	12	24	Yes
Cefoperazone	H	I	Unch	Unch	Unch	Yes
Cefoxitin (may raise creatinine by assay interference)	R	I	8	8–12	24–48	Yes
Ceftazidime	R	I	8–12	24–48	48–72	Yes
Ceftizoxime	R	D	50–100	15–50	10–15	Yes
Cefuroxime	R	I	6	6–10	12–24	Yes
Cephalothin	R	I	6–8	6–8	12	Yes
PENICILLINS						
Amoxicillin	R	I	6	6–12	12–16	Yes
Ampicillin	R	I	6	6–12	12–16	Yes
Azlocillin	R	I	4–6	6–8	8	Yes
Carbenicillin	R	I	8–12	12–24	24–48	Yes
Dicloxacillin	R	I	Unch	Unch	Unch	No
Mezlocillin	R	I	4–6	6–8	8	Yes
Nafcillin	H	D	Unch	Unch	Unch	No
Penicillin G	R	D	Unch	75	25–50	Yes
Piperacillin	R	I	4–6	6–8	8	Yes
Ticarcillin	R	I	8–12	12–24	24–48	Yes
MISCELLANEOUS ANTIMICROBIALS						
Aztreonam	R	D	75	50–75	25	Yes
Chloramphenicol	H	D	Unch	Unch	Unch	No
Ciprofloxacin	H	D	Unch	50	25	Yes
Clavulanic acid	H	D	Unch	Unch	50–75	Yes
Clindamycin	H	D	Unch	Unch	Unch	No
Erythromycin (ototoxic in renal failure)	H	D	Unch	Unch	50–75	No
Imipenem	R	D	Unch	50	25	Yes
Metronidazole	H	D	Unch	50	Avoid	No
Nitrofurantoin (neurotoxic metabolites accumulate)	R	D	Unch	Avoid	Avoid	Yes
Sulfamethoxazole	R	I	6	8–12	12–24	Yes
Tetracyclines (potentiate azotemia, acidosis)	R	I	12	12–18	18–24	No
Trimethoprim	R	I	8–12	18	24	Yes
Vancomycin (ototoxic)	R	I	24–72	72–240	240	No

The main route of drug elimination from the body is noted by *R* for renal, *H* for hepatic, and *NR* for any other route. An important pathway, but not the primary one, is noted by parentheses. For varying levels of renal functions as estimated by measured or calculated creatinine clearance, either the interval between doses is given in hours (interval method, *I*) or the percent of a normal dose (dosage method, *D*) is noted. The notation *Unch* is used to note no change from usual dosage given. *Yes* refers to the loss of enough drug to require a dosage supplement following a dialysis procedure; *No* indicates no need for a dialysis supplement.

Table 12–5. CARDIOVASCULAR DRUGS

Drug	Route of Excretion	Method of Adjustment	C_{cr}> 50	C_{cr} = 10–50	C_{cr}< 10	Dialysis
ANTIARRHYTHMIC DRUGS						
Amiodarone	H	D	Unch	Unch	Unch	No
Disopyramide	R	I	Unch	12–24	24–40	Yes
Flecainide	H	D	Unch	Unch	75	No
Lidocaine	H	D	Unch	Unch	Unch	No
Mexiletine	H	D	Unch	Unch	75	No
Procainamide	H (R)	I	4–6	6–22	8–24	Yes
Quinidine	H	I	Unch	Unch	Unch	Yes
Tocainide	H	D	Unch	Unch	50	Yes
ANTIHYPERTENSIVE DRUGS						
Captopril	R	D	Unch	Unch	50	Yes
Clonidine	H (R)	D	Unch	Unch	Unch	Yes
Enalapril	R	D	Unch	75	50	Yes
Guanabenz	H	D	Unch	Unch	Unch	No
Guanfacine	H	D	Unch	Unch	Unch	No
Hydralazine	H (R)	I	8–12	8–12	12–18	No
Lisinopril	R	D	Unch	50–75	25–50	?
Methyldopa	H (R)	I	6	9–18	12–24	Yes
Minoxidil	H	D	Unch	Unch	Unch	Yes
Nitroprusside (toxic thiocyanate metabolite dialyzable)	H	D	Unch	Unch	Unch	No
Prazosin	H	D	Unch	Unch	Unch	No
Terazosin	H	D	Unch	Unch	Unch	No
β-ADRENERGIC BLOCKERS						
Acebutolol	H (R)	D	Unch	50	30–50	Yes
Atenolol	R	D	Unch	50	25	Yes
Labetalol	H	D	Unch	Unch	Unch	No
Metoprolol	H	D	Unch	Unch	Unch	Yes
Nadolol	R	D	Unch	50	25	Yes
Pindolol	H (R)	D	Unch	Unch	Unch	No
Propranolol	H	D	Unch	Unch	Unch	No
CALCIUM-BLOCKING DRUGS						
Diltiazam	H	D	Unch	Unch	Unch	No
Nicardipine	H	D	Unch	Unch	Unch	No
Nifedipine	H	D	Unch	Unch	Unch	No
Nimodipine	H	D	Unch	Unch	Unch	No
Verapamil	H	D	Unch	Unch	Unch	No
CARDIAC GLYCOSIDES†						
Digitoxin	H	D	Unch	Unch	50–75	No
Digoxin	H (R)	D	Unch	25–75	10–25	No
DIURETICS‡						
Acetazolamide	R	I	6	12	Avoid	No
Amiloride (may produce hyperkalemia)	R	D	Unch	50	Avoid	No
Bumetanide	H (R)	D	Unch	Unch	Unch	No
Furosemide	R	D	Unch	Unch	Unch	No
Metolazone	R	D	Unch	Unch	Unch	No
Spironolactone (may produce hyperkalemia)	H	I	6	6–12	Avoid	No
Thiazides (prototype hydrochlorothiazide)	R	D	Unch	Unch	Avoid	No
Triamterene (may produce hyperkalemia)	H	I	12	12–24	Avoid	No

†Loading dose 50–75% normal in advanced renal disease
‡May produce prerenal azotemia because of ECF volume depletion
See footnote to Table 12–6 for key.

noglycosides accumulate, the risk of nephrotoxicity and ototoxicity increases. Bactericidal efficacy of aminoglycosides correlates with therapeutic peak concentrations. Toxicity, on the other hand, corresponds to rising trough levels. Thus, dosage adjustments for these antimicrobial agents should primarily involve the varying interval format described earlier in this chapter. Individual dose reductions are also occasionally necessary. Assessment of peak and trough aminoglycoside serum levels as well as C_{cr} is necessary to monitor therapy and hopefully avoid toxicity. Concomitant use of loop diuretics, especially ethacrynic acid, greatly in-

Table 12–6. ANALGESICS, SEDATIVES, AND DRUGS USED IN PSYCHIATRY

Drug	Route of Excretion	Method of Adjustment	$C_{cr} > 50$	$C_{cr} = 10–50$	$C_{cr} < 10$	Dialysis
ANALGESICS						
Acetaminophen	H	I	4	6	8	Yes
Acetylsalicylic acid	H	I	4	4–6	Avoid	Yes
Codeine	H	D	Unch	Unch	Unch	Yes
Meperidine	H	D	Unch	Unch	50–75	No
Morphine	H	D	Unch	Unch	50–75	No
Pentazocine	H	D	Unch	Unch	Unch	Yes
BARBITURATES						
Phenobarbital	R	I	Unch	Unch	12–16	Yes
Secobarbital	H	D	Unch	Unch	Unch	No
BENZODIAZEPINES						
Chlordiazepoxide	H	D	Unch	Unch	50	No
Clonazepam	H	D	Unch	Unch	Unch	No
Diazepam	H	D	Unch	Unch	Unch	No
Flurazepam	H	D	Unch	Unch	Unch	No
Oxazepam	H	D	Unch	Unch	Unch	No
Triazolam	H	D	Unch	Unch	Unch	No
Haloperidol	H	D	Unch	Unch	Unch	No
Lithium carbonate (nephrogenic diabetes insipidus; renal tubular acidosis)	R	D	Unch	50–75	25–50	Yes
Phenothiazines (prototype-chlorpromazine)	H	D	Unch	Unch	Unch	No
TRICYCLIC ANTIDEPRESSANTS						
Amitriptyline	H	D	Unch	Unch	Unch	No
Desipramine	H	D	Unch	Unch	Unch	No
Doxepin	H	D	Unch	Unch	Unch	No
Imipramine	H	D	Unch	Unch	Unch	No

The main route of drug elimination from the body is noted by *R* for renal, *H* for hepatic, and *NR* for any other route. An important pathway, but not the primary one, is noted by parentheses. For varying levels of renal functions as estimated by measured or calculated creatinine clearance, either the interval between doses is given in hours (interval method, *I*) or the percent of a normal dose (dosage method, *D*) is noted. The notation *Unch* is used to note no change from usual dosage given. *Yes* refers to the loss of enough drug to require a dosage supplement following a dialysis procedure; *No* indicates no need for a dialysis supplement.

creases the risk of ototoxicity. Aminoglycosides also increase the nephrotoxicity of cyclosporine, a commonly used immunosuppressant.

HEMODIALYSIS AND HEMOPERFUSION IN THE TREATMENT OF DRUG OVERDOSE

Hemodialysis, hemoperfusion, and occasionally peritoneal dialysis can be helpful additions to the management of drug overdose or poisoning. In general, it must be emphasized that these measures are not the primary or sole therapy but rather adjuncts to more standard treatments. Conventional measures including cardiorespiratory support, gastric lavage, and activated charcoal can be combined with forced diuresis (either alkaline or acidic) in patients with intact renal function to treat the majority of drug overdoses.

Criteria to be used when considering dialysis or hemoperfusion for drug intoxication treatment include the following:

1. Unstable vital signs despite fluid replacement, mechanical ventilation, and conventional therapy for drug overdose.
2. Prolonged coma or prolonged ventilator dependence.
3. Progressive deterioration in overall condition despite aggressive care.
4. Prospect of delayed toxicity (*e.g.*, paraquat).

Table 12–7. CLINICAL FEATURES OF NSAID-INDUCED VASOCONSTRICTION

Oliguria
Hyperkalemia
Acute/subacute onset 24 to 48 hours
FE_{Na} nondiagnostic
Typically reversible with early drug cessation

Adapted from Henrich WL: Nephrotoxicity of anti-inflammatory agents. *In* Schrier RW, Gottschalk CW (eds): Diseases of the Kidney, 4th ed. Boston, Little, Brown & Co, 1988, p 1328.

Table 12–8. RISK FACTORS FOR DEVELOPING NSAID-INDUCED VASOCONSTRICTIVE RENAL FAILURE

Intravascular volume depletion
Cirrhosis, nephrosis, congestive heart failure
Shock, sepsis, diuretic use
Advanced age
Hypertension
Preexisting renal disease

Adapted from Henrich WL: Nephrotoxicity of anti-inflammatory agents. *In* Schrier RW, Gottschalk CW (eds): Diseases of the Kidney, 4th ed. Boston, Little, Brown & Co, 1988, p 1328.

5. Overdose with agents known to have toxic metabolites (*e.g.*, methanol, ethylene glycol).
6. Presence of underlying disease that prevents elimination of an offending agent by primary excretory organ.
7. Intoxication with an agent known to be readily extractable by either method at a rate greater than that achieved by endogenous elimination.

Hemodialysis is the primary route of removal for water-soluble agents with low molecular weights and minimal protein binding. Charcoal hemoperfusion is more effective in removing lipid-soluble drugs that are highly protein bound. The charcoal cartridge competes with plasma proteins by absorbing the drug itself and removing it from the blood returning to the patient. If dialysis and hemoperfusion are equally effective in removing an agent, dialysis should be used because of a significant incidence of thrombocytopenia (30%) with hemoperfusion. Table 12–10 categorizes agents into those that are effectively removed by hemoperfusion and those that are not.

Table 12–9. DOSAGE RECOMMENDATIONS FOR DIURETIC USE IN RENAL INSUFFICIENCY

Creatine clearance (ml/min)	20–50	<20
Starting dose	Furosemide, 40 mg IV	80 mg IV
	Furosemide, 80 mg PO	160 mg PO
	Bumetanide, 1 mg IV or PO	4 mg IV or PO
Ceiling dose	Furosemide, 120–160 mg IV	160–200 mg IV
	Furosemide, 240–320 mg PO	320–400 mg PO
	Bumetanide, 4–6 mg IV or PO	8–10 mg IV or PO

Adapted from Brater DC: Use of diuretics in chronic renal insufficiency and nephrotic syndrome. Semin Nephrol 8:333, 1988.

Table 12–10. REMOVAL OF DRUGS AND CHEMICALS BY HEMOPERFUSION

Category	Substance
Effective removal from patients already reported	Acetaminophen
	Acetylsalicylic acid
	Barbiturates
	Carbon tetrachloride
	Chloramphenicol
	Digitoxin
	Digoxin
	Ethchlorvynol
	Glutethimide
	Meprobamate
	Methaqualone
	Methotrexate
	Methyprylon
	Methylsalicylate
	Mushroom toxins (*Amanita phalloides*)
	Paracetamol
	Paraquat
	Penicillin G
	Phenobarbital
	Phenytoin
	Quinine
	Salicylates
	Theophylline
	Thyroid hormone (T_3 or T_4)
Effective removal probable	Amphetamine
	Diphenhydramine
	Quinidine
Effective removal from extracorporeal unit *in vitro*	Codeine
	Isopropyl alcohol
	Paraldehyde
Effective removal *in vitro*, but highly bound to tissue with a large volume of distribution (and/or highly bound to albumin with low free fraction in plasma)	Amitriptyline
	Chlordiazepoxide
	Chlorpromazine
	Diazepam
	Diquat
	Doxepin
	Imipramine
	Oxazepam
	Propoxyphene
Not removed effectively	Bromide
	Ethanol
	Lithium
	Methanol

From Winchester JF: Use of dialysis and hemoperfusion in treatment of poisoning. *In* Dagirdas J, Ing T (eds): Handbook of Dialysis. Boston, Little, Brown & Co, 1988, p 447.

A fourth type of extracorporeal toxin removal system can be achieved with continuous arteriovenous hemofiltration (CAVH) alone or combined with hemodialysis (CAVHD). Because of the permeable membranes involved, hemofiltration relies on convective transport involving elimination of solute (toxin or drug) as solvent is removed. For many solutes, this *solvent drag* phenomenon often offers equivalent clearance rates when compared with conventional hemodialysis because of its continuous time course.[5] Consequently, posttherapy rebound, which may complicate intermittent regimens such as hemodialysis or hemoperfusion, is avoided with CAVH. Unfortunately, relatively little is known regarding drug or toxin removal with this technique. Further studies are necessary before specific recommendations can be made for the use of this therapy in the treatment of drug toxicity or poisonings.

CASE SUMMARY 1

A 50-year-old woman who weighs 55 kg and has chronic renal insufficiency (serum creatinine = 3.0 mg/dl) develops congestive heart failure and atrial fibrillation. Digoxin therapy is indicated. What loading dose would you choose, and at what maintenance dosing regimen?

Calculation of the C_{cr} is the first step in determining loading and maintenance dosages of drugs excreted by the kidneys. Using Cockcroft's and Gault's formula,[1] a significant reduction in C_{cr} would be calculated for this patient (C_{cr} = 18.4 ml/min). Administration of 50 to 75% of a normal loading dose of digoxin would be appropriate at this point. If quinidine is added, a further reduction in digoxin clearance should be expected. A maintenance regimen can be tailored for this patient once her condition has stabilized. A standard maintenance dose could be administered *every other day* if her C_{cr} is less than 10 ml/min. Conversely, providing 25 to 50% of this standard dose on a daily basis would be an alternative if her C_{cr} remains between 10 and 30 ml/min. Frequent measurement of serum digoxin levels will be necessary to ensure therapeutic efficacy while avoiding toxicity.

CASE SUMMARY 2

A 79-year-old man who is a nursing home patient and has an indwelling Foley catheter develops sepsis and is admitted to the hospital for intravenous antibiotic therapy. His serum creatinine level on arrival is 2.4 mg/dl, and he weighs 60 kg. What loading dose of aminoglycoside would you choose in order to achieve therapeutic serum concentrations (8 μg/ml) rapidly, and at what maintenance regimen, given the patient's fluctuating renal function?

A loading dose can frequently be used to establish therapeutic serum levels of a particular drug. A quick rule of thumb for aminoglycoside loading dose calculations involves multiplying the drug's volume of distribution (L/kg) by the patient's weight (in kg) by the serum concentration desired. In this case, using a volume of distribution of approximately 0.25 L/kg and the patient's weight of 60 kg and a peak serum level for either gentamicin or tobramycin of 8 μg/ml would provide a loading dose of 120 mg, or 2 mg/kg, in this particular patient (0.25 L/kg × 60 kg × 8 μg/ml). Given the patient's age and presumed intravascular volume-depleted state, it would be prudent to reduce this loading dose by approximately 20 to 25% to avoid toxicity. Many drugs undergo significant alterations in their volume of distribution in the setting of uremia, which must be considered when performing these quick calculations. Likewise, calculations provide a rough estimate of a loading dose for a given patient and must be tailored to each individual patient appropriately. Designing a maintenance regimen for this patient will be somewhat more complicated because of his fluctuating renal function. Despite the fact that his creatinine level on admission is 2.4, it will most likely continue to rise on a daily basis during the next several days while his condition is stabilizing. It must always be remembered that serum creatinine level is only a rough estimate of true renal function, and, in this particular case, it represents a poor estimate in a very dynamic setting. In adjusting dosage schedules for aminoglycosides because of their significant toxicities, it has generally become standard practice to adjust not only the interval at which a particular dose is administered, but the actual quantity of the individual dose as well. For a C_{cr} of less than 10 ml/min, it would be reasonable to administer 20 to 30% of a standard dose every 24 to 48 hours, depending on peak and trough serum levels as well as the status of the patient's renal function. For a C_{cr} of 10 to 50 ml/min, providing 30 to 70% of a standard dose approximately every 12 hours would be prudent, again following serum levels closely to assure therapeutic peak responses and responding to rising trough levels appropriately with further reductions in dosage.

CASE SUMMARY 3

A 22-year-old mechanic arrives in the emergency room. He is unresponsive; his serum pH

= 7.0, anion gap = 28, lactic acid is normal, serum HCO_3 = 8 mEq/L, and serum creatinine level = 2.5 mg/dl. He is not diabetic. A drug screen is negative for salicylates, ethanol, narcotics, and acetaminophen, although family members relate a history of ethanol abuse and suicidal ideation. What differential diagnoses should be considered? Also, when the causative agent of this patient's condition is identified, hemodialysis is instituted. What other therapeutic measures should be taken?

The diagnoses to be considered in this particular case are those applicable to metabolic acidosis with an increased anion gap. Possibilities include ketoacidosis, uremia, starvation, salicylate overdose, methanol poisoning, ethylene glycol poisoning, lactic acidosis, and paraldehyde overdose. As can be determined from the information provided, many of these possibilities can be ruled out. In this case, ethylene glycol (antifreeze) ingestion should be high on the list, given this patient's alcohol abuse history, occupation, and suicidal ideation. Ethylene glycol is a toxic agent because of its metabolism by the enzyme alcohol dehydrogenase to oxalic acid. This acid is problematic for the kidneys because of precipitation within the tubules, causing obstruction and tubular necrosis, which ultimately delay excretion of this poison. Signs of ethylene glycol toxicity include confusion, seizures, and coma. Later complications that may arise include myositis and myocarditis. If the condition is recognized early, treatment may best be provided with forced diuresis to accelerate renal excretion and to limit oxalate precipitation within the tubules. However, in this patient's case, given his comatose state on arrival and marked acidosis, hemodialysis is in order because of ethylene glycol's readily dialyzable nature. In addition to dialysis, administration of ethanol should be instituted because of the fact that this substrate competes with ethylene glycol for alcohol dehydrogenase's catalytic effect, which ultimately reduces the production of oxalic acid. If ethanol is to be given while the patient is on hemodialysis, it can be administered directly into the dialysis solution to keep the patient's serum ethanol concentration at approximately 100 mg/dl.

References

1. Cockcroft DW, Gault MH: Prediction of creatinine clearance from serum creatinine. Nephron 16:31, 1976.
2. Bennett WM: Use of drugs in the patient with renal insufficiency. *In* Rose BD (ed): Pathophysiology of Renal Disease, 2nd ed. New York, McGraw-Hill, 1987, p 577.
3. Bennett WM, Aronoff GR, Golper TA, et al: Drug prescribing in renal failure. Philadelphia, American College of Physicians, 1987.
4. Henrich W: Nephrotoxicity of nonsteroidal anti-inflammatory agents. *In* Schrier RW, Gottschalk CW (eds): Diseases of the Kidney, 4th ed. Boston, Little Brown & Co, 1988, p 1328.
5. Golper TA, Bennett WM: Drug removal by continuous arteriovenous hemofiltration. Med Toxicol 3:341, 1988.
6. Brater DC: Use of diuretics in chronic renal insufficiency and nephrotic syndrome. Semin Nephrol 8:333, 1988.

CHAPTER 13

CHRONIC RENAL FAILURE

John Badalamenti and Thomas D. DuBose, Jr.

CAUSES

The most common disease causing end-stage renal disease (ESRD) in the United States, as reported by the United States Renal Data Systems Annual Report, is diabetes mellitus (30%). Hypertension (26%) and glomerulonephritis (14%) represent the second and third leading causes of ESRD in adults, respectively. In children, however, reflux pyelonephritis, renal hypoplasia/dysplasia, congenital cystic diseases, and renal tumors (Wilms' tumor) represent the most prevalent causes. These data should be used in any evaluation of patients with chronic renal failure (CRF), taking specific steps to exclude the most common causes in the age-group in question.

APPROACH TO PATIENTS

In the evaluation of patients with an elevated serum creatinine level, it is important to establish the following: (1) the acute or chronic nature of the renal functional impairment, (2) the cause of the renal dysfunction, and (3) the presence of superimposed reversible factors. First, establishing the presence of CRF will influence the long-term renal survival because, by definition, CRF is an irreversible process. Second, identification of a specific pathologic process will influence short- and long-term therapeutic intervention. Aggressive treatment of the primary pathologic process as well as the metabolic derangements of CRF will mitigate, to some extent, the progression to ESRD. Last, the identification and correction of any secondary reversible factors contributing to the renal dysfunction may quickly restore a level of renal function compatible with conservative management and will prevent or modify renal damage from a secondary pathologic process.

Establishing the Diagnosis

The diagnosis of CRF in a patient with an elevated creatinine level is established by (1) defining the coexistence of a disease known to cause renal damage and (2) demonstrating evidence of chronically progressive renal dysfunction.

Diseases Known to Cause Renal Damage. The clinical features of common diseases that cause progressive renal dysfunction are illustrated in Table 13–1. Although the patient is usually the source of the clinical information needed to diagnose CRF, more accurate information can sometimes be found in previous records (school, military, insurance, hospital, or previous physicians). Therefore, these should be routinely searched in the evaluation of patients with renal dysfunction of unknown cause (*e.g.*, evidence of proteinuria on a previous routine urinalysis).

Evidence of Progressive Renal Dysfunction. As a renal pathologic process progresses, changes in excretory function and histopathology will inevitably take place. Consequently, a reliable marker for CRF is a previously documented elevated serum creatinine level, implying sustained renal dysfunction and irreversibility. As this process continues, renal destruction (tubular atrophy and interstitial fibrosis) may result in shrinking of kidney size. Consequently, radiographic search for shrunken kidneys, by either kidney-ureter-bladder imaging (KUB) or renal ultrasonography, is mandatory in any patient with decreased renal function. **In most chronic renal diseases, the demonstration of small kidneys serves as the most reliable distinguishing feature of chronicity.** It should be noted, however, that exceptions do exist. Normal-size kidneys and CRF may be observed in diabetic nephropathy, multiple myeloma, amyloidosis, malignant nephro-

Table 13–1. CLINICAL FEATURES OF DISEASES CAUSING CHRONIC RENAL FAILURE

History
Glomerulonephritis: Macroscopic/microscopic hematuria, proteinuria, renal biopsy, skin rashes, arthralgias/arthritis
Hereditary nephritis: Family history, deafness, lenticular abnormalities (Alport's syndrome)
Diabetes mellitus: Family history, polyuria, polydipsia, retinopathy
Nephrosclerosis: Episodes of accelerated or malignant hypertension, poorly controlled blood pressure for extended periods
Interstitial nephritis: Frequent bladder/kidney infections, enuresis, incontinence, chronic pain, analgesic abuse, gastrointestinal bleeding episodes, macroscopic hematuria, renal colic
Obstructive uropathy: Frequency and/or hesitancy on urination, renal colic, stones, macroscopic hematuria, vaginal bleeding
Cystic disease: Family history, renal colic and stones, macroscopic hematuria
Physical Examination
Glomerulonephritis: Malar rash, arthritis, palpable purpura
Hereditary nephritis: Sensory-neural deafness, ocular abnormalities
Diabetes mellitus: Retinopathy, neuropathy
Nephrosclerosis: Hypertensive retinopathy, elevated blood pressure
Obstruction: Large prostate, palpable bladder and/or kidneys
Laboratory Tests
Chronic glomerulonephritis: Dysmorphic RBCs/RBC casts, oval fat bodies, proteinuria
Diabetes: Hyperglycemia, glycosuria
Interstitial nephritis: Diagnostic intravenous pyelography (IVP) if chronic pyelonephritis
Secondary glomerulonephritis: Positive antinuclear antibody and/or anti-DNA antibody titers, hypocomplementemia
Obstructive uropathy: Dilated renal collecting system on IVP, CT scan, or renal ultrasonography
Hereditary nephritis: Dysmorphic RBCs, RBC casts, abnormal audiogram
Cystic disease: Multicystic kidneys and liver on CT scan, ultrasonography, or diagnostic IVP

Adapted from Miller RB: The patient with chronic azotemia, with emphasis on chronic renal failure. *In* Schrier RW (ed): Manual of Nephrology. Boston, Little, Brown & Co, 1988.

sclerosis, polycystic kidney disease, and rapidly progressive glomerulonephritis. In the presence of normal-sized kidneys, evidence of previous renal dysfunction, histologic chronicity by renal biopsy, or extrarenal organ dysfunction should be sought.

Evidence for extrarenal organ dysfunction in CRF is found in the bone marrow and the skeletal system. As renal mass declines, a decrease in renal erythropoietin (EPO) production will result in the type of anemia observed in chronic disease states (see Anemia of Chronic Renal Failure). In only two chronic renal diseases, polycystic kidney disease and malignant nephrosclerosis, normal blood counts may occur regularly. Furthermore, as renal mass declines, phosphate retention will result in the development of hypocalcemia and secondary hyperparathyroidism (renal osteodystrophy) (see Calcium and Phosphorus Disorders). Subperiosteal reabsorption of the metacarpals and/or phalanges on magnified hand radiographs and/or subperiosteal reabsorption of the distal or medial clavicles on chest x-ray films are the earliest findings of renal osteodystrophy.

In summary, **irreversible renal dysfunction should be established by previous evidence of an elevated creatinine level, the presence of anemia of chronic disease, and radiographic demonstration of shrunken kidneys and/or renal osteodystrophy. Histologic confirmation of CRF by renal biopsy will be necessary in those cases that do not meet these criteria.**

Estimation of the Severity

After the presence of CRF is established, the degree of renal dysfunction must be defined in order to guide further intervention. The degree of intervention may range from aggressive treatment of the primary disease and coexisting hypertension in mild renal insufficiency to conservative follow-up and preparation of patients for dialysis in those with severe renal compromise.

The severity of renal dysfunction is assessed through the recognition of advanced clinical features of CRF (the uremic syndrome) and through the quantitation of the remaining glomerular filtration rate (GFR). The clinical features of advanced CRF are listed in Table 13–2. Although some features may predominate at different levels of renal function, virtually all features will be present at the time ESRD is reached. Quantitation of residual renal function should be performed through studies that directly assess GFR, such as measurement of the clearance of endogenous creatinine or of radionuclide/radiographic agents. These methods will be discussed later (see Monitoring the Progression of CRF).

Identification of Reversible Factors

The importance of identifying potentially reversible factors that may cause or contribute to CRF cannot be overemphasized, because pro-

Table 13–2. CLINICAL FEATURES OF ADVANCED CHRONIC RENAL FAILURE (UREMIC SYNDROME)

Symptoms
- General: Fatigue, weakness, lethargy
- Skin: Itching, easy bruising, skin discolorations, pallor or frost
- Cardiovascular: Dyspnea, orthopnea, edema, pericardial chest pain
- Gastrointestinal: Anorexia, early-morning nausea, vomiting, dysgeusia, uriniferous breath, early satiety, hiccups
- Neuromuscular: Decreased ability to concentrate, restless legs, parethesias, muscle cramps and/or twitching

Signs
- General: Bitemporal wasting
- Skin: Ecchymoses, excoriations, pallor, hyperpigmentation, hyperkeratoses
- Oral: Uriniferous breath, stomatic ulcers
- Cardiovascular: Hypertension with retinopathy and/or S4 gallop, murmur, pericardial friction rub, edema, ejection flow murmur
- Neuromuscular: Sensory/motor peripheral neuropathy, drowsiness, mental confusion, myoclonus, asterixis, seizures, coma

Laboratory Findings
- Elevated BUN and creatinine, decreased GFR
- Metabolic acidosis (hyperchloremic or high anion gap)
- Normochromic normocytic anemia
- Hyperuricemia
- Hyperphosphatemia, hypocalcemia
- Radiographic evidence of shrunken kidneys and/or early renal osteodystrophy
- Proteinuria
- Broad granular casts on urinalysis

Adapted from Miller RB: The patient with chronic azotemia, with emphasis on chronic renal failure. *In* Schrier RW (ed): Manual of Nephrology. Boston, Little, Brown & Co, 1988.

gression to ESRD may be slowed and initiation of dialysis delayed. Common remediable factors in CRF are listed in Table 13–3. Specific factors merit emphasis:

Volume Depletion. Both true and effective volume depletion occur frequently in CRF. As renal function declines, most patients become volume overloaded as a result of sodium retention. Because of volume excess, many patients are placed on diuretics, often resulting in extracellular fluid (ECF) volume depletion. Furthermore, because sodium regulation is tenuous in CRF, any concomitant or superimposed disorder (diarrhea, vomiting), which may be mild when renal function is normal, may result in severe volume depletion in patients with CRF. Therefore, frequent assessment of volume status is necessary in advanced renal failure.

Urinary Tract Obstruction. Obstruction of the urinary collecting system is particularly common in elderly men with benign prostatic hypertrophy and may be corrected by Foley catheter drainage and transurethral prostatectomy. Obstruction in women, on the other hand, may signify the presence of invasive cervical/endometrial carcinoma. **In the evaluation of CRF, therefore, a rectal examination in men and a pelvic examination in women are essential to rule out an obstructive component of the renal dysfunction.** The presence of urinary tract obstruction can be reliably detected by renal ultrasonography, which should be ordered if obstruction is being considered.

Hypertension. Malignant hypertension causes both histologic changes (fibrinoid necrosis) and angiotensin-mediated vasoconstriction, decreasing renal blood flow and renal function. As hypertension is treated, decreased hydrostatic pressure may precede vascular relaxation, causing further compromise of renal blood flow and renal function. **Control of hypertension must be gradual, therefore, to allow vascular relaxation and decreased blood pressure (BP) to coincide.** There is no advantage to decreasing systolic BP below 160 mm Hg acutely. However, the overriding goal in the management of hypertension in CRF is eventually to achieve a normal BP (<145/95 mm Hg).

Drugs. Therapeutic agents may contribute to the compromise of renal function by direct toxicity (aminoglycosides, antifungal agents, chemotherapeutic agents, and fluorinated anesthetics), by hemodynamic alterations (angiotensin-converting enzyme [ACE] inhibitors, prostaglandin inhibitors, diuretics), and by the development of an interstitial inflammatory response (analgesics, nonsteroidal antiinflammatory agents, penicillins, sulfa-derived antibiot-

Table 13–3. COMMON REVERSIBLE FACTORS IN CHRONIC RENAL FAILURE

- True or effective volume depletion: Vomiting, diarrhea, excessive diuresis, congestive heart failure
- Urinary tract obstruction: Papillary necrosis, nephrolithiasis, bladder outlet obstruction (prostatic hypertrophy or cancer, cervical cancer with bladder invasion)
- Vascular disease: Uncontrolled, accelerated, or malignant hypertension; excessive treatment of hypertension; renal artery stenosis; renal vein thrombosis
- Infection: Severe bilateral pyelonephritis
- Nephrotoxic agents: See Table 13–4
- Metabolic disorders: Severe hypercalcemia, hyperphosphatemia, hyperuricemia, potassium depletion, metabolic acidosis
- Glomerulonephritis or vasculitis: Systemic lupus erythematosus, rapidly progressive glomerulonephritis, vasculitis, postinfectious glomerulonephritis
- Interstitial nephritis: Drugs (allergic interstitial nephritis), toxins, and autoimmune diseases (Sjögren's syndrome, sarcoidosis)
- Pregnancy: Especially with toxemia
- Acute renal failure of any cause

ics, and xanthine oxidase inhibitors). **Meticulous monitoring of drug levels of any potential nephrotoxin, with parallel assessment of renal function, is necessary and may demand discontinuing the agent at the first sign of further renal functional compromise.**

Toxins. These substances cause renal injury either by direct renal tubular toxicity (heavy metals, organic solvents, radiographic contrast agents) and/or intratubular precipitation and obstruction (myoglobin, hemoglobin, radiographic contrast agents). Intratubular obstruction can usually be avoided by meticulous volume expansion, coupled with either osmotic agents (mannitol) or loop diuretics (furosemide, bumetanide). Although these therapeutic options are available, radiographic contrast agents should be strictly avoided in high-risk patients, such as patients with preexisting renal insufficiency (CRF with serum creatinine level >3 mg/dl and advanced age), diabetes mellitus with renal involvement, multiple myeloma, true or effective intravascular volume depletion, or a history of prior contrast-induced acute renal failure, as well as in patients receiving other potential nephrotoxins (*e.g.*, aminoglycosides).

Pregnancy. Pregnant patients with CRF are at a high risk for complications such as worsening renal function, preeclampsia, accelerated hypertension, intrauterine growth retardation, and fetal demise. Women with less than 50% of normal renal function are usually discouraged from conceiving. However, the presence of sustained hypertension represents the poorest prognostic sign for both mother and fetus. Patients with systemic lupus erythematosus, stable renal function for 6 months, normotension, and no recent systemic signs of active disease are reported to have no contraindication to pregnancy and may do well. Conversely, women with scleroderma or polyarteritis nodosa fare extremely poorly during pregnancy and should be specifically counseled against it.

Delaying the Progression of CRF

Only by attenuation of the primary etiologic process, by avoidance of nephrotoxic agents, and by control of hypertension can progression of CRF be modified reliably. However, experimental evidence has suggested that secondary hemodynamic alterations caused by the decrease in nephron mass may also contribute to the renal demise. Further experimental evidence has proposed that modification of these factors (especially hyperfiltration in remaining functional nephron units) may delay the onset of ESRD.

Intervention in the Primary Disease. A detailed discussion is beyond the scope of this text. In general, however, intervention should include relief of urinary tract obstruction, normalization of elevated BP, correction of metabolic fluid and electrolyte abnormalities, treatment of autoimmune disorders, discontinuation of nephrotoxins, elimination of infection, and correction of renal vascular stenosis when appropriate.

Avoidance of Potential Nephrotoxins. A comprehensive list of potential nephrotoxins is displayed in Table 13–4. Close monitoring of drug levels and renal function is usually necessary. Discontinuation of nephrotoxic agents should be routine at the first sign of further decline in renal function.

Protein Restriction. Dietary protein restriction had been previously recognized to ameliorate uremic symptoms (see Table 13–2). New evidence has shown a benefit of protein restriction on the secondary hemodynamic changes that occur as nephron mass declines. Such changes include elevation in single-nephron glomerular filtration rate, intraglomerular hyperperfusion, and elevation of intraglomerular capillary pressure, all of which eventually lead to the development of focal segmental glomerulosclerosis and irreversible renal deterioration. The ameliorative effects of protein restriction may be secondary to restoration of tubuloglomerular feedback decreasing afferent arteriolar dilatation, thus preventing systemic hypertension from being transmitted to the glomerular capillary bed. Until the results of a national

Table 13–4. POTENTIAL NEPHROTOXINS

Exogenous Nephrotoxins
Antibiotics: Aminoglycosides, tetracyclines, amphotericin, colistin/polymyxin, cephalosporins, penicillin, rifampicin, sulfa-based antibiotics
Anesthetics: Methoxyflurane
Radiographic contrast agents
Heavy metals: Mercury, arsenic, lead, gold, copper, cadmium
Organic solvents: Carbon tetrachloride, ethylene glycol, methanol
Analgesics: Phenacetin, acetaminophen, prostaglandin inhibitors
Antihypertensive agents: Angiotensin-converting enzyme inhibitors, thiazides, loop diuretic agents
Chemotherapeutic agents: Cisplatin, nitrosureas, methotrexate, mitomycin C
Xanthine oxidase inhibitors
Endogenous Nephrotoxins
Myoglobin
Hemoglobin

cooperative trial of protein restriction in patients with CRF (Modification of Diet in Renal Disease Study) are made available, the benefit of dietary protein restriction in humans with CRF remains anecdotal. **Nevertheless, it has become common practice to initiate protein-restricted diets (*e.g.*, 0.6 g/kg body weight of dietary protein per day) or, alternatively, 20 to 30 g/day of protein supplemented by amino acids or their ketoanalogues.** Because patient compliance is necessary, some investigators recommend verification of compliance by the measurement of 24-hour urinary nitrogen excretion and the application of the following formula:

$$\text{Estimated protein intake} = 6.25 \times (\text{urine urea [g]} + 30 \text{ mg/kg})$$

Control of Hypertension (see Hypertension in Chronic Renal Failure). A correlation between systemic hypertension and renal deterioration was first observed many years ago. It has been appreciated only recently that transmission of systemic pressure to the glomerulus, with resulting intraglomerular hypertension, plays a major role in the progressive renal demise of many forms of CRF. Therefore, control of hypertension emerges as the paramount goal in the preservation of residual renal function in CRF. BP should be kept at the lowest level that enables patients with CRF to continue a daily routine (near or below 140/90 mm Hg if tolerated). Brenner and colleagues have suggested that control of systemic hypertension with ACE inhibitors may be more efficacious in delaying progression to ESRD because of the vasodilatory effect of these agents on the efferent glomerular arteriole. The theoretical increased efficacy of ACE inhibitors has not yet been demonstrated unequivocally in controlled studies of humans. However, trials of these agents are underway in several centers. **Patients on ACE inhibition should be monitored for changes in renal function and hyperkalemia, the most serious side effects of these agents in CRF.** Consequently, ACE inhibitors should be used with great caution in patients with a tendency toward hyperkalemia (diabetes mellitus, tubulointerstitial disease).

Monitoring the Progression of CRF

As renal function declines, the ensuing metabolic disorders associated with CRF will result in clinical manifestations (see Table 13–2) that inevitably will require therapeutic intervention. Consequently, frequent monitoring of patients with CRF for changes in symptoms, physical findings, and laboratory data, including estimates of renal function, should be routine. However, recent criticism of the standard measures of renal function has placed the accuracy of these tests in question.

Limitations of Creatinine in Monitoring Progression of CRF

Time-honored laboratory standards for monitoring renal function in CRF include the serum creatinine level, the measurement of endogenous creatinine clearance, and the Cockcroft and Gault calculation of creatinine clearance based on age, weight, and sex.* Recent literature has also advocated use of the reciprocal of the serum creatinine (1/cr) versus time.

Serum creatinine level is dependent on the balance between creatinine generation and creatinine excretion. During progression of CRF, creatinine generation (muscle mass and diet) and the pathway of excretion (glomerular filtration and tubular secretion) may change. As a result, changes in serum creatinine level are influenced by the following:

1. *Total muscle mass.* Serum creatinine level is directly proportional to muscle mass. The latter is affected by sex (male > female), age (young > old), and the presence of muscle wasting. Any change in muscle mass will affect total body creatinine pool and, therefore, the serum creatinine level.
2. *Protein intake.* Meat is our most important dietary source of creatinine. Decreased meat intake, as in a low-protein diet, may decrease creatinine generation and serum creatinine level by 10 to 30%.
3. *Pathway of creatinine excretion.* Creatinine is filtered (60 to 90%) and secreted (10 to 40%). As renal function deteriorates, the proportion of secreted creatinine increases. As a result, a greater proportion of creatinine excretion will be derived from secretion rather than filtration.

The creatinine clearance, therefore, will overestimate GFR as renal disease progresses to near end stage. It follows that drugs that compete with the tubular secretion of creatinine also will cause an increase in serum creatinine level and a decrease in creatinine clearance.

---

*$C_{cr} = (140 - \text{age}) \times \text{wt (kg)}/P_{cr} \times 72$ (men)
$C_{cr} = (140 - \text{age}) \times \text{wt (kg)}/P_{cr} \times 85$ (women)

However, in this example, GFR will not change. Two of the more frequently used medications that compete with tubular creatinine secretion are trimethoprim-sulfamethoxazole and cimetidine. Therefore, **changes in serum creatinine and creatinine clearance must be evaluated, taking into account changes in weight, diet, and medications.**

The Cockcroft and Gault calculation of creatinine clearance based on age, sex, and weight does not overcome the inherent limitations of the measurement of serum creatinine level. Furthermore, because calculations are based on weight, this formula will overestimate GFR in states of obesity and edema, in which weight gain is not associated with changes in muscle mass.

The use of the reciprocal serum creatinine (1/cr) versus time has been advocated in following progression of CRF and is based on the expectation that the rate of decline will parallel decrements in GFR. A linear decline in 1/cr versus time would then predict the rate of progression of CRF. Any deviation from this linear relationship would suggest either the presence of a superimposed secondary process or stabilization of the renal demise. Because 1/cr is based on the measurement of serum creatinine level, it will also be subject to the same inconsistencies as mentioned previously. Furthermore, studies have suggested that the progressive decline in 1/cr in CRF is not linear, thus questioning the utility of 1/cr in monitoring progression to ESRD.

More accurate assessment of GFR can be achieved through the measurement of the clearance of ^{125}I-iothalamate, ^{99}Tc-DTPA, ^{51}Cr, or iothalamate meglumine. Although more expensive than creatinine clearance, these methods are more rapid, accurate, and possibly better suited to the routine clinical situation, avoiding the pitfalls of creatinine-based laboratory parameters.

TREATMENT

Metabolic Derangements in Chronic Renal Failure

Metabolic Acidosis

Normal acid-base homeostasis is maintained though a balance of endogenous acid production (metabolism of proteins) and net renal acid excretion. The control of net acid excretion is accomplished by (1) the reabsorption of filtered bicarbonate and (2) excretion of acid, which involves the titration of urinary buffers and the production and excretion of ammonium.

As renal failure advances, ammonium production declines largely because of a reduction in functional renal mass. Hyperkalemia may also affect the degree of acidosis by inhibiting renal NH_4^+ production and excretion. Hydrogen ion secretion, by the collecting duct, may also decrease in advancing CRF. This secretion of acid is under aldosterone control and is influenced by systemic acid-base balance, tubular flow rate, sodium delivery to this segment, and potassium balance (hyperkalemia decreases hydrogen ion secretion). Selective aldosterone deficiency, often present in diabetes mellitus and tubulointerstitial renal disease, will aggravate metabolic acidosis by decreasing hydrogen ion excretion both directly and through the development of hyperkalemia. Consequently, **as renal dysfunction progresses to end stage, metabolic acidosis will develop primarily by two pathophysiologic mechanisms: (1) decreased renal production/excretion of NH_4^+ (uremic acidosis) and (2) decreased distal tubular hydrogen ion secretion (hyperchloremic metabolic acidosis).**

Treatment of the metabolic acidosis of CRF has, as its basis, the prevention of the long-term skeletal effects of chronic acidosis. Acid retained in the ECF is buffered by alkali derived from bone salts (calcium carbonate), resulting in progressive loss of bone tissue and skeletal demineralization. The approach to treatment of metabolic acidosis of CRF is based on the administration of alkali ($NaHCO_3$ or Shohl's solution) sufficient to return the serum pH toward normal. In the hyperkalemic form of hyperchloremic metabolic acidosis associated with hypoaldosteronism, concomitant therapy for hyperkalemia may also be necessary (furosemide, fludrocortisone, and/or Kayexalate).

Volume Disorders

As mentioned previously, patients with CRF are prone to either volume overload or volume depletion because of the impaired rate at which these patients are able to achieve salt balance. This is caused by the relatively fixed rate of sodium excretion typical of the advanced stages of renal dysfunction. Thus, patients with CRF walk a tightrope between volume overload and volume depletion. **Consequently, it is important to monitor frequently the volume status of patients with CRF, especially during intercurrent illness or changes in therapeutic inter-**

vention. Parameters to be followed in the assessment of volume status include body weight, BP, jugular venous distention, skin turgor, skin and mucous membrane moisture, peripheral edema, and development of congestive heart failure (CHF).

Other clinical parameters such as the urine sodium concentration, urine osmolality, fractional excretion of sodium (FE_{Na}), or renal failure index may not be useful in distinguishing volume depletion from other causes of renal failure because of the obligate sodium excretion in CRF. However, when volume depletion is severe and superimposed on CRF, an abnormally low FE_{Na} is indicative of volume depletion.

The treatment of ECF volume disorders in CRF is outlined in Table 13–5. **The fundamental principle is to establish euvolemia.** In situations of volume excess, this is best accomplished by decreasing sodium intake (dietary sodium restriction and discontinuation of sodium-containing intravenous fluids) or by increasing renal sodium excretion (diuretic administration). GFR should be taken into account when choosing a diuretic agent because thiazides are usually ineffective at a GFR less than 30 ml/min. Meticulous monitoring of volume status, renal function, and potassium is mandatory when using these agents in CRF. Potassium-sparing diuretics (amiloride, triamterene, spironolactone) should be avoided in CRF. Patients with volume depletion should be treated by discontinuation of any therapeutic agents at fault and/or treatment of gastrointestinal (GI) volume losses (vomiting, diarrhea). Intravenous NaCl should be administered as outlined in Table 13–5.

Table 13–5. TREATMENT OF EXTRACELLULAR FLUID VOLUME DISORDERS IN CHRONIC RENAL FAILURE

Volume Excess	
1. Decrease sodium intake	
Dietary sodium restriction (2–4 g/day)	
Discontinue sodium-containing intravenous fluids	
2. Increase renal sodium excretion	
Thiazide diuretics: Hydrochlorothiazide	
Loop diuretics: Furosemide	
Bumetanide	
Volume Depletion	
1. Decrease volume losses	
Discontinue diuretics	
Treat contributing disorder: antiemetics, antidiarrheal agents	
2. Replace volume lost	
Intravenous NaCl:	Give 0.9% NaCl until orthostasis is improved or urine output is increased. Switch to 0.45% normal saline (with or without D_5W) until oral sodium and fluid intake is resumed.

Potassium Disorders

Potassium excretion is accomplished primarily by renal excretion of potassium secreted by the cortical collecting duct. As renal function declines, urinary potassium excretion will decrease as a result of a severely diminished GRF and a distal tubular defect in potassium excretion. Although potassium balance is preserved until late in CRF, decreased total renal potassium excretion becomes manifest at GFR <10 to 15 ml/min. On the other hand, a distal tubular defect in potassium excretion (hyporeninemic hypoaldosteronism) may exist in certain renal diseases (diabetes mellitus, tubulointerstitial disease), causing elevated serum potassium levels at much higher levels of GFR. As the decrement in renal potassium excretion continues (and potassium intake remains unchanged) the GI tract, particularly the colon, under aldosterone stimulation will adaptively increase fecal potassium excretion. Similarly, the ability of patients with CRF to handle potassium loads (*e.g.*, associated with meals) will depend on intracellular potassium movement, which is promoted by beta-adrenergic stimulation, insulin, and a functioning sodium-potassium adenosine triphosphatase. Therefore, aldosterone deficiency, beta-blockade therapy, insulin deficiency, and digitalis administration may be associated with severe hyperkalemia. In contrast, increased mineralocorticoid elaboration, beta-adrenergic agonists, insulin administration, and the development of diarrhea may reduce the plasma potassium level.

Prompt treatment of hyperkalemia (discussed in Chapter 4) is mandatory when myocardial toxicity exists as evidenced by peaked T waves, decreased R-wave amplitude, widened QRS complex, prolonged PR interval, and eventual disappearance of the P wave on the electrocardiogram (ECG).

Water Balance

As nephron mass decreases, the kidneys become incapable of concentrating and diluting the urine maximally, thus placing patients with CRF at risk for water intoxication (hyponatremia) or dehydration (hypernatremia). Large amounts of solute-free water (5% dextrose in water, 5% dextrose in 0.25% NaCl, 5% dextrose in 0.33% NaCl) should be avoided, especially in states of enhanced arginine vasopressin secretion (volume depletion, CHF, postoperative state). The treatment of asymptomatic hyponatremia requires fluid restriction. Symptomatic hyponatremia (mental confusion, stupor, coma) will require careful hypertonic saline administration (3% NaCl), preferably combined with furosemide therapy to avoid sudden volume overexpansion and osmotic shifts. In contrast, hypernatremia is less often a problem because thirst mechanisms remain intact in most patients with CRF.

Patients at highest risk for serious hypernatremia include debilitated patients with a deranged thirst mechanism (cerebrovascular accident, dementia) or patients with limited access to solute-free water (nursing home patients on high osmotic loads such as tube feedings). Treatment of hypernatremia is by administration of solute-free water (0.45% NaCl with or without 5% dextrose) after euvolemia is restored with 0.9% NaCl. Correction of both hyponatremia and hypernatremia should be gradual (not >2 mEq/L/hr) to avoid the complications of central pontine myelinolysis or cerebral edema, respectively.

Magnesium Disorders

In the advanced stages of CRF, the majority of patients will have modest elevations of serum magnesium level. Magnesium intoxication, however, is unusual unless a magnesium load is administered in the form of magnesium-containing laxatives (milk of magnesia) or antacids (Maalox, Mylanta). For this reason, **magnesium-containing agents should be avoided in patients with CRF with a GFR <30 ml/min.** Hypomagnesemia is rare in CRF and will not be discussed.

Calcium and Phosphorus Disorders

Because the kidneys play a critical role in the regulation of calcium and phosphorus homeostasis, it is not surprising that hyperphosphatemia and hypocalcemia eventually occur in patients with CRF. As renal failure advances, phosphate excretion is impaired, resulting in hyperphosphatemia. This hyperphosphatemia, in turn, will cause hypocalcemia via two principal mechanisms: (1) the formation of $CaPO_4$ and (2) the inhibition of $1,25(OH)_2D_3$ elaboration from the kidneys, decreasing calcium and phosphorus absorption from the intestine. The resulting hypocalcemia stimulates the elaboration of parathyroid hormone (PTH) and bone calcium reabsorption. Thus, secondary hyperparathyroidism resulting in renal osteodystrophy represents a trade-off to maintain calcium balance as renal function declines. Renal osteodystrophy is initiated early in CRF as evidenced by the elevated PTH levels, increased osteoid production, increased osteoclastic reabsorption, and increased bone turnover present in most patients with a GFR of 60 ml/min. Therefore, **early intervention in calcium/phosphorus derangements is essential in preserving the integrity of bone.**

The treatment of calcium/phosphorus derangements in CRF is based primarily on control of serum phosphate with calcium-based phosphate binders and the administration of vitamin D as outlined in Chapter 14. Aluminum-based phosphate binders should be avoided in CRF to prevent chronic aluminum toxicity.

Specific Organ Dysfunction in Chronic Renal Failure

Hematologic Abnormalities in Chronic Renal Failure

Decrements in renal hormonal production and renal excretory function that accompany CRF progression will have profound effects on the three constituent cell types of blood: erythrocytes (RBCs), leukocytes, and platelets, resulting, respectively, in the anemia, immunosuppression, and bleeding tendency of advanced CRF.

Anemia of Chronic Renal Failure. As renal function declines, anemia becomes a universal finding present in virtually all patients with a serum creatinine level >3.5 mg/dl. Of the primary causes of the anemia of CRF (Table 13–6), decreased EPO (erythropoietin) production is the most important. Eschbach and Adamson found that the anemia associated with chronic dialysis was completely corrected by the admin-

Table 13–6. PRIMARY CAUSES OF THE ANEMIA OF CHRONIC RENAL FAILURE

1. Decreased erythropoietin production
    - Loss of viable renal parenchyma
    - Decreased hemoglobin oxygen affinity (increase in 2,3-diphosphoglycerate from acidemia)
2. Inhibitors of erythropoiesis (uremic toxins)
3. Hemolysis (uremic alterations of RBC membrane)

Table 13–7. LABORATORY CHARACTERISTICS OF THE ANEMIA OF CHRONIC RENAL FAILURE

Normochromic normocytic anemia
Echinocytes (burr cells)
Normal or high serum iron concentration, normal or low iron-binding capacity
Normal or high serum ferritin
Decreased reticulocyte index
Normal platelet count, possibly increased bleeding time
Decreased ^{51}Cr RBC survival
Decreased hemoglobin-oxygen affinity (increased 2,3-diphosphoglycerate)

istration of recombinant EPO. Other contributing factors, such as a decreased RBC survival time (hemolysis) and the presence of uremic inhibitors of erythropoiesis, also influence the degree of anemia.

The laboratory characteristics of anemia are described in Table 13–7. The diagnosis of the anemia of chronic renal disease should be made only when the influence of secondary causes (*e.g.*, iron and/or folate deficiency) has been appropriately ruled out.

The treatment of the anemia of CRF (Table 13–8) is based on the correction of contributing factors (vitamin B_{12} and folate deficiency, GI bleeding), the preservation of renal mass (treatment of primary disease, avoidance of nephrectomy), and the avoidance of agents that may accelerate RBC destruction or cause toxicity to the bone marrow. If the anemia is unresponsive to these measures, is causing symptoms (chest pain, severe fatigue), or is requiring regular transfusions, efforts to increase EPO levels and/or decrease the effect of uremia on RBCs (*e.g.*, dialysis) should be initiated.

EPO levels can be increased by the administration of either androgenic steroids or recombinant EPO. Androgenic steroids may result in masculinization in female patients and hepatocellular toxicity and tumors. Consequently, long-acting parenteral agents with a high anabolic to androgenic ratio (*e.g.*, nandrolone phenpropionate) are recommended. Initial dosing should be reduced by 50% in females to avoid unsightly masculinization. EPO administration is the treatment of choice based on recent studies showing a dose-dependent stimulation of RBC production and complete reversal of the anemia of chronic renal disease. EPO is administered parentally in dosages of 50 to 150 units/kg body weight three times per week. However, the high cost of this agent and the limited availability of commercial EPO to the general public limit its use. Chronic dialysis patients with significant anemia (hematocrit <25%) are the targeted recipients of EPO at present.

Table 13–8. TREATMENT OF ANEMIA OF CHRONIC RENAL FAILURE

General Measures
- Correct iron and/or folate deficiency
- Preserve renal mass (treat primary disease, avoid nephrectomy)
- Maintain adequate nutrition
- Avoid exposure to agents affecting RBCs
- Treat causes of coexisting hemolysis or GI blood loss

Specific Measures
- Increase erythropoietin levels
  - Androgens: Nandrolone phenpropionate, 1–3 mg/kg IM weekly or biweekly until desired hematocrit is achieved, then monthly maintenance
  - Erythropoietin: Recombinant erythropoietin, 50–150 units/kg IV, SC, or IM three times per week until desired hematocrit is achieved; optimal maintenance is unknown
- Decrease circulating inhibitors of erythropoietin and/or changes in RBC membrane by the uremic environment
  - Dialysis

Complications of EPO administration in patients with ESRD are listed in Table 13–9. Hypertension, thrombosis of hemodialysis accesses, and decreased dialysis efficiency are secondary to the increased blood viscosity as the anemia is corrected. Hyperkalemia is probably related to decreased efficiency of dialysis, increased appetite resulting from an improvement in well-being, and increased RBC turnover and potassium release. Iron deficiency may develop during treatment as a result of the increased RBC production initiated by EPO therapy.

Platelet Dysfunction. Patients with advanced CRF have an increased bleeding tendency, usually from the GI tract, which is a major cause of morbidity and mortality. Frequent manifestations of this tendency are ecchymoses, purpura, epistaxis, bleeding from venipuncture sites, and mucous membrane lesions. This increased bleeding tendency is associated with an abnormal bleeding time and represents decreased platelet adhesiveness, decreased platelet release reactions (*e.g.*, release of adenosine diphosphate), and decreased platelet aggregation.

Treatment of the hemostatic defect in uremia (Table 13–10) is based on improvement of the

Table 13–9. COMPLICATIONS OF RECOMBINANT ERYTHROPOIETIN THERAPY

Hypertension
Thrombosis of hemodialysis access
Hyperkalemia
Decreased efficiency of dialysis
Iron deficiency

Table 13–10. TREATMENT OF BLEEDING ABNORMALITIES IN CHRONIC RENAL FAILURE

Agent	Dosage	Duration of Action
Cryoprecipitate	10 units IV every 12–24 hours	12–18 hours
1-Deamino-8-D-arginine vasopressin (DDAVP)	0.3 μg/kg IV in 50 ml saline given over 15–30 min	4–8 hours; tachylaxis after 1–2 treatments
Conjugated estrogen	0.6 mg/kg/day IV for 5 days	2 weeks
Dialysis	1–3 treatments	Variable; peritoneal dialysis may be better than hemodialysis

uremic environment through dialysis and replacement of unknown "coagulation factors" through the administration of cryoprecipitate, 1-deamino-8-D-arginine vasopressin (DDAVP), and/or conjugated estrogens. The choice of agent depends on the desired onset and duration of action. Cryoprecipitate and DDAVP are used in states of active bleeding. Disadvantages of these agents are short duration of action and risk of hepatitis B or human immunodeficiency virus infection (with cryoprecipitate). When immediate action is unnecessary and prolonged action is desired, parenteral estrogen should be considered, as well as initiation of maintenance dialysis.

Defects of Granulocyte and Lymphocyte Function. In the granulocyte compartment of the immune system, both a decreased amount of circulating chemotactic factors and a decreased ability of neutrophils to respond to these factors have been demonstrated. In the lymphocyte compartment, absolute lymphopenia may develop in advanced CRF. Functional effects on cellular immunity are demonstrated by a depressed delayed-type hypersensitivity response.

These immunologic abnormalities translate clinically into increased susceptibility to infection and decreased responses to conventional vaccines. Nevertheless, vaccination is recommended for most patients with advanced CRF. Table 13–11 lists the vaccines recommended for patients with advanced CRF. Response after vaccination may be variable, especially with hepatitis B vaccine (rates as low as 30 to 50%). Recent evidence suggests that deltoid administration rather than gluteal administration may improve the responsiveness to hepatitis B vaccine (92% response rate).

Table 13–11. RECOMMENDED IMMUNIZATIONS IN CHRONIC RENAL FAILURE

Vaccine	Dosage	Frequency of Administration
Influenza A and B	0.5 ml (15 μg) via single IM injection	Annually
Pneumococcus	0.5 ml (575 μg) via single SC or IM injection	Booster depending on antibody response and levels
Hepatitis B	2 ml (40 μg HbsAg) at 0, 1, 5, and 6 months; 1 ml IM in each deltoid	Booster depending on antibody response and levels
Tetanus toxoid	0.5 ml single IM injection	Booster every 10 years

Dermatologic Disorders in Chronic Renal Failure

The most common dermatologic disorders associated with CRF and treatment are summarized in Table 13–12.

Pruritus. Uremic pruritus occurs in as many as 85% of patients and can be either generalized or localized to the trunk and/or the extremities. The skin content of calcium, magnesium, or phosphorus has been implicated in uremic pruritus. Although some patients have responded, there has been no consistent improvement of pruritus with parathyroidectomy, lowering dialysate magnesium, or improving hyperphosphatemia.

Xerosis (Dry or Scaling Skin Lesions). This lesion may vary from mild to severe and may be generalized or limited to the extremities. Atrophy of sebaceous glands and of secretory and ductal portions of sweat glands and altered metabolism of vitamin A with increased skin

Table 13–12. SPECTRUM OF DERMATOLOGIC DISORDERS AND TREATMENT IN CHRONIC RENAL FAILURE

Uremic pruritus	Antihistamines: diphenhydramine (25–50 mg PO) or hydroxyzine (25–50 mg PO) Ultraviolet B radiation
Xerosis	Moisturizers (usually ineffective)
Kyrle's disease	Agents that inhibit keratinization and promote epithelial proliferation (usually ineffective)
Discoloration/ pigmentation	Correct anemia (see Table 13–8), correct bleeding tendency (see Table 13–10), and avoid iron overload

and plasma levels may be causative. Moisturizers are recommended but have little effect on this lesion.

Kyrle's Disease (Hyperkeratosis Follicularis et Parafollicularis in Cutem Penetrans). The lesions are pruritic irregular papules, 2 to 8 mm in diameter, with hyperkeratotic plugs that may coalesce, generally sparing the face, mucous membranes, palms, and soles. Topical agents promoting epidermal proliferation and inhibiting keratinization have limited effectiveness.

Skin Discoloration or Pigmentation. Pallor of the skin in CRF is usually related to the anemia of chronic renal disease. Sallow coloring is due to a combination of hypermelanosis and retention of urochrome and/or carotene. Brown discoloration may be related to coexisting malnutrition or hemosiderosis (iron overload). Purpura, easy bruising, and bleeding are attributable to a qualitative platelet defect and increased capillary permeability.

Nervous System Disorders of Chronic Renal Failure

In advanced CRF, nervous system dysfunction remains a major cause of mental and physical disability. Nervous system disorders of uremia can be classified according to the temporal relationship to dialysis. Before the initiation of dialysis, either uremic encephalopathy or uremic neuropathy may be observed in many patients with advanced renal failure. During the initial dialysis or after the institution of maintenance dialysis, the dialysis disequilibrium syndrome and dialysis dementia, respectively, may become manifest. A discussion of these entities is beyond the scope of this chapter and will be addressed in Chapter 18.

Uremic Encephalopathy. Uremic encephalopathy may occur in either acute or chronic renal failure when the GFR falls below approximately 10 ml/min. The symptoms may vary in severity from anorexia and inability to concentrate to frank coma and seizures (Table 13–13). The severity and rate of progression of these symptoms vary directly with the rate of deterioration of renal function. Therefore, the more severe presenting symptoms will be seen in acute renal failure. These symptoms, whatever the severity, are usually alleviated by dialysis and/or successful renal transplantation.

Table 13–13. SIGNS AND SYMPTOMS OF UREMIC ENCEPHALOPATHY

Early:	Anorexia, nausea, insomnia, restlessness, decreased attention span, decreased sexual interest
Moderate:	Vomiting, sluggishness, easy fatigue, drowsiness, sleep inversion, decreased sexual performance
Severe:	Itching, disorientation, bizarre behavior, myoclonus, asterixis, convulsions, stupor, coma

Uremic Neuropathy. Two types of neuropathy exist in advanced renal failure: polyneuropathy and mononeuropathy. **Uremic polyneuropathy is typically manifested by a bilaterally symmetrical disturbance of both sensory and motor functions.** Sensory changes are in the typical stocking and glove distribution, usually more pronounced distally in lower extremities. Motor disturbances usually cause muscle wasting and weakness in arms and legs. The restless legs syndrome and burning feet syndrome may be manifestations of these sensory motor changes. Physical signs pertaining to uremic polyneuropathy include loss of deep tendon reflexes in knees and ankles and/or impairment of vibrational, pain, pressure, light touch and temperature sensations in the stocking and glove distribution. In uremic mononeuropathy, these abnormalities will be found in the distribution of single or multiple isolated nerves.

Dialysis usually stabilizes or improves the peripheral neuropathy. However, **the most important variable determining recovery from peripheral neuropathy is the condition of the patient before the initiation of dialysis.** For example, in patients with severe neuropathy, dialysis may only partially improve this, even after several years. Consequently, **initiation of dialysis early in the course of neuropathy is necessary because clinical disability from neuropathy is rare when dialysis is initiated at a GFR of 10 ml/min.**

Gastrointestinal Disorders

Although GI disorders are common in CRF, significant controversy exists concerning whether there is an increased incidence of these functional disorders over the general population. It is clear, however, that an increased morbidity and mortality due to GI abnormalities exist in the population with ESRD, especially when associated with hemorrhage. GI disorders in CRF can be divided into two broad categories: functional disorders and specific anatomic lesions.

Functional Disorders of the GI Tract. GI symptoms are common with advanced CRF. Anorexia, early-morning nausea, vomiting, hiccups, and a change in taste sensation or the presence of a metallic taste in the mouth (dys-

Table 13–14. GASTROINTESTINAL DRUGS USED IN CHRONIC RENAL FAILURE

Antacids
- Avoid magnesium-containing agents
- Avoid long-term use of aluminum hydroxide
- Calcium carbonate can be used for acid neutralization

Antihistamines (H_2-blocking agents)
- Cimetidine: (reduce 50% in CRF) 300 mg PO twice a day or 400 mg at bedtime
- Ranitidine: 150 mg PO once a day

Laxatives
- Fiber: Bran, apple or pear daily, psyllium hydrophilic mucilloid
- Stool softener: Docusate sodium, docusate sodium plus bowel irritant casanthranol
- Avoid magnesium-containing laxatives
- Sorbitol or mineral oil may be used in refractory cases

Antidiarrheal agents
- Loperamide HCl
- Diphenoxylate/atropine

geusia) are common symptoms as renal function deteriorates to end stage. Symptoms of dyspepsia (early satiety, heartburn, eructation) present in CRF may be related to ingestion of iron supplements, calcium carbonate, or aluminum salts; to metabolic acidosis; or to primary GI pathology (*e.g.*, peptic ulcer disease, diabetic gastroparesis). Constipation is also a frequent complaint and may be due to changes in diet (elimination of fruit in potassium-restricted diets), low fluid intake, inactivity, and the administration of aluminum-based phosphate binders. As constipation may lead to bowel perforation, it is important to intervene early. GI drugs to relieve these functional disorders are summarized in Table 13–14.

Specific Anatomic Lesions of the GI Tract in Chronic Renal Failure. GI tract lesions found in advanced renal failure are summarized in Table 13–15. Stomatitis is characterized by painful ulcerations, coating of the tongue, metallic taste, and uriniferous breath, which are probably due to the liberation of ammonia from the metabolism of urea by urease-containing bacteria. Esophagitis and esophageal tears account for 5 to 20% of upper GI bleeding in hemodialysis patients. Gastritis, on the other hand, is very common, as high as 100%, in patients with advanced CRF and is an important cause of upper GI hemorrhage (20 to 50%).

Table 13–15. GASTROINTESTINAL LESIONS IN CHRONIC RENAL FAILURE

- Oral: Stomatitis, parotitis
- Esophageal: Esophagitis, Mallory-Weiss tear
- Gastric: Gastritis, peptic ulcer, telangiectasias
- Small bowel: Pepic ulcer (duodenum), duodenitis, telangiectasias
- Large bowel: Cecal ulcers, stercoral ulcers, diverticulosis/diverticulitis, telangiectasias
- Pancreatic: Pancreatitis
- Hepatic: Congestive hepatomegaly, hepatitis C, cytomegalovirus

Telangiectasias have been observed throughout the GI tract in advanced renal failure and account for 20% of upper GI and 30% of lower GI hemorrhage. The cause may be recurrent low-grade obstruction, chronic venous hypertension, and/or aluminum binders. Telangiectatic lesions should be localized by endoscopy and either cauterized or photo/cryocoagulated for control of bleeding. However, many lesions are beyond the reach of conventional endoscopes. In these cases, estrogen-progesterone therapy may be used to reduce bleeding.

Lower GI lesions of advanced CRF include telangiectasias, diverticulosis, colonic ulcers, and stercoral (rectal) ulcers. Colonic ulcers and diverticulosis may be complicated by hemorrhage and perforation and result in high mortality. Stercoral ulcers are produced by pressure necrosis from feces on the rectal mucosa. Aluminum-based phosphate binders and autonomic neuropathy have been implicated in the development of these ulcerations.

Dialysis amyloidosis with β_2-microglobulin accumulation may be found in perivascular regions of the GI tract and may predispose to significant GI bleeding.

In the diagnostic evaluation of the GI tract in CRF, it is recommended that patients with GI bleeding and/or persistent dyspeptic symptoms unresponsive to treatment undergo endoscopy. We advise this because GI radiology is less sensitive in CRF as a result of the increased incidence of hypertrophic gastric folds, telangiectasias, and gastritis.

Skeletal Disorders in Chronic Renal Failure

In advanced CRF, two forms of bone disease are observed: osteitis fibrosa cystica (secondary hyperparathyroidism) and aluminum-associated osteomalacia (see Chapter 14). **The maintenance of skeletal integrity in patients with advancing CRF may be achieved through (1) strict control of serum calcium and phosphorus levels (requires dietary phosphate restriction, calcium-based phosphate binders, and calcium supplementation), (2) $1,25(OH)_2D_3$ administration, (3) correction of metabolic acidosis with alkali therapy, and (4) avoidance of aluminum-based phosphate binders.**

Cardiovascular Disorders in Chronic Renal Failure

Cardiovascular disease is the primary cause of death in patients with advanced CRF. The high prevalence of cardiovascular disease exists in CRF because of the frequency of associated risk factors (*i.e.*, hypertension, lipid abnormalities, and diabetes mellitus) in this population. This predisposition to the development of ischemic, hypertensive, and diabetic cardiomyopathies, compounded by the frequent occurrence of uremic pericarditis as ESRD is approached, places patients with advanced CRF at high risk for serious cardiac events (*i.e.*, myocardial infarction, CHF, and acute cardiac tamponade).

Hypertension in Chronic Renal Failure. Hypertension occurs in greater than 80% of patients with ESRD on initiation of dialysis. Hypertension in advanced CRF is a result of either increased cardiac output or increased total peripheral resistance or both. The increase in cardiac output in advanced CRF is predominantly a result of sodium and water overload (increased preload). Other important factors increasing cardiac output include anemia and, possibly, the presence of a high-flow arteriovenous fistula. In contrast, increased total peripheral resistance is secondary to renin-dependent vasopressor release from the kidneys. Consequently, **the most important factors responsible for hypertension in advanced CRF are volume expansion and the vasopressor function of the kidneys.**

Although overlap exists between these syndromes, division of hypertension of CRF into volume-dependent and renin-dependent categories aids in the approach to BP control, as illustrated in Table 13–16. In patients with sustained hypertension (diastolic BP >95 mm Hg), therapy should be initiated. Because most patients with advanced CRF have volume-dependent hypertension, initial therapy should involve the establishment of euvolemia. Dietary sodium restriction (2 to 4 g sodium per day) should be initiated with addition of a loop diuretic (furosemide, bumetanide) if BP remains elevated.

Sustained hypertension, despite achievement of euvolemia, requires initiation of an antihypertensive agent. Initial therapy should consist of adrenergic blockade, calcium channel blockade, and/or ACE inhibition. Particular attention should be paid to the route of excretion of any agent chosen, because some antihypertensive agents will accumulate in renal failure (*e.g.*, nadolol, atenolol, ACE inhibitors), possibly causing serious hypotension. Furthermore, effects on potassium regulation should be considered because potassium excretion is impaired in CRF and hyperkalemia may occur. Agents such as beta-adrenergic blockers and ACE inhibitors should be used in conjunction with potassium restriction and frequent potassium monitoring. Changes in renal function should also be monitored because hypertension control may result in a decline in GFR. If hypertension still persists despite the presence of euvolemia and the addition of adrenergic blockade, calcium channel blockade, and/or ACE inhibition, a vasodilating agent such as prazosin (an alpha-adrenergic blocker with vasodilating effects), nifedipine (calcium channel blocker), or hydralazine should be added. Finally, if hypertension remains uncontrolled despite maximal doses of previous agents, the combination of minoxidil (the most potent vasodilator available) and either a beta-adrenergic-blocking agent or a centrally acting adrenergic-blocking agent may be effective. With minoxidil administration, strict monitoring for hypotension, reflex tachycardia, sodium retention and edema formation, hirsutism, and pericardial effusion will be necessary. In patients not on dialysis, adjustment of diuretics will be necessary to counteract the potent sodium-retaining effect of minoxidil.

Bilateral nephrectomy for refractory hypertension, once used frequently, should be avoided because anemia may worsen significantly after removal of the kidneys. If nephrectomy becomes necessary, EPO administration will aid in ameliorating any further worsening of the anemia.

Table 13–16. APPROACH TO BLOOD PRESSURE CONTROL IN CHRONIC RENAL FAILURE

1. Restore euvolemia
    - Sodium restriction: 2–4 g/day
    - Diuretics: See Table 13–5
2. Antihypertensive therapy
    - Initial therapy
        - Adrenergic blocking agents
            - Beta blockers
            - Centrally acting agents: clonidine, guanabenz, methyldopa
            - Alpha$_2$-blocking agents: prazosin and/or combined alpha and beta blockers: labetalol
        - Calcium channel antagonists
        - Angiotensin-converting enzyme inhibitors
3. If inadequate response, add:
    - Vasodilator: hydralazine, nifedipine (calcium channel antagonist)
4. If inadequate response, substitute:
    - Minoxidil combined with beta-adrenergic or centrally acting adrenergic blocking agent

Ischemic Heart Disease. In the population with ESRD, ischemic heart disease (IHD) is an important cause of morbidity and mortality. The high incidence of the disease exists partially because of the high frequency of risk factors in this population. First, hypertension, as previously mentioned, is present in more than 80% of patients with CRF. Consequently, left ventricular hypertrophy is common. Second, lipid abnormalities, most notably type 4 hyperlipoproteinemia, increased low-density and very low-density lipoprotein cholesterol content, and decreased high-density lipoprotein may begin early in the course of advanced CRF (GFR of 30 ml/min). Third, cigarette smoking has a high prevalence in the population with CRF. This factor together with hypertension significantly increases the frequency of ischemic events. Finally, the influences of the underlying primary disease (*e.g.*, diabetes mellitus) on the heart will also influence the development of IHD.

Clinical manifestations of IHD are no different in CRF than in the general population. Similarly, the mainstay of treatment is also based on nitroglycerin derivatives (sublingual, topical, or oral nitrates) and beta-adrenergic agents or calcium channel blockade. However, diagnosis may be less straightforward in the population with CRF.

Results of creatine phosphokinase (CPK)-MB isoenzymes, exercise, and/or radionuclide stress testing may be altered in advanced renal failure. First, elevations in total CPK and CPK-MB fraction can be noted in patients who have CRF and who exhibit no other evidence of cardiac ischemia or infarction. Second, ECG exercise stress testing is often limited by poor exercise tolerance resulting from polyneuropathy, chronic anemia, and poor physical training, with target heart rate seldom being reached. The addition of thallium radionuclide scanning (exercise or dipyridamole) is helpful in symptomatic patients. However, in the absence of symptoms, the high frequency of resting cardiac abnormalities with thallium scanning makes this test less useful. Finally, coronary angiography, the time-honored standard for defining coronary artery disease, is not without risk in CRF. Both irreversible radiocontrast-induced acute renal failure and blood volume expansion (with pulmonary edema) occur frequently in patients who have advanced renal disease and are subjected to the radiographic dye load of coronary angiography. Consequently, **thallium stress testing and, particularly, coronary angiography should be used in symptomatic patients who have a high risk of IHD, who have failed intensive antianginal therapy, and who are acceptable candidates for coronary angioplasty and/or bypass surgery.** The high-risk population for IHD in CRF will most likely have the following characteristics: age >50 years, white race, male gender, elevated total serum cholesterol, and the presence of symptoms of IHD and/or segmental left ventricular wall motion abnormalities on two-dimensional echocardiography.

Pericarditis. Pericarditis is a frequent and serious complication of advanced renal failure, with a potential for causing serious arrhythmias, cardiac tamponade, and death. Consequently, early recognition and proper management of pericarditis are important in the management of progressive CRF.

Two categories of pericarditis in CRF include uremic and dialysis-associated pericarditis. Uremic pericarditis is encountered in patients who have ESRD but are not yet on maintenance dialysis. Dialysis-related pericarditis, in contrast, occurs in patients who have advanced CRF and are receiving maintenance dialysis.

The clinical features of pericarditis in advanced renal failure are listed in Table 13–17. Fever, chest pain, and a pericardial friction rub are the most frequent manifestations. Chest pain is pleuritic in nature, increased by rotation of the trunk, deep breathing, and the supine position. Relief of pain by sitting forward is also typical. The pericardial friction rub is typically evanescent, scratching in quality, and heard best at the left parasternal border in end expiration with a patient sitting forward. Hypotension is a common manifestation of dialysis-related pericarditis, but it is unusual in uremic pericarditis unless cardiac tamponade is present.

The most common manifestations of cardiac tamponade are dyspnea, tachypnea, chest pain, hypotension with a narrow pulse pressure, jugular venous distention, and pulsus paradoxus. The presence of these symptoms indicates emergent need for pericardiocentesis.

Table 13–17. CLINICAL FEATURES OF PERICARDITIS

Fever
Chest pain, pleuritic in nature
Pericardial friction rub
Hypotension
Cardiomegaly or pleural effusion on chest x-ray film
Diffuse ST-T wave elevations on electrocardiogram (unusual)
Pericardial effusion on echocardiography (diagnostic)

Management of the percarditis of CRF without tamponade begins with the initiation or intensification of dialysis. Regional anticoagulation or limited systemic anticoagulation should be used. Persistence of pericardial fluid after 10 to 14 days of therapy or an enlarging pericardial effusion requires intervention either by pericardiocentesis and introduction of nonabsorbable steroids or by anterior pericardiectomy.

Heart Failure in Chronic Renal Failure. Heart failure is a common complication of advanced CRF, usually precipitated by increased preload, increased afterload, or intrinsic myocardial failure. The main causes of heart failure in CRF are summarized in Table 13–18.

The treatment of CHF in advanced renal failure includes decreasing preload, accomplished by normalizing ECF volume (see Table 13–5), decreasing arteriovenous fistula flow rates, correcting the anemia of chronic disease (see Table 13–8), and initiating certain pharmacologic agents that specifically reduce preload (*e.g.*, nitroglycerin or isosorbide dinitrate, furosemide, prazosin, and sodium nitroprusside).

Afterload reduction can be accomplished, in general, by normalization of hypertension, but vasodilator agents such as nitroprusside, hydralazine, prazosin, and ACE inhibitors may be the agents of choice in patients with severe CHF and advanced renal failure.

Finally, efforts to increase myocardial contractility may be necessary, especially in patients with left ventricular dilatation. Digoxin is the agent of choice. The primary renal excretion of digoxin combined with the narrow therapeutic window of digitalis derivatives indicates that dosage should begin at 0.0625 to 0.125 mg every other day, with frequent monitoring of blood levels to prevent digoxin toxicity.

Table 13–18. CAUSES OF HEART FAILURE IN CHRONIC RENAL FAILURE

Increased preload
Hypervolemia
Anemia
Arteriovenous fistula
Increased afterload
Uncontrolled or accelerated hypertension
Decreased myocardial function
Coronary artery disease
Cardiomyopathy: Uremic, diabetic, hypertensive, ischemic cardiomyopathies
Myocarditis
Pericarditis: Cardiac tamponade, constrictive pericarditis
Acidosis: Serum pH <7.2
Electrolyte abnormalities: Hyper/hypokalemia, hypophosphatemia
Nutritional deficiencies: Vitamin, protein deficiencies
Myocardial calcifications
Systemic diseases: Scleroderma, amyloidosis, polyarteritis nodosa

DEFINITIVE THERAPY FOR END-STAGE RENAL DISEASE: INDICATIONS FOR DIALYSIS*

Preparing Patients for Dialysis

As a patient with CRF approaches ESRD, a smooth transition to renal replacement therapy or dependence on dialysis is important. Preparation of patients should include education and access placement.

Education

Particular emphasis should be placed on the changes in daily routine that will occur once dialysis begins, such as dietary restrictions, daily schedules, amount and types of medications required, and frequency and expectations of follow-up.

Permanent Dialysis Access Placement

Hemodialysis. The permanent access of choice for patients requiring hemodialysis is an endogenous arteriovenous fistula because of the 65 to 75% 3-year survival rate. To aid in preserving arteriovenous fistula survival, the venous system of the chosen arm should be guarded from the trauma of frequent BP measurement and venipunctures before placement of the access. Ideally, the arteriovenous fistula should be placed 2 to 6 months before initiation of dialysis to allow fistula maturation.

When the quality of the arm veins is poor (small caliber, deeply located in the arm), arteriovenous connection must be made via either a graft made from polytetrafluoroethylene (Teflon) or from an autologous saphenous vein. Three-year graft patency rate is 30%, which is substantially inferior to the arteriovenous fistula. A 2- to 3-week delay in using the graft will allow healing of the subcutaneous tunnel and endothelialization of the graft itself.

Peritoneal Dialysis. Insertion of the double-

*See also Chapters 17 and 18.

cuffed Tenckhoff's catheter should be performed at least 2 weeks before the initiation of dialysis to allow for peritoneal membrane closure.

Indications for the Initiation of Dialysis

In the acute uremic state, the indications for dialysis are directed toward preventing life-threatening complications (Table 13–19). In CRF, however, the general rule is to initiate chronic dialysis when conservative management of the patient no longer maintains quality of life and productivity, especially when a patient is emotionally and intellectually prepared to do so. Certain specific indications deserve emphasis:

Central and Peripheral Nervous System Dysfunction. Dialysis should be initiated at the first signs of deterioration of mental status and during the early stages of peripheral neuropathy.

Uremic Pericarditis. Delay of dialysis in patients with uremic pericarditis may cause the development of a hemorrhagic pericardial effusion and cardiac tamponade. Therefore, it is imperative to initiate dialysis when confronted with a pericardial friction rub.

Malnutrition. As renal failure progresses, the development of nausea, vomiting, and changes in taste sensation will interfere with nutritional intake. Consistent declines in body weight unrelated to therapy for volume overload become an indication for initiation of dialysis.

Asymptomatic Indications for Dialysis. Some nephrologists recommend initiation of dialysis, regardless of symptoms, when the decrement in GFR reaches a critical value after which symptoms inevitably develop. Guidelines are depicted in Table 13–19.

Table 13–19. INDICATIONS FOR THE INITIATION OF DIALYSIS

Acute Indications
Uremic syndrome (See Table 13–2)
Volume overload unresponsive to diuretics
Hyperkalemia uncontrolled with therapy
Severe metabolic acidosis
Major bleeding episode
Chronic Indications
Creatinine clearances <0.10–0.15 ml/min/kg lean body weight (GFR <8–10 ml/min). In diabetic, creatinine clearance <0.15–0.20 ml/min/kg (GFR <10–15 ml/min).

Suggested Readings

Anderson S, Rennke HG, Brenner BM: Therapeutic advantage of converting enzyme inhibitors in arresting progressive renal disease associated with systemic hypertension in the rat. J Clin Invest 77:1993, 1986.

Brenner BM, Rector FC (eds): The Kidney, 4th ed. Philadelphia, WB Saunders, 1991.

DuBose TD Jr: Acid-base balance. *In* Eknoyan G, Knochel JP (eds): The Systemic Consequences of Renal Failure. New York, Grune & Stratton, 1984.

Elser AR: Gastrointestinal bleeding in maintenance dialysis patients. Semin Dialysis 1:198, 1988.

Eschbach VW, Adamson VW: Anemia in renal disease. *In* Schrier RW, Gottschalk CW (eds): Diseases of the Kidney, 4th ed. Boston, Little, Brown & Co., 1988.

Eschbach JW, Egrie JC, Downing MR: Correction of the anemia of end-stage renal disease with recombinant human erythropoietin. N Engl J Med 316:73, 1987.

Fraser CL, Arieff AI: Nervous system complications in uremia. Ann Intern Med 109:143, 1988.

Gimenez LF, Solez K, Walker WG: Relation between renal calcium content and renal impairment in 246 human renal biopsies. Kidney Int 31:93, 1987.

Hostetter TH, Meyer TW, Rennke HG, et al: Chronic effects of dietary protein in the rat with intact and reduced renal mass. Kidney Int 30:509, 1986.

Levy AS, Perrone RD, Madias NE: Serum creatinine and renal function. Annu Rev Med 39:465, 1988.

Miller RB: The patient with chronic azotemia, with emphasis on chronic renal failure. *In* Schrier RW (ed): Manual of Nephrology. Boston, Little, Brown & Co, 1988.

Mujais SK, Sabatini S, Kurtzman NA: Pathophysiology of the uremic syndrome. *In* Brenner BM, Rector FC (eds): The Kidney. Philadelphia, WB Saunders, 1985, pp 1587–1630.

Rose BD: Manual of Clinical Problems in Nephrology. Boston, Little, Brown & Co, 1988.

Rostand SG, Rutsky ED: Ischemic heart disease in chronic renal failure: Management considerations. Semin Dialysis 2:98, 1989.

United States Renal Data Report. Bethesda, Md, The National Institutes of Health, The National Institutes of Diabetes and Digestive and Kidney Diseases, Division of Kidney, Urologic and Hematologic Diseases. 1989.

CHAPTER 14

RENAL BONE DISEASES AND ALUMINUM TOXICITY IN RENAL PATIENTS

Jack W. Coburn, William G. Goodman, and Isidro B. Salusky

The kidneys maintain the body's external balance of calcium, phosphorus, and magnesium; they synthesize calcitriol (1,25-dihydroxycholecalciferol or 1,25$(OH)_2D_3$), the active form of vitamin D; they are a major target organ for parathyroid hormone (PTH) action and the site of its clearance and degradation; and they are the major route of excretion for aluminum that enters the body. Therefore, it is not surprising that mineral metabolism is altered as nephron function is lost.

Some degree of bone disease, collectively called *renal osteodystrophy*, nearly always accompanies chronic renal failure. Because several different disorders of bone can develop, they should be called the *renal bone diseases* or the *renal osteodystrophies*, as it is necessary to identify the predominant problem. There are two major types of renal osteodystrophy, but several pathogenic factors are involved. The first type is high-turnover bone disease, due largely to the development of secondary hyperparathyroidism, and the second type is low-turnover bone disease, which exists as osteomalacia in its florid form or as a milder aplastic bone disease. Aluminum toxicity is a major pathogenic factor causing low-turnover bone disease, but reduced PTH secretion, abnormal vitamin D status, iron overload, and other pathogenic factors may also be involved in the pathogenesis. The pathogenesis and laboratory features are described first, followed by a consideration of the clinical syndromes and their management. The metabolism of aluminum and the features of aluminum toxicity are considered, and a unique type of dialysis amyloidosis that causes bone cysts, skeletal and periarticular pain, and fractures is reviewed. Symptoms of the latter disorder are difficult to distinguish from those of metabolic bone diseases.

PATHOGENESIS OF BONE DISEASE

In the course of developing renal failure, several processes contribute to increased PTH secretion and secondary hyperparathyroidism (Table 14–1), although the exact sequence is uncertain. They include phosphate retention (but often with little or no initial rise in serum phosphorus), reduced synthesis of calcitriol, reduced calcemic action of PTH, and a decrease in ionized calcium in the blood. At some point, there is a change in parathyroid physiology so that higher serum calcium levels are required to suppress the PTH secretion by individual cells. This is termed a shift in the set-point for calcium-mediated PTH release; as a result, a higher serum calcium level is needed to suppress PTH secretion. In more advanced renal failure, true hyperphosphatemia and hypocalcemia are observed, and the intestinal absorption of calcium is impaired. Hyperplasia and progressive enlargement of the parathyroid glands occur and greatly amplify the total amount of PTH that is secreted. Complex interactions occur among the regulatory factors. For example, phosphate retention, perhaps at an intracellular level and without an increase in serum phosphorus, can inhibit calcitriol synthesis, and this reduction in calcitriol production may impair the normal feedback suppression of PTH by an elevated serum calcium level. Although there is increased PTH secretion, the

Table 14–1. FACTORS CONTRIBUTING TO HIGH SERUM PTH LEVELS IN RENAL FAILURE AND RESPONSIBLE PATHOGENIC MECHANISMS

Cause of Increased PTH Levels	Pathogenic Mechanism(s)
Hypocalcemia	Hyperphosphatemia, low serum calcitriol levels, ? skeletal resistance to PTH
Low calcitriol levels	Phosphorus retention, nephron destruction, ? acidosis, transtubular phosphate flux
Shift of parathyroid "set-point" (higher calcium needed to suppress PTH secretion per cell)	Low calcitriol level, phosphorus retention, ? other
Parathyroid hyperplasia—marked and slow to involute	Cause uncertain, same factors that stimulate PTH secretion
Skeletal resistance to PTH action	Down-regulation of PTH receptors, low calcitriol, hyperphosphatemia
Reduced degradation of PTH—interpretation of PTH assay	Reduced renal clearance of PTH (fragments)

Modified from Coburn JW, Slatopolsky E: Vitamin D, parathyroid hormone, and the renal osteodystrophies. *In* Brenner BM, Rector FC Jr (eds): The Kidney, 4th Ed. Philadelphia, WB Saunders, 1990.

kidneys' synthesis of calcitriol is not adequate to reverse the process, and even more PTH is required.

Abnormal Metabolism of Vitamin D

The kidneys are the major organs responsible for the synthesis of calcitriol, the most active form of vitamin D. The synthesis of calcitriol is stimulated by PTH, hypocalcemia itself, and a reduced dietary intake of phosphate; calcitriol synthesis is inhibited by opposite changes. The actions of calcitriol include stimulation of intestinal calcium absorption and suppression of PTH synthesis, both by having a direct parathyroid effect and by raising serum calcium levels; calcitriol also affects bone metabolism and modulates the function of the immune system. Although it was initially believed that reduced calcitriol synthesis was a major factor causing osteomalacia in renal failure, evidence now indicates that abnormal vitamin D metabolism contributes in a major way to secondary hyperparathyroidism. Phosphate retention (even without an increase in serum phosphorus level) is of importance in lowering calcitriol synthesis in early renal failure, and increased extrarenal synthesis of calcitriol may occur when plasma $1,25(OH)_2D$ levels are raised substantially with vitamin D or $25(OH)D_3$ therapy. Osteomalacia due to abnormal vitamin D metabolism in a patient with renal failure is unusual and is probably limited to patients with coexistent vitamin D deficiency, as manifested by low serum levels of $25(OH)D_3$.

Aluminum Metabolism

The normal intake of aluminum is 2 to 4 mg/day, and only a minute fraction is absorbed and then excreted in the urine. When renal function is reduced, the absorbed aluminum is retained within the body. Aluminum loading can arise from aluminum-contaminated dialysis solutions and from intravenous solutions, such as casein hydrolysate or albumin, that contain aluminum. It occurs when the oral intake of aluminum is markedly increased (*e.g.*, during therapy with aluminum hydroxide, aluminum carbonate, or sucralfate). Aluminum absorption is markedly augmented by citrate ingestion, whereas other factors have trivial effects. Excessive aluminum in the body is very slowly removed by dialysis alone because most plasma aluminum is bound to transferrin. Aluminum affects bone formation by impairing osteoblast function and/or proliferation, by altering the solubility of calcium-phosphate crystals, and by directly inhibiting the secretion of PTH by the parathyroid glands; thus, aluminum accumulation is the most important cause of osteomalacia or aplastic bone disease in renal failure. **Aluminum toxicity can cause altered brain function (dialysis encephalopathy), anemia, proximal myopathy, and perhaps abnormal myocardial function. Other factors can also lead to low bone formation (Table 14–2).**

Amyloidosis due to β_2-Microglobulin

In patients on dialysis for more than 5 years, a unique type of amyloidosis can cause skeletal and joint symptoms. β_2-Microglobulin is the major constituent of this amyloid. Normally, B_2-microglobulin is filtered at the glomerulus and then degraded by the tubules; in patients undergoing long-term dialysis, the blood levels of B_2-microglobulin increase far above normal. The reason why amyloid deposits develop in some but not all dialysis patients is not clear, nor is it understood why these amyloid deposits have a predilection for periarticular structures and bone. The presence of hyperparathyroidism may favor their development. **Syndromes arising from B_2-microglobulin amyloidosis can be confused with those of renal osteodystrophy, and the disorders can coexist.**

MILD TO MODERATE RENAL FAILURE

In mild to moderate renal failure, bone usually shows features of mild hyperparathyroidism, serum phosphorus levels are normal or even low, and serum calcium levels can be normal or minimally depressed. Skeletal symptoms are generally absent, although they may occur in children and in adults who are younger than 40 years and have long-standing and slowly progressive renal failure due to tubulointerstitial disorders (*e.g.*, polycystic kidney disease). **Aluminum toxicity is unusual, but it can occur when aluminum gels and Shohl's solution (citric acid/sodium citrate) are prescribed concomitantly.** Mild metabolic acidosis may exist and contribute to decreased skeletal mineralization.

ADVANCED AND END-STAGE RENAL DISEASE

In such patients with advanced and end-stage renal disease (ESRD), hyperphosphatemia is usual and metabolic acidosis may be profound. The dietary intake of calcium is often low, and the ingestion of vitamins, including vitamin D, may be reduced. Initiation of dialysis has an effect on these parameters: Serum calcium level often increases, partly because dialysate calcium exceeds the plasma ultrafilterable calcium. This is less evident in patients on peritoneal dialysis (*e.g.*, continuous ambulatory peritoneal dialysis [CAPD]), because of the accompanying hypoalbuminemia. Hyperphosphatemia is affected less by dialysis and is very common, more so in those on hemodialysis than CAPD; **thus, 90 to 95% of patients undergoing hemodialysis require phosphate-binding agents to lower predialysis serum phosphorus level to 1.5 to 1.8 mmol/L (4.6 to 5.6 mg/dl).** Plasma aluminum levels rise within a few weeks if dialysate aluminum levels exceed 0.3 to 0.5 mmol/L (8 to 14 μg/L) but increase more slowly and more variably when the patients are given aluminum gels as phosphate-binding agents. Acidosis usually improves, although serum bicarbonate levels are often subnormal before dialysis.

LABORATORY, RADIOGRAPHIC, AND HISTOLOGIC FEATURES

Serum Calcium

Hypocalcemia is common, particularly during the first few months of hemodialysis, and it persists longer with CAPD because of the lower serum albumin levels. Hyperphosphatemia, if present, contributes to hypocalcemia. Low serum calcium levels (<2.0 mmol/L or 8.0 mg/dl) can be associated with a mixed skeletal lesion with histologic features of both osteitis fibrosa and osteomalacia.

Hypercalcemia is not infrequent in long-term hemodialysis patients. It can occur with severe secondary hyperparathyroidism and osteitis fibrosa or with aluminum toxicity, and it can develop quickly, either with or without symptoms, when patients are treated with $CaCO_3$, calcitriol, or both. Other causes must also be considered (Table 14–3). Because these patients cannot excrete calcium in their urine and because the usual dialysate calcium level prevents calcium loss during dialysis, hypercalcemia may persist until dialysis is done using a low-calcium dialysate (see Case Summary 1).

Table 14–2. FACTORS LEADING TO REDUCED BONE FORMATION IN PATIENTS WITH RENAL FAILURE

Aluminum accumulation (Mechanism: ? aluminum on forming surface, aluminum in osteoblasts, increased serum aluminum, decreased PTH)
Low calcium and phosphorus product in serum: (hypocalcemia common, hypophosphatemia rare)
Low PTH levels (Mechanism: parathyroidectomy, diabetes mellitus, high serum calcium, calcitriol therapy, aluminum loading)
Iron accumulation (rare, can accompany aluminum accumulation)
Diabetes mellitus (mechanism multifactorial, ? low PTH)
Decreased vitamin D: (significant when nutritional vitamin D deficiency coexists)
Miscellaneous and unidentified factors (e.g., immobilization)

Modified from Coburn JW, Slatopolsky E: Vitamin D, parathyroid hormone, and the renal osteodystrophies. *In* Brenner BM, Rector FC Jr (eds): The Kidney, 4th Ed. Philadelphia, WB Saunders, 1990.

Table 14–3. CAUSES OF HYPERCALCEMIA IN DIALYSIS PATIENTS

Severe secondary hyperparathyroidism
Aluminum toxicity
Treatment with $CaCO_3$, calcium citrate, etc.
Therapy with calcitriol or other vitamin D sterol
Dialysate calcium >3 to 3.5 mEq/L
Endogenous calcitriol (sarcoidosis, tuberculosis, or other granulomatous disease)
Malignancy: Renal cell carcinoma; neoplasm: lung, gastrointestinal tract, or other; multiple myeloma
Immobilization
Marked hypophosphatemia (rare)

Modified from Coburn JW, Slatopolsky E: Vitamin D, parathyroid hormone, and the renal osteodystrophies. *In* Brenner BM, Rector FC Jr (eds): The Kidney, 4th Ed. Philadelphia, WB Saunders, 1990.

Blood Ionized Calcium

Although total serum calcium and serum albumin levels generally permit proper patient management, ionized calcium levels can be useful, particularly when serum albumin levels differ from normal (*e.g.*, in patients undergoing CAPD).

Serum Phosphorus

Hyperphosphatemia is common with both hemodialysis and CAPD, although it is not as marked with the latter. Therapy with calcitriol may aggravate hyperphosphatemia because it can increase phosphate absorption. In patients with severe secondary hyperparathyroidism and osteitis fibrosa, hyperphosphatemia can be resistant to phosphate binders as a result of increased phosphate flux out of bone.

Alkaline Phosphatase

When the serum alkaline phosphatase level is elevated, serum gamma-glutamyl transferase (GGT) or 5′ nucleotidase should be determined to rule out a hepatic cause of the elevated level; fractionation of alkaline phosphatase can be done, but it is costly and time-consuming. For practical purposes, an elevated level of alkaline phosphatase with normal GGT level defines *bone alkaline phosphatase.* The alkaline phosphatase originates from osteoblasts, and the levels rise slowly and progressively as osteitis fibrosa develops. With osteomalacia due to aluminum toxicity, the levels can also be increased, although patients with osteomalacia due to very severe aluminum toxicity may have normal levels of alkaline phosphatase.

Parathyroid Hormone Levels

PTH levels are above normal in most patients with ESRD, but the degree of elevation is modified by PTH metabolism, the PTH antiserum used, and the degree of secondary hyperparathyroidism. After its secretion, PTH is quickly degraded into *midregion* and *carboxy-terminal* fragments. With midregion and certain carboxy-terminal PTH assays, the degree of PTH elevation is profound because the renal clearance of these PTH fragments is markedly reduced. In patients who have ESRD with moderate to severe osteitis fibrosa, the midregion PTH levels exceed 15 to 20 times the upper normal limit, whereas the amino-terminal or "intact" hormone assays are at least 4 to 5 times normal. The PTH range that identifies primary hyperparathyroidism in nonazotemic patients cannot be used to indicate osteitis fibrosa in a patient with ESRD. One should use a PTH assay that has been characterized according to the bone histologic features found in patients with ESRD. Because aluminum loading may directly inhibit PTH secretion as well as raise serum calcium levels, PTH levels are often lower than expected in patients with aluminum loading. **The combined use of serum PTH and plasma aluminum determinations can help distinguish patients with aluminum toxicity from those with hyperparathyroid bone disease.**

Serum magnesium levels are usually modestly elevated in patients with ESRD, and they increase strikingly when magnesium-containing laxatives are used. When the levels exceed 2 mmol/L, symptoms of flushing and burning of the skin can occur.

Plasma Aluminum

Plasma aluminum levels are often above normal in patients with ESRD (normal range, <0.3 mmol/L or <10 μg/L), but the levels are usually below 1.5 mmol/L (40 μg/L) unless there is an exogenous source of aluminum (oral aluminum gels or aluminum-contaminated dialysate). Evidence of aluminum toxicity is common when plasma levels exceed 3 mmol/L (80 μg/L) but values of 1.5 to 3 μmol/L (40 to 80 μg/L) can be found in aluminum-intoxicated

Table 14–4. FACTORS PREDISPOSING TO HIGH- OR LOW-TURNOVER BONE DISEASE

High Turnover	Low Turnover
Children; young adults > older patients	Diabetes mellitus
Female > male	Prior parathyroidectomy
Tubulointerstitial > glomerular diseases	Prior transplant (? steroid therapy)
Poor phosphate control (via increased PTH)	Aluminum exposure (dialysate, oral)
	Binephrectomy
	Calcitriol therapy, $CaCO_3$ therapy
	High calcium level in CAPD solutions

patients when aluminum exposure has been withdrawn for longer than 1 to 2 months.

Other Investigations

In the clinical management of patients with renal insufficiency of more than 1 to 2 years duration, other investigations are indicated, particularly in patients with more risk of developing high-turnover bone disease (Table 14–4). These include skeletal radiographs, bone scan, and bone biopsy.

Metabolic Bone Survey

A metabolic bone survey may detect features of osteitis fibrosa (severe secondary hyperparathyroidism) and extraskeletal calcifications. Subperiosteal erosions are most readily seen on the radial surfaces of the phalanges (Fig. 14–1); rarely, they are found in the sacroiliac joints, along the pubic rami, or along the lateral scapulae when hand films are negative. Brown tumors of osteitis fibrosa are rare with "renal" hyperparathyroidism. X-ray findings of erosions do not date their appearance unless an earlier or normal radiograph is available for comparison; old erosions may persist after aluminum toxicity has supervened but with no mineralization of bone surface.

Radiographs can also show thin-walled cysts at the ends of long bones arising from dialysis amyloidosis; these may be mistaken for brown tumors. Pseudofractures due to osteomalacia are uncommon, even in renal patients with documented osteomalacia; hence, negative studies are meaningless. Extraskeletal calcifications of different types can occur (Table 14–5). Calcification of periarticular tissues and about the joints (Fig. 14–2) and large subcutaneous masses that are often around joints can be detected with radiographs and their progress followed. They may be associated with acute or subacute arthritic symptoms and are correlated with high serum calcium and phosphorus product and substantially elevated PTH levels.

Bone Scan

In patients with osteitis fibrosa, the bone scan often shows diffuse and symmetrical uptake of isotope (*e.g.*, a "superscan"). In those with severe aluminum-related osteomalacia, it will typically show less uptake in bone, a finding accentuated by the reduced renal excretion of the radionuclide and increased background activity. The bone scan may show fractures without displacement and pseudofractures that are not detected on radiographs. The scan will often detect soft-tissue calcifications, such as those in the lungs, which are not detectable radiographically. In advanced dialysis amyloidosis, bone

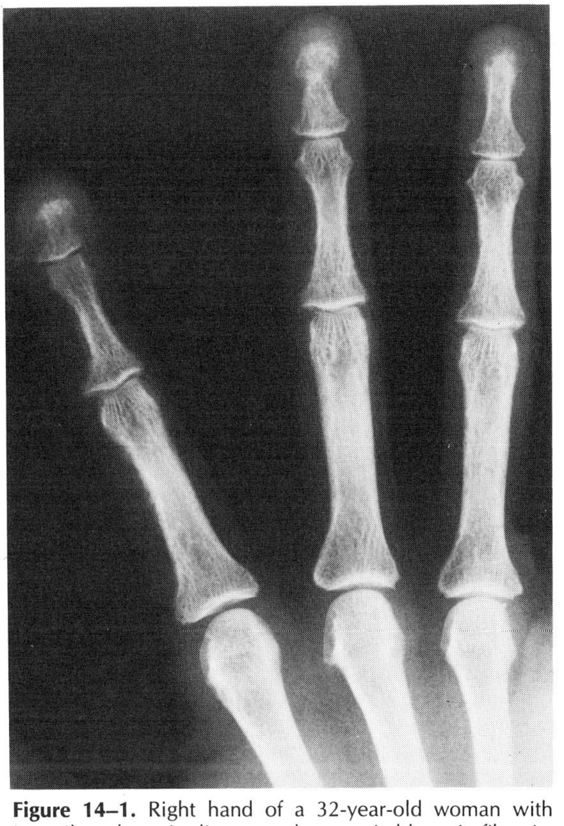

Figure 14–1. Right hand of a 32-year-old woman with juvenile polycystic disease and congenital hepatic fibrosis. During 4 years of hemodialysis, the midregion parathyroid hormone rose slowly from 24,000 to 79,000 pg/ml and alkaline phosphatase increased to 744 IU/ml. She had a ruptured quadriceps tendon in the past, but she otherwise lacked musculoskeletal symptoms. Radiographs show subperiosteal erosions on the radial surfaces of the second and third digits; there were also erosions and bulbar deformities of the distal phalanges, producing pseudoclubbing.

Table 14–5. TYPES OF EXTRASKELETAL CALCIFICATIONS, PATHOGENIC FACTORS, AND THEIR MANAGEMENT

Type/Location	Pathogenic Factor	Consequences	Management
Conjunctival	High pH of eye High Ca × P product	Acute: "red eye" Chronic: "white eye"	Reduce Ca × P product
Periarticular	High Ca × P product	Acute "arthritis" or periarthritis	PO_4 control, PTX
Tumoral	High Ca × P product	Periarticular masses restrict motion Inflammation not common	PO_4 control, PTX
Pulmonary	?*	Pulmonary insufficiency, pulmonary hypertension	
Cardiac	?*	Arrhythmias, cardiac failure	
Vascular	?, low serum Mg *Plus* high PTH and high serum P	Often no symptoms Calciphylaxis (rare)	No treatment PTX for calciphylaxis

*The chemical composition of these visceral calcifications differs from other extraskeletal calcifications. PTX, parathyroidectomy.

Modified from Coburn JW, Slatopolsky E: Vitamin D, parathyroid hormone, and the renal osteodystrophies. *In* Brenner BM, Rector FC Jr (eds): The Kidney, 4th Ed. Philadelphia, WB Saunders, 1990.

scans can show localized uptake at the sites of cystic deposits, but this technique is not highly sensitive.

Bone Biopsy and Histology

A bone biopsy carried out after double tetracycline labeling and with the preparation of undecalcified sections can provide precise identification of the bone disease present. Surface staining for aluminum and in many instances for iron should be done. Such preparations are rarely available in hospital pathology laboratories, and samples must be sent to a specialized laboratory. Tetracycline (0.5 g b.i.d. for 2 days) is given over two periods separated by a 10- to 20-day interval for "double labeling"; this permits measure of bone formation rate and distinction of low, normal, and high turnover states. A biopsy is easily done in an outpatient setting using local anesthetic combined with analgesia similar to that used for gastrointestinal endoscopy (*e.g.*, intravenous low-dose midazolam and meperidine). In general, a bone biopsy is needed only for problem cases or for decision-making with regard to parathyroidectomy.

Several types of skeletal lesions can be seen. Severe hyperparathyroidism leads to peritrabecular fibrosis (osteitis fibrosa) with high bone turnover, whereas mild parathyroid disease may only show high turnover. The osteoid seams may be wide in osteitis fibrosa, but osteomalacia, as defined by a low bone formation rate and delayed mineralization, is absent. Osteomalacia is recognized by a widened osteoid seam and reduced bone formation rate and mineralization, whereas aplastic bone disease is characterized by low bone formation but normal or reduced width of osteoid seams. A mixed lesion is occasionally seen with peritrabecular fibrosis plus features of osteomalacia. The mixed lesion is commonly associated with hypocalcemia and/or a low serum phosphorus level, or it can occur when patients evolve from hyperparathyroidism to aluminum toxicity. Aluminum-related bone disease is defined by >25 to

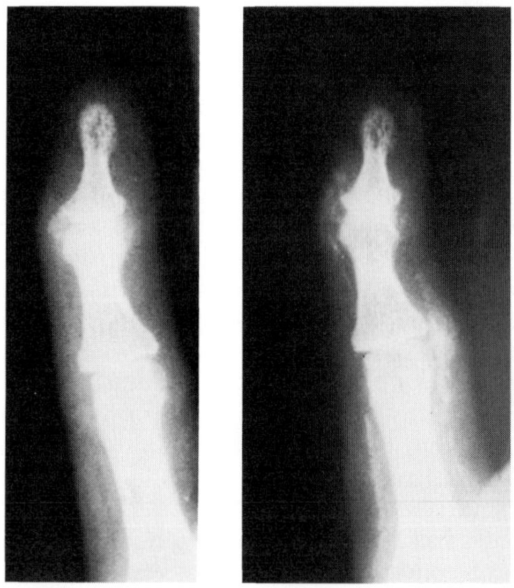

Figure 14–2. The patient is a 31-year-old woman who has end-stage renal disease managed with continuous ambulatory peritoneal dialysis. She developed pain, swelling, and warmth of her right index finger. She had recently become less compliant with the prescribed aluminum hydroxide, and her serum phosphorus level increased from 1.9 to 2.9 mmol/L (5.9 to 9.0 mg/dl), with a serum calcium level of 2.4 mmol/L (9.6 mg/dl). Radiographs showed the development of periarticular and soft-tissue calcifications during a 6-week period. Her pain responded to indomethacin treatment, and the swelling decreased after she had resumed her phosphate-binding agents. Parathyroidectomy was ultimately done because her serum phosphorus level remained elevated.

30% surface staining for aluminum and evidence of aluminum toxicity; this occurs most commonly with the osteomalacic or aplastic lesions and is less common with normal histologic features or a mixed lesion. Surface aluminum staining is rare with osteitis fibrosa, even when the total bone aluminum is substantially elevated. The high rate of bone turnover may limit aluminum deposition on the forming surfaces of bone. Rarely, osteomalacia can be attributed to iron deposition on the bone-forming surface. Patients with ESRD rarely show oxalate deposits and accompanying osseous pathology; primary oxalosis, megadose vitamin C therapy, concomitant regional enteritis, and the addition of ascorbic acid to dialysate have been implicated as pathogenic to cause such deposits in dialysis patients.

GENERAL MANAGEMENT OF CLINICAL PROBLEMS

Mild to Moderate Renal Failure (C_{cr} 30 to 70 ml/min)

Bone disease is mild, and symptoms do not occur except in growing children. Serum biochemical findings are commonly normal, although the serum phosphorus level may be low. If measured, PTH levels are moderately elevated. Theoretically, dietary phosphate restriction or therapy with low doses of calcitriol would be of prophylactic value. If a phosphate-binding agent is given, it should be calcium carbonate or calcium acetate; calcitriol can reverse the secondary hyperparathyroidism and the accompanying skeletal changes, and it appears to be safe as long as the dosage is only 0.25 to 0.5 μg/day and hypercalcemia is avoided. ***If Shohl's solution (sodium citrate/citric acid) is given to treat acidosis, aluminum gels must not be given.***

Advanced Renal Failure Before Dialysis (C_{cr} <15 ml/min)

To manage hyperphosphatemia, dietary phosphate restriction should be initiated (<25 mmol/day) and calcium carbonate or calcium acetate given as a phosphate binder if serum phosphorus level is >1.7 mmol/L (5.3 mg/dl). These should be started at doses of 1 to 1.2 g with each meal, and the dose is adjusted to bring the serum phosphorus level to <1.8 mmol/L (5.6 mg/dl). If the serum phosphorus level exceeds 3 mmol/L (9.3 mg/dl), aluminum carbonate, one capsule with each meal, should be given initially, and then a calcium salt is substituted after the serum phosphorus level declines below 3 mmol/L (9.3 mg/dl). For optimal effectiveness and safety, the phosphate binder should be taken with meals. If metabolic acidosis is significant (serum bicarbonate <18 mEq/L), $NaHCO_3$ tablets, 40 to 80 mEq/day, should be added.

SYMPTOMS AND CLINICAL SYNDROMES ASSOCIATED WITH RENAL BONE DISEASES

Several symptoms or specific syndromes occur in association with the renal bone diseases. Symptoms are often vague and poorly defined, and they develop insidiously. Because there are few objective findings, the clinical condition is often overlooked until it is advanced. Similar symptoms can occur from totally different pathogenetic processes (Table 14–6), yet the

Table 14–6. CLINICAL FEATURES OF THE RENAL OSTEODYSTROPHIES AND THE ASSOCIATED PATHOGENIC PROCESS

Clinical Feature	Pathogenic Mechanisms
Bone pain	Aluminum; β_2-M-amyloid; osteitis fibrosa
Periarthritis, joint pain	β_2-M-amyloid; high PTH; periarticular calcifications
Proximal myopathy	Aluminum; high PTH; reduced vitamin D
Pruritus	High PTH, high serum P, high serum Ca, uremia itself
Fractures	Aluminum; β_2-M-amyloid > osteitis fibrosa
Skeletal deformities	Aluminum > osteitis fibrosa (except in children)
Bone cysts	β_2-M-amyloid > osteitis fibrosa
Osteopenia	Aluminum; ?β_2-M-amyloid
Extraskeletal calcifications	Phosphate excess; high PTH; low serum Mg
Tendon rupture	High PTH

Aluminum = aluminum accumulation; β_2-M = β_2-microglobulin.

management must be tailored to the specific cause.

Muscle weakness affects the proximal muscles of the lower extremities, making it difficult to climb stairs or rise from a low chair. Bone pain may or may not be present. Vague, deep pains in the back, hips, legs, and/or knees are often related to weight-bearing or a change in position. The pain, particularly with dialysis amyloidosis, is worse at night. Occasionally, hyperparathyroidism can cause localized, severe bone pain (*e.g.*, involving a pretibial area, ankle, or hip). There may or may not be localized bony tenderness (see Case Summary 2). Skeletal deformities are much more common in children than adults but can occur in adults as a result of altered bone remodeling or osteomalacia.

Pruritus can occur with uremia *per se,* with secondary hyperparathyroidism, with marked hyperphosphatemia, and with hypercalcemia *per se.* If hypercalcemia is present, lower calcium dialysate may be needed; if hyperphosphatemia exists, efforts at phosphate restriction should be vigorous. **Parathyroid surgery should be performed for pruritus only when evidence of marked hyperparathyroidism is unequivocal.**

Acute periarticular inflammation or true arthritis can develop as a consequence of extraskeletal calcifications or pseudogout. Symptoms and signs can appear over 1 to 2 days, and radiographs often show periarticular calcifications (see Fig. 14–2). Acute symptoms often respond to therapy with antiinflammatory agents. If hyperphosphatemia exists, it should be treated. Patients undergoing dialysis rarely develop acute gouty arthritis.

Spontaneous tendon rupture occurs not infrequently in dialysis patients; the Achilles, quadriceps, and digital tendons are most often involved; the cause is unknown, but its association with evidence of overt secondary hyperparathyroidism and its occurrence in primary hyperparathyroidism suggest that high PTH levels predispose to the process.

Calciphylaxis is an unusual syndrome characterized by peripheral ischemia, skin necrosis, and vascular calcifications that progresses in dialysis patients with a history of uncontrolled hyperphosphatemia and hyperparathyroidism (Fig. 14–3). It may progress quickly and be fatal; at times, its course is often reversed by parathyroidectomy. Patients with diabetes mellitus can show similar features, but the course is little affected by such surgery.

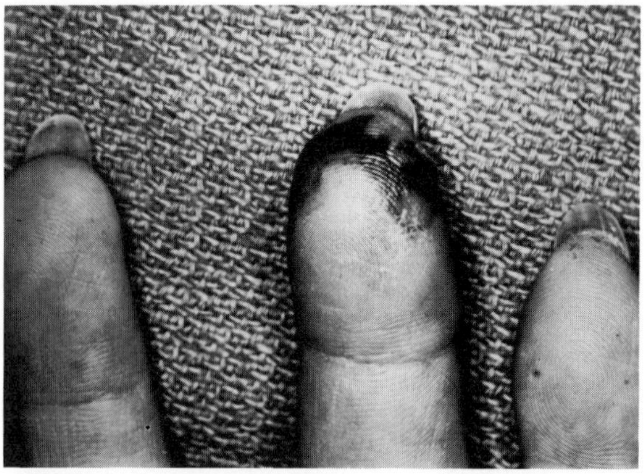

Figure 14–3. This hemodialysis patient developed painful ischemic lesions of his fingers; his serum calcium level had been 2.4 mmol/L (9.6 mg/dl), serum phosphorus level 3.4 mmol/L (10.5 mg/dl), alkaline phosphatase level 335 IU/ml, and parathyroid hormone level 12 times normal with an "intact assay." Because of the progression of the lesion, parathyroidectomy was done, with disappearance of pain within 4 to 5 days and healing of the lesion by 6 weeks.

Aluminum-related bone disease, also called *fracturing osteomalacia,* can present with severe bone pain, fractures, and proximal muscle weakness. Bone biopsy shows either osteomalacia or aplastic bone disease. Laboratory features include normal or elevated serum calcium levels, PTH levels that are often lower than expected, and plasma aluminum levels that generally exceed 3 μmol/L (81 μg/L). Following infusion of the chelating agent, deferoxamine (DFO), 40 mg/kg, plasma aluminum level increases, often by more than 6.0 μmol/L (165 μg/L). When aluminum-loaded patients are withdrawn from aluminum for several months, histologic features of aluminum toxicity can persist, with plasma aluminum levels as low as 0.8 μmol/L (22 μg/L) and an increment of plasma aluminum after DFO that is far less. Features that often help separate aluminum-related bone disease from secondary hyperparathyroidism are listed in Table 14–7.

Overt secondary hyperparathyroidism is defined by the presence of markedly elevated PTH levels and bone biopsy specimens showing severe osteitis fibrosa. These patients may have no bone pain, vague and minor complaints of pain, or severe localized pain limited to one site. Fractures are rare, but muscle weakness may be severe. Pruritus is sometimes severe. Biochemical observations include normal or increased serum calcium levels, serum phosphorus levels that are often elevated and refractory to phosphate binders, and bone alkaline phosphatase levels that show a progressive increase over time. Radiographs commonly show subperiosteal erosions and extraskeletal calcifications (see Figs. 14–1 and 14–2). Plasma aluminum levels are often elevated but generally are less than 3.5 to 5.5 μmol/L (94 to 149 μg/L) (see Table 14–7).

Amyloidosis, which is rare before 5 years of dialysis, is manifested by one or more of the following: carpal tunnel syndrome; pain in the shoulders, hips, and knees (and the pain is characteristically worse at night); trigger fingers; camptodactyly; and a higher incidence of fractures, particularly of the hip. There are no characteristic biochemical features; radiographs often show thin-walled cysts in the ends of long bones (Fig. 14–4).

MANAGEMENT OF MINERAL HOMEOSTASIS IN RENAL FAILURE BEFORE DIALYSIS

Phosphate Restriction and Phosphate Binders. These are used as described earlier. With the use of $CaCO_3$ or calcium acetate as binders, there is adequate supplementation of calcium. Serum phosphorus level should be maintained at 1.2 to 1.5 mmol/L (3.7 to 4.7 mg/dl). Aluminum gels should be avoided or, if essential, limited to three to six capsules per day.

Calcitriol. Calcitriol has definite value with continued hypocalcemia, when skeletal alkaline phosphatase is increasing, or with radiographic features of osteitis fibrosa. Such features are more likely in those at greater risk for high bone turnover (see Table 14–3). The daily oral dose should be 0.25 to 0.5 μg/day, with serum calcium and phosphorus levels monitored at 2- to 4-week intervals. Hypercalcemia should be avoided to minimize the risk of hastening progression of renal disease. Children with renal failure almost always require therapy with calcitriol plus $CaCO_3$, or their secondary hyperparathyroidism will progress.

PATIENTS UNDERGOING DIALYSIS

Dialysate

A dialysate calcium level of 3 to 3.25 mEq/L has been routine for hemodialysis; lowering the dialysate calcium to 2.5 mEq/L can permit the use of $CaCO_3$ or calcium acetate with less risk of hypercalcemia. The dialysate magnesium should be 0.4 to 0.5 mEq/L. The dialysate must be prepared from water with aluminum concentration less than 0.3 μmol/L (8 μg/L); this is best accomplished by reverse osmosis, often in conjunction with deionization. For peritoneal

Table 14–7. FEATURES THAT HELP DIFFERENTIATE ALUMINUM-RELATED BONE DISEASE FROM HYPERPARATHYROID BONE

Feature	Hyperparathyroid Bone Disease	Aluminum-Related Bone Disease
Fractures	Not characteristic	Common
Proximal muscle weakness	Can occur	Common
Periarthritis	Occurs	Uncommon
Tendon rupture	May occur	Not characteristic
Extraskeletal calcifications	Common	Not characteristic
Serum calcium	Low to high; often >2.5 mmol/L	Low to high Often >2.7 mmol/L
Serum phosphorus	Variable May be >2 mmol/L	Variable May be <1.8 mmol/L
Alkaline phosphatase	120 to 800% of normal	70 to 300% of normal
Serum PTH:		
Intact or N-assay*	>3 to 4 times normal†	<4 to 5 times normal†
Midregion assay	>15 to 20 times normal†	<40 to 60 times normal†
Plasma aluminum‡	Rarely >5 μmol/L Often <3 μmol/L	Generally >3 μmol/L Rarely <1.5 μmol/L
Increment of plasma aluminum after deferoxamine‡	Rarely >14 μmol/L Often <4 μmol/L	Generally >6 μmol/L Rarely <3 μmol/L
Microcytic anemia	Unusual	Common in epidemics (dialysate aluminum) Rare in endemic cases (oral aluminum)
Risk factors	Younger age Noncompliance	Diabetes mellitus, prior parathyroidectomy, earlier renal transplant, earlier binephrectomy

*N-assay: amino-terminal assay.
†Increment above PTH level of normal subjects.
‡After aluminum withdrawn (Al-containing drugs & dialysate Al), values are often lower.

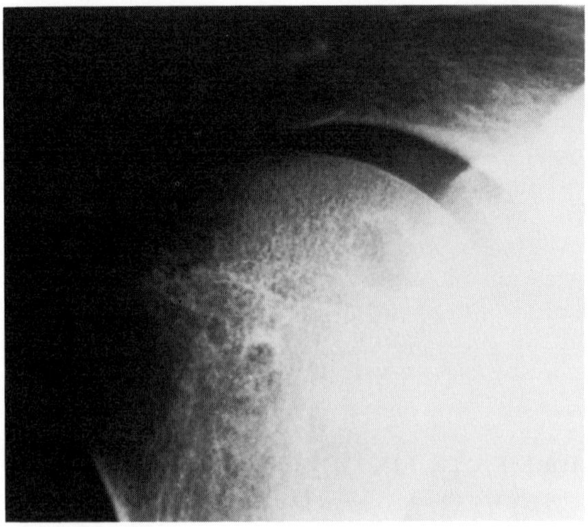

Figure 14–4. The patient is a 56-year-old man who had undergone hemodialysis for 14 years. He had pain in his shoulders, much worse at night; radiographs showed thin-walled cysts of both shoulders and the metacarpals as well. He had had numbness and pain in his hands, with relief of symptoms following carpal tunnel release surgery. The tissue removed showed birefringence characteristic of amyloid, and an immunoperoxidase stain revealed β_2-microglobulin. The pain in his shoulders improved after intraarticular steroid therapy.

dialysis (CAPD solutions), a calcium level of 3.5 mEq/L elevates blood ionized calcium, but total calcium may be normal as a result of hypoalbuminemia. The continued elevation of ionized calcium and excessive lowering of PTH may be responsible for a high incidence of aplastic bone disease observed in CAPD patients, even in the absence of any aluminum loading. The use of CAPD solutions with a lower calcium level (*e.g.*, 2.5 mEq/L) may avoid this problem and permit the use of $CaCO_3$ as a phosphate binder and the suppression of PTH with calcitriol without the need for continued elevation of ionized calcium. With either hemodialysis or CAPD, lower calcium in dialysate (*e.g.*, 2.5 mEq/L) should not be used in a noncompliant patient because of the risk of loss of bone mineral if the patient does not take the prescribed $CaCO_3$ and/or calcitriol. Dialysate magnesium should be 0.5 mEq/L with CAPD.

Phosphate Control

Dietary phosphate intake should be less than 25 to 30 mmol/day, and the dose of phosphate binder ($CaCO_3$ or calcium acetate) should be adjusted to maintain the predialysis serum phosphorus level between 1.5 and 1.9 mmol/L (4.7 to 5.9 mg/dl). If the serum calcium level exceeds 2.6 to 2.7 mmol/L (10.4 to 10.8 mg/dl), the dialysate calcium should be reduced to 2.5 mEq/L. If serum phosphorus exceeds 1.9 mmol/L (5.9 mg/dl) despite these maneuvers, aluminum hydroxide or aluminum carbonate may be needed as well, but the dose should not exceed two capsules with each meal, and the plasma aluminum level should be monitored every 3 to 4 months. **A patient taking aluminum gels must not ingest calcium citrate.** With marked hyperparathyroidism, hyperphosphatemia may arise from excessive phosphorus flux from bone, and parathyroidectomy may be required. If serum phosphorus level declines below 1.5 mmol/L, the dose of binder must be decreased; some dialysis patients, particularly those on CAPD, require no phosphate binders.

Calcitriol (1,25(OH)$_2$D$_3$)

Because it is easier to prevent progressive hyperparathyroidism than treat it once it is established, there is rationale for the earlier use of calcitriol in dialysis patients. **A serum calcium level below 2.3 mmol/L (9.2 mg/dl) and a progressive increase of bone alkaline phosphatase and PTH are more definite indications for such therapy.** Therapy with calcitriol should not be started until the serum phosphorus level is below 2 mmol/L (6.3 mg/dl), and it should not be given if serum calcium level exceeds 2.7 mmol/L (10.8 mg/dl). The initial dose should be 0.25 to 0.5 μg/day; if the bone alkaline phosphatase is elevated and serum PTH is markedly increased, 1 μg/day may be required.

The potential side effects of calcitriol therapy include worsened hyperphosphatemia and the occurrence of hypercalcemia. The former may increase the risk of extraskeletal calcifications, particularly if the calcium and phosphorus product (mmol × mmol) reaches 5 to 5.6 (62 to 70 in mg/dl × mg/dl). **Hypercalcemia during the early course of therapy is more likely to develop in a patient with aluminum-related bone disease** or one with severe hyperparathyroidism and marked parathyroid hyperplasia. Otherwise, hypercalcemia may appear when an elevated alkaline phosphatase level declines to normal (*e.g.*, sometimes after 6 to 12 months of therapy).

Parenteral calcitriol has recently been introduced, and the risk of hypercalcemia may be less with parenteral than oral calcitriol (perhaps because the former has less intestinal action to augment calcium absorption and greater suppression of PTH secretion); however, results of comparative studies of the two modalities are not available. When calcitriol is given parenterally to a hemodialysis patient, the usual intravenous dose is 1 to 2 μg with each dialysis.

With either route of calcitriol administration, hypercalcemia can occur, but it is less evident with intravenous than oral treatment. When serum calcium level exceeds 2.8 to 2.9 mmol/L (11.2 to 11.6 mg/dl), calcitriol should be stopped; after the serum calcium level has returned to normal, it can be restarted at a lower dose. Because calcitriol is more potent than hypercalcemia *per se* in suppressing PTH secretion, one approach to a patient with secondary hyperparathyroidism and hypercalcemia is to lower the dialysate calcium to 2.5 mEq/L, followed by the more aggressive use of parenteral or oral calcitriol. If hypercalcemia occurs despite the use of the low-calcium dialysate, calcitriol must be discontinued and parathyroidectomy should be considered (see below).

Aluminum Toxicity

When patients have biochemical evidence of aluminum loading, they should be managed by withdrawing *all* aluminum-containing drugs and the use of aluminum-free dialysate (*e.g.*, <0.3 μmol/L [<8 μg/L]). Whether chelation therapy with DFO is indicated will depend on the symptoms present. If a patient has symptomatic bone disease or encephalopathy, the symptoms commonly improve after chelation therapy with DFO. The chance of improvement and even survival with encephalopathy is less when treatment is limited to the withdrawal of aluminum exposure. When chelation therapy is indicated, DFO should not be given more frequently than **once weekly** and in the lowest dose possible (*e.g.*, 0.5 to 1 g/week). After giving DFO, 6 to 12 hours are required for optimal chelation of aluminum; then the patient should have dialysis using highly efficient dialysis to remove the chelated aluminum and iron, as well as the free DFO. Plasma aluminum levels should be monitored at regular intervals during DFO therapy. If serum aluminum level exceeds 18 μmol/L (490 μg/L) after DFO, the dose should be reduced, as such patients may develop acute aluminum encephalopathy.

Mucormycosis is an important risk of DFO therapy in dialysis patients. How it develops is uncertain, but DFO chelates available iron and may act as a siderophore to enhance fungal growth. The optimal duration of DFO therapy is unknown; a patient's clinical status and a repeat bone biopsy after 6 to 12 months may provide a guide to the need for further treatment. Hypocalcemia and an increase in PTH levels are common during DFO therapy; some patients develop overt secondary hyperparathyroidism and require parathyroid surgery, and therapy with calcitriol is indicated when serum calcium level declines.

PARATHYROIDECTOMY

Secondary hyperparathyroidism sometimes requires parathyroidectomy. Aluminum-related bone disease must be ruled out, and severe secondary hyperparathyroidism must be documented by biochemical, roentgenographic, and often by bone histologic criteria. The indications include (1) the appearance of calciphylaxis, (2) severe skeletal pain and myopathy, (3) progressive extraskeletal calcifications and refractory hyperphosphatemia, (4) persistent hypercalcemia (serum calcium level >2.9 to 3 mmol/L [11.6 to 12.0 mg/dl]), and (5) pruritus intractable to dialysis or other medical treatment. Other causes of hypercalcemia, including sarcoidosis, hypercalcemia of malignancy, and the excess intake of calcium and vitamin D, must be considered and ruled out. An algorithm to follow in reaching a decision for parathyroidectomy is shown in Figure 14–5.

The optimal surgical procedure (*e.g.*, subtotal parathyroidectomy, total parathyroidectomy plus forearm transplantation of parathyroid fragments, or total parathyroidectomy) depends in part on operative findings. Choice of a surgeon with broad experience with parathyroid surgery in patients with ESRD is critical. Recurrence of hyperparathyroidism from hyperplasia of remnant parathyroid tissue (either in the neck or in transplanted tissue in the forearm) versus induction of aplastic bone disease because of subnormal PTH levels is a factor to consider in a decision regarding the type of surgery. If only three glands are identified, they should all be removed.

Preoperatively, patients should receive calcitriol, 1 to 2 μg/day, for 3 to 5 days before surgery. If serum calcium level decreases below 1.7 to 2 mmol/L (6.8 to 8 mg/dl) during the first 36 hours postoperatively, intravenous calcium gluconate, prepared to provide 2.5 to 5 mmol of calcium per hour, may be needed for 24 to 48 hours until the intestinal absorption of calcium increases. If the postoperative decrease in serum calcium level is less than 0.5 to 0.6 mmol/L (2.0 to 2.4 mg/dl), it is likely that

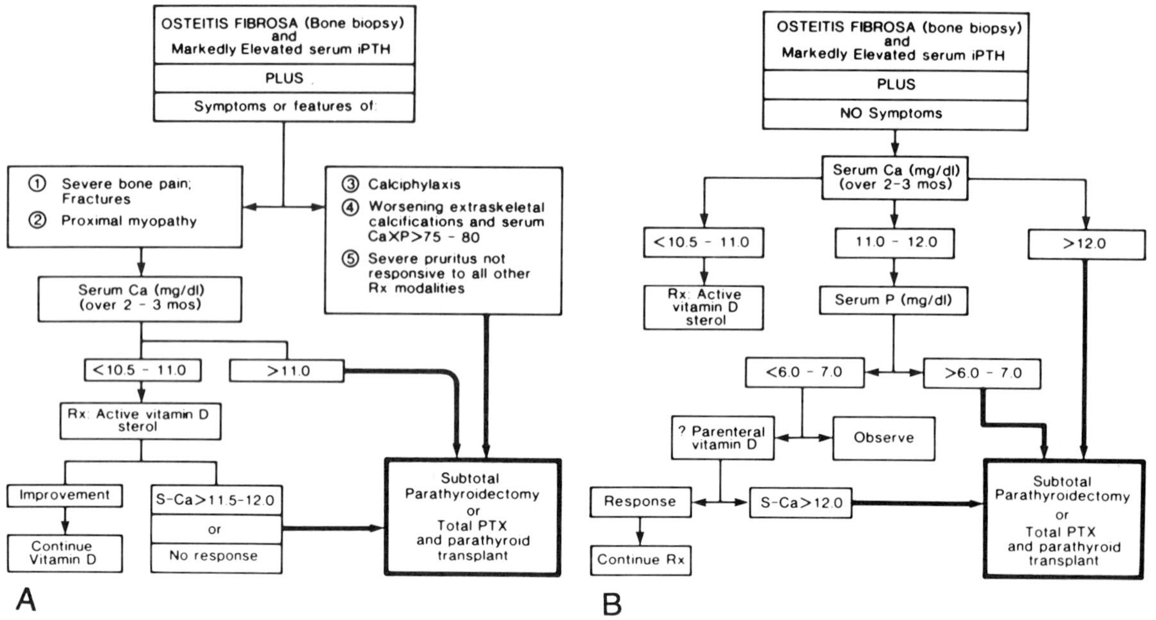

Figure 14–5. Algorithm showing an approach to decision-making for parathyroidectomy in secondary hyperparathyroidism in a patient with end-stage renal disease with symptoms (A) or without symptoms (B). (Reprinted from Salusky IB, Coburn JW: The renal osteodystrophies. *In* DeGroot LJ, et al (eds): Endocrinology, 2nd ed. Philadelphia, WB Saunders, 1989.)

excessive parathyroid tissue remains behind or that the skeletal histology was not that of osteitis fibrosa. Oral $CaCO_3$ or calcium acetate should be given in doses of 1 to 2.5 g 3 to 5 times daily, until the serum calcium level increases, and oral calcitriol may be needed in doses as high as 1 to 3 μg/day. Serum magnesium level occasionally falls as a consequence of the "hungry bone," and magnesium replacement may be needed. Serum phosphorus level often declines after surgery; because of the risk of profound and worsening hypocalcemia, phosphate should be avoided unless the serum phosphorus level falls below 0.6 to 0.7 mmol/L (1.8 to 2.1 mg/dl). Aluminum-containing gels should also be avoided postoperatively because of the risk of aluminum-related bone disease.

CASE SUMMARY 1

A middle-aged woman on hemodialysis for diabetic nephropathy had a serum calcium level of 2.6 mmol/L; a bone biopsy disclosed aplastic bone disease with 35% aluminum staining. She had a history of prior cerebrovascular accidents with minimal residuals. Aluminum gels were discontinued, and she was given $CaCO_3$ as a phosphate binder. Two months later, she came into the dialysis unit showing withdrawal, confusion, and decreased ability to walk for several days. She was hospitalized with a tentative diagnosis of a new stroke. Serum calcium level was 3.2 mmol/L (12.8 mg/dl), and serum albumin level was 33 g/L. No improvement followed a standard hemodialysis (dialysate calcium, 3.25 mEq/L); the next hemodialysis was done using a dialysate calcium of 2 mEq/L, and her neurologic symptoms resolved.

This diabetic patient with "asymptomatic" aluminum loading was managed by changing the phosphate binder from aluminum hydroxide to $CaCO_3$. Two months later, she displayed mental symptoms associated with moderate hypercalcemia; her symptoms disappeared, but not until dialysis was done with a reduced calcium level in the dialysate.

CASE SUMMARY 2

A 47-year-old woman undergoing dialysis for ESRD due to interstitial nephritis developed severe pain in the left pretibial area that was aggravated by weight-bearing. There was localized pretibial tenderness. Her serum calcium level was 2.3 to 2.5 mmol/L (9.2 to 10 mg/dl), serum phosphorus level was 2.9 to 3.5 mmol/L (9.0 to 10.9 mg/dl) despite adherence to $CaCO_3$; alkaline phosphatase level was 350 IU/

L with a GGT of 20 U/L (normal, 15 to 45); and plasma aluminum level was 2 μmol/L (54 μg/L). Serum midregion PTH had increased from 24,000 to 48,000 pg/ml, and a bone scan showed diffusely increased uptake (e.g., a superscan) with additional localized uptake over the left tibia. Skeletal x-ray films showed no subperiosteal erosions. She received intravenous calcitriol with a slow decrease of bone alkaline phosphatase to 145 IU/L, but her PTH level continued to rise. Her tibial pain slowly decreased, but her hyperphosphatemia was resistant to phosphate binders. A bone biopsy specimen showed severe osteitis fibrosa with insignificant aluminum staining. She underwent subtotal parathyroidectomy (five hyperplastic glands were identified); postoperatively, her serum calcium level declined to 1.5 mmol/L (6.0 mg/dl) but then rose to 2.3 mmol/L (9.2 mg/dl) on oral calcitriol and $CaCO_3$. Serum phosphorus level decreased to 1.5 to 1.9 mmol/L (4.6 to 5.9 mg/dl).

This patient displayed refractory hyperphosphatemia despite compliance with her diet and $CaCO_3$; she developed severe localized bone pain without radiographic abnormalities, but she had increased local uptake of bone scan. The disappearance of her symptoms as bone alkaline phosphatase fell during intravenous calcitriol therapy suggested that the pain was related to osteitis fibrosa. After parathyroidectomy, her serum calcium and phosphorus levels fell, with the latter readily controlled with $CaCO_3$. The identification of five parathyroid glands indicates the value of a skilled surgeon who is familiar with the varied parathyroid anatomy in such patients.

CASE SUMMARY 3

An 8-year-old boy with reflux nephropathy and progressive azotemia (C_{cr}, 25 ml/min/1.75 m^2) was seen because of bone pain, skeletal deformities, muscle weakness, and hypercalcemia. Parathyroidectomy had been done 3 years earlier because of a radiographic diagnosis of secondary hyperparathyroidism, and repeat neck exploration was done 1 year later with removal of a small remnant of parathyroid tissue. The patient received $A1(OH)_3$ gel for 4 years to maintain serum phosphorus level between 1.2 and 1.4 mmol/L (3.7 and 4.3 mg/dl). Midregion PTH was 1980 pg/ml (normal, 80 to 330 pg/ml); plasma aluminum level was 4.8 μmol/L (130 μg/L); and bone biopsy disclosed osteomalacia, "absent" bone formation, and 65% surface staining for aluminum. After infusion of 1 g of DFO, urinary aluminum excretion rose from 2.4 to 18.5 μmol/24 hr (65 to 500 μg/24 hr). (Normal urinary aluminum, 0.4 to 1.5 μmol/24 hr [11 to 40 μg/24 hr].) He received weekly DFO injections for 6 months. Hypercalcemia disappeared, his muscle weakness improved, and he was able to walk after undergoing corrective orthopedic surgery. His renal function was unchanged. Further history disclosed that he had received therapy with Bicitra (Shohl's solution or sodium citrate/citric acid) for the management of metabolic acidosis for the 4 years before the bone biopsy.

This patient showed hypercalcemia and radiographic features of secondary hyperparathyroidism that represented earlier erosions that had not mineralized when aluminum-related bone disease replaced the osteitis fibrosa. These manifestations of aluminum-related bone disease have been called *pseudohyperparathyroidism.* The therapy of metabolic acidosis and hyperphosphatemia of chronic renal failure with a combination of sodium citrate/citric acid and aluminum-containing gels markedly augmented the absorption of aluminum and led to the serious sequelae of aluminum toxicity.

Selected Readings

Alfrey AC: Phosphate, aluminum and other elements in chronic renal disease. *In* Schrier RW, Gottschalk CW (eds): Diseases of the Kidney, 4th ed. Boston, Little, Brown & Co, 1988, p 3371.

Andress DL, Norris KC, Coburn JW, et al: Intravenous calcitriol in the treatment of refractory osteitis fibrosa of chronic renal failure. N Engl J Med 321:274, 1989.

Coburn JW, Salusky IB: Control of serum phosphorus in uremia. N Engl J Med 320:1140, 1989.

Felsenfeld AJ, Rodriguez M, Coleman M, et al: Desferrioxamine therapy in hemodialysis patients with aluminum-associated bone disease. Kidney Int 35:1371, 1989.

Kaye M, D'Amour P, Henderson J: Elective total parathyroidectomy without autotransplant in end-stage renal disease. Kidney Int 35:1390, 1989.

Kleinman KS, Coburn JW: Amyloid syndromes associated with hemodialysis. Kidney Int 25:267, 1989.

Llach F, Coburn JW: Renal osteodystrophy and maintenance dialysis. *In* Maher JF (ed): Replacement of Renal Function by Dialysis, 3rd ed. Dordrecht, Holland, Kluwer Academic Publishers, 1989, p 912.

Norris KC, Goodman WG, Howard N, et al: Iliac crest

bone biopsy for diagnosis of aluminum toxicity and a guide to the use of deferoxamine. Semin Nephrol 6 (Suppl 1):27, 1986.

Salusky IB, Coburn JW: The renal osteodystrophies. *In* DeGroot LJ, Besser M, Cahill GF Jr, et al (eds): Endocrinology, 2nd ed. Philadelphia, WB Saunders, 1989, p 1032.

Sherrard DJ, Andress DL: Renal osteodystrophy. *In* Schrier RW, Gottschalk CW (eds): Diseases of the Kidney, 4th ed. Boston, Little, Brown & Co, 1988, p 3035.

CHAPTER 15

NUTRITIONAL THERAPY IN PATIENTS WITH RENAL FAILURE

Raimund R. Hirschberg and Joel D. Kopple

There are three major goals for the nutritional therapy of patients with renal disease: (1) to maintain good nutritional status; (2) to arrest or retard further progression of renal failure; and (3) to prevent or ameliorate uremic toxicity and other metabolic disorders that occur with advanced renal failure.

Although the evidence is not conclusive, data from clinical and experimental studies indicate that a reduction of dietary protein and phosphorus may retard the progression of chronic renal failure (CRF). Therefore, diets for patients with renal disease are designed to be low in protein and phosphorus content. Such diets will also reduce uremic toxicity in patients with advanced renal failure. However, feeding a low-protein diet to renal patients bears the risk of inducing malnutrition. As patients progress toward end-stage renal disease (ESRD), the risk for wasting increases. Hence, to achieve the goals previously listed, a patient's nutritional intake and status should be managed by both a nephrologist and a renal dietician.

MONITORING THE NUTRITIONAL STATUS AND DIETARY INTAKE

Patients who have CRF and a creatinine clearance <30 ml/min/1.73 m^2 should be evaluated periodically for malnutrition. A nephrologist should take a history and conduct a physical examination, and a renal dietitian should evaluate a patient's nutrient intake and perform anthropometric measurements to assess nutritional status. Selected serum biochemical measurements are also helpful to evaluate for malnutrition (Table 15–1).

Wasting may occur in patients with CRF because their intake of essential nutrients is inadequate (particularly protein and/or calories) or because of superimposed or underlying catabolic diseases. A catabolic state in patients with renal failure may be indicated by a high blood urea nitrogen (BUN):creatinine ratio (Table 15–2). A high BUN:creatinine ratio may also be caused by high protein intake, gastrointestinal bleeding, inadequate removal of urea by dialysis, or a high renal fractional reabsorption of urea, which can occur in prerenal acute renal failure (ARF) and with low renal perfusion (see Case Summary 1).

NUTRITIONAL REQUIREMENTS IN CHRONIC RENAL FAILURE

Protein and Energy Requirements

The dietary prescription for patients with renal failure must address both the quantity of protein and the source of protein ingested daily. In a low-protein diet, the proteins ingested should be of high biologic value. Such proteins, commonly found in meats and animal products rather than in plants, contain amino acids in a mixture similar to that found in human protein.

Two types of low-protein diets are used for patients with CRF: (1) A mildly protein-restricted diet provides about 0.55 to 0.60 g/kg/day of protein. About 0.35 g/kg/day of protein should be of high biologic value (i.e., from animal sources). (2) A more severely protein-restricted diet provides about 0.28 g/kg/day of protein and is supplemented with a mixture of essential amino acids or a mixture of both essential amino acids and the ketoacids and hydroxyacid analogues of the essential amino acids. The amino acid mixtures available for

Table 15–1. ANTHROPOMETRIC AND BIOCHEMICAL PARAMETERS THAT INDICATE PROTEIN-CALORIE MALNUTRITION

Anthropometry
- ↓ body weight
- ↓ height (children)
- ↓ growth rate (children)
- ↓ skinfold thicknesses (body fat)
- ↓ midarm muscle circumference (muscle mass)

Biochemistry
- ↓ serum transferrin
- ↓ serum albumin
- ↓ serum prealbumin
- ↓ serum total protein
- ↓ serum cholinesterase
- ↓ serum pseudocholinesterase
- ↓ certain plasma amino acids (leucine, isoleucine, tryptophan, valine, tyrosine)
- ↑ plasma total nonessential amino acids
- ↑ plasma glycine
- ↓ plasma valine/glycine ratio
- ↓ plasma ratio of essential/nonessential amino acids

supplementing renal diets contain the nine essential amino acids (Table 15–3). Ketoanalogues or hydroxyanalogues of amino acids contain a ketogroup or hydroxygroup in place of an amino group. Ketoacids or hydroxyacids are rapidly transaminated in the liver into their respective amino analogues. **Hence an advantage of using ketoacid and hydroxyacid supplements is the reduced nitrogen load, which reduces urea production.**

In several European countries, ketoacid formulas containing calcium salts are commercially available (Table 15–4). Because these diets have a high calcium content, hypercalcemia may develop in some patients. The risk of hypercalcemia is much lower with the use of other ketoacid mixtures that contain amino acid-ketoacid complexes and smaller amounts of calcium (Table 15–5). In the United States, ketoacid supplements are currently only available for clinical studies and are not approved for general use by the Food and Drug Administration.

Several lines of evidence indicate that protein- and phosphorus-restricted diets may reduce the rate of progression of CRF. The most dramatic examples of the effect of protein restriction reducing the rate of progression have been described with very low-protein diets supplemented with ketoacids, especially with the formulation EE (see Table 15–5). However, there is currently no definitive evidence regarding whether these ketoacid-supplemented diets are more protective against progression of renal failure than less restrictive low-protein diets (*e.g.*, providing 0.55 to 0.60 g/kg/day of protein). Large multicenter trials currently under way are expected to answer this question.

Table 15–2. CLINICAL CONDITIONS ASSOCIATED WITH AN INCREASED OR REDUCED BLOOD UREA NITROGEN TO CREATININE RATIO IN PATIENTS WITH RENAL FAILURE

BUN:Creatinine Ratio >15
- High protein intake
- Gastrointestinal bleeding
- Volume depletion, decreased perfusion of the kidneys, prerenal renal failure
- Low urine flow
- Urinary tract obstruction

BUN:Creatinine Ratio <10
- Low protein (nitrogen) intake
- Chronic liver failure (cirrhosis)
- High urine flow (water diuresis)

Table 15–3. AMINO ACID FORMULATION FOR SUPPLEMENTATION OF VERY LOW-PROTEIN DIETS (AMINESS N, KABIVITRUM, SWEDEN)*

Amino Acid	g/60 kg Body Weight/Day
Histidine	0.81
Isoleucine	1.08
Leucine	1.62
Lysine acetate (equivalent to lysine 1.17 g)	1.64
Methionine	1.62
Phenylalanine	1.26
Tryptophan	0.45
Tyrosine	1.35
Valine	2.43
Total amino acid intake (g/60 kg body weight/day)	13.43
Total nitrogen intake (g/60 kg body weight/day)	1.59

*Recommended daily quantity for a 60-kg patient.

Table 15–4. CALCIUM AMINO-KETOACID FORMULATION FOR SUPPLEMENTATION OF VERY LOW-PROTEIN DIETS*

Amino Acid/Ketoacid	g/60 kg Body Weight/Day
Calcium-α-ketoisovalerate	2.88
Calcium-ketoisocaproate	4.00
Calcium-α-keto-β-methylvalerate	2.92
Calcium-L-phenylacetate	2.00
Calcium-D,L-hydroxymethionine	2.12
L-Lysine acetate	0.80
L-Histidine	0.54
L-Threonine	0.66
L-Tryptophan	0.34
Total amino/keto/hydroxyacid intake (g/60 kg body weight/day)	16.30
Calcium intake (g/60 kg body weight/day)	1.60
Total nitrogen intake (g/60 kg body weight/day)	0.39

*Recommended daily quantity for a 60-kg patient.

Table 15–5. AMINO-KETOACID FORMULATION EE FOR SUPPLEMENTATION OF VERY LOW-PROTEIN DIETS*

Amino Acid/Ketoacid	mmol/60 kg Body Weight/Day
Histidine-α-ketoisocaproate	4
Lysine-α-ketoisocaproate	7
Lysine-α-ketoisovalerate	7
Lysine (R,S)-α-keto-β-methylvalerate	7
Threonine	15
Tyrosine	20
Ornithine-α-ketoisovalerate	7
Ornithine-α-ketoisocaproate	7
Ornithine (R,S)-α-keto-β-methylvalerate	7
Calcium D,L-α-hydroxy-γ-methylthiobutyrate	2
Total amino/keto/hydroxyacid intake (mmol/60 kg body weight/day)	83
Total nitrogen intake (g/60 kg body weight/day)	1.78

*Recommended daily quantity for a 60-kg patient.

Until more definitive information is available, we use the following approach to the dietary protein intake of patients with chronic renal disease: **When a patient has evidence of chronic progressive renal failure, we prescribe either the 0.55 to 0.60 g protein/kg/day diet or the ketoacid supplement diet providing the ketoacid formula EE (see Table 15–5).** Because this latter diet is not available in the United States, except for use in research studies, the former diet is normally prescribed. Patients are informed that there is yet no definitive evidence that these diets will retard the rate of progression of renal failure, but that the current evidence is strongly suggestive. Phosphorus restriction is employed concomitantly (see below). Evidence indicates that these diets will not engender malnutrition as long as patients adhere carefully to these diets and maintain a high-calorie intake (see below). To achieve good dietary compliance, patients must be seen at least monthly by both a dietitian who is experienced in renal dietetics and a physician.

The recommended protein intake for maintenance hemodialysis patients is 1.1 to 1.2 g/kg/day. For patients undergoing continuous ambulatory peritoneal dialysis (CAPD), slightly more protein, 1.2 to 1.3 g/kg/day, is recommended because of their daily losses of protein and peptides. In protein-malnourished CAPD patients, up to 1.5 g protein/kg/day may be prescribed. With both hemodialysis and CAPD patients, at least 50% of the dietary protein should be of high biologic value.

Special attention must be devoted to maintaining sufficient calorie intake. **Recent clinical research indicates that patients with CRF, whether treated conservatively or with maintenance dialysis, have the same energy expenditure as normal individuals.** Therefore, most patients with CRF need approximately 35 kcal/kg/day to maintain neutral nitrogen balance and acceptable nutritional status. During periods of transient superimposed illnesses, the calorie intake may need to be increased.

The proportions of the calorie intake that should be provided as carbohydrates or fat are not well defined. **We currently prescribe a fat intake of about 30 to 40% with a ratio of polyunsaturated to saturated fatty acids of about 1:1.** The remaining nonfat and nonprotein calories are provided by complex carbohydrates. Some but not all studies indicate that patients on long-term hemodialysis may develop low serum or tissue (skeletal muscle, red blood cells) levels of carnitine. Because carnitine enhances the transport of fatty acids into mitochondria, carnitine deficiency may contribute to the development of hyperlipidemia in ESRD. In some reports, oral or intravenous carnitine treatment may decrease plasma cholesterol, low-density lipoprotein cholesterol, and triglycerides and may increase high-density lipoprotein cholesterol and a patient's exercise tolerance and general sense of well-being. However, other reports show no lipid-lowering effects of carnitine, and an increase in plasma triglycerides or anemia has occasionally been described with carnitine therapy. Maintenance dialysis patients with hypertriglyceridemia that is unresponsive to dietary therapy may be given a trial of L-carnitine in a dose of 0.5 g/day orally or 1 to 1.5 g IV three times weekly, after hemodialysis.

CASE SUMMARY 1

A 69-year-old woman was referred for evaluation of a high BUN level and BUN:creatinine ratio. Her BUN level was 123 mg/dl, which had persisted for several weeks. Her serum creatinine level was 1.5 mg/dl, and the BUN/creatinine ratio was 82. She had congestive heart failure (New York Heart Association class 3) and a history of three myocardial infarctions. Her medicinal intake included nifedipine, nitroglycerin, propranolol, prazosin, and furosemide (160 mg twice daily). During the previous 6 months, she had lost 11 kg of edema-free body weight. Her 24-hour creatinine clearance was 20 ml/min; the fractional excretion of urea was 6%. She had metabolic alkalosis with a serum bicarbonate level of 29 mmol/L. Results of renal ultrasonography were unremarkable and showed normal kidney size. Her urinalysis results were within normal limits. She was 5 feet 3 inches tall and weighed 52 kg. Serum albumin and total protein concentrations were within normal limits. Midarm muscle circumference was 196 mm, placing the patient at the 10th percentile of her age and sex group; her serum transferrin concentration was 110 mg/dl (normal range 250 to 300 mg/dl). A dietary recall performed by a dietitian revealed an average protein intake of about 21 g/day (0.4 g/kg/day) and a calorie intake of approximately 20 to 25 kcal/kg/day. Her main food sources were vegetables, fruit, and dairy products, and she avoided meats. Hence, her dietary protein was to a large extent of low biologic value (low content of essential amino acids).

Reviewing the findings in this patient, there seem to be two causes for her high BUN level and BUN:creatinine ratio. First, her serum creatinine level was unusually low for her degree of renal failure. The disproportionately low serum creatinine level was a result of the following factors: She was malnourished, as indicated by the loss in body weight and the low relative body weight and arm muscle circumference. Malnutrition in this patient was probably caused by a low intake of protein and calories, possibly augmented by catabolism often observed in patients with severe congestive heart failure. In addition, because of her avoidance of meat, her intake of essential amino acids may have been especially low, further adding to her tendency to become protein malnourished. Her low nutrient intake, as well as her age and sex, resulted in a low muscle mass, which reduces creatinine synthesis. Thus, for any degree of renal failure, she will have a disproportionately low serum creatinine level and a higher BUN:creatinine ratio. Second, she had a high renal tubular net reabsorption of urea, as indicated by the low fractional excretion of urea (*i.e.*, a disproportionately low urea clearance in comparison to her creatinine clearance or glomerular filtration rate [GFR]). High renal tubular urea reabsorption is observed in patients who have poor renal perfusion in comparison to their GFR (*i.e.*, they have a high filtration fraction). In this woman, this is most likely the result of low cardiac output as well as low intravascular volume. The low intravascular volume may be induced by the large dosage of furosemide that probably caused the metabolic alkalosis. Very low rates of urine flow can also lead to a decline in the renal tubular reabsorption of urea (see Table 15–2).

This patient was treated as follows: prazosin was discontinued, the propranolol and furosemide dosages were reduced, and treatment with the angiotensin-converting enzyme (ACE) inhibitor captopril was begun. The patient was encouraged to increase her protein intake to 0.55 to 0.60 g/kg/day (including ≥0.35 g high-biologic-value protein) and her calorie intake to 35 kcal/kg/day. Compliance with the dietary regimen was encouraged at biweekly visits with a dietitian. The patient's edema-free body weight increased, and serum transferrin levels rose to normal within 3 months. The fractional excretion of urea increased to 26 to 31%. Serum creatinine concentration initially increased slightly and stabilized at about 1.7 mg/dl. BUN level decreased gradually to values varying between 39 and 45 mg/dl.

To achieve the treatment goals outlined earlier, the diet prescribed to patients with renal failure should be high in calories and low but adequate in protein (nitrogen) content. Good dietary compliance by a patient is essential for successful nutritional therapy. Compliance must be encouraged at each visit by both the dietitian and nephrologist. In addition, instruments to monitor the dietary protein intake should be used. One such method involves an estimate of nitrogen output. In patients who are in neutral or almost neutral nitrogen balance, the nitrogen losses equal the nitrogen (protein) intake. Thus, the measurement of nitrogen losses from the body usually gives an accurate measurement of nitrogen (protein) intake.

Most nitrogen output occurs in urine and stool; in addition, there are losses of about 0.5 g/day primarily from sweat, respiration, blood drawing, and growth of skin, hair, and nails. To avoid laborious measurements of nitrogen, one can take advantage of the fact that urea is the major product of protein and amino acid degradation. **Hence, the urea nitrogen appearance (UNA) can be used to estimate the total nitrogen output and, thus, the nitrogen intake, provided that a patient is in almost neutral nitrogen balance, as are most patients with CRF. UNA is the amount of urea that is lost in all outputs (*i.e.*, urine, dialysate, fistula drainage, and so on) and that accumulates in the body's fluids.**

Table 15–6 provides the formulas used to calculate the UNA and the total nitrogen intake

Table 15–6. ALGORITHM TO ESTIMATE THE UREA NITROGEN APPEARANCE (UNA) AND THE TOTAL NITROGEN OUTPUT AND INTAKE

1. UNA (g/day) = urinary urea nitrogen (g/day) + change in body urea nitrogen (g/day) + R
2. Change in body urea nitrogen (g/day) = $(BUN_f - BUN_i$, g/L/day$) \times BW_i$ (kg) $\times$ (0.6 L/kg) + $(BW_f - BW_i$, kg/day$) \times BUN_f$ (g/L)
3. Total nitrogen output (g/day) = 0.97 × UNA (g/day) + 1.93
4. Dietary nitrogen intake (g/day) = 0.69 × UNA (g/day) + 3.30

BW = body weight; BUN = blood urea nitrogen.
R = The urea nitrogen of other fluid losses (such as fistulas, drainages, or peritoneal dialysate in g/day).
i, f = initial and final values at beginning and end of collection period.
0.6 L/kg = estimate for the fractional total body water (urea is equally distributed in this volume).

and output. The formulas for calculating the total nitrogen intake and output have been determined empirically in patients with CRF. For patients not undergoing dialysis, the BUN level (and, hence, body urea nitrogen) is usually rather constant. Thus, the change in body urea nitrogen is zero (N = 0) and the formula for calculating UNA can be reduced to UNA = urine urea N (Equation 1 in Table 15–6). In patients undergoing hemodialysis, the collections for urea nitrogen measurements should be made during a dialysis-free interval; because in patients treated with CAPD there is no such interval, the urea nitrogen content of the peritoneal dialysate should be measured during the period of the UNA determination and should be added to equation 1 in Table 15–6. For patients undergoing CAPD, a separate adjustment is also necessary for the calculation of total nitrogen losses to adjust for daily dialysate losses of total protein (about 9 g/day), peptides, and free amino acids (about 3 g/day).

Vitamin Requirements

There is a high incidence of certain vitamin deficiencies in patients with renal failure unless they take vitamin supplements. These deficiencies may result from reduced intake, increased losses (as with water-soluble vitamins during hemodialysis, with the exception of vitamin B_{12}, which is protein bound) or from a low production rate, such as for 1,25-dihydroxyvitamin D_3. The most commonly observed vitamin deficiencies in patients who have CRF and are not taking supplements are probably in pyridoxine (B_6), ascorbic acid (C), folic acid, and 1,25-dihydroxyvitamin D_3. **Hence, vitamin supplements are routinely prescribed for patients with CRF, especially for those undergoing maintenance dialysis.** Supplements should provide the water-soluble vitamins, including folic acid, vitamin B_6 (pyridoxine), vitamin C, vitamin B_1 (thiamine), vitamin B_2 (riboflavin), and nicotinic acid. Treatment with 1,25-dihydroxyvitamin D_3 may be started early in the course of CRF to prevent the development of secondary hyperparathyroidism (see Chapter 14). Some nephrologists routinely give vitamin D_3 (10,000 IU daily for 5 consecutive days every 3 months) to patients on maintenance dialysis. This treatment may also be indicated in elderly nondialyzed patients in whom a nutritional and social history reveals evidence of vitamin D deficiency. Retinol (vitamin A) is not routinely prescribed, because even small doses have been reported to cause bone toxicity in some patients. Table 15–7 gives more details concerning doses of vitamin supplements.

Mineral Requirements

Nutritional therapy may help to prevent certain disorders of mineral metabolism. Hyperphosphatemia is often associated with advanced CRF and poses the risk of inducing secondary hyperparathyroidism, soft-tissue calcification, and possibly more rapid progression of chronic renal disease. **Foods rich in protein usually are also high in phosphate; therefore, low-protein diets also reduce the phosphate intake and decrease plasma phosphate levels.** For nondialyzed patients with CRF, the phosphorus prescription is 5 to 10 mg/kg/day with the diet that

Table 15–7. RECOMMENDED VITAMIN SUPPLEMENTATION FOR PATIENTS WITH RENAL FAILURE

Vitamin D	See text
1,25-Dihydroxyvitamin D_3	See text
Vitamin K	None
Vitamin K, about 10 mg should be given every other day to patients who are treated with antibiotics and who are not eating food.	
Vitamin E	10 IU/day
Niacin	20 mg/day
Thiamin HCl (vitamin B_1)	2 mg/day
Riboflavin (vitamin B_2)	2 mg/day
Pantothenic acid (vitamin B_3)	10 mg/day
Pyridoxine HCl (vitamin B_6)	5 mg/day (10 mg/day for dialysis patients)
Ascorbic acid (vitamin C)	60 mg/day
Biotin	200 mg/day
Folic acid	0.8–1 mg/day
Vitamin B_{12}	3 μg/day

includes protein in the amount of 0.55 to 0.60 g/kg/day; 4 to 10 mg/kg/day of phosphorus is ingested with the ketoacid diet. For patients on maintenance hemodialysis or CAPD, the dietary phosphorus intake should be maintained below 800 mg/day.

Phosphate binders may be given to reduce the intestinal absorption of phosphate. Several different types of phosphate binders are used, most of which have side effects that may occasionally outweigh their advantage. Aluminum hydroxide, which has relatively effective phosphate-binding capacity, may lead to aluminum accumulation and bone disease, anemia, and possibly a rare form of dementia when used for long periods. Calcium carbonate and calcium citrate may cause hypercalcemia. Combined prescription of citrate and aluminum-containing salts should strictly be avoided, because the former enhances the intestinal aluminum absorption and enhances aluminum toxicity. Because low-protein, low-phosphorus diets are also low in calcium and patients with CRF usually have impaired intestinal calcium absorption, calcium carbonate or calcium citrate supplements may be preferred to bind intestinal phosphate. These calcium binders have the advantages of maintaining more normal calcium pools as well as reducing intestinal phosphate absorption. Certain calcium salts of amino acids and ketoacids present in the ketoacid diet (such as calcium-ketoisovalerate) bind phosphate and reduce intestinal absorption and prevent or reduce hyperphosphatemia in CRF. This action may provide a further advantage for the use of low-protein diets with ketoacid supplementation.

Calcium supplements should be prescribed carefully to prevent hypercalcemia, especially when used in conjunction with 1,25-dihydroxyvitamin D_3. Chronically uremic patients need about 1200 to 1600 mg of calcium per day to maintain calcium balance. With hemodialysis, there is usually no calcium loss into the dialysate, because the dialysate contains equal or higher concentrations of calcium ions than plasma ionized calcium. Some calcium losses may occur in CAPD with the use of the more hypertonic dialysate. The protein-restricted, low-phosphorus diets used for nondialyzed patients with CRF or for patients treated with maintenance hemodialysis or CAPD should be supplemented with about 1000 mg of calcium per day. Calcium carbonate (calcium content 40%), calcium lactate (calcium content 18%), calcium gluconate (calcium content 9%), or, for nondialyzed patients with CRF, calcium ketoacid salts are suitable. Calcium chloride should be avoided because it provides an acid load.

Patients with advanced CRF often develop mild to moderate metabolic acidosis with an elevated anion gap, mainly as a result of retention of protons and anionic acid groups, such as sulfate. In addition, some patients with CRF develop hyperchloremic nonanion gap metabolic acidosis such as in renal tubular acidosis. Long-standing acidosis may contribute to bone disease, malaise, and other symptoms. Furthermore, there is experimental evidence that acidemia promotes renal interstitial injury and thus contributes to further progression of renal failure. We therefore prescribe sodium bicarbonate as needed to maintain blood bicarbonate concentrations between 20 and 24 mmol/L. A dose of 0.5 to 1 mmol/kg of sodium bicarbonate per day may be given, followed by frequent plasma bicarbonate measurements to adjust the dose.

The magnesium requirement in CRF is about 200 mg/day. This is usually achieved or surpassed with a patient's dietary intake. Although some losses of magnesium may occur with hemodialysis and peritoneal dialysis, there is usually no need for magnesium supplements. **When severe hypermagnesemia occurs, it is almost always associated with a large intake of magnesium compounds from such sources as magnesium-containing antacids or laxatives.** Serum magnesium measurements should be part of routine laboratory monitoring.

Tolerance to a large sodium intake is often reduced in CRF. Similarly, the ability to conserve sodium is frequently impaired in patients who have CRF and are not in need of dialysis therapy. The prescribed sodium intake should be determined according to individual needs. Patients with CRF often do well with 1.5 to 4 g/day of sodium. Those with sodium-retaining states (*e.g.*, edema, congestive heart failure, nephrotic syndrome) or poorly controlled hypertension are more likely to require the lower quantities. Those individuals with larger obligatory losses will require more. Water intake is generally allowed *ad libitum* until patients commence maintenance dialysis treatment.

Patients on maintenance hemodialysis are prescribed about 1.5 to 2.5 g sodium per day. Larger amounts promote increased thirst and water intake leading to large interdialytic weight gain. Patients on maintenance hemodialysis are generally restricted to 700 to 1000 ml of water per day plus urine losses. Patients on CAPD may use hypertonic dialysate to remove

Table 15–8. POTASSIUM CONTENT OF SOME FOODS

Foods	Potassium (mg/100 g)
Dairy Products	
Yogurt	149–187
Milk	147–155
Cheese	
Swiss	~100
Butter cheese	~ 78
Camenbert	~110
Eggs	147
Margarine	7
Butter	20
Meat	
Roast beef	348
Pork	~350
Meatloaf	~228
Chicken	~250
Turkey	~300
Fish	
Catfish	282
Salmon	371
Crabmeat	266
Bread	~132
Potatoes	~443
Potato chips	1000
Vegetables	
Broccoli	464
Cauliflower	328
Beans, green	256
Cucumber	141
Lettuce	224
Tomatoes	297
Sauerkraut	288
Catsup	~1160
Fruits	
Apples	137
Avocados	503
Bananas	393
Strawberries	142
Grapefruits	181
Oranges	170
Prunes	221
Watermelons	158
Dried fruits	
Apples	622
Apricots	1700
Peaches	1340
Prunes	824
Raisins	630
Miscellaneous	
Honey	47
Mayonnaise	18
Olive oil	1
Chocolate	397
Coca cola	1
Beer	38
Wine, white	82
Wine, red	102

large quantities of salt and water and can tolerate greater sodium intake. CAPD patients may be allowed more water intake (*e.g.*, 1000 to 1500 ml/day plus urine losses) because of the greater ease of removing water each day in most CAPD patients. Water intake refers to the intake of water from all sources (*i.e.*, oral, intravenous) regardless of whether the water is in coffee, milk, soft drinks, juices, or alcoholic beverages or food.

Hyperkalemia is a major risk for patients with advanced renal failure or ESRD. To prevent hyperkalemia, the daily potassium intake should not exceed 70 mEq (about 2800 mg). Hence, foodstuffs rich in potassium (Table 15–8) should, at most, be allowed only in small quantities. Patients with renal failure must be counseled with regard to potassium intake, and their serum potassium concentration should be monitored. Patients with hyperkalemia may occasionally require cationic ion exchange resins, usually in their calcium form, to reduce intestinal potassium absorption. These resins may cause constipation, and rarely, a mechanical ileus may occur, with an acute abdomen. Hence, the use of exchange resins should be accompanied by small amounts of 50 to 70% sorbitol or a similar laxative.

CASE SUMMARY 2

A 19-year-old man was treated with maintenance hemodialysis for 11 years because of ESRD secondary to congenital bilateral vesicoureteral reflux. His compliance with medical and dietary prescription was poor despite repeated intensive counseling. Two days after his last hemodialysis, he was found unconscious in his car and was brought to the emergency room by paramedics. Examination revealed a bradyarrhythmia with widened QRS-complexes on electrocardiography (ECG). The patient's serum potassium level was 10.3 mmol/L. Immediate cardiopulmonary resuscitation and hemodialysis were instituted, and an exchange resin was given by enema. The patient's heart rate became rhythmic with a normal ECG tracing, and he gained consciousness after about 30 minutes. He later revealed that he ate a large serving of a banana split in a restaurant, containing chocolate and strawberry ice cream, one whole banana, strawberries, fruit sauce, chocolate sauce, and nuts. Almost all of the individual foods in this mixture are high in potassium (see Table 15–8). Hence, this nearly fatal complication was brought on by dietary potassium overload. The acute hyperkalemia was probably superimposed on an already elevated serum potassium level caused by chronically excessive potassium intake and by the fact that his most recent hemodialysis had occurred 2 days previously.

Trace Elements

Little is known about the trace element requirements in CRF. Deficiencies of most trace elements are probably not common. In general, we do not recommend supplementation of the diet with trace elements, with the exception of iron; only certain patients with CRF will need iron supplements. **The best routine marker to indicate low body iron stores is a reduced serum ferritin concentration.** In such patients, oral iron supplements should be given daily; 100 mg of ferrous sulfate daily or a comparable dose of ferrogluconate is often prescribed. Some patients with ESRD require blood transfusions for anemia. Because red blood cells contain large amounts of iron, patients receiving many blood transfusions are at risk for iron overload, which may be ascertained by very high serum ferritin levels. The need of patients on maintenance hemodialysis for blood transfusions has become uncommon since erythropoietin has became available. **When erythropoietin is used, most patients require iron supplements until the blood hemoglobin has stabilized at its higher level, because the increased erythropoiesis will consume the iron stores.**

Table 15–9. RECOMMENDED DIETARY NUTRIENT INTAKE FOR PATIENTS WITH CHRONIC RENAL FAILURE NOT TREATED WITH DIALYSIS

Protein	
Low-protein diet	0.55–0.60 g/kg/day (≥0.35 g/kg/day of high-biologic-value protein)
Very low-protein diet	0.28 g/kg/day of protein of any biologic value, supplemented with amino acids or ketoacids (see Tables 15–4, 15–5, 15–6)
Calories	≥35 kcal/kg/day
Fat	30–40%
Polyunsaturated/saturated fatty acid ratio	1:1
Carbohydrates	rest of nonprotein calories
Total fiber intake	20–25 g/day
Minerals	
Sodium	1000–3000 mg/day
Potassium	≤70 mEq/day
Phosphorus	4–10 mg/kg/day
Calcium	1400–1600 mg/day
(Calcium supplements are needed in virtually all patients)	
Magnesium	200–300 mg/day
Iron	10–18 mg/day
Zinc	15 mg/day
Vitamins	Supplements as in Table 15–7

Table 15–10. RECOMMENDED DIETARY NUTRIENT INTAKE FOR PATIENTS WITH MAINTENANCE HEMODIALYSIS

Protein	1.1–1.2 g/kg/day; ≥50% of high-biologic-value protein
Energy	≥35 kcal/kg/day
Fat	30–40%
Polyunsaturated/saturated fatty acid ratio	1:1
Carbohydrates	rest of nonprotein calories
Total fiber intake	20–25 g/day
Minerals	
Sodium	750–2000 mg/day
Potassium	≤70 mEq/day
Phosphorus	≤12 mg/kg/day
Calcium	1400–1600 mg/day
(Calcium supplements are needed in virtually all patients)	
Magnesium	200–300 mg/day
Iron	10–18 mg/day
(Supplemented iron salts are sometimes needed; see text)	
Zinc	15 mg/day
Vitamins	Supplements as in Table 15–7

Zinc deficiency has been described in some patients on hemodialysis. Deficiency of this trace element is implicated in impaired taste perception and, in males, impotence. In such patients, a daily supplement of zinc (15 mg) may be tried.

Tables 15–9 to 15–11 summarize the suggested dietary treatment in patients with chronic renal failure and ESRD undergoing hemodialysis or CAPD.

NUTRITIONAL CONSIDERATIONS IN PATIENTS WITH THE NEPHROTIC SYNDROME

The nephrotic syndrome is characterized by proteinuria (≥3 g/day), hypoalbuminemia, hyperlipidemia, and edema. A number of nutritional deficiencies may result from the large protein losses in nephrotic patients. Protein wasting in the nephrotic syndrome results from increased filtration of protein by the glomeruli, some degradation of the filtered protein in the proximal tubular cells, and urinary protein losses. The increased glomerular filtration of

Table 15–11. RECOMMENDED DIETARY NUTRIENT INTAKE FOR PATIENTS ON CAPD

Protein	1.2–1.5 g/kg/day; ≥50% of high-biologic value protein (see text)
Energy	≥35 kcal/kg/day, not including calorie intake from dialysate
Fat	30–40%
Polyunsaturated/saturated fatty acid ratio	1:1
Carbohydrates	rest of nonprotein calories
Total fiber intake	20–25 g/day
Minerals	
Sodium	1000–2500 mg/day
Potassium	≤70 mEq/day
Phosphorus	≤12 mg/kg/day
Calcium	800–1000 mg/day
Magnesium	200–300 mg/day
Iron	10–18 mg/day
(Supplemented iron salts are sometimes needed; see text)	
Zinc	15 mg/day
Vitamins	Supplements as in Table 15–7

protein is caused by a glomerular basement membrane defect that is induced by the underlying renal disease. Although this defect **causes** the proteinuria, the magnitude of the urinary protein loss also seems to be determined by the glomerular capillary blood pressure. Hence, treatment with pharmacologic agents that reduce the glomerular capillary pressure (such as ACE inhibitors) may reduce urinary protein losses and thereby help to maintain or improve nutritional status.

Although the rate of protein synthesis may be increased in the nephrotic syndrome, it is not sufficient to counterbalance the losses. High-protein diets were formerly prescribed (up to 2.3 g/kg/day) to nephrotic patients in order to maximize protein synthesis and improve body protein mass. However, such protein diets promote proteinuria, probably by increasing the glomerular capillary pressure. Protein synthesis does not rise commensurately with the protein losses; therefore, these diets do not increase the low serum protein levels. In addition, high protein intake may accelerate the rate of progression of CRF (see above). Hence, at present, lower-protein diets are advocated. **In short-term studies, these diets have been shown to reduce urinary protein losses to a greater extent than they reduce protein synthesis.** Thus, plasma protein levels remain stable or increase. A low-protein diet used in the treatment of nephrotic patients should contain about 0.55 to 0.60 g/kg/day of protein, with at least 50% of high biologic value; in addition, the protein intake should be increased by 1 g of high-quality protein for each gram of proteinuria. Alternatively, a diet providing 0.80 g/kg/day of protein (with about 50% high-biologic-value protein) may be used. There is no clear indication about the amount of calories needed with such a diet. Indirect evidence indicates that probably 35 to 40 kcal/kg/day is optimal, unless a patient is obese or at risk for becoming so.

Although these moderately low-protein diets have reduced urine protein losses and maintained or improved protein nutriture in short-term studies, the long-term outcome with such diets is yet unknown. For this reason, the nutritional status of nephrotic patients should be monitored very carefully to ensure that protein depletion does not progress with these moderately protein-restricted diets. Some nephrologists recommend combined treatment with these moderately restricted-protein diets and ACE inhibitors. **ACE inhibitors may independently reduce urine protein losses, and animal studies suggest that these compounds may also retard the rate of progression of renal failure.**

In association with the marked losses of urinary albumin, several protein-bound nutrients (trace elements such as iron and copper, vitamins such as 25-hydroxyvitamin D_2, and 1,25-dihydroxyvitamin D_3) might be lost in sufficient quantities in the urine to cause nutritional deficiencies. **Although few studies have evaluated the potential benefits of supplements of these nutrients to nephrotic patients, it would seem prudent to give these supplements.** Some studies suggest that nephrotic patients are more likely to become vitamin D deficient and develop vitamin D-deficient bone disease. Although not all studies have confirmed these observations, some nephrologists recommend the prescription of small doses of 1,25-dihydroxyvitamin D_3 (0.125 to 0.25 μg/day) to nephrotic patients. The hypocalcemia in nephrotic patients is mainly a result of a reduction in the non-ionized (protein-bound) fraction; hence, calcium supplements should be used carefully. For each gram per deciliter by which the albumin plasma levels are below the lower end of the normal range, a reduction of the total plasma calcium by 0.8 mg/dl is to be expected. Hence, only serum calcium concentrations below this adjusted value are considered to reflect hypocalcemia. A similar adjustment of the expected upper range of normal is necessary. Thus, a normal serum total calcium level in a

Table 15–12. RECOMMENDED DIETARY NUTRIENT INTAKE IN PATIENTS WITH THE NEPHROTIC SYNDROME WITHOUT RENAL FAILURE

Protein	
Option A:	0.55–0.60 g/kg/day; ≥0.35 g/kg/day of high-biologic-value protein plus 1 g high-biologic protein/day for each g/day of urinary protein loss.
Option B:	0.80 g/kg/day; ≥50% high-biologic-value protein
Energy	≥35 kcal/kg/day
Fat	30–40%
Polyunsaturated/saturated fatty acid ratio	1:1
Carbohydrates	rest of nonprotein calories
Total fiber intake	20–25 g/day
Minerals	
Sodium	≤2000 mg/day (unless edema is well controlled)
Potassium	as in normals
Phosphorus	≤12 mg/kg/day
Calcium	1400–1600 mg/day
(Calcium supplements are needed in some patients)	
Magnesium	200–300 mg/day
Iron	10–18 mg/day
Zinc	15 mg/day
Vitamins	Supplements as in Table 15–7

severely nephrotic patient indicates an elevated ionized plasma calcium level and is to be treated as hypercalcemia. If the nephrotic syndrome is accompanied by renal failure, the guidelines for dietary therapy as outlined earlier, as well as in Tables 15–9 and 15–12, should be applied.

The generation of edema in nephrotic patients seems to involve renal sodium retention and an increased total body sodium content. The plasma sodium concentration is usually low even when a patient is hypervolemic. For diuretic-resistant nephrotic patients, the sodium intake should be restricted to about 2 g/day, and the total fluid intake to about 1000 to 1500 ml/day. Nephrotic patients occasionally are hypovolemic; in these circumstances, salt and water loss cannot be undertaken until plasma volume is increased by reducing urine protein losses and increasing plasma albumin levels.

NUTRITIONAL TREATMENT IN PATIENTS WITH ACUTE RENAL FAILURE

The prognosis for patients with ARF is largely determined by the associated illnesses. When ARF is caused by medicines (*e.g.*, radiocontrast media, antibiotics), transient hypovolemia (*e.g.*, placenta previa), or uncomplicated rhabdomyolysis, it is often mild and of short duration. Moreover, the patient is frequently not very ill or catabolic and is able to eat. These patients may be prescribed a low-protein, high-calorie diet—0.55 to 0.60 g/kg/day of protein (≥0.35 g/kg/day of the protein should be of high biologic value) and 35 kcal/kg/day (Table 15–13). Alternatively, for short periods of time not lasting more than several days, 0.30 to 0.40 g/kg/day of the nine essential amino acids may be prescribed as the nitrogen source. **These diets are used to decrease the ureagenesis and to reduce or obviate the need for hemodialysis, but they should not be used if a patient is very wasted, is catabolic, or requires frequent dialysis.** The daily potassium intake may need to be maintained at 50 to 70 mEq/day or lower to prevent hyperkalemia. Phosphorus, sodium, and water intake also may be restricted. When the ARF is of short duration, there may be no need to supplement diets with vitamins or trace elements (see Table 15–13).

Patients with ARF caused by shock, sepsis, or other highly stressful underlying illnesses tend to be very catabolic and have, in general, a poor prognosis. Such patients may have pro-

Table 15–13. RECOMMENDED DIETARY NUTRIENT INTAKE FOR PATIENTS WITH ACUTE, UNCOMPLICATED, SHORT-TERM ACUTE RENAL FAILURE WHO CAN EAT

Protein	
Low-protein diet	0.55–0.60 g/kg/day (≥0.35 g/kg/day of high-biologic-value protein)
RDA for dietary protein	0.80 g/kg/day (for noncatabolic patients with substantial residual renal function)
Hemodialysis diet	1.0–1.2 g/kg/day
Energy	≥35 kcal/kg/day
Fat	30–40%
Polyunsaturated/saturated fatty acid ratio	1:1
Carbohydrates	rest of calories
Total fiber intake	20–25 g/day
Minerals	
Sodium	1000–2000 mg/day
Potassium	≤50–70 mEq/day
Phosphorus	4–12 mg/kg/day
Calcium	800–1000 mg/day
Magnesium	200–300 mg/day
Iron	10–18 mg/day
Zinc	15 mg/day
(Trace element supplements are generally not needed)	
Vitamins	Supplements as in Table 15–7

Table 15–14. ESTIMATION OF BASAL ENERGY EXPENDITURE (BEE) AND ENERGY REQUIREMENTS IN SEVERELY ILL PATIENTS, INCLUDING PATIENTS WITH ACUTE RENAL FAILURE

Male:
BEE = 66.5 + (13.8 × weight (kg)) + (5.0 × height (cm)) − (6.8 × age (years))
Female:
BEE = 65.1 + (9.8 × weight (kg)) + (1.8 × height (cm)) − (4.7 × age (years))
Energy requirements = estimated BEE × adjustment factor × 1.25
Note: Adjustment factors are shown in Table 15–15.

tracted ARF (not resolving within 3 weeks of onset). Protracted ARF is sometimes also observed after open-heart surgery. These latter patients may be less catabolic, but the prognosis for recovering normal kidney function is also rather poor. Such patients will almost always require dialysis for at least several weeks. **As a rule, for the more catabolic individuals, the nutritional therapy (*i.e.*, total parenteral nutrition [TPN], intragastric tube feeding, or oral intake) should be directed at providing needed nutrients.** Fluid and electrolyte balance and the accumulation of metabolic waste products should be controlled by adjusting the intensity of dialysis treatment. If patients with complicated ARF are fed orally, the protein intake should be about 1 to 1.2 g/kg/day. The optimal energy intake varies according to the underlying disease. ARF *per se* probably causes little or no increase in energy expenditure. However, in septic patients, the energy expenditure increases by an average of about 26%. The basal daily energy expenditure (BEE) can be estimated from the Harris-Benedict equation (Table 15–14). The energy requirements in a given

Table 15–15. ADJUSTMENT FACTORS FOR CATABOLIC CONDITIONS COEXISTING WITH ACUTE RENAL FAILURE

Type of Stress	Adjustment Factor
Malnutrition (chronic, severe)	0.70
Nondialyzed chronic renal failure	1
Maintenance hemodialysis	1–1.05
Elective surgery (early, 1–4 days)	1
(late, 18–21 days)	0.95
Peritonitis	1.15
Soft-tissue trauma	1.15
Fractures	1.20–1.25
Infections, mild	1
moderate	1.20–1.40
severe (including sepsis)	1.40–1.60
Burns, 0–20%	1.00–1.50
20–40%	1.50–1.85
40–100%	1.85–2.05

patient can be estimated from the product of the estimated BEE, an adjustment factor for the underlying disease (Table 15–15), and the factor 1.25, which is used to increase the calories administered by 25% to ensure that energy needs are met (see Table 15–14).

Although the vitamin requirements for pa-

Table 15–16. RECOMMENDED TOTAL PARENTERAL NUTRITION FOR PATIENTS WITH ACUTE RENAL FAILURE ASSOCIATED WITH CATABOLIC ILLNESSES

Amino acids	Essential and nonessential free crystalline amino acids including branched-chain amino acids as 4.25–5% solutions. 0.55–0.60 g/kg/day (nondialyzed) 1–1.2 g/kg/day (hemodialysis) 1.2–1.3 g/kg/day (peritoneal dialysis)
Calories	35–50 kcal/kg/day or as calculated (see Tables 15–14 and 15–15) Energy sources: Dextrose monohydrate: 3.4 kcal/g Amino acids: 3.5 kcal/g 20% fat emulsion: 2 kcal/ml
Fat	20% lipid emulsion: 250–500 ml/day, 500–1000 kcal/day
Carbohydrates	70% dextrose monohydrate at a daily dose to complete the energy needs not provided by amino acids and fat
Minerals	
Sodium	40–50 mmol/L
Chloride	25–35 mmol/L
Potassium	about 35 mmol/day
Phosphorus	8 mmol/day
Calcium	5 mmol/day
Magnesium	4 mmol/day
Iron	2 mg/day
Vitamins	
Vitamin D	See text
Vitamin K	7.5 mg/week (may be doubled during antibiotic therapy)
Vitamin E	10 IU/day
Niacin	20 mg/day
Thiamin HCl	2 mg/day
Riboflavin	2 mg/day
Pyridoxine HCl	10 mg/day
Pantothenic acid	10 mg/day
Ascorbic acid	60 mg/day
Biotin	200 mg/day
Folic acid	1 mg/day
Vitamin B_{12}	3 μg/day

Note: Patients must be monitored frequently for serum glucose and mineral levels and body water content, and the daily intake or use of insulin must be adjusted accordingly. When hyperkalemia, hyperphosphatemia, or plasma concentrations of other minerals are elevated at the onset of total parenteral nutrition, the intake of that mineral may be reduced or discontinued transiently.

tients who have complicated ARF and who undergo hemodialysis are not well defined, it would seem prudent to prescribe vitamin supplements in the same amounts given to patients on maintenance hemodialysis (see Table 15–7). Some patients with sepsis and ARF develop severe hypocalcemia, largely as a result of a reduction in their plasma ionized calcium, caused in part by elevated plasma calcitonin levels. In hypocalcemic patients, small doses of 1,25-dihydroxyvitamin D_3 (about 0.25 μg/day) and calcium may be given. **Patients with rhabdomyolysis may develop hypocalcemia because of calcium binding to muscle protein and reduction in vitamin D levels.** Such patients often become transiently hypercalcemic during or after recovery of renal function, and the use of vitamin D compounds or prolonged calcium therapy is usually not indicated. Table 15–16 depicts proposed daily intakes of vitamins and minerals in patients who have ARF and severe underlying illness; they most often will be fed by TPN. It is recognized that these recommendations are based on limited scientific data, and they will almost certainly be modified as more information becomes available.

Many patients who have ARF associated with severe, catabolic underlying disease are not able to ingest food. **They may occasionally be given intragastric feeding, but TPN is often necessary.** The nine essential amino acids (0.3 to 0.4 g/kg/day) may be administered. Patients should not be given more than 40 g/day of the essential amino acids unless nonessential amino acids are also given. For patients who are more catabolic, are malnourished, or are receiving dialysis treatments, TPN providing 1 to 1.2 g/kg/day of both essential and nonessential amino acids is preferable, as it may reduce the degree of negative nitrogen balance. A higher proportion of the essential amino acids and, particularly, the branched-chain amino acids (*i.e.*, isoleucine, leucine, and valine) may be advantageous because it may have a special anabolic effect. As much as 40% of the total amino acid intake has been given as the branched-chain amino acids. These latter formulations of amino acids tend to be more expensive than more standard mixtures that contain essential and nonessential amino acids in a 1:1 ratio.

The energy content of TPN solutions is usually provided as 70% glucose monohydrate, amino acids, and lipid emulsions, usually 20%. The energy released from glucose monohydrate is about 3.4 kcal/g. With 70% dextrose solutions, the available energy is about 2.38 kcal/ml of the 70% solution. Amino acids provide about 3.5 kcal/g. Patients fed by TPN for more than 1 week should receive a portion of their calories from lipids. Preferably, about 20 to 40% of total daily energy intake should be given as lipids. The 10% and 20% fat solutions provide 1.1 and 2 kcal/ml, respectively (see Table 15–16).

Selected Readings

Blumenkrantz M, Kopple J, Gutman R, et al: Methods for assessing nutritional status of patients with renal failure. Am J Clin Nutr 33:1567, 1980.

Feinstein E, Blumenkrantz M, Healy M, et al: Clinical and metabolic responses to parenteral nutrition in acute renal failure. A controlled double-blind study. Medicine (Baltimore) 60:124, 1981.

Ihle B, Becker G, Whitworth J, et al: The effect of protein restriction on the progression of renal insufficiency. N Engl J Med 321:1773, 1989.

Kopple J, Blumenkrantz M: Nutritional requirements for patients undergoing continuous ambulatory peritoneal dialysis. Kidney Int 24 (Suppl 16):S295, 1983.

Kopple J, Monteon F, Shaib J: Effect of energy intake on nitrogen metabolism in nondialyzed patients with chronic renal failure. Kidney Int 29:734, 1986.

Mitch W, Walser M, Steinman T, et al: The effect of a keto acid–amino acid supplement to a restricted diet on the progression of chronic renal failure. N Engl J Med 311:623, 1984.

Rosman J, Meijer S, Sluiter W, et al: Prospective randomized trial of early dietary protein restriction in chronic renal failure. Lancet 2:1291, 1984.

CHAPTER 16

PSYCHIATRIC ASPECTS OF RENAL CARE

Norman B. Levy

When asked what it is like to be a dialysis patient, a 52-year-old pathologist said, "It isn't any fun, but it sure beats being dead!" Obviously, nobody wants to be sick or burdened by a lifelong treatment, let alone dialysis with its dietary and other restrictions. Nevertheless, over 100,000 North Americans find themselves in such a situation, and tens of thousands are recipients of renal transplants. Before discussing some of the psychologic problems encountered in the treatment of patients who are on dialysis or have undergone renal transplantation, we will consider the general aspects.

People who develop renal failure do not represent a cross section of the general population. Rather, this syndrome often afflicts drug addicts and noncompliant hypertensive patients. Another general factor to consider in caring for these people is the unusual demands made on a person with renal failure. Dialysis requires that patients be restricted to a particular form of treatment, usually three times a week, or in the case of continuous ambulatory peritoneal dialysis (CAPD), a few times a day. Those involved in center and satellite dialysis must return to a particular place. All patients on dialysis are asked to adhere to a very demanding diet, which, if followed reasonably well, either removes all of the "fun" foods or makes their portions negligible. These patients are also told to restrict their intake of fluids to a severe degree.[1] Renal transplant recipients live under the threat of organ rejection and must take prednisone and cyclosporine.

In summary, renal patients tend to constitute a somewhat uncooperative population on whom unusual demands are made. It is therefore not surprising that psychologic problems afflict them and that a disparity exists between what physicians want from these patients and what many of them are able to deliver.

PSYCHIATRIC PROBLEMS

Uncooperativeness

CASE SUMMARY 1

The weight gain of a 24-year-old former heroin addict varies between 3 and 5 kg between each dialysis treatment. While being dialyzed, he sings loudly and against the wishes of those around him, screams at nurses when he thinks they are making errors, and is overtly insolent to his fellow patients. At times he misses dialysis runs altogether, offering provocative explanations such as "I didn't show up because it interfered with my social life." He carries a switchblade knife. A psychiatric consultation was called when he threatened a nurse with it because she did not give him mannitol. The consultant found that he was a product of child abuse who had great difficulty with frustration tolerance throughout his life. This made his education very spotty. He did not complete his secondary education, and by the time he quit school, he had major behavioral difficulties, was addicted to marijuana, and was a "pill popper." He supported his habit, which progressed into intravenous heroin, by engaging in petty thievery. When he developed renal failure, he withdrew from street life and severely curtailed his dependency on drugs, but in all likelihood currently continues to use crack cocaine occasionally. This case represents an extreme of behavior and will be used to exemplify what is subsequently said about noncompliant patients.

Uncooperative patients challenge our patience and, at times, even our sanity. They are responsible for the high rate of burnout among dialysis staff, who find that they can work in this environment for only a limited time.

Causes of Uncooperativeness

Frustration Intolerance. Infants and young children cannot tolerate frustration. With maturity, one should gain the ability to delay immediate gratification in favor of more long-term advantages. Adults vary greatly in their attainment of this aspect of maturity. Immature adults usually feel angry about not getting what they want when they want it. Virtually every form of medical treatment involves a delay in gratification and frustration, and its benefits are not immediately realized. The 24-year-old drug addict whose case is presented above had major difficulties in this respect. Being able to sit still, to stop what he was doing, and to come to a dialysis unit was a major task for him—one that he was periodically unable to fulfill.

Depression. Depression will be discussed as a separate entity but also contributes to uncooperative behavior in two ways.

Severely depressed patients with poor self-esteem may have major difficulty mobilizing sufficient energy to be constructive in their lives. Their self-destructiveness may be at odds with and overcome the positive effects of medical treatment. The ultimate reflection of this problem is suicide, which will be discussed later. **However, slower forms of self-destruction may be manifested by not adhering to diet and missing dialysis runs.** Although depression is an expression of anger that is directed inwardly, the anger sometimes spills out, subjecting those around depressed persons to their hostility. This may take the form of screaming at nurses and insolence to fellow patients. The behavior is interpreted as uncooperative.

Anger at Being Sick. Good health is ordinarily taken for granted, and when we recover from an illness we expect that good health will continue. Although we acknowledge our mortality, each of us harbors a combined wish/fantasy that we will somehow continue life in good health and indefinitely. The news media tend to promote such an attitude by announcements of medical and surgical "cures." The public has almost begun to expect that major diseases have been or are on the verge of being cured.

For every individual, the recognition and acceptance of having a serious illness is a major task. Our expectation of entitlement to good health may result in a great degree of anger when we become sick. This anger is often connected with a sense of injustice, rationalized around ideas such as "I'm a married woman with two children. It's not fair that I have kidney disease and that nurse who is single has normal kidney function."

Authority Intolerance. Medical management involves adherence to a hierarchy of authority figures. **Physicians, nurses, and other medical personnel all are authority figures, and patients react to medical personnel as they do to others in authority.** At times this attitude even shows itself by slips of the tongue. I have on many occasions accidentally been called "Father" by my Catholic patients. Many patients cope well with dependent situations. They may derive satisfaction from the regression involved in looking to a parental figure for guidance, comfort, and protection. However, for a significant minority, physicians and other medical personnel are the focus of their anger, as other authority figures have been in their past.

Depression and Suicide

CASE SUMMARY 2

A 44-year-old man who has been diabetic since the age of 19 developed renal failure at age 43. With the progression of symptoms, he stopped work as a school teacher. A few months after renal failure, his wife left him for another man. The patient had been married for 15 years, during which he had progressive difficulty achieving and maintaining an erection. He has been totally impotent for the past 5 years. His visual difficulties responded very well to laser therapy. However, he has recently suffered rapid progression of his peripheral neuropathy, causing him to go from being cane-dependent to being wheelchair-bound. The profundity of his depression caused the nurses to solicit my consultation. I saw him in a once-weekly psychotherapy session for 3 weeks, placed him on nortriptyline (an antidepressant), and psychologically prepared him for my 3-week vacation. During my vacation, I called him once to find out how he was doing and to adjust the medication. When I returned, I learned that he had shot and killed himself 2 or 3 days after my telephone call.

This case is an example of an extreme form of depression.

Depression, described earlier as anger reflected inwardly, occurs as a response to loss. The loss may be real, symbolic, threatened, or fantasized. The lives of patients with chronic illnesses, no less than people with renal failure, are full of losses. Two thirds of dialysis patients never return to full-time work activity. With loss of a job, there is also loss of income and possibly loss of self-esteem and of gender identity. Among these patients, losses are many and extend beyond employment. Patients with renal failure, especially those on dialysis, may lose their freedom, longevity, and sexual function.

Depression is an uncommon syndrome, although it is not an uncommon mood among these individuals. **A small but significant percent of patients with renal failure are clinically depressed (*i.e.*, have the syndrome and require treatment for it).**[2] In the case just cited, the patient lost his job, his sexual functions, his wife, his mobility, his strength, and his longevity, to name the most evident losses. His response was extreme despite medication and psychotherapy. Unfortunately, suicide is more common among dialysis patients than in the general population.[3, 4] It is not known whether patients on dialysis also have a greater incidence of suicide than do persons with other severe chronic diseases. Among persons who are medically ill, the incidence of suicide has been adequately studied only in diabetic individuals and those undergoing dialysis. Perhaps having an easy way to commit suicide predisposes the dialysis population to suicide. About 1:1000 dialysis patients commits suicide. A larger number engage in other forms of behavior that are self-destructive and may lead to death, such as severe dietary indiscretions. **It is therefore important for physicians to identify clinically depressed individuals who are prone to suicidal behavior so that adequate measures may be instituted.**

Less is known about depression and suicide in renal transplant patients than in persons undergoing dialysis.[5] There have been no studies of suicide and few of depression in this population. Suicide is probably no more prevalent among renal transplant recipients than among other groups medicated with prednisone, whose most common psychologic complication is depression. Therefore, physicians should carefully monitor depression in these individuals, especially during periods in which they are receiving large doses.

Anxiety

CASE SUMMARY 3

R.A. was a 21-year-old college student who showed all behavioral signs of anxiety while undergoing dialysis and expressed the feeling that being on hemodialysis was "like watching a Dracula movie." He attempted to diminish his anxiety by operating his radio and television set while writing letters during hemodialysis.

The process of hemodialysis is more anxiety provoking than peritoneal dialysis because it involves greater immediate potential threat to life and well-being. Although such mishaps are rare, they do occur, and virtually all patients in center hemodialysis have seen others in such situations. Anxiety may manifest itself in a number of different ways. Some people experience it directly and are able to identify it as anxiety. When hemodialysis runs took several hours and patients usually stayed overnight at their units, anxiety was commonly encountered as insomnia. Masturbation, especially among men, is common in patients on hemodialysis. Although experienced as a sexual phenomenon, it is essentially a method of reducing anxiety.

Anxiety is often encountered in renal transplant recipients, especially in two situations. Having a transplant and awaiting organ rejection is equated with having the Sword of Damocles hanging over one's head. However, patients tend to acclimate themselves to the situation. They do become anxious when and if early signs of rejection occur. Anxiety is also a side effect of prednisone.

Rehabilitation Problems

CASE SUMMARY 4

A.L. was a 30-year-old carpenter who felt that the physicians and nurses in his hemodialysis unit would strongly disapprove of him if he did not reestablish himself in his work after being on dialysis for several weeks. When he went out for the first time since being sick to subcontract for a major carpentry job, he developed a medical problem. Asked how he felt about returning to work, he said, "I didn't know whether I could do it. . . . I felt down in the dumps. . . . I was willing to try. . . . You never know until you try. . . . I'll have to try again." He continued to have medical problems for several months after this. In the 3 years that he was monitored since then, he never returned to carpentry and worked only intermittently as a bartender.

Medical success is often measured in terms of "full rehabilitation," which usually means return to full-time premorbid work activity. Unfortunately, such a model is not feasible for these patients. Their feeling of ill-health in addition to the treatment itself and its sequelae, may directly interfere with full return to household, school, and outside work. The obvious reason is that dialysis is an intermittent procedure and differs greatly from having normal kidneys, which operate constantly. Also, certain aspects of normal kidney function cannot be replicated by the dialysis machine. For example, before the availability of erythropoietin, all patients had fairly moderate to severe anemia. This and other reasons for diminished vitality such as secondary hyperparathyroidism and partial azotemia present formidable problems, especially to persons involved in manual work. Also, manual workers have more difficulty returning to work than white collar workers, professionals, and business people because their work tends to be less flexible and less likely to be able to accommodate the requirements of life on dialysis. **Therefore, rehabilitation, seen as a function of work activity, favors those occupations connected with higher socioeconomic status.**

Our current economic system, in an attempt to diminish the "punishment" of illness, provides monetary and other compensations to those it considers to be unable to work because of sickness. Thus, it encourages partial or full retirement, especially among those for whom work was never a highly prized activity. Furthermore, one may generalize that even healthy manual and blue collar workers are encouraged to retire younger than individuals in business and the professions.

Men and women differ with respect to rehabilitation, and work for most is a significant factor in self-esteem. Even in these days of greater gender equality, women who are married still have more flexibility (but less so than their mothers did) regarding either engaging in outside work or devoting their energy to the household. Such an option, not available to men and single women, allows women on dialysis to leave the outside work force and become homemakers, which is much more compatible with life on dialysis than most outside work.

Sexual Problems

Men and women on dialysis not only have less sexual function than they did before renal failure, they have less than patients with other chronic physical illnesses. Before systematic investigation of the sexuality of these people, clinicians observed that men on dialysis had more problems with impotence than could be explained on the basis of their apparent medical findings such as fatigue, anemia, and intermittent azotemia. When inquiries were made about the sexual function of these patients, it was discovered that both men and women had marked diminution in the frequency of sexual intercourse in comparison with that before renal failure. **About 70% of men on dialysis and 43% of renal transplant patients are partially or totally impotent.** Both men and women on dialysis and renal transplant recipients have diminution in their sexual interest.[7] Investigations into the origins of these sexual problems largely incriminate organic as opposed to psychologic causes. The main method of ascertaining this differential is by measures of nocturnal penile tumescence, based on the fact that men normally have erections during phase 1 rapid-eye-movement (REM) sleep. Those who complain of impotence but have erections during the night have psychologic causes of this problem, whereas those who are impotent and show no ability to get an erection during the night have an organic cause. The precise organic reason for impotence among those on dialysis as well as renal transplant recipients is not fully understood. A number of metabolic and other factors have been incriminated. These include high levels of prolactin, low levels of testosterone, diminished ability to produce sperm, cessation of menstruation, and hyperparathyroidism. One psychologic cause of sexual dysfunction is depression, in which diminution of libido is a somatic concomitant. Compromise in the sense of gender identity is another cause of impotence. Men who have total cessation of urination may perceive this as a loss of function of the penis, which is the organ of urination as well as of sexuality. Cessation of menstruation, as well as a less attractive appearance, may be perceived by women as defeminizing. Failure to continue work and reversal of the family role may be interpreted by both sexes as a compromise in their gender identity. Organic causes may produce secondary psychologic impotence. If an organically caused episode of impotence is felt to be a major blow to an individual's sense of masculinity, he may withdraw from sexual situations and feel less manly, leading to psychological dsyfunction and further deterioration in his sexual function.

Treatment of the sexual problems of these patients is directed at the underlying cause. **For example, hyperprolactinemia may be treated with bromocriptine, hyperparathyroidism may require surgical therapy, and psychologic difficulties should be appropriately treated as discussed in the section on treatment.**

PSYCHIATRIC FITNESS FOR TRANSPLANTATION

Although it is difficult to prognosticate human behavior, one of the few semireliable indicators is past performance. The variables are great and either an individual's maturity or his or her regression can place the person in a path that is deviant from past behavior pattern.

Transplantation should be avoided in individuals who are seriously depressed or borderline psychotic. Steroids may be unsettling in either group and produce a very stormy course. Individuals who have demonstrated a reluctance to take medicines regularly while on dialysis may refuse to take immunosuppressants and hence ruin their transplanted organ. Surgeons know from their own experience and that of their colleagues that it is best not to operate electively on individuals who predict their own demise or who do not expect to survive after their intended operative procedure.

Another relative indicator of adaptation is the nature and strength of the family/friend supportive system. If such a system is strong, it will help patients work through the adversities of a situation. Lack of such a strong system may leave patients with little to rely on.

In general, the presence or absence of deviant personalities or of mild or moderate psychologic syndromes is not a good predictor of adaptation and should not be used to determine fitness for transplantation.

TREATMENT OF PSYCHIATRIC PROBLEMS

Preventive Therapy

Many measures can diminish or minimize the incidence of psychologic problems among renal patients. Such maneuvers include the careful assessment of patients before a therapy is selected so that the treatment can be tailored to an individual's psychologic needs. **For example, more independent patients should be on a form of self-therapy or should undergo transplantation.** It is also important to identify individuals who are at greater risk for psychologic difficulties, based on their past history and their current presentation. These people should be monitored more closely than others, especially by psychologically trained practitioners, so that if problems arise they may be treated early.

Group Therapies

The most successful group therapies have been those in which the major focus has not been on the psychologic aspects. This focus tends to scare participants away. The groups that have been able to attract relatively consistent attendance have focused on "coping," have a limited number of sessions, are sometimes held in centers while patients are being dialyzed, and invite partners of patients to attend these meetings. The more successful groups tend to have an educational aspect, which may be accomplished by inviting guest professionals such as dietitians, social workers, nephrologists, and transplant surgeons to offer useful information.

Environmental Manipulations

Environmental manipulations comprise relatively simple to more complex activities that sensitive physicians initiate to ameliorate conflicts, avoid difficulties, and otherwise promote a patient's coping with illness and treatment. Included are such activities as setting up days and hours with compatible fellow patients and compatible staff, engaging in reasonable compromises concerning dietary restrictions, and offering sound advice, when appropriate, about activities outside of the medical situation.

Psychotherapy

As a group, renal patients tend to resist formal psychotherapy. They already feel "overdoctored" and, as a group, use denial extensively in facing their psychologic problems. However, selected well-motivated patients may be suitable for and helped greatly by psychotherapy. This treatment, although usually the domain of psychiatrists or psychologists, may also be performed by adequately trained social workers. Generally, both dialysis and renal transplant patients respond to supportive therapies that are focused on particular symptoms and tend to use psychoactive medications. A few patients have undergone extensive psychoanalyses involving several visits per week over periods of years. These are psychologically minded, younger, and very well motivated individuals.

Pharmacotherapy

The symptoms associated with anxiety, depression, mania, and psychosis can usually be either eradicated or markedly ameliorated by the use of psychoactive medications. Fortunately, most of these medicines are not removed by the kidneys and are not dialyzable. The exceptions are the barbiturates, which should be avoided, and lithium, which involves special considerations, mentioned later. **The large family of major tranquilizers, all the antidepressants, and the benzodiazepines pass the blood-brain barrier, are fat soluble, and are metabolized by the liver.**[8] The general rule is to use no more than two thirds of the dosage that would be given to persons with normal kidney function. The reasons for this are encompassed in Chapter 12 and include such considerations as absorption, distribution in the body, and protein binding among patients with renal failure. Lithium, a relatively simple salt, is removed by the kidneys and is dialyzable. It can be used by giving a single dose after each dialysis run. Without kidney function, relatively little of it will be removed until the next dialysis. Also, blood levels of lithium can be easily monitored.

Behavioral Sexual Techniques

A method of treating sexual dysfunctions that was originally described by Masters and Johnson and modified by Helen Singer Kaplan and others has potential wide use in patients on dialysis. The basis for its efficacy lies in the fact that people who have sexual dysfunctions tend to withdraw from intimate contact with their partners. This therapy is practiced by trained social workers and other professionals and involves the use of sensate focusing, which is a method of sexual stimulation, and the setting of sexual goals that are feasible and that do not necessarily include actual intercourse. It favors a progressive, relaxed intimacy that can be successful in markedly improving the sexual function of patients—even those with the severest degree of organically caused sexual dysfunction.

CONCLUSIONS

It is important for medical professionals to be cognizant of the stresses and psychologic complications encountered in patients undergoing dialysis and renal transplantation. Although prevention may be the most important aspect, a number of treatment modalities may offer patients cure or improvement.[9]

References

1. Reichsman F, Levy NB: Problems in adaptation to maintenance hemodialysis: A four-year study of 25 patients. Arch Intern Med 130:850, 1972.
2. Burton HJ, Kline SA, et al: The relationship of depression to survival in chronic renal failure. Psychosom Med 48:261, 1986.
3. Abram HS, Moore GL, et al: Suicidal behavior in chronic dialysis patients. Am J Psychiatry 127:1199, 1971.
4. Haenel T, Brunner F, et al: Renal dialysis and suicide: Occurrence in Switzerland and in Europe. Compr Psychiatry 21:140, 1980.
5. Steinberg J, Levy NB: Psychiatric factors in renal transplantation. *In* Chaterjee SN (ed): Manual of Renal Transplantation. New York, Springer-Verlag, 1979, pp 167–173.
6. Levy NB: Renal transplantation and the new medical era. *In* Guggenheim F (ed): Psychological Aspects of Surgery. Basel, Karger, 1986, pp 167–179.
7. Levy NB: Sexual adjustment to maintenance hemodialysis and renal transplantation: National survey by questionnaire. Trans Am Soc Artif Intern Organs 19:138, 1973.
8. Levy NB: Psychopharmacology in patients with renal failure. Int. J. of Psychiatry in Medicine 20:303–312, 1990.
9. Levy NB: Psychosomatic medicine and consultation-liaison psychiatry: Past, present, and future. Hosp Community Psychiatry 40:1049, 1989.

CHAPTER 17

PERITONEAL DIALYSIS

Ramesh Khanna and Dimitrios G. Oreopoulos

The wide acceptance of continuous ambulatory peritoneal dialysis (CAPD) throughout the world has renewed the interest in peritoneal dialysis in general. Better understanding of peritoneal membrane ultrastructure and the kinetics of fluid and solute transport across the membrane has enabled clinicians to rationally prescribe peritoneal dialysis. Connector technology has reduced the complication rates, especially the incidence of peritonitis. A decade of experience with CAPD has shown that for comparable patients, CAPD and hemodialysis are equally effective in terms of patient survival, quality of life, hospitalization rates, rehabilitation, and results of subsequent transplantation. Technique survival (*i.e.*, the percentage of patients remaining on the same treatment after a certain period) is still lower on CAPD than on hemodialysis, probably because of the ease with which CAPD can be instituted in almost any patient and the potential for discontinuation if a patient is not doing well.

PERITONEAL ULTRASTRUCTURE AND PHYSIOLOGY

The peritoneal cavity is lined by a continuous serous membrane with a simple squamous mesothelium underlain by connective tissue. At any given time, under normal circumstances, the closed peritoneal cavity contains a small amount of fluid (<100 ml). This fluid, along with the surfactant phosphatidylcholine secreted by the mesothelial cells, provides lubrication in the peritoneal cavity, as in the pleural and pericardial spaces, in which the internal organs can move. The peritoneum covers the visceral organs (visceral peritoneum) and lines the inner surface of the abdominal wall (parietal peritoneum). The mesothelium, a single layer of flattened elongated cells of 0.6 to 2 μm thickness, lines the peritoneal membrane. The luminal side of the mesothelial cells has numerous cytoplasmic extensions, the microvilli. Mesothelial cell boundaries are tortuous, and adjacent cells often overlap. The luminal side of the intercellular space is closed by tight junctions and desmosomes. The submesothelial basement membrane exists under the mesothelial cell layer. As elsewhere in the body, the interstitium is composed of collagen fiber bundles and proteoglycan filaments. These filaments form a mat of very fine reticular formation filling the spaces between the collagen fibers and almost all the other minute spaces of the tissues. The fluid in the interstitium is entrapped in the minute spaces among the proteoglycan filaments and flows through the interstitial tissue only very poorly. However, this interstitial fluid diffuses through the gel tissue, allowing rapid transport of not only water molecules, but also electrolytes, nutrients, oxygen, carbon dioxide, and so forth through the interstitium.

Blood Supply of the Peritoneum

The superior mesenteric artery supplies the bulk of the visceral peritoneum and the underlying structures. The intercostal, epigastric, and lumbar arteries supply the parietal peritoneum. The venous blood of the visceral peritoneum is returned to the portal circulation. However, the venous drainage of parietal peritoneum is into caval circulation. This is important because drugs introduced intraperitoneally will be partly subjected to liver handling during their first pass. The capillaries of the parietal and visceral circulation exhibit a complex branching pattern. The capillaries of the peritoneum have a continuous endothelial layer with a supporting continuous basement membrane.

Lymphatic Drainage

Lymphatic drainage from the peritoneal cavity is mainly through specialized openings (lymph stomata) that measure up to 22.5 μm and are located in the subdiaphragmatic peritoneum. The stomata are formed by the separation of adjacent mesothelial cells in the surrounding mesothelium. At the stomata, the mesothelial basement membrane and the underlying lattice of connective tissue become fenestrated and so allow the mesothelial cells and endothelial cells to join together to form a channel from the peritoneal cavity to the lymphatic lumen. The lymph vessels from the subdiaphragmatic area drain into collecting lymphatics within the muscular portion of the diaphragm. From the diaphragm and the diaphragmatic lymph nodes, most of the lymphatic trunks accompany the internal mammary vessels to the anterior mediastinal lymph nodes and thereafter return almost 80% of the lymphatic drainage to the venous circulation via the right lymph duct. In both the parietal and visceral peritoneal interstitium, a rich network of lymphatic vessels is observed. They drain mainly into the thoracic lymph duct. Inspiratory and expiratory diaphragmatic movements appear to open and close the stomata, which provide access to the lymphatic lumen from the peritoneal cavity. Intrathoracic negative pressure and lymphatic contractility, aided by the presence of valves, maintain the forward flow in the lymphatics. **The lymphatics draining the peritoneal cavity act as a one-way system returning excess intraperitoneal fluid and protein to the systemic circulation.** The other major function of the lymphatics is their contribution to the host defenses of the peritoneal cavity. Although the lymphatics carrying fluids and solutes from the intestinal mucosa traverse the mesentery before draining into the thoracic duct, they do not contribute in any significant way to absorption of fluid from the peritoneal cavity. The lymphatics draining the peritoneal cavity are the only pathway for absorption of intraperitoneal biologically inert particles, colloids, cells, and isosmotic–iso-oncotic fluid. Several physiologic factors such as respiration rate, intraperitoneal hydrostatic pressure, body posture, and peritonitis influence the lymphatic flow rate.

Solute Transport Across the Peritoneum

> Solute transport across a membrane occurs either by diffusion or bulk flow.

Solutes are transported to and from the peritoneal microcirculation and peritoneal cavity mainly by diffusion. The greater the solute concentration gradient and the smaller the size of a molecule, the greater is the diffusion. Substances such as oxygen, carbon dioxide, alcohol, and fatty acids, which are both water and lipid soluble, diffuse in the dissolved state through the lipid portion of the membrane; therefore, their rates of transport through membranes are about two times the rate for water. Substances such as water and many of the dissolved ions appear to pass easily through membrane pores and intercellular clefts. Although the exact nature of these pores is unknown, the substances with sizes considerably smaller than the pores pass through them with great ease. Electrical charges lining the pores in both the capillary endothelium and mesothelial cell layer and interstitium are shown to be negative. Therefore, the electrical charge of various ions often markedly affects their ability to diffuse through pores. Pinocytotic transport of solutes (*i.e.*, through vesicles) through cells is an important mechanism of diffusion for solutes with sizes greater than the pore sizes and macromolecules such as proteins. Small amounts of plasma proteins do leak through the pores and perhaps are transported from the vessels through endothelial vesicles into the interstitial space and from there through mesothelial vesicles into the peritoneal cavity. However, there is yet no evidence to indicate that macromolecules are returned to the blood across the capillary wall. The major route for macromolecule absorption from the peritoneal cavity and interstitium is through the lymphatic system.

Bulk or convective flow (*i.e.*, transport of solutes along with osmotically moved water) is an important transport mechanism during peritoneal dialysis when dialysis solutions containing osmotic agents are used. Because of either a hydrostatic or an osmotic pressure gradient across a membrane, during bulk flow, solutes and water move along this gradient at a rate often many times that which can be accounted for by net diffusion. A substance with a molecular weight too great for it to move through the pores of a membrane creates osmotic pressure across the membrane. This pressure then causes bulk flow of water through the pores of the membrane. During convective flow, the concentrations of sodium and potassium in the ultrafiltrate are usually lower than those in the extracellular fluid because of the sieving effect. The possible explanation for such an electrolyte sieving effect is the interaction between the charges of free electrolytes and surface charges in the intercellular gaps, interstitial gel matrix, and mesothelial cells.

In adult humans, during peritoneal dialysis, maximum urea clearances usually do not exceed 40 ml/min even with the most rapid cycling. Although it is suggested that maximum urea clearance is restricted by the effective peritoneal blood flow, indirect evidence indicates that this may not be the case, but multiple factors such as interstitium and stagnant fluid films may limit it. Furthermore, continuous lymphatic absorption during a 4- to 6-hour exchange reduces the small solute clearances by an average of 17%.[1]

Solute Equilibration During Peritoneal Dialysis Exchange

When a solution is dwelled in the peritoneal cavity, solutes from blood and dialysis solution slowly equilibrate with each other. The rate at which different solutes equilibrate depends on the solute size. Also, different patients equilibrate at different rates and consequently have different equilibration ratio and clearance rates. Mass transfer area coefficient (MTAC) expresses peritoneal permeability for a given surface area and is expressed as ml/min/m². This measurement was recommended as an index of peritoneal membrane function. However, because of the complex calculations involved in estimating MTAC, it is seldom used in routine clinical practice. Instead, Twardowski[2] proposed the use of dialysate-to-plasma ratios obtained during a peritoneal equilibration test (see the section on clinical methods to assess the adequacy of dialysis).

Forces That Govern Fluid Transport Across Peritoneal Membrane

Fluid transport across the peritoneum is governed by hydrostatic and colloid osmotic pressures in the capillaries and interstitium. The hydrostatic pressure in the capillaries tends to force fluid and its dissolved substances through the capillary pores and into the interstitial spaces. This process is aided by the colloid osmotic pressure due to small amount of proteins in the interstitial spaces, but the colloid osmotic pressure caused by the plasma proteins aided by the hydrostatic pressure of the interstitial fluid tends to cause fluid to move into the blood from the interstitial spaces. Under physiologic conditions, in the tissues around the peritoneal cavity, the sum of hydrostatic pressures across the capillary membrane is greater than the sum of colloid osmotic pressures of plasma and interstitial proteins, causing a net driving pressure to be slightly positive and to be directed from the capillary lumen toward the surrounding tissue. This outward net driving pressure causes continuous leakage of ultrafiltrate out of the capillaries. It is this ultrafiltrate that becomes interstitial free fluid. Lymph is derived entirely from this interstitial fluid. A small amount of this fluid constantly enters the peritoneal cavity to lubricate the organs protruding into the cavity. Turnover of this fluid is maintained by the continuous uptake of this fluid by the subdiaphragmatic lymphatics.

Peritoneal transport of solutes from the capillaries through the interstitium and the mesothelial cells into the dialysis solution in the peritoneal cavity occurs by diffusion, because of the difference in concentration. **The overall peritoneal clearance of substances from the blood increases with dialysate flow rate up to 6 L/hr.** Further increases in flow rate do not affect the clearance.

Kinetics of Ultrafiltration During Peritoneal Dialysis

During peritoneal dialysis, glucose is used as an osmotic agent to enhance ultrafiltration. Glucose generates a high osmotic pressure, which induces ultrafiltration from the blood. **When 2 L of dialysis solution containing glucose are introduced in the peritoneal cavity during peritoneal dialysis, the forces that normally operate across the capillary are modified in favor of enhanced ultrafiltration.** Studies done in patients on continuous ambulatory peritoneal dialysis (CAPD) have shown that hypertonic (4.25%) dialysis solution when infused and dwelled for 4 hours in the peritoneal cavity causes about 800 to 1200 ml of cumulative net transcapillary ultrafiltration (Fig. 17–1). During the same period, cumulative lymphatic absorption would be about 350 ml. Thus, the net measurable ultrafiltration would be appreciably reduced to 450 to 850 ml. Peak intraperitoneal volume is observed at about 2 hours after the dwell, when lymph flow rate equals the transcapillary ultrafiltration rate. From then on, the intraperitoneal volume will begin to decrease, because lymph flow rate, being constant, exceeds the transcapillary ultrafiltration rate, which begins to decline as a result of glucose absorption and gradual dissipation of osmotic gradient.

Indications and Contraindications for Peritoneal Dialysis

Four main indications for peritoneal dialysis are acute renal failure, chronic renal failure, refractory congestive heart failure, and intraperitoneal chemotherapy. The types of patients who are reportedly candidates for CAPD are listed in Table 17–1. However, the situations in which CAPD is preferred over hemodialysis are not clearly established; many prefer peritoneal dialysis for patients with unstable cardiovascular status, with acute bleeding, on home dialysis, living at a considerable distance from a facility, with diabetic end-stage renal disease (ESRD), with access problems (such as children), or with the potential for reversibility of renal function. Many infrequent uses of peritoneal dialysis are listed in Table 17–2. The contraindications for peritoneal dialysis are listed in Table 17–3.

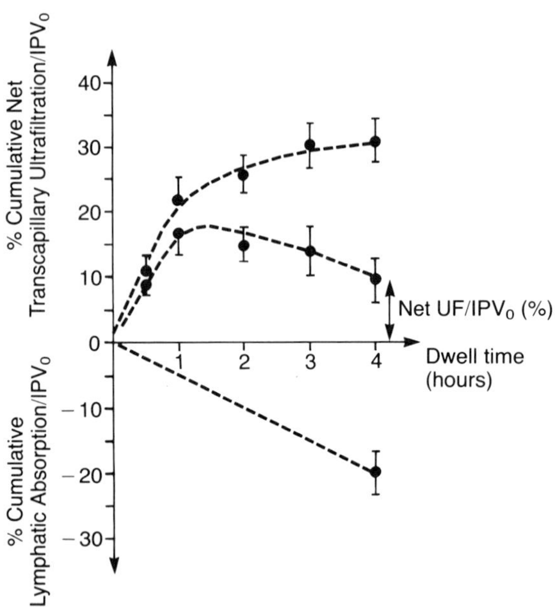

Figure 17–1. Cumulative lymphatic absorption, net ultrafiltration, and cumulative net transcapillary ultrafiltration (mean + SEM) during 4-hour exchanges in 18 CAPD patients using 2 L of 2.5% dextrose dialysis solution. IPV$_0$, intraperitoneal volume at zero time. (Reproduced with permission from Mactier RA, Khanna R, Twardowski ZJ, et al: Contribution of lymphatic absorption to loss of ultrafiltration and solution clearances in CAPD. J Clin Invest 80:1311, 1987.)

Table 17–1. PATIENTS WHO ARE REPORTEDLY TREATED PREFERENTIALLY WITH CAPD

Patients preferring home dialysis
Older patients with complicating cardiovascular disease
Children with small body size and poor vascular access
Diabetic patients with end-stage renal disease
Patients with uncontrollable hypertension during dialysis
Patients with malignant hypertension with renal failure
Patients refusing or requiring frequent blood transfusions
Patients with pretransplant maintenance dialysis
Patients with acute renal failure with prolonged anuria

Current Regimens and Techniques of Peritoneal Dialysis

Intermittent and continuous ambulatory peritoneal dialysis are the regimens in current use. One intermittent peritoneal dialysis (IPD) treatment usually lasts 10 to 24 hours, and several such treatments per week are given to patients to dialyze them adequately. IPD is generally used in hospitals to provide acute dialysis using rapid exchanges. It may be used after catheter placement to control uremia. Skilled nurses are required to place the patient on and off the machine and to handle troubles during treatments. It may be performed manually or with the assistance of a cycler.

Manual or octopus dialysis (also referred to as the carousel, umbrella, or multispiked system) is used at the bedside mainly for acute indications. Nurses trained in peritoneal dialysis

Table 17–2. SOME REPORTED INFREQUENT USES OF THE PERITONEAL CAVITY OR PERITONEAL DIALYSIS

Hypothermia	Hypercalcemia
Psoriasis	Hyperuricemia
Hyperammonia	Hyperoxaluria
Hepatic coma	Hyperkalemia
Exogenous poisoning	Thyrotoxicosis
Metabolic acidosis	Insulin therapy
Refractory nephrotic syndrome	Radiopaque contrast toxicity
Pancreatitis	Blood transfusion in infants
Chemotherapy	

Table 17–3. CONDITIONS IN WHICH PERITONEAL DIALYSIS MAY NOT BE FEASIBLE

Absolute Contraindication
Severe loss of peritoneal surface due to adhesion or recurrent peritonitis
Relative Contraindications
Presence of ostomies (colostomies, ileostomies, nephrostomies)
Recent abdominal surgery or trauma
Unusual peritonitis, e.g., tuberculous, fungal
Extreme obesity
Very large space-occupying mass in the abdomen, e.g., large polycystic kidneys
Contraindications to Continuous Ambulatory or Continuous Cycling Peritoneal Dialysis
Conditions worsened by raised intraperitoneal pressure
Hernias, hemorrhoids
Low back pain
Pleuroperitoneal communication
Midline abdominal incision for fear of ventral hernia
High peritoneal membrane transport
Excessive peritoneal cavity lymph absorption
Limitations to Self-Therapy
Physical handicaps: Blindness
Quadriplegia
Crippling arthritis
Mental retardation, psychosis, poor motivation

are responsible for setting up the octopus (a connecting tubing with eight prongs connected with eight bags). Ward nurses can drain the dialysis solution by lowering an empty bag. They then infuse a fresh solution by simply unclamping the tube of a hanging bag. On-call peritoneal dialysis nurses are responsible for troubleshooting.

A cycler dialysis setup can be used both for acute and chronic dialysis. If it is used for chronic maintenance therapy, two to seven treatments per week for a total of 48 to 80 hours are provided. The features of a cycler machine are (1) pump-assisted or gravity delivery of dialysis solution to a heating bag, where the solution is warmed to the body temperature before infusion by gravity into the peritoneal cavity and drainage of dialysate from the drainage bag to disposal, (2) an infusion volume that can vary from 100 to 3000 ml in 100-ml increments, (3) variable cycle time, (4) per exchange and cumulative ultrafiltration readouts, (5) optional instantaneous displays of fill and drain volumes, (6) gravity flow into and out of a patient, (7) overheating and overfilling regulation, and (8) self-diagnostics. The cycler uses dialysis solution from a 3- or 5-L bag and warms the solution to the desired temperature. An alarm incorporated in the cycler will sound when any of the monitored parameters are disrupted. The usual cycle time from the beginning to the end of drainage is 30 to 60 minutes, and the usual volume of infusion per cycle is 2 L.

PERITONEAL ACCESS

> Access to the peritoneal cavity is either temporary, when return of renal function is anticipated, or permanent with use of a chronic catheter.

Temporary Access to the Peritoneum

A straight, semirigid plastic catheter with multiple side holes or a soft Tenckhoff's catheter is usually inserted at the bedside. The rigid catheter is easily inserted but needs frequent manipulation to maintain a good in-and-out flow. Once it is inserted, it can be used safely for a maximum of 72 hours, beyond which risk of peritonitis increases greatly. Therefore, many prefer a straight Tenckhoff's, which can be left in place for a prolonged period. The steps of catheter insertion for acute or stylet catheter are as follows:

Preinsertion Patient Assessment and Preparation

Bedside insertion should be offered to patients who are cooperative, are not obese, and have not had previous major abdominal surgery. Patients should receive preoperative mild sedation and have an empty stomach before the procedure. The bladder and rectum should be emptied before the procedure. The hair on the lower abdomen is clipped and the skin prepared with povidone. Equipment required for paracentesis is all that is needed for bedside catheter insertion.

All observers and persons in the immediate area, including the patient, should wear surgical masks. It is useful to familiarize the patient with the Valsalva's maneuver. A nurse should be present to assist. A site 2 to 3 cm below the umbilicus in the midline is chosen (this places the site of entry at the linea alba, a point of minimal vascularity and tissue resistance) and anesthetized with a subcutaneous infiltration of 1 or 2% lidocaine without epinephrine; anesthesia is extended to deeper tissue with a larger needle. With a Tenckhoff's catheter, the anesthetized area should include the desired area of subcutaneous tunnel and the exit site.

Rigid Catheter Insertion

The two most widely used rigid catheters in North America are the Stylocath (Abbott Laboratories, North Chicago, Ill.) and the Trocath (Baxter Healthcare System).

Taking all sterile precautions, a small stab wound (2 to 3 mm) is made in the site chosen and anesthetized. The extent of the stab wound should be the size of the outer diameter of the catheter so that it holds the catheter firmly. To help the insertion procedure, some prefer at this time to prefill the peritoneal cavity with 2 L of dialysis solution using a 6- to 8-cm-long 16-gauge angiocath. The catheter with a stylet in place is forced through the abdominal wall by a short thrust or preferably with a rotary motion while the patient tenses his or her abdominal wall. Entry into the peritoneal cavity is recognized by the sudden loss of resistance to catheter penetration. It is very important to direct the catheter tip toward the coccyx while the catheter is being thrust through the abdominal wall.

Once the peritoneal cavity has been entered, the sharp stylet tip is pulled up a few centimeters inside the catheter lumen to avoid accidental viscus injury. The catheter is advanced in the direction of the coccyx to position it deep in the pelvis. The stylet is withdrawn, the catheter is connected to the sterile infusion tubing, and 2 L of dialysis solution are infused and drained out immediately to check the patency of the catheter. After the catheter patency is assured, it is firmly secured to the skin with the aid of the metal disk or by suturing the wings to the skin.

If repeated dialysis is expected, the catheter is removed after 3 to 4 days of dialysis and the track between the skin and peritoneal cavity is maintained patent through a naillike prosthesis called a Deane's prosthesis. When this prosthesis is removed, a new catheter can be inserted without the need for a trocar.

Bedside Tenckhoff's Catheter Insertion

A 2- to 3-cm incision is made in the skin at the insertion site (*e.g.*, the midline 2 to 3 cm inferior to the umbilicus). The lateral margins of either rectus muscle are acceptable alternative sites.

Through the skin incision, the wound is extended to the linea alba with blunt dissection using a curved hemostat. The peritoneal cavity is prefilled with 2 L of dialysis solution using an angiocath or a stylet catheter as described before. At this time, an anchoring purse-string suture is inserted in the fascia. Precaution is taken to avoid preperitoneal infusion of dialysis fluid, which should be suspected if infusion of the dialysis solution produces pain.

While the dialysis solution is being instilled, the Tenckhoff's catheter should be prepared by wetting it with a small volume of normal saline or solution containing antibiotics. Air from the cuffs is removed by rolling them between the fingers while immersed in the solution. A wetted obturator is inserted into the catheter, thus straightening and stiffening it to permit introduction into the Tenckhoff's trocar and beyond it into its correct intraabdominal position.

It is useful to start perforation of the linea alba with a smaller trocar or dilator rather than a needle, thereby facilitating introduction of the larger Tenckhoff's trocar. With firm but gentle pressure and a twisting action, the trocar with its obturator in place is pushed into the peritoneal cavity. To achieve pelvic placement of the catheter, the trocar should be pointing toward the coccyx while it is being advanced. Immediately after the resistance ceases (indicating entrance into the peritoneal cavity), the obturator is removed. The true intraperitoneal placement should be recognized by the welling up of dialysis solution into the barrel of the trocar. The large barrel of trocar is designed to accommodate not only the Tenckhoff's catheter, but also the Dacron cuffs. The catheter stiffened with a stylet is introduced into the peritoneal cavity and positioned in the pelvis. The patient usually complains of rectal pressure when the catheter is in the pelvis.

Once the catheter is positioned in the pelvis, the detachable trocar barrel is removed, leaving the split side pieces in place until the final positioning. At this point, the catheter stylet is removed while the catheter is held firmly in place. The trocar is separated into its two longitudinal sections and withdrawn, leaving the catheter cuff in proper position. The ideal location for the internal cuff is at the preperitoneal level. The catheter is connected to an infusion set, and its patency is tested in the manner described previously. If the function is deemed satisfactory, the catheter is secured in place to the posterior rectus fascia with the previously placed anchoring purse-string suture. The internal cuff is positioned over the linea alba or within the bulk of the muscle at an angle of 45 degrees caudally. After the catheter exit site is chosen, a stab wound (not an incision) is made using a blade, taking care to penetrate only the skin. The opening should be just the size of the catheter. A site that will permit the creation of a tunnel of an appropriate length and shape of the catheter should be chosen. Care is taken to ensure that the subcutaneous cuff is at least 2 cm below the skin. A subcutaneous tunnel is created using a malleable uterine sound or a Faller guide, being careful to manipulate the catheter gently.

For the initial few exchanges, it is best to avoid using hypertonic dialysate, especially if a patient is acutely dyspneic. Such patients are using predominantly their abdominal muscles for respiration, and ultrafiltration from a hypertonic solution will further distend the abdomen and thus decrease the efficiency of the abdominal muscles. Furthermore, if a patient should develop an outflow obstruction of the catheter, the retention of dialysis solution in the peritoneal cavity would be disastrous to an acutely dyspneic patient.

The complications during and after the acute catheter placement and their suggested management are listed in Table 17–4. **Perforation or laceration of internal organs is infrequent but is the most feared complication of catheter insertion.** Organs reported to have been perforated or lacerated include the bowel, bladder, liver, polycystic kidney, aorta, mesenteric artery, and hernia sac. Perforation is most likely to occur in those patients who have had previous abdominal operations with intraabdominal adhesions. Clinical evidence of bowel perforation includes sudden onset of severe abdominal pain, watery diarrhea due to infusion of dialysis solution into the bowel lumen, poor drainage,

Table 17–4. COMPLICATIONS DURING ACUTE CATHETER INSERTION AND THE SUGGESTED MANAGEMENT

Complication	Causes	Suggested Management
Abdominal pain	Inflow	Reduce rate of inflow and/or alkalize the solution
	Outflow	Irrigate the catheter
	Overdistention	Decrease the volume of exchange
	Catheter pressure	Reposition the catheter
	Referred pain	Analgesic
	Air entrapment	Requires no specific treatment
Bleeding	Skin bleeder	Local pressure
	Major vessel "bleed"	Stop dialysis temporarily
	Bleeding disorder	Fresh blood transfusion
Dialysis leak External	Frequent catheter manipulation	Discontinue peritoneal dialysis
	Poor catheter fixation to skin	Discontinue peritoneal dialysis
	Elderly patient	Discontinue peritoneal dialysis
	Raised intraabdominal pressure	Discontinue peritoneal dialysis
	Large intraabdominal mass, e.g., polycystic kidneys	Discontinue peritoneal dialysis
Into the layers of abdominal wall	Previous peritoneal dialysis in the immediate past	Discontinue peritoneal dialysis
	Previous abdominal incision	Discontinue peritoneal dialysis
	Wrong placement of catheter in the abdominal wall	Discontinue peritoneal dialysis
Poor drainage	Loss of siphon effect	Refill the system with dialysate
	Fibrin clot	Irrigate the catheter
	Blood clot	Streptokinase infusion
	Omental entrapment	Replace catheter
Perforation or laceration of internal organs (bowel, bladder, liver, polycystic kidney, aorta, mesenteric artery, hernial sac)	Uncooperative patient Inexperienced operator	Temporarily discontinue dialysis and monitor patient continuously for 24 hours
	Uncooperative patient	Temporarily discontinue dialysis and monitor patient continuously for 24 hours
Intraperitoneal loss of catheter	Frequent manipulation	Laparotomy to remove catheter

and foul-smelling dialysis fluid drainage, which may be mixed with fecal material. The management of such an accident includes removal of the catheter and close observation under the supervision of a surgeon. Laparotomy is not usually required.

Long-Term Peritoneal Access

A Tenckhoff's catheter or one of its modifications (Toronto Western Hospital or swan-neck catheters) is commonly used for long-term peritoneal access (Fig. 17–2), although many different types are available.[3] These catheters are inserted either at the bedside or by a surgeon in an operating room.

> An experienced surgeon who is deeply committed to peritoneal access surgery is a great asset to any peritoneal dialysis program.

Before a permanent catheter is implanted, patients should be examined to rule out those conditions that may require treatment or repair. Active peritonitis from previous acute dialysis must be treated and cured before implanting a permanent catheter. Similarly, a Deane's prosthesis must be removed at least 24 hours before insertion of the catheter. Infected abdominal incisions and stomata predispose to the development of peritonitis during CAPD. Therefore, if possible, catheter insertion should be delayed or avoided as long as either of these conditions is present.

Preinsertion Patient Preparation

Abdominal hair is usually removed 1 day before surgery, preferably with an electric shaver. The belt line of the patient is identified, preferably in the sitting and/or standing position, with slacks and belt as usually worn. Depending on the size and shape of the abdomen, the presence of previous scars, and a patient's preference, the skin is marked to indicate the catheter insertion site and shape and the desired location of the tunnel. The ideal site of the exit hole should be at least 2 cm away from the belt line so that it will not be subjected to scraping with a patient's garments at the waist. Pressure on the catheter tunnel is also thus averted when a patient bends forward. Patients who have a belt line below the umbilicus may not have enough space for catheter insertion below the belt line, and in such cases a catheter insertion site above the belt line may be preferred. In patients requiring high catheter insertion, it is necessary to use a catheter with a long intraperitoneal segment (approximately 20 cm). For those who have a belt line above the umbilicus, it is desirable to insert catheters below the belt line. In an obese individual with a pendulous abdomen, it is necessary to insert the catheter above the fat fold; otherwise, in the standing position when the fat folds hang out, the intraperitoneal segment would be dragged out of the true pelvis, causing drainage problems.

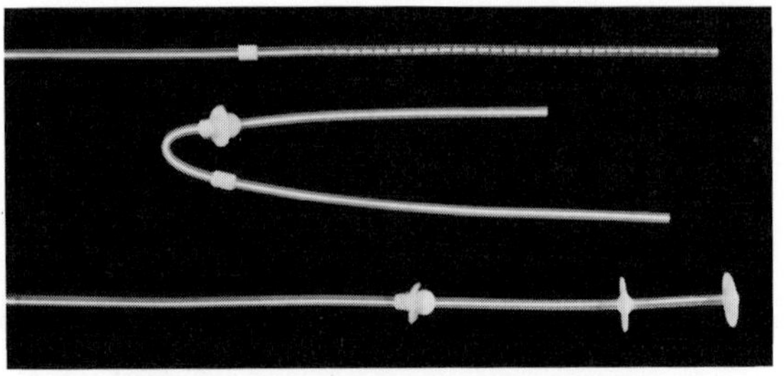

Figure 17–2. Commonly used catheters.

Vancomycin, 1 g (slow intravenous infusion) within 24 hours before surgery or a first-generation cephalosporin (*e.g.*, cephalothin, 1 g) 1 or 2 hours before operating room call is given prophylactically to protect against perioperative infections. Before operation, patients should empty the bladder. Tap water enemas may be required in constipated patients to avoid outflow obstruction.

General anesthesia is avoided if possible, because vomiting and constipation often occur during the postoperative period. Also during this period, voluntary coughing prevents pulmonary atelectasis; coughing, vomiting, and straining markedly increase intraabdominal pressure and may increase the risk of dialysis solution leak.

Surgical Technique

The paramedian approach through the rectus muscle is currently the preferred approach. After surgical preparation of the abdomen, the skin and subcutaneous tissue of the tunnel site are anesthetized with 1% lidocaine. A 3- to 4-cm lateral paramedian transverse incision is made through the skin and the subcutaneous tissue. Perfect hemostasis, preferably using cauterization, is mandatory. An incision is made in the anterior rectus sheath, and the rectus muscle fibers are dissected bluntly in the direction of the fibers down to the posterior rectus sheath. More anesthesia may be required during muscle fiber dissection. A purse-string suture is placed through the posterior rectus sheath, the transversalis fascia, and the peritoneum. A 5-mm incision reaching the peritoneal cavity is made with a scalpel. Care is used to protect the viscera from injury during this maneuver. The catheter is threaded on a wetted straight stiffening stylet and introduced deep into the true pelvis. At this point, a patient may feel some pressure on the bladder or rectum. The radiopaque stripe on the catheter is kept facing anteriorly. The stylet is removed, and then sterile saline is injected through a 50-ml syringe into the peritoneal cavity. If the solution flows freely, the internal cuff (in the case of Tenckhoff's catheters) is brought into the field, and the peritoneum is closed tightly with absorbable suture under direct vision. At this point, the cuff is laid longitudinally, parallel to the rectus muscle, and a stab wound is made in the anterior rectus fascia 3 cm cephalad to the transverse skin incision. The external segment of the catheter is brought through the fascia, and the cuff is positioned deep in the rectus muscle. With the Toronto Western Hospital catheter and the swan-neck Missouri catheter, the bead is placed in the peritoneal cavity, with the flange on the posterior rectus sheath, and the purse-string suture is tightened between them. The flange is sewn to the posterior rectus sheath with four sutures.

Creation of a Subcutaneous Tunnel

The catheter tunnel extending from the cuff to the skin exit should have a diameter close to that of catheter tubing. If the tunnel is too tight, it will not allow free drainage of necrotic tissue and may cause pressure necrosis with skin sloughing. On the other hand, a large tunnel prolongs healing relative to the volume of tissue repair required and allows movement of the catheter within the tunnel. This mechanical stress further delays the healing process. Thus, the last portion of the tunnel (from external cuff to the exit) should be made with a trocar of external diameter similar to that of the catheter tubing.

For Tenckhoff's and Toronto Western Hospital catheters, a subcutaneous tunnel is then made with a tunneler or other instrument, taking care to prevent excessive angulation or bleeding. The tunnel should be next to the abdominal wall musculature, deep to the subcutaneous tissue. The external cuff should be at least 1 cm from the skin exit site, which should be determined during tunneling.

For swan-neck catheters, a superior subcutaneous pocket is made to the level of skin markings to accommodate the bent portion of the catheter. The area between the subcutaneous pocket and the skin exit is anesthetized, and the pocket is extended by blunt probing with the hemostat up to the point where the external cuff will lodge. A small stab wound is made in the anterior rectus sheath above the transverse incision. The catheter is grasped with the hemostat and pulled through the wound. The transverse incision in the anterior rectus sheath is sutured. The bent portion of the catheter is positioned carefully in the subcutaneous pocket. A trocar is attached to the catheter and directed through the exit site. The external cuff is positioned about 1 cm from the skin surface. Care is taken to keep the radiopaque stripe facing forward.

Catheter Patency Testing and Postoperative Care

An adapter is attached to the catheter, and a sterile infusion tube is connected to the adapter. One liter of dialysis solution containing 1000 units of heparin is infused via the infusion tubing and drained immediately. At least 200 ml of solution should drain within 1 minute. Slow drainage usually indicates improper location of the catheter tip or capture of the catheter segment by the active omentum. If good flow is obtained, the skin incision is closed with absorbable subcuticular sutures. The operative site is covered with several layers of gauze dressings and secured with Microfoam surgical tape. Care is taken to keep the radiopaque stripe facing anteriorly.

The position of the intraperitoneal catheter segment is checked on plain x-ray film of the abdomen, and the patient is sent to the ward. The catheter is anchored with several layers of Microfoam tape and dressings, which should be left in place for a week. Additional in-and-out 1-L exchanges are performed to check the patency of the catheter and remove any residual blood from the peritoneal cavity. The exchanges are continued until the effluent dialysis solution is clear. **If the catheter is not functioning, surgical catheter repositioning is required.** Drainage is usually slow (<150 ml/min) if the catheter tip is not in the true pelvis. If the catheter tip is in the true pelvis but is nonfunctional even after 2 to 3 days, omental wrapping is most likely, and omentectomy may be required for correction. Analgesics with constipating side effects (opiates) should be avoided in the postoperative period.

Abdominal scars, a loose abdominal wall from old age or multiple pregnancies, and steroid treatment are associated with poor wound healing and may predispose to postinsertion dialysis leakage. In patients with such lesions, dialysis should be delayed for 24 to 48 hours after catheter insertion, and the initial exchange volume should be as low as possible (*i.e.*, 500 to 1000 ml per exchange). Hernias, when present, should be repaired at the time of catheter insertion. If clinical condition permits, dialysis should be delayed for a week to permit wound healing. It may even be desirable to support such patients with hemodialysis through a subclavian or internal jugular catheter until satisfactory healing takes place. **Carriers of hepatitis B antigen should be isolated from other patients on dialysis, and all necessary precautions should be taken in handling their blood and dialysate.**

Catheter Break-in and Catheter Care

The break-in period for a peritoneal catheter immediately follows catheter insertion.

> In order to achieve optimum long-term catheter function and low rates of complications, strict adherence to break-in procedure is essential.

The different steps suggested in the break-in procedure allow sufficient time for the incision to heal before standard CAPD is begun, at the same time taking care to maintain the catheter patency. During the healing period, undue stress exerted on the incision by the high intraabdominal pressure with 2 L of dialysis solution (especially in the upright position) may traumatize the healing tissue and predispose to dialysis solution leakage. Leaks not only delay ingrowth of fibrous tissue into the cuffs, but also provide a medium for bacterial growth and movement, thus increasing the risk of peritonitis and exit site infection. It is therefore desirable to delay CAPD for at least 10 to 15 days after catheter implantation.

Catheters inserted at the bedside usually require no break-in period, although some physicians use reduced volume (500 ml, then 1000 ml) for the initial four to eight exchanges before proceeding to the normal 2000-ml exchange volume (in a patient with a small abdomen or with respiratory embarrassment, a reduced exchange volume may be required indefinitely).

In patients who have ESRD and in whom a catheter is inserted for long-term use, the catheter may also be used for acute dialysis in the supine position because the intraabdominal pressure during filling in the supine position is limited and leakage is not usually a problem. Peritoneal dialysis in the supine position is usually started immediately after in-and-out exchanges are completed. One-liter volumes of dialysis solutions are used for the first supine peritoneal dialysis. Usually cycler settings are 10-minute inflow, 10-minute dwell, and 12-minute outflow. The outflow time may be prolonged to 15 minutes in case of slow drainage. Each liter of dialysis solution contains 1000 units of heparin. Despite clear dialysate in postimplantation washouts, the dialysate is usually blood tinged during the first cycler dialysis. Some practitioners set the exchange volume at 500 ml for the first four exchanges, 1000 ml for the next four, then proceed to the desired exchange volume if tolerated. Heparin (500 units/L) is added to each dialysis solution bag for at least the first 72 hours. Several sessions of supine dialysis may be given until the incision is well healed and ready to commence standard CAPD.

When a catheter is replaced in a patient who is already on CAPD, it may be tempting to modify the break-in procedure to allow CAPD with lower volumes per exchange. However, such a practice may expose patients to risk of a leak and delayed wound healing. It is our policy to provide them peritoneal dialysis only in the supine position with a cycler until the incision is well healed, which usually takes 1 to 2 weeks. Alternatively, hemodialysis is provided using a subclavian or internal jugular catheter as an access until standard CAPD can be resumed.

When a catheter is inserted at the time of another abdominal surgery, such as hernia repair or cholecystectomy, no change in break-in procedure is recommended except that standard CAPD may be delayed longer than 15 days depending on the surgeon's recommendation.

Subsequent Catheter Care

The surgical dressing placed at the time of insertion is removed after 1 week. Care is taken to avoid pulling or twisting the catheter. The exit site and skin surrounding the catheter are cleansed with povidone-iodine scrub, rinsed with sterile water, patted dry with sterile gauze, covered with several layers of gauze dressings, and secured with Microfoam surgical tape. Weekly dressing changes are continued until the healing process is completed. There are no data in humans with respect to the time needed for firm fibrous tissue ingrowth into the cuff and completion of epidermal growth into the sinus tract. We assume that it may take as long as 6 weeks. Patients may shower only before the dressing change or otherwise must take sponge baths.

Protection of the catheter from mechanical stress seems to be extremely important, especially during the break-in period. A catheter should be anchored in such a way that patients' movements are only minimally transmitted to the exit site. The method of catheter immobilization is individualized, depending on exit location and shape of the abdomen. We think that careful exit site protection prevents infections in most patients.

Special care of the exit site after the healing process is completed is essential to prevent infection. **Routine exit site care includes (1) examining the exit site and tunnel for signs of infection, (2) cleaning the skin to remove dirt and decrease bacteria, and (3) securing the catheter to avoid tension and tugging movements.** Routine exit site care should be performed daily and any time the exit site is red or dirty. Several methods of exit site care are currently practiced. The three commonly used methods are (1) daily cleaning and leaving the exit site exposed, (2) daily cleaning and topical application of povidone-iodine, or (3) daily cleaning, topical application of povidone-iodine, and covering the exit site with sterile gauze.

After satisfactory healing (6 to 8 weeks after implantation) patients may, if they wish, swim in the ocean or private swimming pools, preferably covering the exit site with a colostomy bag with the catheter spike and dialysate bag or capped spike within the same colostomy bag. Bathing in other surface waters such as rivers, lakes, public pools, and whirlpool hot tubs should be discouraged, as should skin diving. After swimming, patients should shower to clean the exit site and then cover it with a sterile dry dressing. Patients should avoid tub bathing but are allowed to shower.

The early complications of permanent catheter insertion are similar to acute catheter insertion, except that their occurrence rates are considerably lower. **Late catheter complications are mainly related to exit site infections; their management is outlined in the decision-making tree for peritonitis (see Fig. 17–9).** Another complication is dialysis solution leakage, which may occur months or even years after catheter insertion. Management of late leakage is similar to that described for acute catheter leakage. However, most cases of late leakage are refractory to conservative management and require surgical repair. External cuff extrusion is a late complication that is usually due to placing a catheter in a shape that does not conform to its natural design. The resilience force of Silastic causes the catheter to assume its original shape. During this process, the external cuff usually extrudes. The design of the swan-neck catheter has completely eliminated this problem. Late catheter nonfunction is extremely uncommon; and when it does occur, it is usually in association with peritonitis.

Indications for Catheter Removal

The need for catheter removal occurs under various conditions. **These may be broadly categorized under two headings: catheter malfunction and complicating medical conditions with a functioning catheter.**

A poorly functioning or nonfunctioning catheter may be removed under the following conditions: 1) Intraluminal obstruction with blood or fibrin clot or omental tissue incarceration. The decision to remove the catheter is usually made only when conservative measures to dislodge the obstruction have failed. 2) Catheter tip migration out of the pelvis with poor drainage. 3) A kink along the catheter's course. 4) Catheter tip caught in adhesions following severe peritonitis. In these situations, there usually are both inflow and outflow draining problems.

A functioning catheter with a complication may have to be removed under the following conditions: 1) Recurrent peritonitis with no identifiable cause. 2) Peritonitis due to exit site and/or tunnel infection. 3) Persistent exit site infection. 4) Tunnel infection and abscess. 5) Late recurrent dialysate leak through the exit site or into the layers of the abdominal wall. 6) Unusual peritonitis (*e.g.*, tuberculosis, fungal). 7) Bowel perforation with multiple-organism peritonitis. 8) Refractory peritonitis due to other causes. 9) Severe abdominal pain either resulting from the catheter impinging on internal organs or during solution inflow. 10) Catheter cuff erosion with infection. 11) Accidental breakage in the continuity of the catheter.

A functioning catheter may be removed because it is no longer needed, such as after successful renal transplantation or peritoneal dialysis, when dialysis is no longer needed, or when a patient transfers to another form of dialysis.

Prescription and Technique of Acute Intermittent Peritoneal Dialysis

The prescription of acute dialysis is usually tailored to a patient's need, such as illustrated by the following case summary.

CASE SUMMARY 1

A 40-year-old man with known chronic renal failure secondary to chronic interstitial disease is admitted to the hospital with a 2-day history of persistent nausea, vomiting, and weakness. Physical examination reveals blood pressure of 190/115 mm Hg in the supine position, pitting edema around both ankles, and fine rales at both lung bases. The electrocardiogram reveals peaked T waves and some widening of the P wave and QRS complex. The following blood test results are obtained: plasma creatinine = 17.3 mg/dl, sodium = 130 mEq/L, potassium = 8.1 mEq/L, chloride = 98 mEq/L, HCO_3^- = 12 mEq/L.

The patient was administered glucose and insulin intravenously. To avoid fatal arrhythmia as a result of hyperkalemia, it was decided to peritoneally dialyze this man acutely to correct the biochemical abnormalities. A Tenckhoff's catheter was inserted at the bedside by the renal fellow. The peritoneal dialysis orders were as follows:

Rx: Peritoneal dialysis for 24 hours using a cycler

Exchange volume 1000 ml

Inflow time 5 min Outflow time 10 min Dwell time 15 min	Cycle time 30 min for first three cycles or a flow rate of 2 L/hr

Use dialysis solution containing 1.5% dextrose with no potassium added.

If no problems occur with inflow and outflow, continue exchanges as follows:

Exchange volume 2000 ml

Inflow time 10 min Outflow time 20 min Dwell time 10 min	Cycle time 40 min or a flow rate of 3 L/hr

Use dialysis solution containing 1.5% alternating with 2.5% dextrose with no added potassium.

Weigh the patient every shift (8 hr); plan for a weight loss of about 2 kg during 24 hours. If this is not achieved, use 2.5% solutions more frequently.

Use exclusively dialysis solutions containing 1.5% dextrose after the desired body weight loss.

Check serum electrolytes 4 hours from the start of dialysis and then every 8 hours during the dialysis. Add potassium 2 mEq/L of dialysis solution if serum potassium level is less than 3.5 mEq/L.

The initial exchange volume preferably should not exceed 1000 ml to minimize the risk of dialysis solution leakage and the patient's discomfort.

The dialysis solution should be left in the peritoneal cavity for 10 to 15 minutes to equilibrate, thus achieving a flow rate of 2 to 3 L/hr.

To minimize infection and blockage of the catheter, 1 g of cephalothin is given 1 to 2 hours before the catheter insertion, and cephalothin (100 mg/L) and heparin (500 units/L) are added to the dialysis solution for the first 24 to 36 hours.

The dextrose concentration of dialysis solution is proportional to the amount of fluid needed to be removed. It should be emphasized, however, that unless a patient has severe pulmonary edema, the removal of the excess fluid should be gradual (over 2 to 3 days).

A potassium-free dialysis solution is used in peritoneal dialysis for most patients with renal failure because the peritoneal membrane clears potassium slowly, and these patients have a tendency toward hyperkalemia. However, if a patient is receiving digoxin, especially during the initial dialysis, potassium should be added to the dialysate to avoid sudden changes in serum potassium level and prevent myocardial irritability and potentially fatal arrhythmia. The

Table 17–5. SPECIAL COMPOSITION OF SOLUTION FOR CASES OF HYPERCALCEMIA AND LACTIC ACIDOSIS

	Amount Added
$NaHCO_3$ (7%)	75 ml
⅔ + ⅓ (dextrose-saline)	1000 ml
NaCl (0.9 g/100 mg)	1000 ml
Dextrose 50%	50 ml
This Mixture Will Contain:	**Concentration**
Bicarbonate	35 mEq/L
Sodium	135 mEq/L
Chloride	100 mEq/L
Dextrose	12 g/L

amount added is usually 3 to 4 mEq/L of potassium chloride.

Occasionally, patients unable to metabolize lactate (*e.g.*, those in hepatic failure or with severe lactic acidosis) may need a dialysis solution containing bicarbonate. Table 17–5 shows the composition of this solution. This bicarbonate solution, if used for more than 24 hours, may induce serious calcium and magnesium losses; hence, these ions should be replaced intravenously. On the other hand, this type of dialysate may be used for treatment of hypercalcemia.

A peritoneal dialysis treatment for acute renal failure should typically last for 48 to 72 hours. It is important that the dialysis orders for acute treatment be written for 24 hours only. At the end of each 24 hours, patients should be reassessed, and a modified order should be written if necessary. Acutely sick patients with unstable vital signs will need more frequent reevaluation.

CONTINUOUS AMBULATORY PERITONEAL DIALYSIS

CAPD is mainly used as a chronic therapy for patients with ESRD. It can be used for acute renal failure but is not as efficient as cycler IPD therapy because of inadequate ultrafiltration.

CAPD is performed manually by the patient or a helper. In adults, 2 L of dialysis solution is usually instilled into the peritoneal cavity for each exchange. CAPD is a self-care home dialysis therapy that requires intensive patient education with respect to procedures, theory, and management of problems.

Mechanics

Continuous dialysis occurs for 24 hours/day, 7 days/week, using a 1- to 3-L volume with two to five cycles (or passes) of fluid per day. A single cycle includes inflow, dwell time, and outflow.

Inflow (5 min/L). Fluid moves from the bag containing dialysis solution into the peritoneal cavity via gravity flow.

Dwell Time. Dwell time accounts for 4 to 8 hours during the day, 6 to 12 hours during the night. Removal of fluid and solutes occurs at this time.

Outflow (7 to 12 min/L). Fluid moves from the peritoneal cavity into an empty bag by means of gravity flow.

Exchange Procedure

The exchange procedure requires access to the tubing system, with a potential for contamination; therefore, it must be performed by trained staff/patients only. Two connecting systems of fluid delivery from the dialysis solution bag into the peritoneal cavity are used: a single-pronged connecting tube attached to the peritoneal catheter and a dialysis solution bag, and a Y-set bagless system (Fig. 17–3).

Steps in exchanging a single-pronged spike system are as follows:

1. A fresh bag of dialysis solution is connected to one end of the connecting tube.
2. Fluid is instilled into the peritoneal cavity during a 10-minute period.
3. The tubing is clamped, and the bag with the connected tubing is folded and carried under the clothing.
4. The solution is left in the peritoneal cavity for 4 to 8 hours. During this period, patients are free to carry on their normal activities.
5. At the end of the prescribed dwell time, the solution is drained by gravity as completely as possible into the attached empty bag.
6. Using aseptic precautions, the bag containing the drained solution is disconnected from the connecting tube and discarded.
7. A new bag of dialysis solution warmed to body temperature is connected, and the cycle is repeated. Dry heat such as microwave is an acceptable method of warming solutions. Water baths should not be used. Hot dialysis solution should never be used.

Steps in the exchange procedure with a Y-set system are as follows:

The Y set has two limbs; one is attached to a drainage bag or container, and the other to a bag of fresh, unused dialysis solution. The remaining end of the system is attached to the catheter. In the beginning of an exchange and

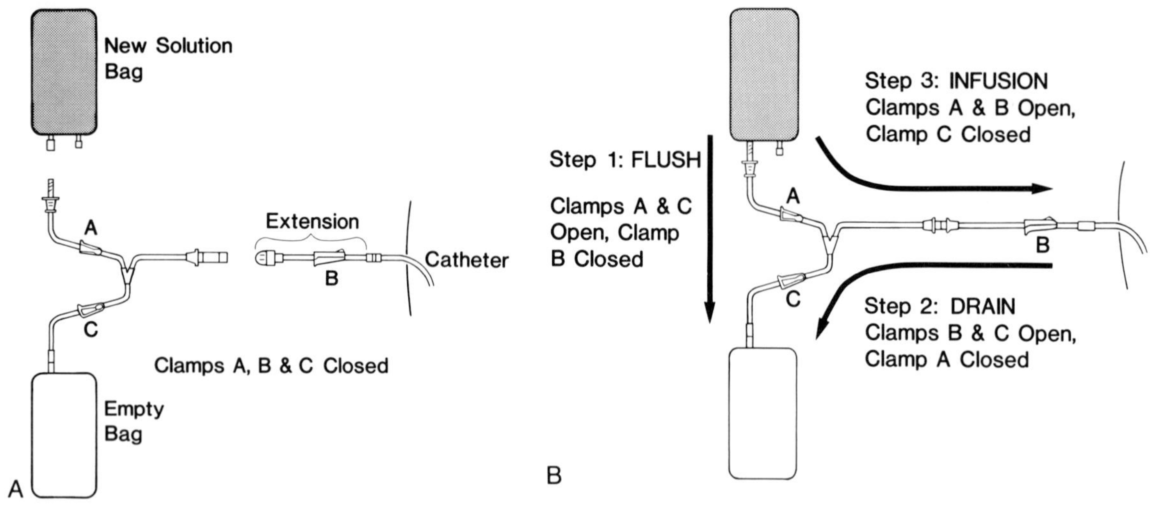

Figure 17–3. Y-set system for solution exchange for CAPD. (*A*) Setup before exchange. (*B*) Steps during exchange.

after connection with a new bag, a small volume of dialysis solution is used to flush the system by draining into the drainage bag, to wash out any bacteria that accidentally may have been introduced into the system during the connection and to remove the antiseptic, if a Y set with antiseptic is used. The rest of the exchange cycle is almost identical to the one described for the single-pronged system. At the end of the exchange, the bag is removed and the patient carries the Y set filled with the antiseptic, or the whole set is removed and the catheter is capped with an antiseptic-containing cap. The long-life connection tube is used for 3 to 6 months and is then changed under sterile conditions by a nurse.

Patients with an average peritoneal membrane transport require four bags per day, each with a volume of 2 L. The timing of their exchange is tailored to a patient's convenience. Some patients, especially those who have high membrane permeability and significant residual renal function, can be maintained satisfactorily on CAPD with only 6 L/day. On the other hand, anuric patients with body surface area greater than 2 m^2 usually require 10 L or more per day for adequate dialysis (see also the section on the peritoneal equilibration test). This can be achieved by five daily exchanges or by using larger volumes in those patients who can tolerate them.

Guidelines for the Choice of Dialysis Solution for Adequate Ultrafiltration

The following suggestions are general guidelines only and are applicable to CAPD patients with average peritoneal membrane transport characteristics. **The rate of fluid removal varies among individual patients, depending on the membrane permeability.** The choice of dextrose concentrations is based on body weight and on lying and standing blood pressure. If a patient's current weight is 0.5 kg or more below the determined dry weight, use 0.5% dialysis solution if available. If not, use 1.5% solution and prolong the dwell time to over 8 to 10 hours to allow significant fluid absorption. If a patient's weight is at dry weight (±0.5 kg) use 1.5% solution. If a patient's weight is between 0.5 and 2 kg above dry weight, use 2.5% solution. If a patient's weight is greater than 2 kg above dry weight, use 4.25% solution. Patients with poor cardiac function may have difficulty in tolerating rapid ultrafiltration with hypertonic dialysis solutions because of ensuing symptomatic hypotension. Similarly, diabetic patients who are on CAPD and who have autonomic dysfunction may become severely orthostatic on rapid ultrafiltration. If a patient is receiving hypotensive medications or a coronary vasodilator, use hypertonic solutions with great caution. Small individuals, those with large cystic kidneys, and those with hernias may require volumes less than 2 L. Management of these complex problems is discussed further in the section on assessment of adequacy of dialysis.

Continuous Cycling Peritoneal Dialysis

Continuous cycling peritoneal dialysis (CCPD) can be a self-care dialysis program and is chosen by those patients desiring to be free of dialysis procedures during the day. It is also used in children, thus liberating patients and parents during the daytime. CCPD requires a cycler machine that warms and measures dialysis solution and delivers solution into the peritoneal cavity. A cycle time is usually set at 2 to 3 hours. The cycler drains the solution from the patient into a disposable plastic reservoir. At the end of cycler dialysis, a fresh 2-L volume of dialysis solution is instilled for a long daytime exchange. Sterile connect and disconnect procedures are performed by a trained patient or nurse. This technique requires intensive education of patients.

Nightly Peritoneal Dialysis

Nightly peritoneal dialysis (NPD) is IPD performed every night with the daytime free of dialysis. Unlike CCPD, in NPD the peritoneal cavity is without dialysate during the day. NPD requires a cycler machine and may be performed in hospitalized patients or at home. In the hospital, nurses trained in peritoneal dialysis place patients on and off the machines and troubleshoot during treatments. Home NPD treatment requires patient education similar to that for CCPD. Home NPD is the preferred peritoneal dialysis technique in patients with poor ultrafiltration due to rapid glucose absorption and in patients prone to abdominal leaks and hernias. However, this treatment is expensive because of the larger volumes of dialysis solutions required.

Dialysis Solution

Dialysis solutions are available in different glucose concentrations (0.5%, 1.5%, 2.5%, and 4.25% dextrose) and are available in many different sizes of containers (0.5-, 1-, 2-, and 3-L volume). The electrolyte concentrations of the solution are kept to match the normal serum value (sodium = 132 mEq/L, chloride = 96 to 102 mEq/L, calcium = 2.5 to 3.5 mEq/L, magnesium = 0.5 to 1.5 mEq/L, and potassium = 0). Because of technical difficulties with preparation and storage of bicarbonate-containing solution, peritoneal dialysis solutions contain lactate as a bicarbonate-generating agent. The usual concentration of lactate in the dialysis solution is 35 to 40 mEq/L. To avoid caramelization of sugar during the sterilization procedure, the pH of these solutions is brought down to 5.5.

TRAINING IN CONTINUOUS AMBULATORY PERITONEAL DIALYSIS

All patients receive CAPD training on an outpatient basis unless their medical condition requires hospitalization. **Patients suitable for training must be in good fluid balance and should not be suffering from uremic symptoms.** A primary care nurse is usually assigned to train and monitor patients. During training, patients receive intensive instruction on renal disease, skills required for maintenance of peritoneal dialysis, medications, and complications encountered through peritoneal dialysis with appropriate actions to take.

> The technique of CAPD should not be applied in a uniform manner to every patient but should be adjusted to the individual patient's abilities.

Some reliable patients may be taught the whole procedure—the bag, dressing, and tubing changes. Others are taught only part of it, such as the bag and dressing changes or even only the bag changes. In the latter case, the nurses change tubing in the hospital. Finally, in certain circumstances, as in blind or very old patients, the entire or part of the procedure should be taught to a family member who is willing to undertake this task.

The time that it takes to train a patient on peritoneal dialysis is variable and depends on many factors; it may range from 5 to 30 days, with an average of 7 days.

BIOCHEMICAL CONTROL AND FLUID BALANCE DURING CONTINUOUS AMBULATORY PERITONEAL DIALYSIS

Because CAPD is a continuous process, it does not produce the "pre-post" biochemical and hemodynamic changes characteristic of other forms of intermittent dialysis. With regard to clearance of various-sized molecules, CAPD is more effective than hemodialysis in removing middle-sized and large molecules. Peritoneal clearance increases with hypertonic solutions, not only because of the ultrafiltration volume, but also because of the solvent drag effect. Because of increased protein losses with this treatment (6 to 12 g/day), most patients on CAPD have hypoproteinemia, and some of them may be in negative nitrogen balance.

CAPD removes a significant amount of sodium (100 to 200 mEq/day), especially if hypertonic solutions are used. Similarly, CAPD achieves excellent control of serum potassium in most patients. **About 10% of patients on CAPD may develop hypokalemia and hence should receive oral potassium supplements.** Potassium should not be added to the bag because it would violate the sterile system. Also, addition of potassium does not raise the serum potassium substantially. **When hyperkalemia appears, as it may in about 5 to 10% of patients, potassium should be restricted and a potassium exchange resin given by mouth.**

During peritoneal dialysis, glucose is used as an osmotic agent to enhance ultrafiltration. Peak intraperitoneal volume is observed at about 2 hours after the infusion of solution. From then on, the intraperitoneal volume starts decreasing as a result of gradual dissipation of glucose-induced osmotic gradient and constant lymphatic reabsorption. Thus, four 4- to 8-hour exchanges a day during CAPD are not the most efficient way of inducing ultrafiltration. For clinical purposes, however, this scheme is practical and achieves adequate fluid balance. In patients with low ultrafiltration, reducing the dwell time to less than 2 hours allows for capture of peak ultrafiltration and achieves better fluid removal.

CHOICE AND ASSESSMENT OF A PERITONEAL DIALYSIS REGIMEN

Inadequate dialysis and ultrafiltration failure cause patients to drop out from CAPD. Although such problems are not frequent, it is important to understand their pathophysiology, which will help in the prescription of an appropriate dialysis regimen or help modify therapy. Adequately dialyzed patients feel well (absence of anorexia, nausea, emesis, dysgeusia, and insomnia), their blood pressure is well controlled, and they maintain a stable lean body mass. Their blood chemistry shows normal amounts of electrolytes, serum creatinine levels well below 15 mg/dl, and hematocrit above 25%. In order to provide adequate dialysis, total creatinine clearance (residual + peritoneal)/1.73 m^2 should be 4 to 5 ml/min (5.8 to 7.2 L/day; 40 to 50 L/week). To achieve such clearances, a patient on CAPD may need 8 to 12 L of dialysis solution per day, depending on the peritoneal membrane permeability. **Patients are said to generate adequate ultrafiltration when they are able to ultrafiltrate at least 5.5 ml of fluid per g of glucose absorbed (1500 ml of ultrafiltrate per 270 g of glucose), or 700 to 1000 ml of ultrafiltration with 2 L of 4.25% solution left in the peritoneal cavity for 4 hours.**

To assess optimum peritoneal dialysis clinically, the following peritoneal equilibration test (PET) has been designed. The steps of the standardized test are as follows:

1. Patients perform an overnight exchange, which should dwell for 8 to 12 hours.
2. Pretest exchange fluid is drained completely over 20 minutes in the sitting position.
3. Two liters of 2.5% dialysis solution are infused at a rate of 200 ml/min. Patients should be in supine position during infusion and for better solution mixing should roll over from side to side after each 400-ml infusion.
4. At the completion of infusion (0 dwell time), 200 ml of dialysis solution is drained into the bag and mixed well; a 10-ml sample is taken, and the remaining 190 ml is reinfused back.
5. Patients are ambulatory during the dwell time.
6. After 120 minutes of dwell time, another sample of dialysis solution is taken and a blood sample is drawn.*
7. After a 4-hour dwell time, the dialysis solution is drained out completely with patients in sitting position, total volume is measured, and a sample is taken.
8. Concentrations of creatinine and glucose are measured in the dialysis solution and blood samples. Because glucose interferes with the Jaffe reagent for creatinine, the creatinine value in the dialysis solution is overestimated. Our laboratory assumes that every 1 mg/dl of glucose overestimates creatinine concentration by 0.0005 mg/dl. Creatinine values are corrected before any calculations are made.
9. Dialysate-to-plasma ratios (D:P) of creatinine at 2 and 4 hours and simultaneous ratios of dialysate glucose to dialysis solution glucose at 0 dwell time ($D:D_0$) are calculated. Based on

*For clinical purposes steps 4 and 6 may be omitted.

more than 100 tests on patients on CAPD, we have categorized patients into low, low average, high average, and high peritoneal membrane transport (Fig. 17–4).

Interpretation of Peritoneal Equilibration Test Results

> The results of the peritoneal equilibration test can be used for prognostication and for diagnosis of CAPD complications.

Patients with high peritoneal membrane transport rates have poor ultrafiltration rates on standard CAPD (4- to 6-hour dwell) because of rapid glucose absorption from the peritoneal cavity into the blood. For the same reason, the solute transport is above average. These patients may have inadequate ultrafiltration despite using all hypertonic solutions during the 24 hours. Therefore, these patients will do well on daily NPD, in which short dwell exchanges are possible. Shortening the exchange time allows for capturing peak ultrafiltration and hence increases net ultrafiltration.

Patients with high average peritoneal membrane transport can achieve adequate dialysis with 8 L of infusion volumes and sufficient ultrafiltration with moderate dialysis solution glucose concentrations, even if they are anuric. These are the ideal patients for standard CAPD.

Most patients with low average transport rates can achieve adequate dialysis with standard CAPD (8-L volumes); however, some may require additional dialysis volume, particularly if they have a high body surface area. In general, these patients have very good ultrafiltration with moderate dialysis solution glucose concentrations.

Patients with low peritoneal membrane transport rates usually have very good ultrafiltration but are likely to develop symptoms of inadequate dialysis on standard CAPD, especially when their residual renal function is negligible.

The PET is frequently used for deciding the appropriate regimen of peritoneal dialysis for a given patient (Fig. 17–5). The following case summary illustrates an example of such a use:

CASE SUMMARY 2

A 70-year-old woman with ESRD of unknown cause was started on CAPD. A PET showed creatinine D:P ratio of 0.97 and glucose D:D_0 of 0.12. The patient was advised that she would experience fluid retention on standard CAPD and therefore should consider alternate therapy. However, at the patient's insistence, CAPD was started. During the first month of CAPD, she gained 14 kg of body weight, mainly as a result of fluid retention. Four 2-L 4.25% glucose dialysis solution exchange could not generate

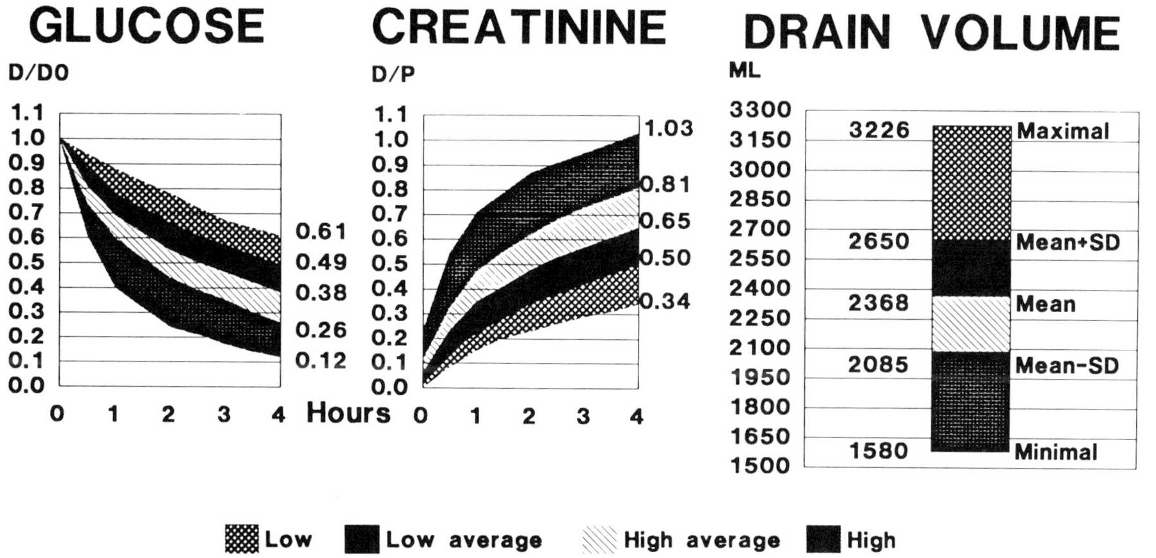

Figure 17–4. The equilibration test results in a study population. The area shaded in different patterns depicts results representing high, high average, average, low average, and low peritoneal transport rates. The bar graph depicts the drain volumes after 4-hour study in the same study population. Patients with high solute transport rates usually have low drain volumes and vice versa.

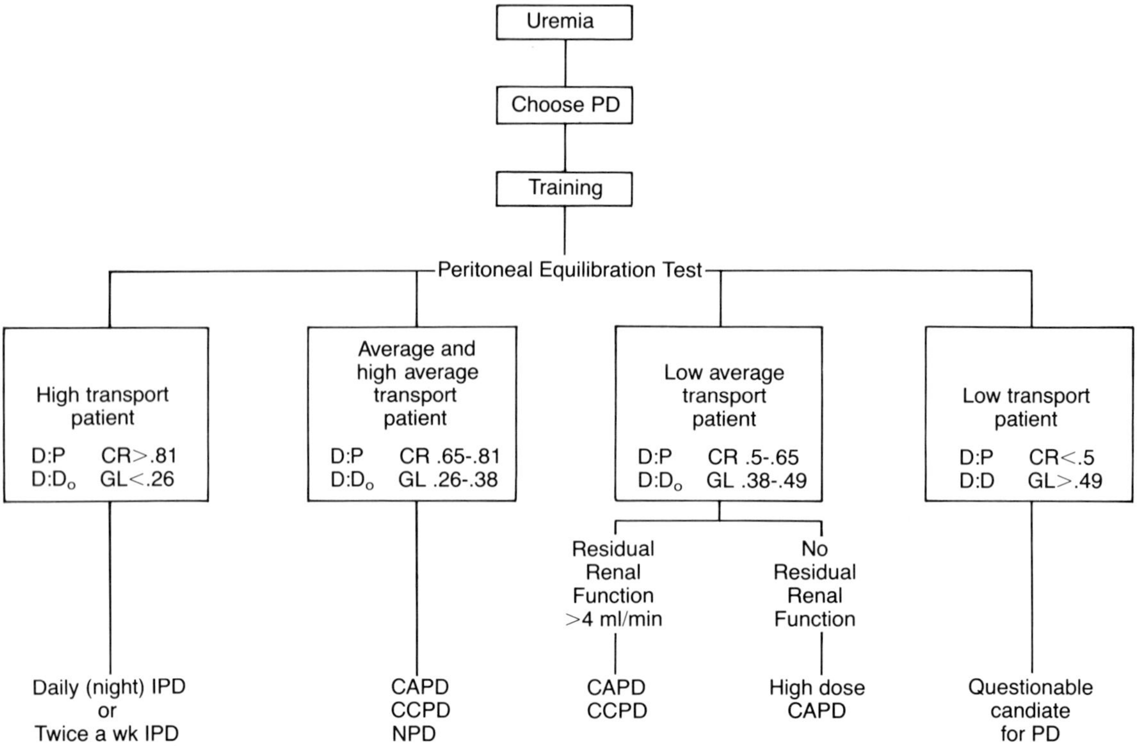

Figure 17–5. Decision-making algorithm for choosing an appropriate dialysis regimen based on the peritoneal equilibration test. (CAPD, continuous ambulatory peritoneal dialysis; CCPD, continuous cycling peritoneal dialysis; CR, creatinine; D:P, dialysate to plasma ratio; D:D$_O$, dialysate effluent glucose to dialysate glucose concentration at zero time; GL, glucose; IPD, intermittent peritoneal dialysis; NPD, nightly peritoneal dialysis.)

any net ultrafiltration. Catheter function was good. Investigations revealed no signs of dialysis solution leakage. The patient was transferred to every-night IPD, with four 2-L exchanges over 8 hours. Ultrafiltration during a session was about 1200 ml. Within 2 weeks of NPD, the patient achieved dry body weight. Dialysis creatinine clearance and serum chemistries were adequate.

The PET can also be used for diagnostic purposes, as shown in Figures 17–6 and 17–7. The following case summary illustrates the use of the PET for diagnosis:

CASE SUMMARY 3

A 35-year-old anuric woman with membranous glomerulonephritis was maintained on standard CAPD. The initial PET showed creatinine D:P ratio of 0.71 and glucose D:D$_0$ of 0.46. Seven months later, she reported weight gain and low dialysis solution drainage volumes. Clinical examination revealed good catheter function and no external evidence of dialysis solution leak. Repeat PET revealed unchanged D:P creatinine and D:D$_0$ ratios. The results indicated loss of dialysis solution from the peritoneal cavity. Computed tomographic scan of the abdomen revealed posterior retroperitoneal space dialysis solution leakage, which was surgically repaired and resolved the problem.

COMPLICATIONS OF PERITONEAL DIALYSIS

The complications observed during peritoneal dialysis are due to one of the following four causes: (1) catheter malfunction, (2) raised intraabdominal pressure by the continuous presence of dialysis solution in the peritoneal cavity, (3) peritoneal response to unphysiologic solution in the peritoneal cavity and contamination, and (4) systemic metabolic complications. Table 17–6 presents a comprehensive list of problems encountered during CAPD. Catheter-related complications are discussed under Peritoneal Access. Management of exit site infection is shown in Figure 17–8.

The continuous presence of dialysis solution in the peritoneal space increases intraabdominal pressure, which worsens with activity such as

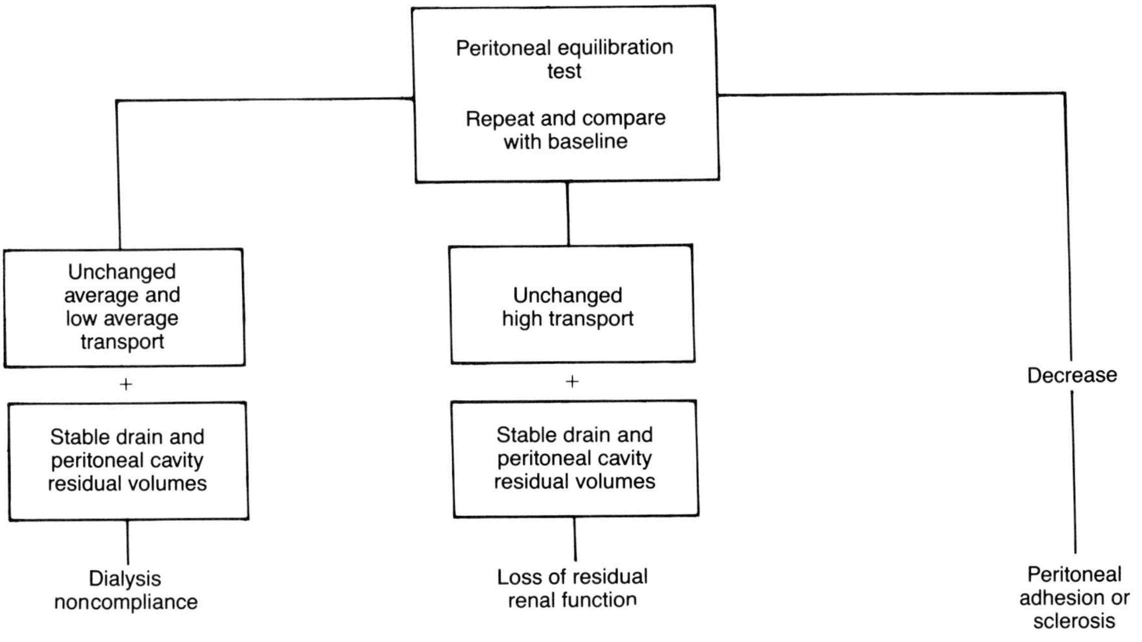

Figure 17–6. Diagnostic use of the peritoneal equilibration test when inadequate dialysis is observed in a patient on CAPD.

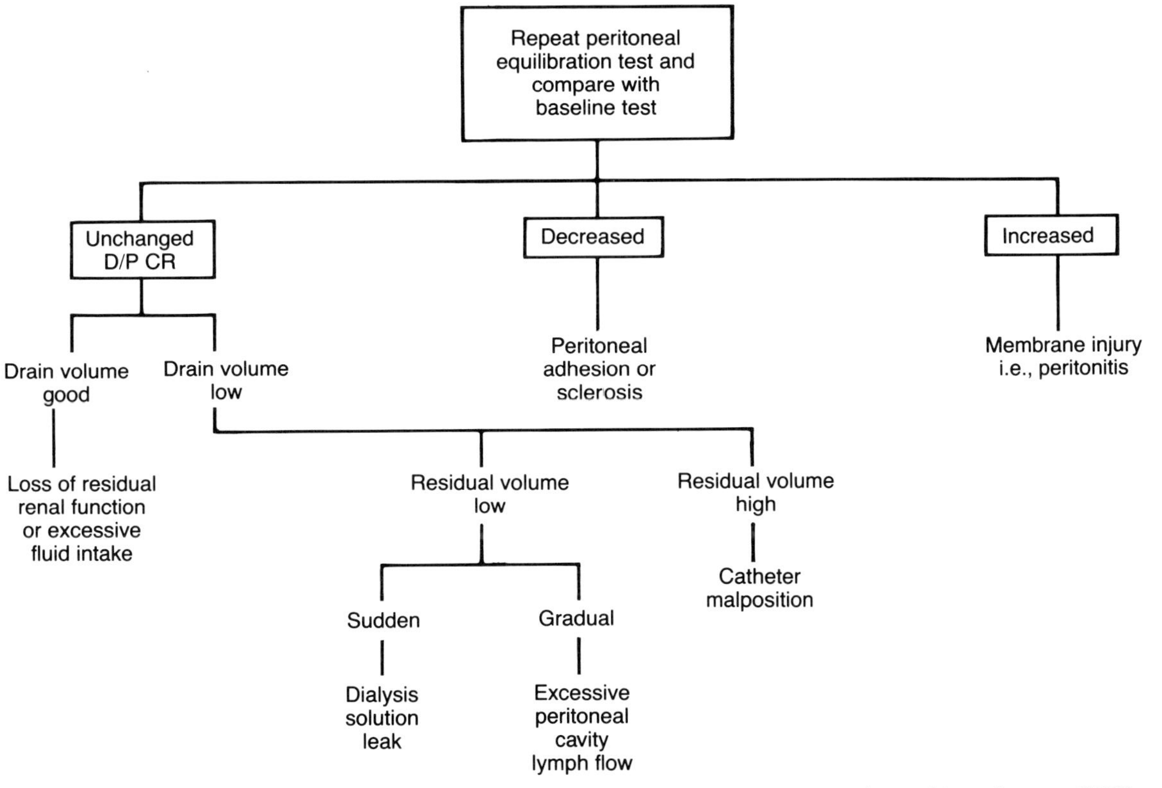

Figure 17–7. Diagnostic use of the peritoneal equilibration test when fluid retention is observed in patients on CAPD.

Table 17–6. FREQUENTLY OBSERVED COMPLICATIONS DURING PERITONEAL DIALYSIS

Causes	Complications
Catheter related	Exit site infection Tunnel infection Peritonitis Pericatheter leakage Poor drainage External cuff extrusion
Raised intraabdominal pressure	CAPD/CCPD: Exacerbation of hernia, hemorrhoids Dialysis solution leakage Pleuroperitoneal communication
Unphysiologic solution and contamination	All types of peritonitis
Metabolic	Obesity and lipid disorders Carbohydrate intolerance Protein depletion

in the peritoneal space increases intraabdominal pressure, which worsens with activity such as walking and jogging. Coughing and straining generate the highest intraabdominal pressure. Elevation of intraabdominal pressure predisposes to abdominal hernias (incisional, inguinal, diaphragmatic, or umbilical). Older patients with or without previous surgical scars are prone to develop these complications. Women may develop a rectocele or a cystocele, with or without uterine prolapse. Persistently raised intraabdominal pressure may also aggravate the symptoms of hiatus hernia and hemorrhoids.

In patients with vertebral disease, the exaggerated lordosis adopted while holding dialysate in the abdomen tends to aggravate the pain and other symptoms. In such a situation, CAPD may have to be discontinued.

A rare but serious complication is transdiaphragmatic dialysate leakage into the pleural cavity. High-glucose and low-protein concentrations in the pleural fluid is diagnostic. To explain this complication, some have blamed enhanced movement of peritoneal fluid to the pleural space via the diaphragmatic lymphatics. In addition, there probably is a preexisting structural defect in the diaphragm. In the presence of massive effusion, peritoneal dialysis has to be discontinued. Such patients who wish to remain on CAPD may be offered pleurodesis with talc or tetracycline, but this may be a painful procedure. Less painful pleurodesis can be achieved with intraperitoneal infusion of a fibrin glue or the patient's own blood (20 to 40 ml).

Peritonitis

Peritonitis is the most frequent complication during CAPD. Peritonitis during CAPD is quite different from surgical peritonitis. Experience during the years has defined several separate subgroups of peritonitis. The incidence of peritonitis has improved from one episode every 12 months to approximately one episode every 16 to 24 patient months as a result of the improved connector technology.

Most episodes of peritonitis in patients on CAPD (about 70%) are due to indigenous skin flora (*i.e.*, *Staphylococcus epidermidis* and *Staphylococcus aureus*). Peritonitis with *S. epidermidis* is usually mild and has a favorable prognosis. In contrast, peritonitis due to *S. aureus* has a much more severe and prolonged course, with a tendency for abscess formation. *Streptococcus viridans* causes severe peritonitis with marked constitutional symptoms, but it can be controlled with antibiotics and has a favorable prognosis.

A smaller fraction of peritonitis episodes (20%) are caused by gram-negative organisms, some of which originate from the bowel. Bowel origin of the organism may be indicated by the presence of two or more species of gram-negative organisms during an episode of peritonitis or the presence of *Bacteroides*. Peritonitis due to unusual organisms such as mycobacteria is rare but has been reported. True culture-negative (aseptic) peritonitis, which also is uncommon (2%), may be due to chemicals, plasticizer, endotoxin, and coincidental administration of antibiotics. However, in the presence of inadequate laboratory facilities, a higher percentage of peritonitis (10 to 20%) may be culture negative. Eosinophilic peritonitis is an asymptomatic, culture-negative condition of unknown cause; it is associated with a cloudy dialysate consisting mainly of eosinophils. It usually occurs in the beginning of CAPD and disappears after 1 to 3 months without any specific treatment.

There are many routes through which organisms may gain entry into the peritoneum and cause peritonitis (Table 17–7).

Diagnosis of Peritonitis

In order to make a clinical diagnosis of peritonitis, two of the following three criteria in any combination are required:

1. Signs and symptoms of peritoneal inflammation, such as sudden onset of abdominal pain and rebound tenderness.

2. Cloudy dialysis effluent containing predominantly polymorphonuclear cells. The total cell count in an uninfected dialysis solution drained from a patient on CAPD is usually less than 50 cells/mm^3. The majority of these cells are macrophages and monocytes. In patients on IPD, the fluid removed at the initiation of dialysis (ascites) usually has higher cell counts (up to 1000 cells/mm^3) than a CAPD patient's fluid.

3. Isolation of organisms either on Gram stain or culture from the drained dialysis solution.

Because it is unusual to find bacteremia during CAPD-associated peritonitis, positive blood cultures during an episode of peritonitis are uncommon. Most peritonitis episodes are mild and can be treated at home. Hypotension is a sign of serious peritonitis and requires aggressive management. The incubation period for bacterial peritonitis is usually 24 to 48 hours from the time of contamination. The symptoms and signs subside very quickly after the therapy is begun. **Slow abatement or nonresolution of peritonitis after the therapy is begun usually indicates either an inappropriate choice of antibiotic, or peritonitis due to a focus of infection in the vicinity such as exit site or tunnel infection.**

Management of Peritonitis

The Peritonitis Management Advisory Committee[4] recommendations for the management of peritonitis are depicted in Figure 17–8.

Establishing a Diagnosis

In order to establish an accurate diagnosis, a large volume of cloudy dialysis solution should

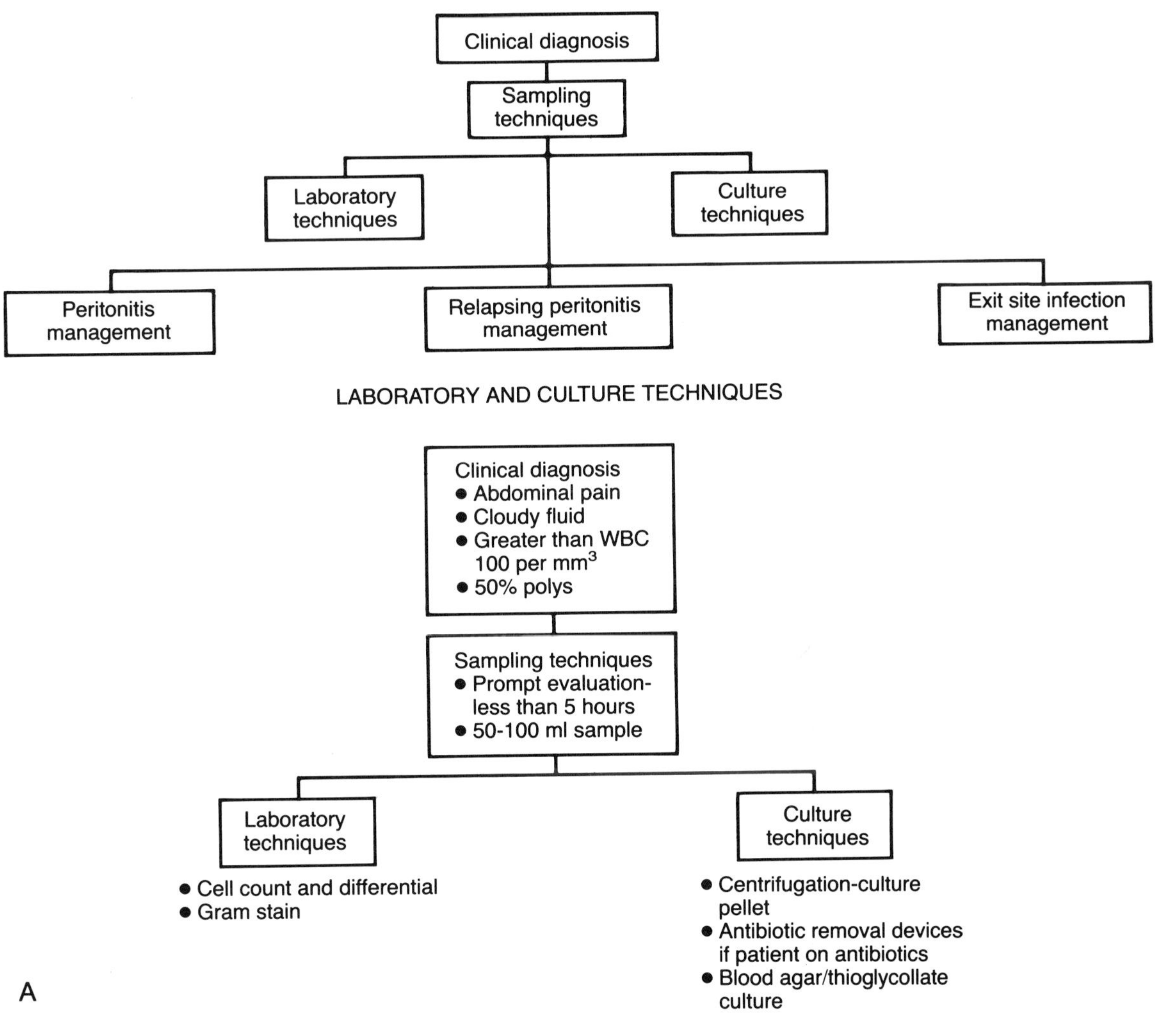

Figure 17–8. Peritonitis management decision algorithm. (*A*) Overview of areas covered.

Illustration continued on following page

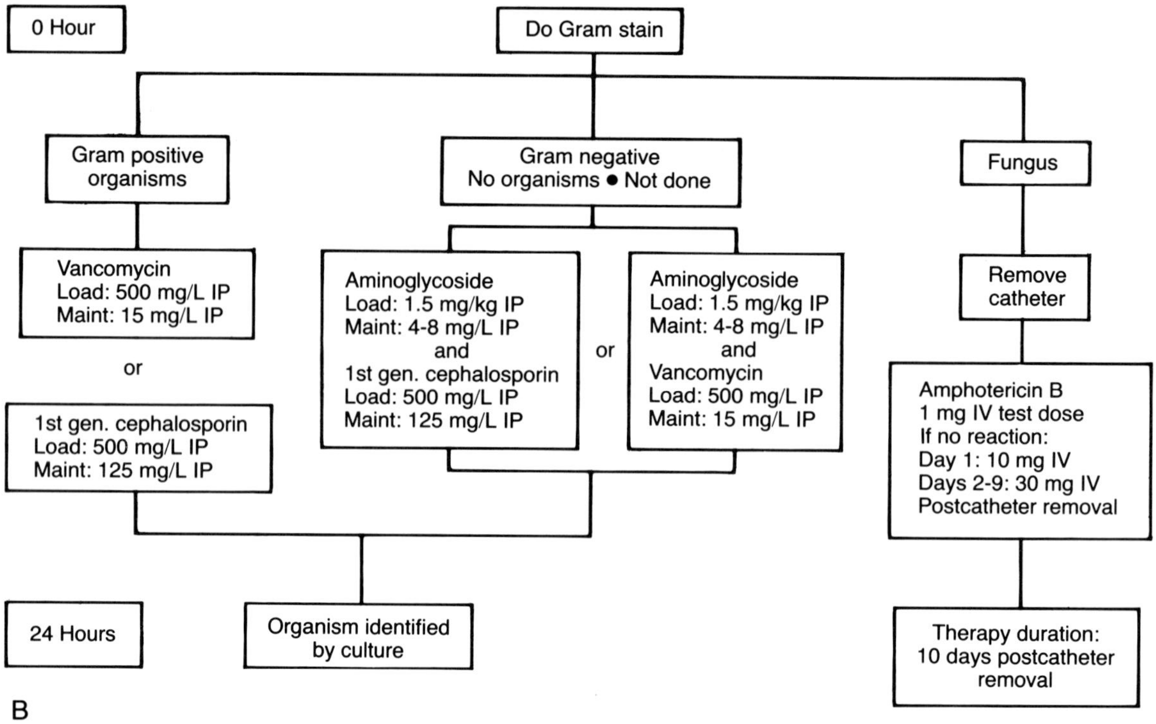

B

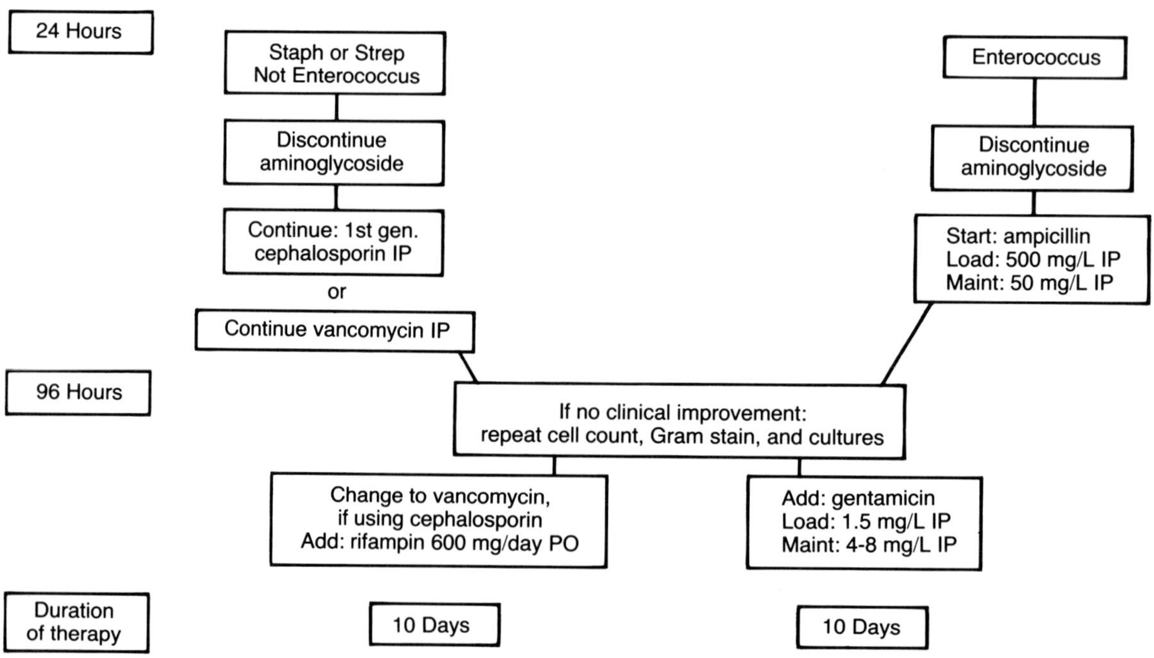

C

Figure 17–8 Peritonitis management decision algorithm *Continued* (*B*) On clinical presentation of peritonitis. (*C*) Gram-positive organism on culture.

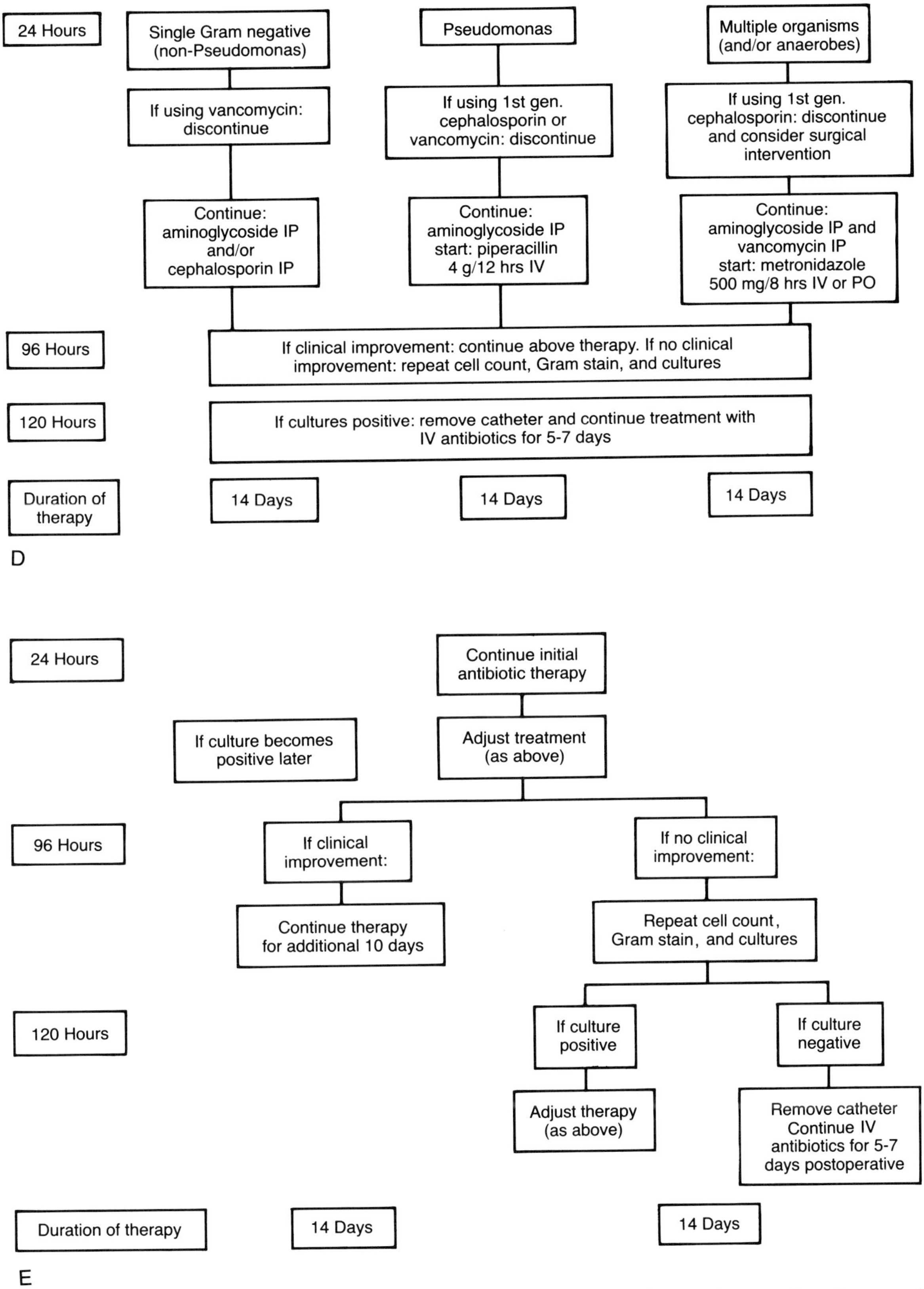

Figure 17–8 Peritonitis management decision algorithm *Continued* (*D*) Gram-negative organism on culture. (In cases of rare gram-negative organisms, therapy should be guided by antibiotic sensitivity patterns.) (*E*) Culture negative.

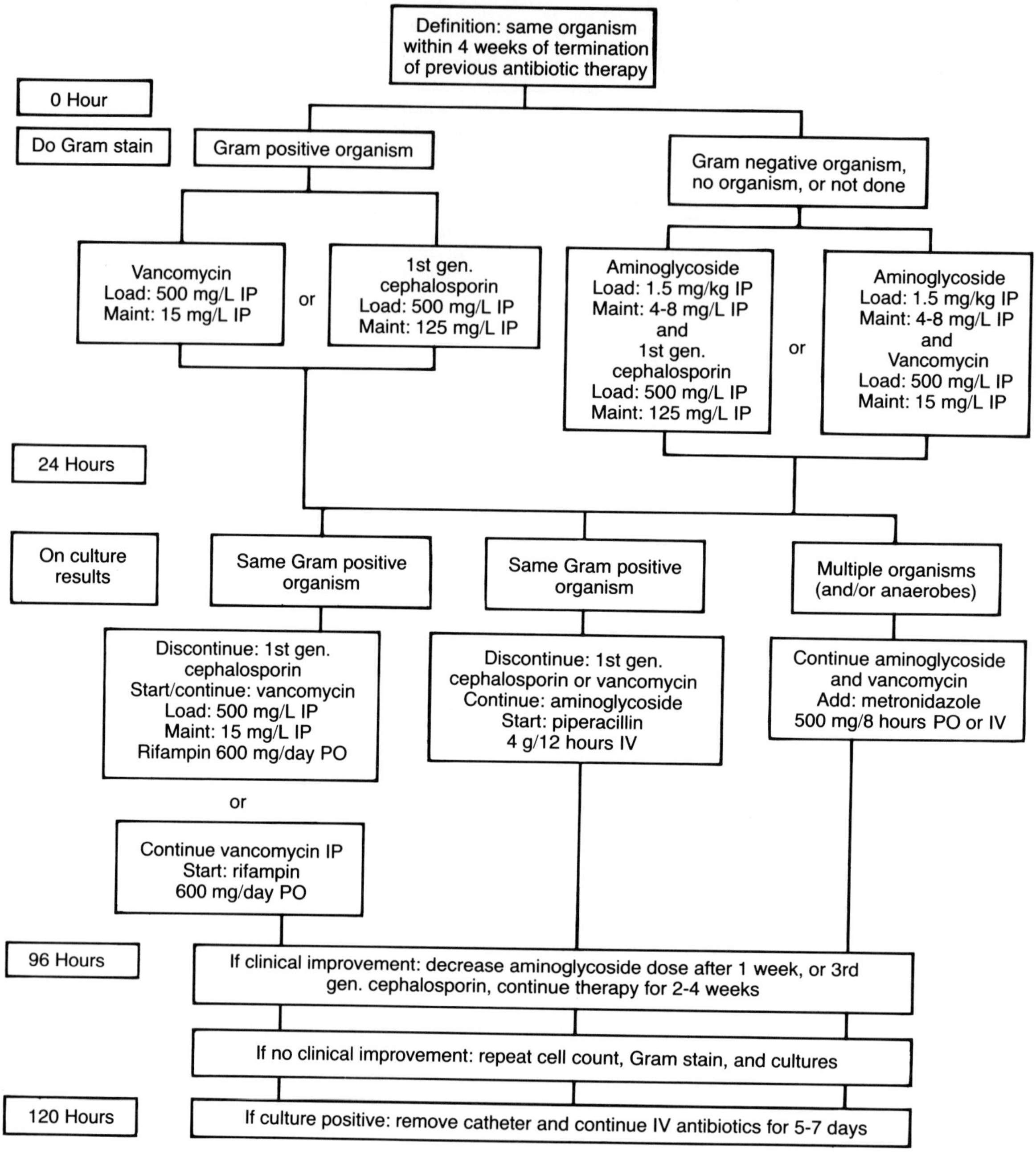

F

Figure 17–8 Peritonitis management decision algorithm *Continued* (*F*) Relapsing peritonitis. (From Keane WF, Everett ED, Fine RN, et al: CAPD related peritonitis management and antibiotic therapy recommendations: Travenol Peritonitis Management Advisory Committee. Peritoneal Dialysis Bulletin 7:55, 1987.)

be sent for both Gram stain and culture as early as possible. Gram stain from the sediment of cloudy dialysis solution identifies microorganisms in only 20 to 30% of cases. Most culture methods currently use a filtration or centrifugation method. Standard culture methods have to be modified by filtration or centrifugation to remove antibiotics from the solution if a patient is being treated with an antibiotic at the time of collection of the dialysis solution.

Early Treatment

Once the diagnosis of peritonitis is suspected and the previously mentioned diagnostic work is completed, the following steps of treatment

Table 17–7. PORTALS OF ENTRY OF INFECTIOUS ORGANISMS INTO THE PERITONEAL CAVITY

Route	Organism
Transluminal	Skin flora: *Staphylococcus epidermidis* *Staphylococcus aureus*
Periluminal	Skin flora Pathogens of exit site
Transmural	Enteric organisms Anaerobes
Hematogenous	*Streptococcus* *Mycoplasma tuberculosis*
Endogenous (per vaginam, intrauterine device, or other source)	Yeast Lactobacillus

are initiated either at home by a patient or in the hospital by a dialysis nurse.

Three exchanges (preferably using 1.5% dextrose dialysis solution) are carried out in succession as rapidly as possible, without the addition of antibiotics or insulin in the case of diabetic patients. These rapid exchanges allow for washout of mediators of inflammations from the peritoneal cavity and rapid relief of peritoneal pain.

The connection tube should be changed within the first 24 hours after the onset, although there is no strong evidence to support such a step.

Fresh dialysis solution is medicated with an aminoglycoside (tobramycin, 1.7 mg/kg body weight), a cephalosporin (cephalothin or cephazolin, 1 g/2-L solution), and heparin (1000 units/2 L) and infused into the peritoneal cavity and allowed to remain for 6 hours. Alternatively, a loading dose of antibiotics may be given intravenously. A gram of intravenous vancomycin infused slowly is an equally effective alternative to cephalosporin. The initial choice of antibiotics is made to cover for a wide spectrum of microbials.

CAPD exchanges are continued as dictated for control of uremia and fluid balance. Each subsequent bag of 2-L dialysis solution for exchanges contains 16 mg of tobramycin, 200 to 500 mg of a cephalosporin, and 1000 units of heparin. Tobramycin and cephalosporin should not be mixed in the same syringe but can be mixed safely in the same dialysate bag.

This regimen is continued until the results of culture and antibiotic sensitivity are available. Appropriate changes in the antibiotics are then made if necessary. In the case of a gram-positive organism peritonitis, it is not necessary to continue with the administration of the aminoglycoside. The half-lives and the loading and maintenance doses of different antibiotics are listed in Table 17–8. Alternative antibiotic dosing guidelines for the treatment of CAPD peritonitis are listed in Table 17–9.

The resolution of peritonitis is monitored clinically and by serial effluent white blood cell counts.

If the peritonitis is resolving, antibiotics are empirically discontinued 7 to 10 days after the start of therapy.

This protocol is modified for fungal, tuberculous, "surgical," or multiple-organism peritonitis or peritonitis following tunnel abscess or severe exit site infection. In most of these special situations, treatment includes removal of the peritoneal catheter, systemic administration of the appropriate antibacterial or antifungal agents, and drainage of the abscess, if present.

An exit site management algorithm is shown in Figure 17–9.

Peritonitis during IPD and CCPD is treated with loading doses of intravenous antibiotics. Additionally, during the dialysis exchanges, maintenance antibiotics and heparin in the dosage recommended for CAPD patients are added to the dialysis solution. Resolution of peritonitis is monitored with predialysis cell counts. For IPD patients between the days of dialysis, antibiotics (other than aminoglycosides) are administered either intravenously or orally. Patients on CCPD receive intraperitoneal antibiotics in every exchange including the long-dwell daytime exchanges.

Recurrent peritonitis not responding to appropriate antibiotics is treated with catheter removal. In such cases, a new catheter is usually inserted after 10 to 15 days. In the interim, these patients are maintained on hemodialysis using a subclavian access.

Absorption of antibiotics from the dialysis solution to the serum is good and rapid. Therefore, in most cases it is not necessary to give the antibiotics intravenously. The outcome of peritonitis treatment with intraperitoneal or intravenous antibiotics is comparable; therefore, the choice of one method versus another should be tailored to the facilities available in a given center.

During peritonitis, probably because of the inflammation, peritoneal clearances of large and small molecules increase and glucose absorption also increases. As a result, **patients may develop hypophosphatemia, hypokalemia, and hypoproteinemia and also have difficulties with ultrafiltration.** If peritonitis leads to extensive adhesions, as can occur after fecal, *Pseudomonas*, or *S. aureus* peritonitis, the peritoneum

Table 17–8. ANTIBIOTIC DOSING GUIDELINES FOR THE TREATMENT OF CAPD PERITONITIS

	Half-Life (hr)			**Dose***			
				Initial		***Maintenance***	
Antibiotic	***Normal***	***ESRD***	***CAPD***	***mg/kg***	***mg/2-L Bag***	***mg/L***	***mg/2-L bag***
Aminoglycosides							
Amikacin	1.6	39	ND	5–7.5	350–500	6–7.5	12–15
Gentamicin	2.2	53	32	1.5–1.7	120	4–6	8–12
Netilmicin	2.1	42	ND	1.5–2	140	4–6	8–12
Tobramycin	2.5	58	36	1.5–1.7	120	4–6	9–12
Cephalosporins							
Cefamandole	1	10	8	—	1000	ND	ND
Cefazolin	2.2	28	27	—	500–1000	125–250	250–500
Cefoperazone	1.8	2.3	2.2	—	2000	500	1000
Cefotaxime	0.9	2.5	2.4	—	2000	250	500
Cefoxitin	0.8	20	15	—	1000	100	200
Ceftazidime	1.8	26	16	—	1000	125	250
Ceftizoxime	1.6	28	11	—	1000	125	250
Ceftriaxone	8	15	13	—	1000	ND	ND
Cefuroxime	1.3	18	15	—	1500	250	500
Cephalothin	0.2	3.7	ND	—	2000	250	500
Moxalactam	2.2	20	16	—	1000	ND	ND
Cephradine	0.9	12	ND	—	500	125–250	250–500
					1000 PO	NA	NA
Cephalexin	0.8	19	9	—	1000 PO	NA	NA
Penicillins							
Ampicillin	1.3	15	ND	—	500	50	100
Azlocillin	0.9	5.1	ND	—	500	250	500
Mezlocillin	1	4.3	ND	—	3000 IV	3000/12 hr IV	ND
Piperacillin	1.2	3.9	ND	—	4000 IV	4000/12 hr IV	ND
Ticarcillin	1.2	15	ND	—	2000 IV	2000/12 hr IV	ND
Vancomycin and others							
Vancomycin	6.9	161	83	—	1000	15	30
Aztreonam	2	7	7.1	—	1000	250	500
Ciprofloxacin	4	8	13	—	750 PO	ND	ND
Clindamycin	2.8	2.8	ND	—	300	150	300
Erythromycin	2.1	4	ND	—	300	75	150
Metronidazole	7.9	7.7	11	—	500 PO/IV	ND	ND
Rifampin	4	8	ND	—	600 PO	NA	NA
Sulfamethoxazole	10	13	14	—	1600 PO	100–200	200–400
Trimethoprim	14	33	34	—	320 PO	20–40	40–80
Antifungal							
Amphotericin	360	360	ND	—	0.5	0.5	1
Flucytosine	4.2	115	ND	—	3000 PO	NA	NA
					200	50–100	100–200
Ketoconazole	2	1.8	2.4	—	400 PO	NA	NA
Miconazole	24	25	ND	—	100	50	100

*All doses are calculated for a 70-kg person who is using standard 2-L bags.

The route of administration is intraperitoneal unless otherwise specified.

These data should only be used as initial guidelines. Individualized dosing is recommended when possible.

The pharmacokinetic data and dosing recommendations presented here are based on published literature reviewed through January 1987 and personal experience. Those dosage recommendations that differ from product labeling are based on more recent experience.

There is no evidence that mixing different antibiotics in dialysis fluid (except for aminoglycosides and penicillins) is deleterious for the drugs or patients.

Do not use the same syringe to mix antibiotics.

CAPD, continuous ambulatory peritoneal dialysis; ESRD, creatinine clearance @ 10 mg/min, patient not on dialysis; NA, not applicable; ND, no data; IV, intravenous; PO, oral.

(From Keane WF, Everett ED, Fine RN, et al: CAPD related peritonitis management and antibody therapy recommendations: Travenol Peritonitis Management Advisory Committee. Peritoneal Dialysis Bulletin 7:55, 1987.)

Table 17–9. ALTERNATIVE ANTIBIOTIC DOSING FOR THE TREATMENT OF CAPD PERITONITIS

	Dose*		
	Initial		Maintenance
	mg/kg	*mg/2-L bag*	*mg/2-L Bag/ Dosing Interval*
Aminoglycosides			
Amikacin	5–7.5	350–500	140/24 hr
Gentamicin	1.5–1.7	120	40–60/24 hr
Netilmicin	1.5–2	140	50–70/24 hr
Tobramycin	1.5–1.7	120	40–60/24 hr
Cephalosporins			
Cefamandole	—	1000	1000/24 hr
Cefazolin	—	500–1000	ND
Cefoperazone	—	2000	2000/12 hr
Cefotaxime	—	2000	2000/12 hr
Cefoxitin	—	1000	1000/24 hr
Ceftazidime	—	1000	1000/24 hr
Ceftizoxime	—	1000	1000/24 hr
Ceftriaxone	—	1000	1000/24 hr
Cefuroxime	—	1500	ND
Cephalothin	—	2000	NA
Moxalactam	—	1000	1000/24 hr
Cephradine	—	500	ND
		1000 PO	500/6 hr PO
Cephalexin	—	1000 PO	500/6 hr PO
Penicillins			
Ampicillin	—	500	ND
Azlocillin	—	500	ND
Mezlocillin	—	3000 IV	3000/12 hr IV
Piperacillin	—	4000 IV	4000/12 hr IV
Ticarcillin	—	2000 IV	2000/12 hr IV
Vancomycin and others			
Vancomycin	—	1000	1000/5–7 days
Aztreonam	—	1000	ND
Ciprofloxacin	—	750 PO	750/12 hr PO
Clindamycin	—	300	ND
Erythromycin	—	300	ND
Metronidazole	—	500 PO/IV	500/8 hr PO
Rifampin	—	600 PO	600/24 hr PO
Sulfamethoxazole	—	1600 PO	1600/24 hr PO
Trimethoprim	—	320 PO	320/24 hr PO
Antifungal			
Amphotericin	—	0.5	1–3/12 hr
Flucytosine	—	3000 PO	1000/24 hr PO
		200	400/24 hr
Ketoconazole	—	400 PO	400/24 hr PO
Miconazole	—	100	ND

*Because serum levels of potentially oto- and vestibular toxicity antibiotics are relatively constant when administered in each exchange, alternative dosing approaches are being developed. One such approach uses a longer dosing interval, thereby allowing peak and trough serum levels to be achieved. In this table, after the initial loading is administered intraperitoneally, the amount of antibiotic given and the time interval for maintenance dose is presented. Clinical experience with this approach is limited. All doses are calculated for a 70-kg adult who is using standard 2-L bags. The route of administration is intraperitoneal unless otherwise specified. These data should only be used as initial guidelines. Individualized dosing is recommended when possible.

The pharmacokinetic data and dosing recommendations presented here are based on published literature reviewed through January 1987 and personal experience CAPD, continuous ambulatory peritoneal dialysis; NA, not applicable; ND, no data; IV, intravenous, PO, oral.

(From Keane WF, Everett ED, Fine RN, et al: CAPD related peritonitis management and antibody therapy recommendations: Travenol Peritonitis Management Advisory Committee. Peritoneal Dialysis Bulletin 7:55, 1987.)

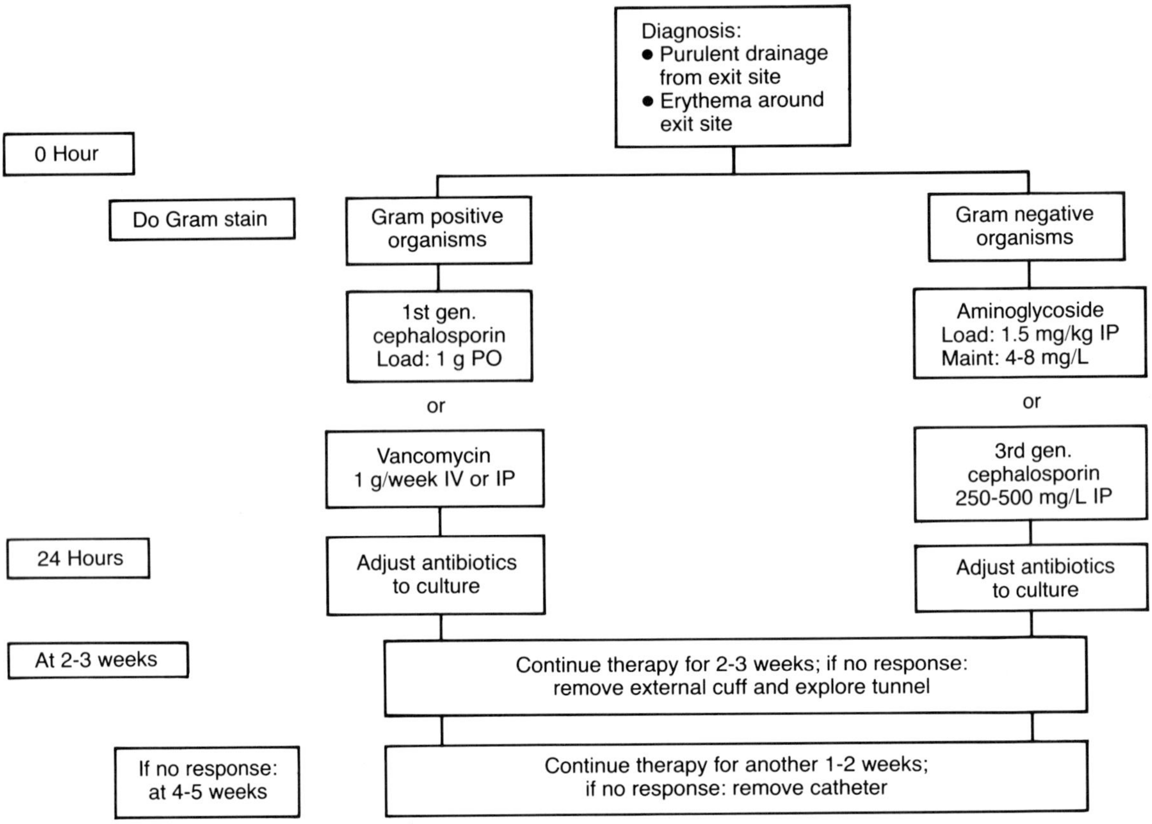

Figure 17–9. Exit site management algorithm. The recommended antibiotic therapy is over and above the local exit site care, which is an important part of its management. (From Keane WF, Everett ED, Fine RN, et al: CAPD related peritonitis management and antibiotic therapy recommendations: Travenol Peritonitis Management Advisory Committee. Peritoneal Dialysis Bulletin 7:55, 1987.)

may lose its capacity for ultrafiltration and peritoneal dialysis may have to be abandoned.

Antibiotic prophylaxis for peritonitis is not recommended because it favors the emergence of resistant organisms. For patients severely ill with peritonitis, hospitalization is indicated. A course of oral or intravenous rifampin is indicated for patients with persistent or recurrent *S. aureus* infection. In these patients, defective intracellular bactericidal properties of peritoneal macrophages allow persistence of viable organisms inside the cells. Rifampin penetrates these cells and eradicates the bacteria.

Accidental contaminations are treated with tube change followed by either a course of cephalosporin or a single intravenous injection of a gram of vancomycin.

After treatment of peritonitis and before the patient goes home, a CAPD nurse should review the patient's technique in an attempt to determine whether errors in techniques have contributed to the peritonitis.

Complications

Fibrous adhesions with the loss of dialyzing surface area occur frequently as a sequela of severe peritonitis resulting from bowel perforation, *S. aureus*, and *Pseudomonas* infection. It is unclear at this time if severe recurrent peritonitis could lead to sclerosing peritonitis.

Encapsulating or sclerosing peritonitis (*i.e.*,the formation of a dense layer of fibroconnective tissue on the membrane) may appear during or several months or years after cessation of either IPD or CAPD. The disease progresses slowly and may remain asymptomatic for a long time; however, rapid progression also has been described. Presenting symptoms may include loss of ultrafiltration capacity (with rapid glucose absorption initially and with slow glucose absorption later), recurrent abdominal pain, intermittent vomiting, and eventually partial or complete small bowel obstruction. Peritoneal clearances of solutes usually remain at an acceptable level but may decrease in the later stages. Such sclerosis is a serious complication with a high incidence of fatal outcomes. Most deaths result from severe malnutrition, sepsis, and bowel-related surgical complications.

The cause of encapsulating peritonitis is unknown. Afflicted persons have a higher frequency of certain risk factors—namely, recurrent severe peritonitis treated with numerous antibiotics, use of acetate-containing solution, increased use of hypertonic solutions because of loss of ultrafiltration capacity, use of chlorhexidine antiseptic solutions, and use of beta-blockers. It is noteworthy that this complication is extremely rare in those who have used only lactate-containing dialysis solutions manufactured in North America. Because we lack a proper understanding of this disease process, no definitive strategy has evolved to prevent it.

Systemic metabolic complications during CAPD are a result of either the use of glucose in the dialysis solution or the continuous loss of nutrient in the drained dialysis solution. In patients on CAPD, daily glucose absorption of 100 to 200 g may cause lipid derangement. Serum triglyceride levels increase in most of these patients, but hypertriglyceridemia develops only in those who are hypertriglyceridemic at initiation of therapy and are exposed to drugs known to produce hypertriglyceridemia, such as androgens or beta-blockers. High-density lipoprotein (HDL) cholesterol level is low in these patients. Diabetic patients develop hypertriglyceridemia but not at the same rate as nondiabetic persons.

During CAPD, daily losses of protein range between 6 and 12 g and of amino acids between 1 and 2 g. Therefore, in patients on CAPD, most of the essential and nonessential amino acids in the plasma are lower than normal. With daily dietary protein intake of 1 g/kg body weight or more, the serum protein and albumin levels are maintained in the low normal range. Vitamin B complex, vitamin C, and folic acid are lost during CAPD, and the blood levels of these compounds are therefore low if not supplemented in the diet. Patients on CAPD should receive supplements of these vitamins. Also, blood levels of vitamin A, retinol-binding protein, and vitamin E are high.

Uremic Complications During Continuous Ambulatory Peritoneal Dialysis

Anemia during CAPD is less severe than in hemodialysis, probably because patients on CAPD do not lose blood. Transfusion requirements of patients on CAPD are lower than for those on chronic hemodialysis. During CAPD, improvement in anemia is striking, and in some patients the hemoglobin may reach normal or even above-normal levels. The mechanism of this improvement is unknown, but it may represent removal of toxic substances that have suppressed the bone marrow's response to erythropoietin.

Hypertension is common in patients starting dialysis, and it can usually be controlled by reducing total body sodium and by ultrafiltration. On IPD, predialysis blood pressure can be controlled if one can maintain the patient close to dry weight at all times. The control of hypertension with CAPD is excellent. Most patients, even those suffering from malignant hypertension, become normotensive within 1 to 2 months of starting CAPD, and many, especially the elderly, may become hypotensive. (Interestingly, the blood pressure returns to normal at a time when body weight is increasing, probably as a results of sodium depletion on CAPD.) If a patient becomes hypotensive, administration of sodium by mouth while simultaneously keeping the body weight normal by dialysis usually returns the blood pressure to normal.

CAPD removes some parathyroid hormone fraction (iPTH), but does not reduce the plasma levels of parathyroid hormone. The iPTH decreases only when its secretion is suppressed by an increase in serum calcium. Osteitis fibrosa persists despite treatment with $1,25(OH)_2D_3$. If a physician wishes to decrease the serum iPTH and stimulate healing of the osteitis fibrosa, the serum calcium must be maintained at slightly hypercalcemic levels (10.5 to 11 mg/dl) at the cost of risking kidney stone formation or other soft tissue calcifications. By itself, CAPD does not maintain the serum phosphate at a normal level, and these patients require small amounts of phosphate binders. In the past few years, it has become clear that long-term use of aluminum-containing phosphate binders may cause significant aluminum accumulation in the body, leading to aluminum toxicity (aluminum-induced osteomalacia or dialysis dementia). To avoid such problems, it is recommended that calcium carbonate be used as a phosphate binder. It is very important that patients take calcium with the meal; otherwise, calcium binding may be minimal, but hypercalcemia may occur more frequently. When serum phosphorus level is 6 ml/dl or more, one must avoid using vitamin D or its metabolites to minimize soft-tissue calcification.

Nerve conduction velocities do not decrease in patients undergoing either hemodialysis or peritoneal dialysis, except in those who are underdialyzed or severely malnourished. Studies in patients on CAPD for periods up to 2 years show no deterioration in nerve conduction velocities. However, there is no improvement either.

The frequency of pericarditis in patients who have chronic renal failure and are undergoing any form of dialysis has ranged from 15 to 20%. Clinically, pericarditis presents with chest pain, a pericardial friction rub, low-grade fever, and mild leukocytosis. Tamponade can be controlled by needle pericardiocentesis, but if it is recurrent, one proceeds to surgical pericardiectomy or the formation of a pericardial window and communication with the pleural cavity. **Pericarditis without tamponade generally responds to conservative management—namely, increased dialysis, salt restriction, and strict control of fluid intake.** The incidence of pericarditis on CAPD is extremely low. When pericarditis does occur, it is usually due to underdialysis by a noncompliant patient.

Reduced perfusion as a result of hypotension, which is not uncommon during CAPD, can provoke ischemic complications in patients with generalized atherosclerosis. Such patients may require corrective or palliative surgery to relieve their symptoms. These patients are noted to have a large number of cardiovascular and cerebrovascular problems, such as recurrent angina, arrhythmias, acute myocardial infarction, transient ischemic attacks, and complete strokes, but no one has yet defined the contribution of CAPD to their pathogenesis or progression.

Some researchers have suggested that the increased incidence of cardiovascular and cerebrovascular complications in dialysis patients is due to accelerated atherosclerosis associated with hypertriglyceridemia and low levels of HDL fractions. However, many patients beginning CAPD are older and hence have complications in the heart and brain; even so, it is possible that CAPD may accelerate these complications. However, a short (6-month) preliminary study of a small number of patients carried out in our center showed that CAPD does not have an aggravating influence on atherogenic factors related to lipoprotein—namely, decreased HDL cholesterol and elevated low-density lipoprotein cholesterol levels. In fact, some patients had increased concentrations of HDL cholesterol.

Patients on CAPD have frequent episodes of herpes zoster and candidal infections, suggesting that they may have a significant degree of immunosuppression.

PERITONEAL DIALYSIS IN DIABETICS WITH END-STAGE DISEASE

Diabetic patients approaching dialysis suffer from numerous complications such as peripheral vascular disease, autonomic neuropathy, hypertension, cardiovascular disease, and visual disturbances. **In caring for such a complicated patient, peritoneal dialysis offers the potential advantage of reduced cardiovascular stress, a steady biochemical state, better control of hypertension and extracellular fluid volume, and intraperitoneal administration of insulin. In diabetic patients, peritoneal access is easier to establish and less troublesome.** Heparinization and access-related complications, which are a major cause of morbidity while on hemodialysis, are avoided. Moreover, CAPD offers freedom from a machine and enables travel without upsetting facility dialysis schedules. Another advantage is good control of blood glucose by intraperitoneal administration of insulin, eliminating the need for multiple subcutaneous insulin injections.

Blood Glucose Control in Diabetic Patients on Intermittent Peritoneal Dialysis

Blood glucose control while on IPD is achieved with a combination of subcutaneous and intraperitoneal administration of an amount of insulin adjusted to individual requirements. On dialysis days, blood glucose is controlled by giving the patient's usual daily dose of insulin by subcutaneous injection, and in addition regular insulin is added to the dialysis solution until the last five exchanges of dialysis, when insulin is omitted to prevent postdialysis hypoglycemia. At the initiation of each patient's dialysis program, dialysis insulin requirements are determined. The amount of insulin required is directly proportional to the amount of glucose load given to the patient during dialysis to achieve ultrafiltration. Insulin is added to the dialysis solution bags during intermittent dialysis, depending on the strength of dextrose infused. Insulin requirements on dialysis in a given patient depend on a patient's sensitivity to insulin and have to be determined on an individual basis.

Blood glucose is monitored every 4 to 6 hours, and the dose of insulin is adjusted accordingly. During the last six exchanges, no insulin is added to the dialysate bag to avoid rebound hypoglycemia when the dialysis is stopped. In between dialysis days, only subcutaneous insulin is given as per standard practice. It takes as long as 2 weeks after initiation of dialysis to determine the exact amount of insulin required by an individual patient. **Once established, the insulin requirements do not generally change unless new complications are encountered.**

Blood Glucose Control in Diabetic Patients on Continuous Ambulatory Peritoneal Dialysis

The aim of treatment is to achieve a fasting blood glucose level of around 140 mg/dl, 1-hour postmeal (breakfast, lunch, and supper) levels below 200 mg/dl at all times, and a glycosylated hemoglobin of 7% or below.

Because of the physiologic similarities between normal insulin secretion and the intraperitoneally administered insulin, intraperitoneal administration of insulin during CAPD appears to achieve a tighter control of blood glucose than do other forms of insulin administration. Most of the insulin secreted by the pancreas is transported to the liver by the portal vein, and 50% of the portal venous insulin is extracted by the liver before reaching systemic circulation. This relatively high concentration of insulin in the liver promotes metabolic modulation of absorbed nutrients before they enter the systemic circulation and is likely to be important in normal glucose homeostasis. Insulin administered into the peritoneal cavity is absorbed by diffusion across the visceral peritoneum into the portal venous circulation and directly through the capsule of liver, thus simulating physiologic insulin secretion more closely than does systemic insulin therapy. Intraperitoneal insulin also reaches the systemic circulation by convective transfer via the peritoneal cavity lymphatics.

The absorption kinetics of intraperitoneal administration of regular insulin promote the control of glycemia throughout the dwell time. Intraperitoneal insulin is absorbed along with the obligatory glucose load from the dialysis solution, and insulin absorption continues until the end of the dwell. Peak insulin levels in the serum are observed 30 to 45 minutes after its administration into an empty peritoneal cavity and delayed until 90 to 120 minutes, when insulin is added to the dialysis solution. Approximately 50% of the insulin instilled into the peritoneal cavity is absorbed after an 8-hour dwell time.

All patients are dialyzed with four 2-L exchanges a day. The bags are exchanged during the day, 20 minutes before the major meals (*i.e.*, breakfast, lunch, and supper). The fourth exchange is made at around 11 PM. At this time, a patient has a snack consisting of a sandwich and a small drink.

Patients are advised to consume a diet providing 20 to 25 kcal/kg of body weight per day and containing 1.2 to 1.5 g/kg of body weight of protein. During the initial control, blood glucose level is measured four times a day (*i.e.*, fasting, and before breakfast, lunch, and supper). Using a syringe with a long needle, regular insulin is added to each dialysate bag just before the fluid is infused intraperitoneally. The bag is inverted two or three times to aid mixing. The dose of insulin is proportional to the concentration of glucose in the dialysis solution.

Despite great interpatient variation in intraperitoneal insulin requirements of diabetic CAPD patients, the daily intraperitoneal insulin dose in a given patient is usually greater than twice the pre-CAPD daily subcutaneous dose. At the initiation of CAPD, 150% of the pre-CAPD daily subcutaneous insulin dose can be safely divided among all four exchanges, with a reduced insulin dose added to the overnight dwell to avoid nocturnal hypoglycemia. Intraperitoneal insulin therapy must be individualized, and review of morning fasting, 2-hour postprandial, and preexchange blood glucose levels of the previous day allows stepwise changes in insulin added to each cycle until desired blood glucose control is achieved. Each peritoneal dialysis exchange with intraperitoneal insulin should be performed before meals to promote peak insulin absorption at the time of food intake in order to minimize meal-related hyperglycemia. Strict aseptic technique using a long needle should be used to add insulin to the dialysis solution through the injection port. If blind diabetic patients are unable to use an assist device for the injection of insulin into the bag (Inject-Aid), a partner or nurse can premix insulin with the dialysis solution for up to 24 hours without any significant insulin adsorption to the plastic bags. Increments in insulin are required for each additional hypertonic dialysis cycle incorporated into the daily routine. Intraperitoneal insulin requirements during episodes of peritonitis are widely believed to be increased, but hypoglycemia has been reported when the usual dose of intraperitoneal insulin was continued during peritonitis. Blood glucose level during peritonitis is likely to be determined by the relative importance of increased insulin absorption and reduced carbohydrate intake due to anorexia versus increased glucose absorption and infection-related catabolic state. The need for follow-up monitoring of blood glucose level and subsequent modification of insulin dosage is thus emphasized, especially during changes in a patient's routine treatments.

The following case summary illustrates blood glucose control in a typical diabetic patient on CAPD:

CASE SUMMARY 4

A 32-year-old insulin dependent man with ESRD began peritoneal dialysis. During the catheter break-in period, he required a total of 24 units of regular insulin to maintain a fasting blood glucose level of 132 mg/dl and a 1-hour postmeal blood glucose level of 167 mg/dl. Fifteen days later, he started CAPD training. The following insulin doses were prescribed for the first day of CAPD:

Rx: Four CAPD exchanges during the next 24 hours. Use 1.5% alternating with 2.5% dialysis solution to lower body weight by 1 kg.

Timings of exchanges: 8:00 AM, 12:30 PM, 6:00 PM, and 10:00 PM.

Diet: 1500-calorie diabetic diet.

Breakfast and meal times: 8:15 AM, 12:45 PM, and 6:15 PM.

May have a snack at 10:15 PM.

Using aseptic precaution, add insulin to the dialysis solution bags with a long needle into the injection port and mix thoroughly.

Dose of insulin per bag:

1.5% solution 6 units of regular insulin
2.5% solution 8 units of regular insulin

Check finger-stick blood glucose level before each exchange.

Report blood glucose levels below 80 or over 300 mg/dl.

The following blood glucose levels were reported for the first day:

8:00 AM, 82 mg/dl
12:00 noon, 284 mg/dl
6:00 PM, 296 mg/dl
10:00 PM, 267 mg/dl

The following insulin doses were prescribed for the second CAPD day:

Rx: Add regular insulin to each bag (except 10:00 PM) as follows:

1.5% solution, 8 units
2.5% solution, 10 units

10 PM exchange bag of solution, add insulin as follows:

1.5% solution, 5 units
2.5% solution, 6 units

The following blood glucose levels were reported for the second day:

8:00 AM, 109 mg/dl
12:00 noon, 146 mg/dl
6:00 PM, 286 mg/dl
10:00 PM, 278 mg/dl

This patient's insulin dose for the 12:00 noon exchange was increased by 2 units, and the blood glucose level for the subsequent days were at the targeted levels.

Patients are trained to check their blood glucose levels with the finger-stick method. This method, which gives quick results and correlates reasonably well with the venous blood glucose levels, helps to detect unexpected fluctuations in blood glucose. The finger-stick test is performed 5 to 10 minutes before each bag exchange, and whenever necessary, the dose of insulin added in the next bag is adjusted according to the guidelines taught to individual patients at the time of training.

Intraperitoneal insulin therapy has been shown to reduce the mean glucose level, meal-related hyperglycemia, and daily glucose exertions when compared with subcutaneous insulin. In diabetic patients on CAPD, such treatment objectives as maintaining morning fasting glucose level less than 140 mg/dl, postmeal hyperglycemia less than 200 mg/dl, and hemoglobin A_{1c} levels less than 9% have been achieved with intraperitoneal insulin administration. **If care is not exercised and a physician has an overzealous desire to control glucose levels to nearly normal, severe or even fatal hypoglycemia can occur with intraperitoneal insulin administration.**

Not all patients can be maintained on intraperitoneal insulin because of individual patient variations, preferences, and insulin responsiveness. A recent survey of blood glucose control during CAPD was conducted by the National CAPD Registry. Approximately 47% of the 487 surveyed patients on CAPD use intraperitoneal insulin for their blood glucose control, 30% use

Table 17–10. REMOVAL OF PERITONEAL CATHETER IN A PATIENT RECEIVING A TRANSPLANT

Clinical Situation	Management
Cadaveric transplantation	
No exit site infection	Remove before hospital discharge
Exit site infection	Remove at the time of transplantation
Living related transplantation	
Two-haplotype match	Remove at the time of transplantation
One-haplotype match	Same as cadaveric transplantation
Splenectomy	Remove at the time of surgery
Posttransplant dialysis	Intermittent or continuous ambulatory peritoneal dialysis if peritoneum is intact

subcutaneous insulin, and the rest of the patients either require no insulin or are on subcutaneous insulin and oral hypoglycemic agents.

RENAL TRANSPLANTATION IN PATIENTS RECEIVING PERITONEAL DIALYSIS

Analysis of our experience of transplantation demonstrated no significant differences in patient or graft survival between those receiving hemodialysis or peritoneal dialysis during the pretransplant period. Also similar in the two groups were the causes of death; the incidence of wound infection; bacterial sepsis (positive blood culture); pneumonia, cytomegalic virus infection, and other infections such as those of the urinary tract; and the pattern and incidence of episodes of rejection during the first year after transplant. Episodes of peritonitis were observed in the group on peritoneal dialysis, but as mentioned before, they were treated successfully with the conventional protocol. Guidelines for removing the catheter at appropriate times are given in Table 17–10.

References

1. Mactier RA, Khanna R, Twardowski ZJ, et al: Contribution of lymphatic absorption to loss of ultrafiltration and solute clearances in CAPD. J Clin Invest 80:1311, 1987.
2. Twardowski ZJ: New approaches to intermittent peritoneal dialysis therapies. *In* Nolph KD (ed): Peritoneal Dialysis. Dordrecht, Netherlands, Kluwer Academic Publishers, pp 133–151, 1989.
3. Oreopoulos DG, Helfrich GB, Khanna R, et al: Peritoneal catheters and exit site practices: Current recommendations. Peritoneal Dialysis Bulletin 7:130, 1987.
4. Keane WF, Everett ED, Fine RN, et al: CAPD related peritonitis management and antibiotic therapy recommendations: Travenol peritonitis management advisory committee. Peritoneal Dialysis Bulletin 7:55, 1987.

CHAPTER 18

HEMODIALYSIS

Nuhad Ismail and Raymond Hakim

Hemodialysis is by far the most prevalent treatment for both acute renal failure and end-stage renal disease (ESRD). In 1986, 330,000 patients were on renal replacement therapy worldwide; of these, 70% were on hemodialysis, 9% were on peritoneal dialysis, and 21% had functioning renal allografts. The United States had the largest proportion (37%) of these patients. The proportion of patients who are over 55 years and are being accepted for hemodialysis is increasing, and probably around 50% of patients on hemodialysis now are older than 60 years. In many cases, these patients have many other morbid conditions that complicate their dialysis procedure.

Advances in dialysis technology and recent economic pressures on dialysis units, coupled with patient preference for shorter dialysis treatment times, have recently led to the implementation of high-efficiency and high-flux dialysis. Successful application of these treatment modalities has been demonstrated in short-term clinical experiences with no detrimental impact on morbidity, and the majority of chronic hemodialysis patients may prove to be candidates for this mode of therapy. The long-term effects of such treatments on patient survival still need further elucidation.

Although an artificial kidney sustains the life of patients with ESRD, the morbidity and mortality of these patients is substantially higher than in the age-adjusted population. Although we know how to dialyze patients, we still do not know exactly what constitutes adequate dialysis, perhaps in part because our knowledge of the molecular basis of uremia is still very incomplete and at this time it is impossible to model the dialysis prescription for all toxic solutes.

The uremic syndrome is complex and multifactorial and remains only partially responsive to adequate dialysis.

PHYSIOLOGIC PRINCIPLES OF HEMODIALYSIS

The basic physiologic principles of hemodialysis have been known for many years. In simple terms, dialysis represents the interaction of a patient's blood and a balanced solution (the dialysate) across a semipermeable membrane. **During hemodialysis, two physical processes operate simultaneously: diffusion and ultrafiltration.**

Diffusion (or clearance) is the movement of solutes such as urea from the blood compartment to the dialysate across a semipermeable membrane and the movement of substances such as acetate or bicarbonate from the dialysate to the blood. The driving force for this movement is the concentration gradient across the membrane. **The amount of material that diffuses or fluxes is a function of the concentration gradient, the surface area of the membrane, and the permeability of the membrane, as well as the size and charge of the solute, the blood flow rate, and the dialysate flow rate.** Clearance of small molecules is flow dependent, whereas the clearance of large molecules is far less dependent on blood and dialysate flow (Fig. 18–1). The contribution of charge of a solute is exemplified by phosphate, in which the charge and water of hydration surrounding the molecule may decrease its net clearance. Phosphate has a smaller molecular weight than creatinine, yet it has an effective clearance approximately two thirds that of creatinine. Finally, membrane resistance to solute flux is higher if the membrane is thick or if the number of pores is small.

Ultrafiltration (or convective transport) involves the bulk movement of solvent across the membrane. The driving force in this circumstance is the hydrostatic pressure gradient across the dialysis membrane (called the transmembrane pressure [TMP]). Solutes will also

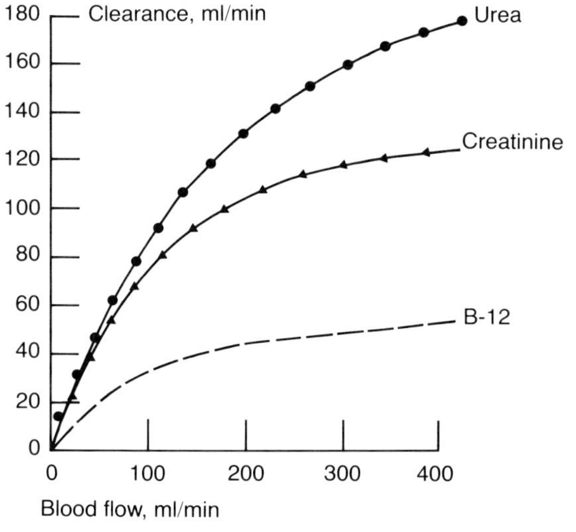

Figure 18–1. Dialyzer clearance of substances of different molecular weights as a function of blood flow (solute clearance during hemodialysis). Clearance is inversely related to molecular size. The clearance of large molecules is not as flow dependent as the clearance rate of small molecules. (From Gibson RL: Dialysis. *In* Stone WJ, Rabin PL (eds): End-Stage Renal Disease. New York, Academic Press, 1983, p 189.)

be removed in this process, in the same concentration as they exist in solvent, in this case plasma water. Hence both processes, diffusion and convection, contribute to the removal of solute. However, the convective transport is quantitatively much less important than diffusion for solute transfer, particularly for small molecules that have a high diffusion coefficient.

Clinical Terms

Transmembrane pressure is the hydrostatic pressure gradient between the blood and the dialysate compartment that determines ultrafiltration (and convective solute transfer). Algebraically, it is equal to the pressure in the blood compartment minus the pressure in the dialysate compartment, which is usually a negative pressure.

Both blood compartment pressures and dialysate pressure decrease as they flow inside a dialyzer, because of decreases in pressure. Therefore, by convention, TMP is taken as the sum of the blood outlet pressure (venous pressure [VP]) and dialysate inlet pressure (DP).

Example: TMP = VP + DP

If VP = 75 mm Hg and DP = −200 mm Hg

Then TMP = 75 − (−200) = 275 mm Hg

The *ultrafiltration coefficient* (KUF) reflects the permeability of a particular membrane to water and is defined as the number of milliliters of fluid that can be transferred across the membrane per 1 mm Hg in 1 hour.

Example: If the KUF of a dialyzer is 4 ml/mm Hg/hr, then at the above TMP, this dialyzer will result in net ultrafiltration of 4 × 275 = 1100 ml/hr.

Dialyzer clearance refers to the volume of blood cleared of a particular substance per unit time. Dialyzer clearance is a useful measure of dialyzer performance that can be used to compare the performance of various dialyzers. Dialyzer clearance is usually given as *in vitro* data and is specified in the manufacturer's pamphlet supplied with the dialyzers.

Types of Dialyzers

An artificial kidney (dialyzer) is made of up two compartments, the blood and the dialysate compartments, separated by a semipermeable membrane. The dialyzer has four ports: two inlets for blood and dialysate and two outlets. A blood pump pushes blood through to the blood compartment; blood leaves the dialyzer from the opposite end after it is partially cleared. The flow is usually in a countercurrent direction for maximum diffusion gradient (Fig. 18–2). Dialyzers can be manufactured in different configurations, but they all have the same operating principles described earlier.

The hollow-fiber dialyzer is the most recently developed type of dialyzer and the most

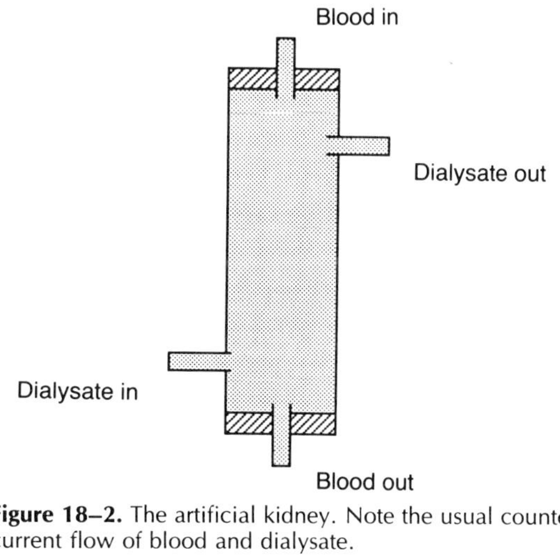

Figure 18–2. The artificial kidney. Note the usual countercurrent flow of blood and dialysate.

commonly used. It consists of 10,000 to 15,000 capillary tubes, each 200 to 300 μm in diameter, tightly bound in a bundle. Blood flows inside the capillary tubes, and the dialysate circulates around the outside of the fibers. These dialyzers have a high ratio of membrane surface area to blood volume. An advantage of these dialyzers is that they have low compliance, and the extracorporeal blood volume does not increase with changes in the TMP, blood flow, or dialysate flow. Another advantage of the hollow-fiber dialyzers is their lower priming volume, usually less than 100 ml, and small compliance compared with parallel-plate dialyzers.

Parallel-plate dialyzers consist of sheets of membranes laid on top of one another over supporting structures. Blood flows inside the membranes and dialysate between the membranes.

Coil dialyzers are essentially not in use now because of their high compliance and coil volume, which make their clearance and ultrafiltration characteristics unpredictable.

In addition to their structural differences, dialyzers also vary in the composition of the membrane material and can be made from cellulose that is derived from cotton fibers (*e.g.*, cuprophane) or substituted cellulose (*e.g.*, cellulose acetate). They may also be synthetic membranes such as polysulfone, polyacrylonitrile, and polymethyl methacrylate. **Physicians caring for patients on hemodialysis should become familiar with the different characteristics of the dialysis membranes for proper dialysis prescription.** Such information as the surface area of the membrane, its *in vitro* clearance, and its ultrafiltration coefficient are usually available with the dialyzer package insert or appropriate tables in textbooks of dialysis.

A typical dialysis setup starting from the arterial needle in the vascular access of the patient and back to the venous needle is schematically shown in Figure 18–3. Pertinent parameters of the dialysis procedure are described below the figure. An important aspect of the hemodialysis machine is its monitoring function. The monitors on the blood circuit are discussed in Table 18–1. The segment between the arterial access and blood pump is a high-risk segment and is the only source of passive entry of air into the circuit. In addition to the arterial and venous pressure monitors, the overall purpose of which is to stop the roller blood pump, the air-foam detector not only stops the roller pump but also clamps the venous line, preventing further return of blood to the patient.

The *dialysate* circuit monitors assure the safety of dialysis against improperly mixed dialysate concentrates, overheated dialysate, or blood leaks. Dialysate monitors include the conductivity, pH, temperature, dialysate pressure, and blood leak monitors.

PERMANENT VASCULAR ACCESS FOR CHRONIC HEMODIALYSIS

One of the most important aspects in the total management of patients with ESRD is the planning and creation of a permanent vascular access for hemodialysis. Careful planning and a skillful and meticulous operative procedure are the most important determinants of this lifeline for patients with ESRD. **Clotting, stenosis, and low flow not only cause inefficient dialysis and poor control of uremia, but together with access site infections constitute the most common causes of morbidity and hospitalization of patients with ESRD. Planning of vascular access must start with strong emphasis on preservation of extremity veins, particularly those of the forearms and especially those of the nondominant arm vessels where the initial access is inserted.** Early placement of the permanent vascular access prevents loss of forearm veins and allows time for proper maturation of the fistula. This generally should occur when the serum creatinine level is approximately 8 mg/dl or when the creatinine clearance is <15 ml/min.

Access Planning

The upper extremity is preferred, as the incidence of infection is less and development of arterial steal syndrome is less frequent and less critical than in the lower extremity. The nondominant arm is used preferentially to keep the dominant arm free while a patient is on dialysis. The lower extremity is used as a last resort only when all other sites for access placement have been exhausted.

The most distal site available should be used first to reserve maximal vessel length for future revision.

An endogenous arteriovenous (AV, or Cimino fistula) is always preferable to a synthetic graft AV shunt because of its long-term patency rate and lower incidence of infection. The vein should be of adequate size preoperatively for

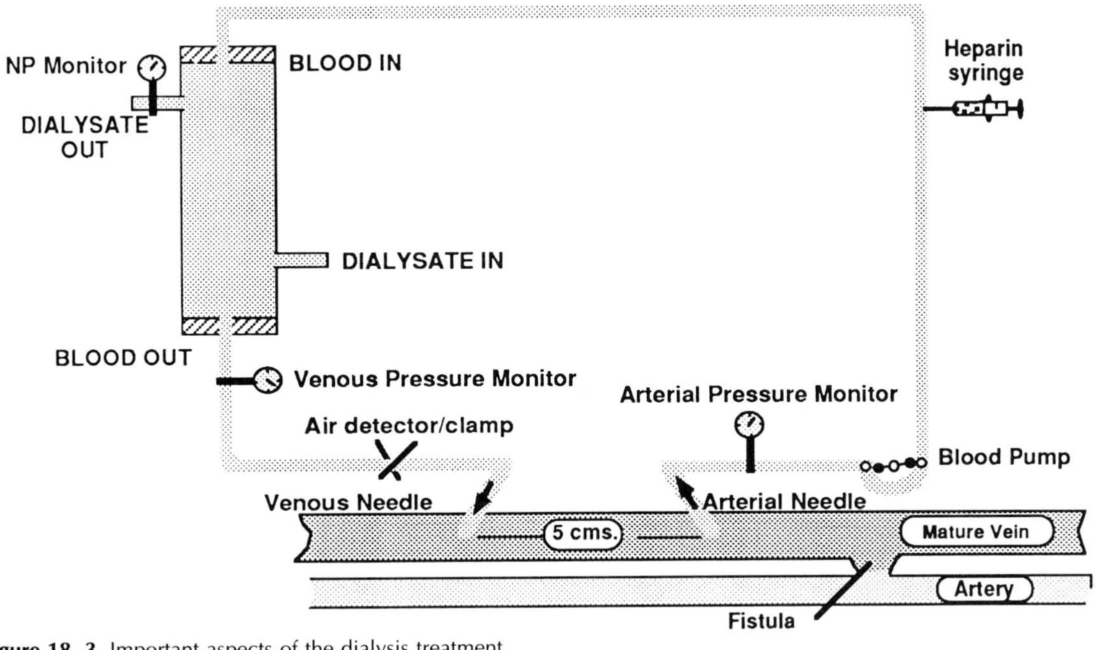

Figure 18–3. Important aspects of the dialysis treatment.

1. Note that both the arterial and venous needles stick the mature vein of the fistula.
2. The ends of the needles should be separated by about 5 cm to lessen recirculation. Recirculation formula = 100% × P − A/P − V = % recirculation.
   P = BUN concentration in systemic circulation
   A = BUN concentration at dialyzer blood inlet (arterial)
   V = BUN concentration at dialyzer blood outlet (venous)
   Recirculation results in inadequate dialysis (when R > 20%). May be a sign of poor flow in fistula.
3. Note the usual *countercurrent* flow of blood and dialysate into the dialyzer.
4. TMP = VP + NP. Controls rate of ultrafiltration. VP is usually +50 to +100 mm Hg. NP is the negative pressure: Hydrostatic pressure across the membrane adjusted by varying resistance to inflow of dialysate.
5. Typical Q_D = dialysate flow is 500 ml/min. Typical Q_B = blood flow is 300 ml/min. These flows are higher in high-flux dialysis.

Table 18–1. BLOOD CIRCUIT MONITORS

	Role	Causes of Alarm*
"Arterial" pressure monitor Usual location: preblood pump (sometimes postpump) Normal range: −20 to −80 mm Hg (subatmospheric)	Guards against excessive suction on vascular access Shuts blood pump (with automatic venous line clamping)	Decreased blood flow or pressure through access Lines between needle and pump kinked Faulty arterial needle position Stenosis graft arterial anastomosis Access clotting Air bubbles High blood pressure (high-limit alarm) Disruption of circuit between pump and access Saline infusion line unclamped Blood pump has torn pumping segment
"Venous" pressure monitor Usual location: distal to dialyzer Normal range: ±50 mm Hg of venous pressure (arteriovenous grafts may be up to 200 mm Hg)	Protects against excessive resistance to blood return Shuts blood pump Calculation of transmembrane pressure	High blood flow with small venous needle (gauge #16) Venous line clotting Stenosis of venous limb of access Faulty position of venous needle Venous line kinking Clot in venous drip chamber Clot in venous limb of access

*If no obvious causes, always evaluate vascular access.

the creation of a Cimino fistula. If a patient has small, thin-walled veins lying deep in the subcutaneous fat, fistulas are impractical and prosthetic grafts should be the first choice. Likewise, diabetics and patients with arteriosclerosis may not have suitable vessels for a successful Cimino fistula. **In general, an AV Cimino fistula should ideally be placed at least 3 months before anticipated dialysis,** whereas for a synthetic graft, at least 3 weeks is needed for maturation and subsidence of the inflammatory response that inevitably accompanies the placement of a foreign substance subcutaneously.

Types of Access

Two major kinds of vascular access are discussed here. Discussion of detailed surgical techniques is beyond the scope of this chapter.

Endogenous Arteriovenous Fistula

The basic requirement for creation of a Cimino fistula is an adequate artery and vein close to each other for anastomosis. The most commonly used site is at the wrist, usually connecting the cephalic vein to the radial artery (Brescia-Cimino fistula). Recent modification of the forearm fistula placed even more distally in the anatomic snuffbox has been reported. Fistulas can also be constructed between the brachial artery and cephalic vein; however, higher cardiac output often results in these cases, and this arrangement may not be suitable for all patients. During a period of maturation of the fistula over 3 months, the venous limb of the fistula dilates and its wall thickens ("arterializes"), permitting repeated insertions of dialysis needles. The anastomosis is done as side of artery to side of vein (side to side), end of artery to end of vein, end of artery to side of vein, or end of vein to side of artery. With the side-to-side method, venous hypertension and swelling of the hand may result. Edema of the entire hand (sometimes with ulceration and varicosities) and painful thumb (sometimes with eczema and oozing from under the nail bed) are manifestations of venous hypertension. Converting from side to side to an end of vein to side of artery anastomosis produces better flow in forearm veins. Another complication is the steal syndrome, which manifests as coolness, pallor, pain, and cyanosis in the hand or fingers distal to the fistula. Patients with diabetes and elderly patients with atheromatous peripheral vascular disease are more prone to this complication. In the steal syndrome, blood is "stolen" from the digital vessels (ulnar artery) to the lower-resistance fistula (radial artery) by retrograde perfusion. Ligation of the distal radial artery is the treatment of choice. Occasionally, banding of the fistula is done by placing polytef bands around the fistula. Other complications of the endogenous fistula include thrombosis, which can be an early or a late complication. Early thrombosis is due to surgical technical factors. Late thrombosis is due to poor flow, hypotension, or hypercoagulability. Successful thrombectomy with a Fogarty balloon-tipped catheter should be accomplished as soon as possible after the event to avoid the onset of fibrosis. When stenosis occurs at or near the anastomotic site secondary to arterial fibrosis or fibrous intimal hyperplasia, a new fistula should be created proximally using the already dilated vein. A short stenotic segment found in the vein itself can be repaired locally using a small vein patch. If stenosis is more diffuse, an entirely new access will be required or a new fistula must be created proximally. Balloon dilations for stenosis and the use of streptokinase have been successfully used to treat thrombosis of a vascular access.

The endogenous AV fistula has excellent long-term function and a low rate of infection. Cumulative patency rate at 1 year is about 85%, and 50% at 4 years. Infections are usually due to *Staphylococcus aureus* and are successfully treated with local care and systemic antibiotics. With severe abscess or septicemia secondary to an infected fistula, the infected vein should be excised and the subcutaneous tunnel drained. Congestive heart failure is a very unusual complication of the endogenous fistula but may occur with upper arm and femoral fistulas.

> Native vein fistulas are the access of first choice.

When the fistula matures, the vein proximal to the anastomosis is used for both the afferent (usually called the *arterial*) needle, as well as the venous needle. The arterial needle is the most distal and is placed about 3 cm from the anastomosis. The venous needle is placed proximal to the arterial needle and at least 5 cm away from it to lessen the problem of recirculation (a portion of blood leaving the efferent needle being aspirated by the afferent needle).

After the fistula is successfully created, specific instructions are given to the patient (Table 18–2).

Prosthetic Grafts

Biologic Grafts. These include bovine grafts prepared from the carotid artery or human umbilical veins. The rate of infection with these grafts is high, and they have a tendency to form multiple aneurysms.

Synthetic Grafts. The most popular of these is the polytetrafluoroethylene (PTFE) or Teflon graft. These grafts may be straight and placed between the radial artery at the wrist and the basilic vein near the antecubital fossa. Both ends of the graft are anastomosed to sides of the artery and the vein. The straight grafts may be satisfactory for young patients but not diabetic patients, in whom the distal radial artery may be small or arteriosclerotic. The more common is the loop graft placed in the forearm between the basilic vein and brachial artery or cephalic vein and brachial artery. They can also be placed in the upper arms or thighs. **The 6-mm-diameter PTFE prosthesis provides adequate flow for hemodialysis and a low incidence of high-output congestive failure or peripheral steal syndrome.** Two to 3 weeks is allowed for healing of the subcutaneous tunnel after surgical implantation of the graft. Elevation of the arm above the cardiac level hastens the resolution of the edema and inflammation, and an intravenous stand and elevation of the arm with a stockinette are at times required. Early puncture of the graft may result in a hematoma that may compress the graft or become a nidus for infection. The dialysis needles should be at least 5 cm from each other, the arterial needle placed at about 3 cm from the arterial anastomosis and the venous needle at about 3 cm from the venous anastomosis. Infection is more common with prosthetic grafts than native vein fistula. *S. aureus* or *Staphylococcus epidermis* is the most common organism responsible for infection, but *Escherichia coli* is also a common pathogen. **Septicemia may occur without local signs of infection.** Patients should receive antimicrobial prophylaxis whenever they undergo a surgical procedure that may result in bacteremia, such as dental extraction. When the graft is infected, local revision of the infected segment with aggressive antibiotic therapy may salvage the graft. More often, removal of the graft is necessary.

Table 18–2. ARTERIOVENOUS FISTULA PATIENT INSTRUCTIONS

1. Begin developmental exercises 7 to 10 days postoperatively. These are done by squeezing and relaxing a rubber ball or a rolled wash cloth for 5 minutes every hour when awake, with a tourniquet placed on the arm 10 to 12 inches above the anastomosis.
2. Check for pulsation and bruit several times a day. A buzz should be heard over the fistula. If the buzz disappears, call your doctor.
3. Do not have blood pressure taken or let anyone do needle sticks in the extremity that has the fistula.
4. Bruising or swelling over the fistula can be caused by needle sticks during dialysis or from bumping the fistula. If this happens, apply ice for the first 12 hours; then apply moist, warm soaks for the next 12 hours. Wrapping the arm with an elastic (Ace) bandage for 3 to 4 hours after dialysis will help the swelling and bruising caused by dialysis. Elevate the extremity to reduce swelling.
5. No heavy lifting with the affected extremity.
6. Do not sleep on the affected extremity, as pressure can cause clotting.
7. No showers until incisions are healed.

Early graft thrombosis is usually due to technical surgical problems, hypotension, premature graft use with a subsequent tunnel hematoma formation, or anatomic causes of low flow through the graft.

Late graft thrombosis is usually due to stenosis at the venous outflow tract and is often due to neointimal proliferation at the graft vein anastomosis.

For a stenosis localized at the venous anastomosis or in the vein immediately proximal to it, a patch angioplasty can be used. If a stenotic segment is large, a jump graft is used. Percutaneous transluminal angioplasty is gaining popularity in treating venous stenosis.

> Septicemia may occur from a synthetic AV graft without local signs of infection.

Injection of streptokinase directly into clotted shunts and manually massaging the clot may be successful in 60 to 70% of thrombosed grafts. However, thrombolytic therapy has not been effective in all series.

Recurrent graft thrombosis may be empirically treated with oral anticoagulation. The role of prophylactic antiplatelet and coumadin anticoagulation, however, is unclear.

Access for Acute Hemodialysis

Frequently, an access is urgently needed to treat patients with acute renal failure, patients with newly recognized uremia, patients with ESRD during the maturation period of a recently created permanent access or revision of a permanent access, or patients on peritoneal dialysis needing temporary hemodialysis.

Percutaneous

Access to circulation in these patients can be accomplished by the percutaneous cannulation of the femoral, subclavian, or internal jugular veins. Two types of catheters are available: single or double lumen. The double-lumen catheter is more commonly used. In this type of catheter, there are two openings at the tip at different sites along the length of the cannula, and blood inside is partitioned. The advantage of the double-lumen catheter is that recirculation is lessened because the openings of the inflow and outflow ports are at different sites. In the single type, a Y adapter is used at the distal end of the catheter and blood is alternately pushed from the patient to the dialyzer and then back to the patient.

A soft catheter similar to the one that surgeons place intraoperatively has become available. It can be placed percutaneously in the internal jugular vein by trained nephrologists.

Technique for Percutaneous Cannulation of the Internal Jugular Vein

The right side of the neck is preferred for venipuncture for three reasons: the dome of the right lung and pleura is lower than the left; there is a more-or-less straight line to the atrium; and the large thoracic duct is not endangered.

There are three approaches to cannulating the internal jugular vein: posterior, central, and anterior. In trained hands, each is an effective means. The route chosen depends on the experience and preference of the operator. In general, the central approach is easiest to learn and to do.

In the central approach, the surgeon locates the triangle formed by the two heads (sternal and clavicular) of the sternomastoid muscle and the clavicle. It may be helpful to have awake patients lift their head slightly off the bed to make this triangle more visible. In some patients with a large or obese neck, it may be difficult to identify the triangle.

The needle is inserted at the apex of the triangle formed by the two heads of the sternomastoid muscle and the clavicle.

The needle is directed caudally and laterally, parallel to the medial border of the clavicular head of the sternomastoid muscle, toward the ipsilateral nipple at a 45 to 60% angle with the frontal plane.

If the vein is not entered after the needle has been inserted a few centimeters, the needle should be slowly withdrawn, maintaining negative pressure on the syringe. If the vein is still not entered, the needle is withdrawn completely; it is then reinserted and directed 5 to 10 degrees more in the lateral direction. If the vein is still not entered, the needle should be directed more in line with the sagittal plane. **However, do not direct the needle medially (across the sagittal plane), because the carotid artery will be punctured.**

Subclavian Catheter

Advantages, Disadvantages, and Contraindications. The subclavian catheter can be left in place several weeks (up to 6 to 8 weeks with meticulous care). It allows patients to be ambulatory and to be dialyzed as outpatients.

One disadvantage of subclavian catheterization is thrombosis or stenosis of subclavian vein, which can affect the venous outflow of subsequent accesses in the arm. Manifestations of subclavian vein thrombosis include swelling in the arm on the side of the subclavian catheter. Treatment of stenosis includes angioplasty followed by antiplatelet agents. Also, a subclavian catheter should not be inserted in a bacteremic patient before initial treatment of the bacteremic state. It is not suitable for patients with pulmonary edema who cannot lie flat or in Trendelenburg's position. Finally, major life-threatening complications may occur. Complications include puncture of the subclavian artery, pneumothorax, pericardial tamponade, arrhythmias, brachial plexus injury, superficial infections, and bacteremia. However, the frequency of these complications is low in the hands of an experienced nephrologist.

When placing a subclavian catheter, one should avoid the side where a new fistula has been placed or is to be placed. Subclavian vein thrombosis may also follow prior transvenous pacemaker insertions. Upper extremities previously used for transvenous pacemaker insertions should be investigated for venous patency prior to creation of permanent vascular access. The contralateral arm should be used for placement of permanent access if a subclavian vein stenosis or thrombosis is discovered during venography. Finally, subclavian catheters should not be placed in presence of severe coagulopathy.

Technique for Catheter Placement. Patients should be placed in slight Trendelenburg's position, with a rolled towel placed longitudinally between the scapulae. The selected area should be prepared and draped.

The surgeon should locate the clavicular notch and anesthetize with xylocaine in the area of insertion and into the clavicular periosteum, then probe for the subclavian vein with a small-gauge needle. An introducer catheter or subclavian catheter needle is inserted under the clavicle and anterior to the first rib in the direction of the contralateral shoulder.

Once the subclavian vein is cannulated, the surgeon withdraws the inner trocar and immediately occludes the plastic cannula with a finger, while the patient performs a Valsalva's maneuver. The surgeon passes the guide wire through the short catheter and into the superior vena cava, then removes the introducer catheter and establishes hemostasis.

The hemodialysis catheter is fed over the guide wire, and a hemostat is clamped on the wire as it exits the distal end of the catheter; then, the catheter is advanced into the superior vena cava (tip of the catheter just inside the right atrium).

The surgeon withdraws the guide wire and flushes the catheter at clamp sites with dilute heparin saline solution. The catheter is occluded at clamp sites with dilute heparin solution in the catheter. The catheter is securely sutured at at least two sites.

An upright PA and lateral chest film is obtained to ascertain the correct position of the subclavian catheter (the catheter tip should not cause tenting of the superior vena cava, especially double-lumen catheters). No patient can be dialyzed until the chest film is checked by the renal fellow.

For outpatients, 5000 units of sodium heparin is placed in the catheter, which is then clamped. The site is dressed with a hyperalimentation dressing kit.

A subclavian catheter should be removed if a patient is septic and there are no other obvious sources of infection, if blood cultures are positive, or if there is a purulent discharge at the exit site.

> Do not push a subclavian catheter back if it becomes dislodged. This may result in a high rate of bacteremia. A new catheter can be inserted over a guide wire.

When the catheter is used, and after each hemodialysis, heparin is placed in each port and left in place until the next dialysis to prevent clotting. Heparin (5000 units) plus additional saline to fill the dead space is placed in each port. The dead space is usually 1.2 to 1.3 cm.

Clotting of a subclavian catheter can be treated with urokinase or streptokinase. Urokinase (5000 units) is used in each port of the double-lumen catheter and left in place for 20 minutes before aspiration. Caution should be exercised to minimize the streptokinase or urokinase infusion into the circulation.

INTERNAL JUGULAR CATHETER (HEMOCATH)

This catheter, placed in the operating room by a surgeon, has a cuff at the skin exit site. It is a suitable catheter for patients who need a temporary hemodialysis access for 2 to 3 months.

FEMORAL CATHETER

Advantages, Disadvantages, and Contraindications. A femoral catheter is easy to place, and complications are minor and not life-threatening. Insertion is possible in semirecumbent patients. Also, it may be used in bacteremic patients (new catheter for each dialysis).

With use of a femoral catheter, however, patients must remain hospitalized and must stay in bed and the catheter needs to be changed within 5 to 7 days.

There should be no prior history of surgery or thrombosis of the femoral vein on the side of insertion of the catheter. Aortofemoral and femoropopliteal bypasses are specific contraindications to femoral vein cannulation. There should be no severe coagulopathy before inserting the catheter.

Technique for Catheter Placement. Patients should be lying flat. The leg in which the femoral catheter is going to be placed is rotated outward. The groin is shaved, cleansed with an antiseptic, and draped.

The femoral pulse is located. The femoral vein is then located 2 cm below the inguinal ligament, approximately 1 cm medial to the femoral pulse. The area of insertion is anesthetized with 1% lidocaine and probed with a small-gauge needle for the femoral vein. The needle is withdrawn once the femoral vein is located, and an introducer catheter is inserted into the femoral vein, maintaining negative pressure and slight angulation throughout the procedure.

Once the femoral vein is cannulated, the inner trocar is withdrawn and the plastic cannula is immediately occluded with a finger. The guide wire is passed through the short catheter into the femoral vein. **It is important for the guide wire to be freely movable back and forth after its insertion. If the guide wire feels tight, catheter insertion should not be attempted.** Rather, the guide wire should be withdrawn completely, the angle of the needle in the vein changed (sometimes the needle hub has to be lowered to the skin level to almost parallel the vein) and the guide wire reinserted. The introducer catheter is removed, and hemostasis is established. Then the hemodialysis catheter is fed over the guide wire.

A hemostat is clamped on the wire as it exits the distal end of the catheter, and then the catheter is advanced into the inferior vena cava, using a rotary motion. The guide wire must be held at all times. The guide wire is then withdrawn. At the clamp sites, the catheter is flushed with a dilute heparin saline solution, and the catheter is sutured to the skin. The area should be observed for local hematoma, and pressure is applied as needed. If the catheter is inadvertantly inserted into the femoral artery instead of the vein, the surgeon should withdraw it, apply firm pressure for 15 minutes, and then reattempt femoral vein cannulation.

Complications include puncture of the femoral artery, traumatic AV fistula, retroperitoneal hemorrhage, and femoral vein thrombosis and phlebitis.

Care of the Femoral Catheter and Subclavian Catheters. Strict aseptic technique must be applied to femoral and subclavian catheters placed for hemodialysis. Exit sites should be inspected daily for signs of infection. Dressings should be changed by the sterile technique, using procedures identical to those designed for hyperalimentation catheters. There should be minimal manipulation of the catheter in order to decrease the chances of accidental dislodgment or infection. **Femoral and subclavian catheters placed for hemodialysis should not be used for any purpose other than hemodialysis.** No blood samples should be obtained or medications or fluids administered through them. The longevity of the subclavian catheters is much greater than that of the femoral catheters, which are usually left in place for 1 week. Patients must remain flat and at bed rest when the femoral catheter is in place. In general, femoral catheters should only be placed in patients who are in intensive care units. Subclavian catheters allow patients more mobility and may be placed in patients outside the intensive care unit, as well as in outpatients. Subclavian catheters can be changed as infrequently as every 3 to 6 weeks.

Complications include puncture of the femoral artery, traumatic AV fistula, retroperitoneal hemorrhage, and femoral vein thrombosis and phlebitis.

External

Scribner's Shunt

Scribner's shunt, an external AV shunt, is mainly used in acute renal failure. It is becoming less popular with the advent of percutaneous access devices. It has a limited life span and poses a high risk of infection and clotting. Accidental hemorrhage or hemorrhage from arterial rupture secondary to an infected shunt may be fatal. A Scribner's shunt is placed either in the forearm (distal radial artery to cephalic vein) or in the leg (posterior tibial artery to the long saphenous vein at the ankle). When a Scribner's shunt is clotted, a number 3 Fogarty balloon is used for declotting. After successful declotting, a constant heparin infusion should be started to prevent reclotting. Salvaging vessels used in Scribner's shunts for future permanent access is possible.

ADEQUACY OF DIALYSIS

The prescription of dialysis remains empiric. Until recently, the length of dialysis was determined primarily by the clinical judgment of the attending nephrologist. Although several proposals were made to guide clinicians, these suffered from a lack of correlation between the prescription and patient outcome. A multicenter study to investigate this issue has been completed, and the results have allowed the quantitation of dialysis prescription.

The National Cooperative Dialysis Study (NCDS) was designed to investigate the effect of altering dialysis prescription to change either the ambient urea level or the dialysis time. Because there was no universal agreement concerning the timing of the urea measurement (pre- or postdialysis, at the beginning of the week or at the end of the week), the concept of a *time-averaged concentration* (TAC) of urea was developed to represent the surrogate parameter for small molecules, whereas time on dialysis was used as a surrogate parameter of the middle molecules. TAC_{urea} can be defined as

$$TAC_{urea} = \frac{(C_1 + C_2) \times td + (C_2 + C_3)\, Id}{2\,(td + Id)}$$

where td = time on dialysis
Id = interdialytic time
C_1 = predialysis blood urea nitrogen (BUN)
C_2 = post dialysis BUN
C_3 = next predialysis BUN

The patients participating in the NCDS were divided into four groups:

Group 1: Long dialysis time (4½ to 5 hours) + TAC = 50 mg/dl
Group 2: Long dialysis time (4½ to 5 hours) + TAC = 100 mg/dl
Group 3: Short dialysis time (2½ to 3 hours) + TAC = 50 mg/dl
Group 4: Short dialysis time (2½ to 3 hours) + TAC = 100 mg/dl

No difference in mortality was found among the four groups during the study period; however, withdrawal from the study for medical reasons was significantly greater in patients in the high-BUN groups than in the low-BUN groups. Hospitalization rate was also greater in the high-BUN groups. Although time on dialysis was not a statistically significant parameter, it nevertheless was an important parameter. Similarly, although there was no difference in mortality between different groups during the study, there was a higher mortality rate in the high-BUN groups after termination of the study.

This prospective study therefore indicated that the dialysis prescription had an effect on the occurrence of medical complications and hospitalization rates, and that TAC_{urea} was a useful target for monitoring and prescribing dialysis.

One possible definition of adequate dialysis is a treatment prescription that ameliorates and prevents complications of uremia. Although there may be no single measure of the adequacy of dialysis treatment, patients who are adequately dialyzed must have satisfactory blood pressure control and achieve reasonable overall rehabilitation. Patients must have adequate nutritional status, with improvement in the degree of platelet function, cardiovascular status, musculoskeletal function, and neurobehavioral status.

Another index that was partly derived from the results of the NCDS study is generally labeled the *KT/V parameter*. To understand this, it is important to recollect that the cycle of changes of blood urea and nitrogen in a patient on chronic hemodialysis, as represented in Figure 18–4, indicates a sharp decrease during the dialytic treatment and a gradual increase during the interdialytic period.

During dialysis, BUN concentration decreases as a function of three parameters: dialyzer urea clearance (K_u), dialysis treatment time (td), and the volume of distribution of urea (V).

> Despite having the same BUN level as a smaller patient, a large patient will require more dialysis because of differing total body urea content and urea volume of distribution.

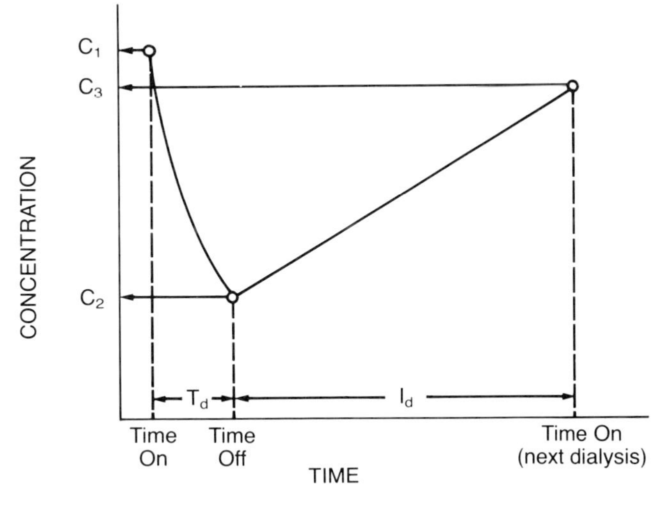

Figure 18–4. Change in solute concentration during and between dialyses. (From Sargent JA: Kinetic modeling in the guidance of dialysis therapy. Dial Transplant 8:1101, 1979.)

On the other hand, the increase in BUN during the interdialytic period depends on the following:

1. Rate of generation of urea. This is a function of the protein catabolic rate, which in a stable noncatabolic patient reflects dietary protein intake.
2. The volume of distribution of urea.
3. Residual renal function.

> KT/V is the most accepted index for determining adequacy of dialysis.

KT/V of 1 to 1.4 constitutes adequate dialysis.
KT/V of <0.8 is definitely inadequate.

Guidelines for adequate dialysis are shown in Table 18–3. In the NCDS, a protein catabolic rate of at least 1 gm/kg/day correlated with a lower morbidity.

DIALYSIS PRESCRIPTION

Writing a dialysis prescription requires the expertise of a physician who is knowledgeable about the physiologic principles of hemodialysis, the differing characteristics of the dialyzer membrane with which he or she is acquainted, and the proper choice of the dialysate solution most suitable for a patient's medical condition and perturbed biochemical profile. Patients who have ESRD and are on maintenance hemodialysis primarily need regular assessment of their dry weights and, most importantly, the most adequate dialysis prescription as discussed earlier. Patients with acute renal failure and those in whom hemodialysis for chronic renal failure is being initiated require close and often frequent assessment of their general medical condition and more careful supervision of their dialysis. The efficiency of dialysis in these special patients should be gradually increased.

Table 18–3. GUIDELINES FOR ADEQUATE DIALYSIS PRESCRIPTION

1. Target
   KT/V = 1 for thrice-weekly sessions
   KT/V = 1.5 for twice-weekly sessions
2. Assume V = 55% of body weight in females and 60% of body weight in males.
3. Assume K to be 20% less than the reported manufacturer's clearance.

e.g., 60 = kg man
K = 200 ml/min
∴ Actual K = 150 ml/min
V = 60 × 60% = 36 L
to get KT/V = 1 (on thrice-weekly schedule) requires:

$$\frac{(160 \text{ ml/min}) \times T}{36{,}000 \text{ ml}} = 1$$

$$\therefore T = \frac{36{,}000}{160} = 225 \text{ min} = 3 \text{ hr } 45 \text{ min}$$

4. Protein catabolic rate = 1 g/kg/day
5. TAC_{urea} = 50 mg/dl or midweek predialysis BUN = 60 to 80 mg/dl

Indications for Hemodialysis

Hemodialysis is indicated in patients with pericarditis; uremic encephalopathy; pulmonary edema refractory to diuretics; neuropathy; uremic bleeding; or a compromised nutritional state with anorexia, nausea, or vomiting. Biochemical indications include BUN close to 100 mg/dl; serum creatinine level of 10 mg/dl; creatinine clearance of 5 to 7 ml/min; and hyperkalemia and acidosis.

For patients with acute renal failure, the indications for dialysis often include volume overload, acidosis, and hyperkalemia that cannot be managed medically. **For patients who develop azotemia from chronic renal failure, rapid corrections of urea, fluid, and electrolytes may result in a disturbance in the pathophysiologic adaptation that occurs slowly in the response to renal failure, and a disequilibrium syndrome may arise.** In this case, the prescription for dialysis should be increased gradually from a KT/V of 0.5 during the first dialysis to a KT/V of 1 or greater by the third dialysis. This can occur over 3 to 5 days. **Reduction of the dose of dialysis can be achieved either by maintaining blood flows <200 ml/min, using a dialyzer with a smaller surface area, or administering blood and dialysate in a cocurrent fashion.**

In general, because patients with acute renal failure usually receive medical attention early in their disease, very few present with uremic encephalopathy. However, if this occurs, phenytoin at a loading dose of 1 g and maintenance dose of 300 mg should be given before the first dialysis but can be safely tapered after 2 to 3 weeks of dialysis. This treatment would prevent potential seizure activity. The composition of the dialysate is generally uniform in many electrolytes but needs to be specified in some others.

Dialysate sodium is typically 140 mEq/L except in patients with severe hyponatremia or hypernatremia. The dialysate sodium should be adjusted to prevent rapid correction of hyponatremia to avoid risk of central pontine myelinolysis and to avoid exacerbation of the disequilibrium syndrome by avoiding rapid correction of hypernatremia. Ultrafiltration itself will correct dilutional hyponatremia to a great extent. As a general guideline, hyponatremia should not be corrected at a rate faster than 0.7 to 1 mEq/L/hr, and hypernatremia should not be corrected at a rate faster than 1 mEq/L/hr.

The dialysate potassium level should be tailored according to the plasma potassium level and in general should not be lower than 1 mEq/L. Zero-potassium baths are not recommended. However, whenever they are used, serum potassium should be checked very frequently; otherwise, unrecognized dangerous hypokalemia may ensue, particularly as the metabolic acidosis is also corrected by dialysis.

The dialysate dextrose should be 200 mg/dl, particularly in patients with sepsis or diabetes mellitus or in patients receiving beta blockers.

Typical dialysate calcium is in the range of 3 to 3.5 mEq/L, which is equivalent to 6 to 7 mg/dl of ionized calcium. It then is in equilibrium with the ionized calcium in the serum, which generally is approximately 5 mg/dl. Therefore, in most cases, there will be a positive calcium balance in patients during every dialysis. A dialysate calcium of 2.5 mEq/L may be used for patients who are taking high doses of calcium containing phosphate binders and who are prone to or develop hypercalcemia during treatment with calcium supplements or vitamin D.

Dialysis Prescription in Acute Renal Failure

If the indication is solely fluid overload without significant azotemia or other electrolyte abnormalities, isolated ultrafiltration or continuous arteriovenous hemofiltration is the procedure of choice.

Three to 4 L of fluid removal would be sufficient to relieve the manifestations of pulmonary edema. **For hemodynamically unstable patients with volume overload, azotemia, hyperkalemia, or other metabolic abnormalities, sequential ultrafiltration followed by dialysis is more hemodynamically physiologic. If hyperkalemia is life-threatening, start hemodialysis initially to control the high potassium level, and remove fluid on dialysis by adjusting the TMP accordingly. Use a bicarbonate bath instead of an acetate bath.**

If a patient has severe azotemia, particularly if he or she is hyponatremic, and **if there is concern about the disequilibrium syndrome, then the initial dialysis should be short and should result in a reduction of the BUN to no more than 50% of predialysis level.** This is achieved by using initial blood flows of 150 to 200 ml/min and a dialyzer of smaller surface area (around 0.7 to 1 m^2) in a concurrent fashion. Duration of dialysis is gradually increased to 3 and then 4 hours. Patients with BUN >150 mg/dl may be given phenytoin prophylactically before dialysis. Phenytoin is continued for several days thereafter until they are stable.

Dialysis in Patients on Chronic Hemodialysis

Patients should be admitted to the hospital for initiation of dialysis and observed for a number of days during their first three dialyses, because the risk of disequilibrium and seizures is greatest during those periods. Patients with no other active medical problems can be discharged once they achieve a KT/V of 1.

A typical prescription for patients on chronic dialysis should specify the frequency of dialysis per week (usually 3 times a week); the time on dialysis, target KT/V = 1 to 1.4; the dialyzer; the blood flow rate (usually ≥300 ml/min); the dialysate flow rate (usually 500 ml/min); and the estimated dry weight. **This weight is the weight at which hypotension begins to occur, and it generally cannot be estimated until hypotension or severe cramps develop in the patient.** This estimated dry weight should be reassessed frequently, particularly at the beginning of dialysis initiation, because patients who present for dialysis often are malnourished. Once dialysis is initiated, their nutritional status may gradually improve, with a consequent increase in their dry weight.

Dialysate composition is usually determined by the composition of the central delivery system. Most modern facilities use bicarbonate as the base, because it is associated with fewer adverse symptoms and complications on dialysis. The concentration of bicarbonate in the typical dialysate is approximately 35 mEq/L, so that it can diffuse into the blood across a positive concentration gradient. Potassium is generally maintained at a concentration of 2 mEq/L in the dialysate. For patients who are maintained on digoxin, an increase in the potassium concentration to 3 mEq/L may be necessary to avoid the risk of digoxin toxicity associated with hypokalemia.

The prescription should also include the anticoagulation regimen—standard heparin, tight or no heparin, and regional or citrate anticoagulation.

Finally, the permanent vascular access diagram and instructions on needle placement should be specified.

COMPLICATIONS OF HEMODIALYSIS

Hemodialysis-Related Hypotension

Approximately 20% of hemodialysis patients experience hypotension during a regular hemodialysis procedure. The sequelae of this hypotension are protean and include nausea and vomiting, decreased mental status, particularly in the elderly, and postdialysis malaise and easy fatigability. Seizures, when they occur, are usually self-limited. Seizure activity more often occurs in patients who are being initiated on dialysis or are acutely ill with other conditions such as sepsis, myocardial infarction, hypoxia, or electrolyte imbalance. **The sequelae of hypotension in a patient on dialysis are not necessarily benign and may be accompanied by neurologic complications such as stroke; cardiac ischemia manifesting as angina, myocardial infarction, or arrhythmias; aspiration pneumonia; or vascular access clotting.** To understand the pathophysiologic basis of this hypotension, it is important to examine the determinants of blood pressure.

Mean arterial pressure is determined by peripheral vascular resistance (PVR) and cardiac output. Cardiac output is a function of stroke volume and heart rate, and stroke volume in turn depends on plasma volume and myocardial contractility. During hemodialysis, reduction of plasma volume will result in hypotension if the compensatory changes in heart rate, PVR, or myocardial contractility do not occur. The extent to which plasma volume decreases with ultrafiltration depends not only on the rate of ultrafiltration, but also on the *plasma refilling rate* of the vascular compartment from the intracellular and interstitial fluid compartments.

> The major problem underlying development of dialysis-induced hypotension is more rapid removal of fluid from the intravascular space than can be replaced, coupled with an inability to adequately increase PVR.

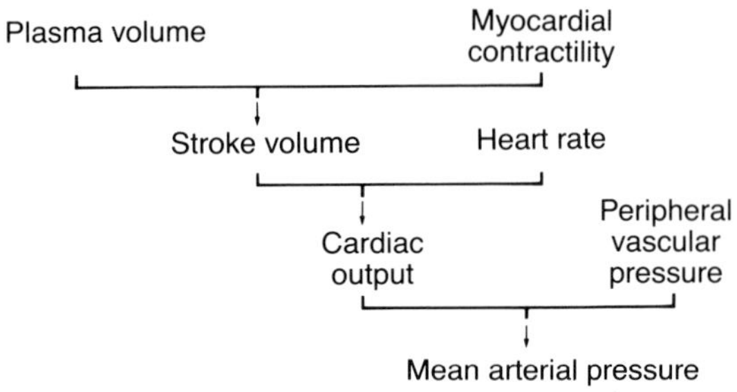

Figure 18–5. Determinants of systemic blood pressure.

Causes

The etiology of dialysis-associated hypotension is multifactorial. Regardless of the cause, the initial pathophysiologic event is a relative depletion of the vascular volume and decreased cardiac output. A glance at Figure 18–5 will quickly reveal the most common causes of dialysis hypotension, which are listed in Table 18–4 and briefly reviewed here.

Plasma Refilling Rate. The reduction in plasma volume produced by ultrafiltration leads to an increase in plasma oncotic pressure and a decrease in capillary hydrostatic pressure. Both promote mobilization of fluid from the extravascular space. The degree to which plasma volume declines depends on the relative ultrafiltration rates and plasma refilling rates from the intracellular and interstitial fluid compartments. The rate of ultrafiltration required during dialysis is determined by the interdialytic weight gain and duration of dialysis. Greater weight

Table 18–4. CAUSES OF HYPOTENSION DURING DIALYSIS

- Excessive or rapid removal of fluid greater than *plasma refilling rate*
  - High ultrafiltration rates, large interdialysis weight gain, and short therapy time.
  - Low estimated dry weight.
  - Low dialysate sodium concentration
  - Low plasma protein level
- Dialysate buffer
  - Sodium acetate
- Autonomic nervous system dysfunction
- Antihypertensive medications
- Cardiac factors
  - Hypertension
  - Pericardial effusion
  - Coronary artery disease
  - Cardiomyopathy
  - Negative inotropic agents
  - Anemia and arteriovenous fistula
- Warm dialysate solution
- Hypoxemia
- Blood-membrane interactions
- Miscellaneous: anemia, eating on dialysis, dialysate calcium, magnesium and potassium, depletion of catecholamines, interleukin-1

gains and shorter treatment times often cause hypotension. Patients should restrict interdialytic weight gains to 3% of their body weight. Too low an estimated dry weight also results in ultrafiltration rates that can exceed the rate of plasma refilling. **The first measure in chronic dialysis patients who were previously stable and who develop recurrent hypotension, particularly toward the end of their dialysis, is reassessment of their dry weight.** If a patient has a good appetite and there are no manifestations of fluid overload such as peripheral edema or predialysis hypertension, it is possible that muscle mass has increased. This type of hypotension would be particularly evident toward the end of dialysis as patients near their estimated dry weight. Evaluation of dry weight should be only gradual (0.5 to 1 kg at a time).

Other Factors. Other factors, particularly in the dialysate, also affect the frequency of hypotension. In particular, **dialysate sodium appears to be a major factor determining blood pressure stability during dialysis.** Low dialysate sodium (<136 mEq/L) reduces serum sodium level and promotes movement of extracellular sodium intracellularly, further exacerbating the plasma volume reduction induced by ultrafiltration. The effect of low dialysate sodium will be most pronounced during the early part of dialysis, when plasma sodium is decreasing most abruptly.

The hemodynamic response to volume depletion also varies with the dialytic process used. During conventional hemodialysis (*i.e.*, combined dialysis and ultrafiltration), there is a decrease in cardiac index and stroke volume index similar to that found during ultrafiltration alone. However, systemic vascular resistance does not change or decreases, leading to reductions in blood pressure. During isolated ultrafiltration, systemic vascular resistance increases and there is no significant change in blood pressure, although stroke volume and cardiac output decrease. Several lines of evidence suggest that serum osmolality changes account for the difference between these two dialytic procedures.

Acetate Buffer. The role of acetate buffer in cardiovascular instability is most notable in elderly dialysis patients who metabolize acetate slowly. Use of dialyzers with large surface area allowing a large influx of acetate, which may exceed a patient's ability to metabolize it to bicarbonate, is an important factor predisposing to hypotension. Although acetate causes vasodilation, vasodilation may not be the only basis for its effects on blood pressure. Data on the effect of acetate on myocardial function are conflicting. The hypoxemia associated with acetate dialysis is more severe than that with bicarbonate dialysis, and hypoxemia may play an important role in the pathogenesis of hypotension. Some investigators have noted that oxygen supplementation can correct hypoxemia and decrease the incidence of hypotension in patients on dialysis. **It is interesting to note that even when dialysis is performed against a dialysate sodium of 140 mEq/L, bicarbonate buffer with dialysate offers significant hemodynamic advantages over acetate, even in many stable patients on dialysis.** It has also been shown that plasma refilling rates with acetate dialysate are slower than with bicarbonate, and this effect is unrelated to osmotic changes.

Autonomic Nervous System. The role of autonomic nervous system dysfunction has been highlighted by some investigators, but others believe that this role is overemphasized. It is possible that there is impairment of vascular response to norepinephrine and that this impairment may be caused by acetate, hyponatremia, or hypokalemia. Autonomic neuropathy remains a common finding in patients on chronic dialysis, especially those with diabetes or, as some investigators believe, with severe secondary hyperparathyroidism. **The influence of autonomic neuropathy on the pathophysiology of hypotension results from patients' inability to respond appropriately to vascular volume depletion by increasing the PVR and/or heart rate.** Dilation of the capacitance vessels may also occur in autonomic neuropathy, with resultant peripheral pooling of blood and a decrease in central vascular volume. In addition, peripheral vasoconstriction may be pathologically altered by atherosclerosis or vasodilatory factors present during the procedure. An increased dialytic clearance and a reduced end-organ response to catecholamines may potentiate the hypotension in patients on chronic hemodialysis.

Antihypertensive Medications. Many antihypertensive medications impair vasoconstriction (*e.g.*, hydralazine). Beta blockers decrease cardiac contractility and limit the increase in heart rate in response to sympathetic influences. Because hypotension due to these medications is associated with predialysis hypertension, a therapeutic dilemma often arises. Hypertensive patients are often advised not to ingest these medications until after the dialysis session. A specific family of drugs that do not seem to predispose to hypotension during dialysis, even if ingested before dialysis, are the converting enzyme inhibitors, which are effective in the absence of renal function. Long-acting nitrates also decrease venous return and predispose to dialysis hypotension. Narcotic analgesics and anxiolytic agents also have hypotensive effects and should be avoided.

> Most antihypertensive medications, long-acting nitrates, and narcotics/anxiolytics should be withheld for 4 hours before dialysis if at all possible.

Cardiac Factors. The heart's ability to maintain or increase cardiac output in response to volume depletion plays a major role in the prevention of hypotension. Hypertrophy and dilatation of the left ventricle, increased age, atherosclerosis, and coronary artery disease all can limit this response. Decreased cardiac reserve may also be due to the chronic high-output state secondary to the anemia and presence of arteriovenous fistula. Pericardial effusions are usually small and not clinically significant. In the presence of congestive heart failure or pericarditis, which may be clinically silent, the pericardial effusions may increase and thus impair ventricular filling. Long-standing calcium and phosphorus abnormalities may predispose to ectopic calcification in the myocardium or conduction system, leading to decreased contractility or arrhythmias.

Warm Dialysate Solution. During hemodialysis, blood comes in contact with warmed dialysate and returns to the patient at a slightly increased temperature. Vasodilation and hypotension may occur.

Hypoxemia and Blood-Membrane Interactions. See separate sections.

Miscellaneous Causes. Postprandial hypotension is common and may aggravate the risk of hypotension during dialysis. Other causes include dialysate pyrogens, which may cause monocyte activation, increase interleukin-1 levels, and promote hypotension. Refractory hypotensive episodes have also occurred with severe hypermagnesemia. Table 18–5 lists the steps that are useful in the management of patients with frequent hypotensive episodes, and Table 18–6 summarizes the treatment of a hypotensive episode once it has occurred. Recently, several studies have examined the effects of dialysate calcium on myocardial performance during dialysis. These studies have suggested that a low dialysate calcium may be associated with increased incidence of hypotension but further studies are required.

Table 18–5. MANAGEMENT OF FREQUENT DIALYSIS HYPOTENSION

Reassessment of estimated dry weight. Gradual elevation of estimated dry weight (0.5–1 kg at a time).
Avoid antihypertensive drugs before dialysis. Reduce as much as possible other medications (narcotic analgesics, sedative/hypnotics, nitrates).
Increase hematocrit if very low (to above 25–30%)
Evaluate for silent pericardial effusion.
Patient participation
Avoid excessive interdialytic weight gains.
No eating during dialysis.
Increase dialysate sodium to 140 mEq/L.
Switch to bicarbonate dialysis (especially with high blood flow rates).
In selected patients, use a cool dialysate.
Prophylactic oxygen, particularly in elderly or patients with low predialysis paO_2.
Sequential ultrafiltration/dialysis is occasionally necessary when high ultrafiltration rates are required.

Muscle Cramps

Muscle cramps occur in approximately 10% of dialysis treatments. Cramps tend to occur more frequently after large amounts of ultrafiltration and/or at the end of dialysis if the weight has been allowed to decrease below the estimated dry weight. Muscle cramps most commonly occur in association with hypotension. In a minority of cases, cramps during dialysis occur without antecedent hypotension. Although the pathophysiology of cramps is not well understood, volume contraction of the extracellular fluid due to rapid ultrafiltration, particularly when associated with a rapidly changing plasma osmolality, is thought to be the major cause of dialysis-induced muscle cramps. In one study, cramps were associated with ultrafiltration rates of >700 ml/hr, whereas during treatment with ultrafiltration rates <400 ml/hr, cramps did not occur. The use of low-sodium dialysate solution is associated with a high incidence of muscle cramps.

Table 18–6. TREATMENT OF THE HYPOTENSIVE EPISODE

Trendelenburg's position
Reduce ultrafiltration pressure and flow rates
0.9% saline solution (100–200-ml boluses)
Hypertonic albumin (avoid in last 1 hour on dialysis) when serum albumin is low (<2.5)
Intranasal oxygen
Avoid pressor agents

Prevention

Prevention of muscle cramps is best achieved by reduction of interdialytic weight gains and hence the consequent need for rapid ultrafiltration. Repetitive dietary counseling may be helpful in some cases. In general, weight reductions of <3 to 5% of estimated dry weight can be easily tolerated. Higher interdialytic weight gains are also associated with more pronounced hyponatremia before dialysis; thus osmolality changes during dialysis are also accentuated.

Treatment

Several procedures are used to treat muscle cramps.

The **ultrafiltration rate can be decreased** temporarily.

Intermittent administration of **normal saline in 100-ml boluses** or hypertonic sodium chloride, 10 ml of 23% solution, can help. The disadvantage of administration of hypertonic or isotonic saline is that the net weight reduction during the dialysis procedure will be less. The repetitive use of hypertonic sodium chloride, particularly when given toward the end of dialysis, may lead to hyperosmolarity and increased thirst and weight gain in the interdialytic period.

Administration of 50 ml of **50% hypertonic glucose solution** or 10 ml of hypertonic saline is equivalent in terms of partial or complete relief of cramps.

A dialysate sodium of 140 mEq/L also helps treat cramps.

For patients with modest interdialytic weight gains and frequent cramping during dialysis, **quinine sulfate** may be beneficial. Quinine acts on skeletal muscle by increasing the refractory period and decreasing the excitability of motor end plate. It is degraded in the liver. A 260-mg dose given 2 hours before initiation of dialysis can decrease the frequency of intradialytic cramps.

Stretching muscles and standing up also helps. The treatment of muscle cramps should be tempered with the knowledge that although they are painful, they are not life-threatening. Thus, preventive measures based on assessment of the patient and the dialysis procedure are preferable to hasty overtreatment, which decreases the compliance required of the patient.

Assess the projected weight loss and estimated dry weight.

Nausea and Vomiting

Nausea and vomiting occur in about 5 to 10% of dialysis treatments. Most episodes are related to hypotension. They may also be an early manifestation of the dialysis disequilibrium syndrome in a newly initiated patient. Diabetic gastroparesis may also play a role. To treat nausea and vomiting, a physician should correct hypotension, if present. In addition, patients should receive promethazine (25 mg PO or IV), metoclopramide (5 mg PO), or cyproheptadine (4 mg PO).

Uremic Pruritus

Pruritus frequently complicates ESRD, occurring in approximately 25% of patients. In most cases, elevated parathyroid hormone and phosphate levels are common biochemical findings and presumably reflect the deposition of calcium phosphate crystals in the skin. Most commonly, patients become symptomatic coincident with the terminal stages of renal failure and before beginning dialysis. The institution of either hemodialysis or peritoneal dialysis frequently has little or no impact on itching. There is no consistent temporal relationship between pruritus and dialysis treatments. Some patients itch mostly during dialysis; others are most symptomatic on off-dialysis days. Most patients have worsening of itching during the summer. Pruritus is often episodic. The etiology of uremic pruritus in patients with normal calcium and phosphorus concentrations remains obscure. There is evidence suggesting a role of dermal mast cells in its etiology. In a small group of patients, the mast cell stabilizer ketotifen offered dramatic improvement. Dryness of the skin, allergens such as heparin and ethylene oxide, and histamine release from mast cells have all been implicated in the production of pruritus.

Treatment

To control pruritus, one must first control hyperphosphatemia and hyperparathyroidism. Topical emollients containing lanolin or camphor are relatively ineffective (only 18% of patients respond) but should be tried. The heparin formulation should be changed (beef to pork heparin or vice versa). Ultraviolet B phototherapy, twice weekly for 2 to 6 weeks, may offer relief. Repeat courses may be given. Oral antipruritics such as diphenhydramine (25 to 50 mg PO b.i.d.) and hydroxyzine HCl (10 mg PO t.i.d.) are sometimes effective. Oral activated charcoal (6 g daily) has also been suggested.

Bullous Dermatoses of Hemodialysis

This entity has been called *pseudoporphyria*. Like porphyria cutanea tarda, which has become a well-recognized phenomenon in patients undergoing chronic hemodialysis, pseudoporphyria is also characterized by cutaneous fragility and blistering of sunlight-exposed skin. Individuals typically have no history of porphyria cutanea tarda or cutaneous photosensitivity before beginning hemodialysis. Iron overload is often encountered. Hemoperfusion, in series with hemodialysis, may be effective.

Drug-induced bullous photodermatoses have to be ruled out; these drugs include tetracycline, furosemide, naproxen, vitamin B_6, dapsone, and nalidixic acid.

Complications Related to Anticoagulation

Clinical bleeding represents a major complication of acute and chronic renal failure and appears to be most directly related to a functional platelet disorder. It has been suggested that uremic patients have an abnormal platelet–vessel wall interaction. The capability of the vessel wall to generate a potent antiaggregatory substance, prostacyclin, increases in uremia, whereas endothelial cells seem to generate an abnormal Factor VIII: von Willebrand's factor. The hemorrhagic tendency in uremic patients is also influenced by the presence of anemia. A low hematocrit negatively influences the rheologic component of platelet–vessel wall interaction.

Treatment of uremic platelet dysfunction is outlined in Table 18–7.

Table 18–7. TREATMENT OF UREMIC PLATELET DYSFUNCTION

Red blood cell transfusions	Keep hematocrit >30%
Recombinant erythropoietin	
1-deamino-8-D-arginine vasopressin (DDAVP)*	0.3 μg/kg IV over 15–30 min (in 50 ml saline)
Cryoprecipitate†	10 units IV every 12–24 hr
Conjugated estrogens‡	0.6 mg/kg IV daily for 5 days

*Useful for acute bleeding before surgery; releases Factor fVIII/vWF from vascular endothelium; onset of action <1 hr, duration 4–8 hr; tachyphylaxis may develop after 1–2 doses.

†Useful for acute bleeding; risk of viral hepatitis and acquired immunodeficiency syndrome; rich in Factor fVIII/vWF and fibrinogen; onset of action 1–4 hr, duration 24–36 hr.

‡Not useful for acute bleeding; onset of action in 6 hr with progressive shortening of bleeding time over next 5–7 days; duration of action of about 2 weeks; mechanism of action unknown.

> The best laboratory hallmark of clinical bleeding caused by uremia is the bleeding time.

Heparin-Induced Bleeding

Although institution of dialysis corrects the functional platelet disorder that is encountered in uremic patients, the use of heparin plays an additional role in the bleeding complications related to hemodialysis. Heparin is required during hemodialysis to prevent extracorporeal blood clotting. Patients differ in their sensitivities to the anticoagulant action of heparin as well as their ability to metabolize heparin.

In addition to its effect on clotting parameters (enhancement of antithrombin III effect), bleeding complications from heparin may be due to heparin-induced thrombocytopenia, which has been reported in as many as 25% of patients receiving heparin. The highest incidence of thrombocytopenia is associated with heparin from bovine lung, whereas that from bovine intestinal mucosa appears to have a lower incidence. Thrombocytopenia may also occur during dialysis from blood-membrane interactions, leading to platelet aggregation, and is maximum at 1 hour into dialysis, with platelet counts declining to <100,000 after 1 hour from normal values at the start of dialysis.

Bleeding complications in patients on dialysis are not related only to the amount of heparin used but are also strongly influenced by the underlying risk factors of the patient. Such patient categories are listed in Table 18–8.

Hemorrhagic episodes in uremic patients range from mild disturbances such as ecchymoses, epistaxis, and purpura to more dramatic episodes such as gastrointestinal bleeding, retroperitoneal bleeding, hemopericardium, and subdural hematomas. These hemorrhages are often spontaneous and not associated with any overt trauma or invasive procedures. Many other episodes of hemorrhage are related to ill-timed diagnostic or therapeutic procedures.

> Diagnostic or therapeutic procedures (lumbar puncture, pleural tap, biopsy) should be avoided on dialysis days.

Gastrointestinal Bleeding. Lesions such as telangiectasia, gastritis, and duodenitis occur more frequently in patients on maintenance dialysis than in the general population. Peptic ulcers do not appear to be significantly more common in patients on hemodialysis in the absence of hypercalcemia. Hypergastrinemia is present in patients on dialysis but does not appear to be ulcerogenic in this setting. **Endoscopy is an essential part of a patient's evaluation, because many lesions are missed by x-ray studies.** Guaiac-positive stools are commonly noted in patients on dialysis. Unselected patients on chronic hemodialysis have been reported to have twice the blood loss than a group of azotemic nondialyzed patients (6.3 vs. 3.2 ml/day). Causes of lower gastrointestinal bleeding in dialyzed patients include telangiectasias and angiodysplasia, cecal colonic ulcers, stercoral ulcers (rectal ulcers produced by pressure necrosis by feces on the rectal mucosa), and diverticular disease (especially in patients with polycystic kidney disease). Constipation caused by phosphate binders and the presence of autonomic neuropathy may exacerbate diverticular disease.

Subdural Hematoma. Subdural hematoma has been reported to occur in up to 1% of patients on dialysis. **It should be suspected in any patient who experiences a change in mental status or an unusually persistent headache or neurologic disturbance.** Subdural hematomas are reported to be more common in patients who experience the dialysis disequilibrium syndrome because of the associated increase in cerebrospinal fluid pressure and brain swelling. Computed tomographic scanning is particularly helpful in establishing the diagnosis.

Table 18–8. CONDITIONS IN WHICH CITRATE ANTICOAGULATION IS RECOMMENDED

Conditions
Any active bleeding
Recent surgery with bleeding complications
Surgery in which bleeding is deleterious
Cardiovascular surgery
Ophthalmic surgery
Renal transplantation
Brain surgery
Pericarditis
Intracerebral hemorrhage
Thrombocytopenia
Coagulopathy

Retroperitoneal Bleeding. Spontaneous retroperitoneal bleeding may present as occult acute anemia or may be associated with acute abdominal distress, obstructive jaundice, or femoral nerve palsy. The bleeding may be very insidious, delaying the correct diagnosis. Nonspontaneous retroperitoneal hemorrhage is likely to be more common and is associated with iatrogenic causes such as diagnostic angiography or inadvertent puncture of the femoral artery during placement of a femoral vein dialysis catheter.

Anticoagulation Regimens

During dialysis, heparin is given to prevent clotting in the extracorporeal circuit. Activated clotting time (ACT) is assessed at frequent intervals to determine the safest amount of heparin needed and to prevent prolonged bleeding. Several methods of heparin administration are possible, and familiarity with these methods is important in the management of patients.

Systemic Heparinization. Heparin is administered either by the infusion pump method or by the bolus method. A bolus dose of heparin, usually 50 units/kg of lean body weight, is given; then an infusion pump is started, delivering around 500 to 1000 units of heparin per hour. The loading dose is increased to 75 units/kg if the patient is on erythropoietin. The infusion pump is usually stopped 30 minutes to 1 hour before the end of dialysis. The ACT is monitored and aimed at twice the baseline values during heparin administration. ACTs should be obtained on each new admission and once a month before dialysis, 1 hour after initiation of dialysis, and ½ hour before the end of dialysis.

Toward the end of dialysis, ACTs in the range of 170 seconds are appropriate.

The following actions are suggested (based on clotting times and depending on individual patient):

ACT	Action to be Taken
<1 minute	Push 2000 units heparin
1–2 minutes	Push 1000 units heparin
2–3 minutes	Push 500 units heparin
3–4 minutes	No action
>5 minutes	Hold heparin

Patients with external shunts, subclavian catheters, and hemocaths should have their ACT kept at 3½ to 4 minutes during dialysis.

Additional ACT measurements should be

done when clot or fibrin formation is observed in the venous trap; when a patient has an infection; when a patient has recently had a bleeding problem; or when a patient had dialyzer clotting during the treatment.

Tight Heparin Regimen. Indications include moderate bleeding risk such as pericarditis or recent surgery. Target clotting times are 150 to 160 seconds with the ACT method. To avoid fluctuations in heparin levels, the continuous infusion technique rather than the bolus method is recommended.

Heparin-Free Regimen. This is the method used in patients with active bleeding, in patients in whom heparin is contraindicated, or in patients who are at high risk of bleeding (Table 18–9). This regimen uses initial rinsing of the extracorporeal circuit with saline and heparin, but without infusing this saline into the patient. After initiation of dialysis, periodic saline rinse with 300 ml every 15 minutes is needed. This technique is not recommended with subclavian or femoral catheters or for patients in whom a blood flow of at least 300 ml/min cannot be achieved. The risk of clotting of the dialyzer is about 15% with this regimen. Blood products or hyperalimentation lipids should not be administered during heparin-free dialysis.

Citrate Anticoagulation Regimen. This is the method of choice for patients who are at high risk for bleeding or who are actively bleeding. In this technique, blood in the extracorporeal circuit is anticoagulated by chelating its calcium with sodium citrate and by using a zero-calcium dialysate bath. At the same time, an infusion of calcium chloride is given to the patient through the venous limb distal to the dialyzer. About two thirds of the citrate returns to the patient and is metabolized. A modified method of citrate anticoagulation is infusion only of citrate. No zero-calcium bath or calcium reinfusion is used. Risk of clotting with citrate anticoagulation is low, and the advantage over heparin-free dialysis is that high blood flows are not necessary. Serum calcium level should be monitored, and risk of alkalemia should be considered because citrate is also metabolized to bicarbonate. Citrate infusion rate is adjusted according to the ACT.

Regional Heparinization. In this technique, protamine sulfate is used distal to the dialyzer to neutralize the heparin administered proximal to the dialyzer. This technique is rarely used now.

Hemodialysis-Associated Hypoxemia

Hemodialysis with acetate dialysate is accompanied by the development of hypoxemia, occurring within 15 minutes of initiation of dialysis in up to 90% of patients, and decreasing the arterial oxygen tension (paO_2) from 5 to 35 mm Hg. The decrease in paO_2 typically is 10 to 20% of baseline. In many patients, this reduction is of no clinical significance, but it may be critical in patients with limited cardiac or pulmonary reserve. The type of dialyzer membrane and the dialysate bath (acetate) are major factors in the development of this hypoxemia.

Cellulosic dialyzer membranes (particularly cuprophane) activate the alternative complement pathway. Within minutes after contact with the blood, they induce leukoagglutination and neutropenia. Pulmonary sequestration of white blood cell aggregates causes intrapulmonary diffusion defects and widening of the alveolar-arterial oxygen difference, causing early (5 to 15 minutes) modest hypoxia. Minimal complement activation is also caused by polysulfone, polyacrylonitrile, and polymethyl methacrylate membranes. The duration of complement activation is longer with the cellulosic membranes (up to 90 minutes). With reuse process, cuprophane's ability to activate complement is decreased. Complement activation leads in addition to leukoagglutination to release of vasoactive substances that may raise pulmonary artery pressure. This rise in pulmonary artery pressure has been documented with cellulose membranes at times of neutropenia but not with polyacrylonitrile membranes, which do not activate complement and may scavenge vasoactive substances.

With acetate buffer, the hypoxemia is more severe and additive to that resulting from the dialysis membrane and usually occurs later in dialysis (15 to 60 minutes). Acetate-containing dialysate causes hypoventilation and subsequent hypoxemia by three mechanisms: (1) Hypocapnia results from loss of carbon dioxide to the dialysis solution. (2) During acetate dialysis, the respiratory quotient (carbon dioxide produced/oxygen consumed) is decreased. This results in hypocapnia with subsequent hypoxemia. (3) Consumption of oxygen by the metabolism of acetate.

Bicarbonate dialysate solutions can also result in hypoventilation, particularly when bicarbonate in the dialysate is >35 mEq/L. The resulting metabolic alkalosis may cause hypoventilation.

Preventive measures such as the use of bicarbonate buffer, a noncomplement-activating membrane, and supplemental oxygen can lessen the incidence of dialysis hypoxemia and is important to patients with an already compromised cardiopulmonary status, such as patients with predialysis pO_2 levels <80 mm Hg.

Dialysis-Associated Pericarditis

Pericarditis occurs in 8 to 12% of patients on hemodialysis. Tamponade has been reported to occur in a high percentage of dialyzed patients developing pericardial disease. Pericardial effusion is frequently present and is almost consistently hemorrhagic. An identifiable period of inadequate dialysis was found in 56% of patients in one large series. Antecedent viral or bacterial infection antedated 36% of pericarditis episodes in the same series, but purulent pericarditis was identified in none of these patients. Evidence from several studies negates any possible etiologic role of anticoagulation. Volume overload and malnutrition, possibly a reflection of inadequate dialysis, are also predisposing factors. **Hypotensive episodes early during dialysis and thrombosis of dialysis access can be early warning signs and must alert physicians to impending tamponade.** Constrictive pericarditis has been reported in 12% of patients with dialysis-associated pericarditis.

Chest pain is the most frequent complaint (76%) and is pleuritic in 46% of cases. Dyspnea occurs less frequently. About 8% of patients are asymptomatic. A pericardial friction rub occurs at some point during the clinical course in the majority (85%) of patients. The absence of these signs does not rule out the presence of a large pericardial effusion. Fever occurs in about one fourth of cases. The chest x-ray film shows pericardial fat pad in only 7% of patients with large pericardial effusions. Cardiomegaly is present in 96% of patients. Manifestations of volume overload (pleural effusion and pulmonary edema) are present in 25 to 50% of cases. The echocardiogram demonstrates pericardial effusion in 90% of cases. Although small-volume posterior fluid collection is commonly seen, anterior effusions are indicative of large effusions. Electrocardiogram shows ST-T changes indicative of pericarditis in 30% of patients. Most commonly associated arrhythmias are atrial fibrillation and flutter (in approximately 18%). Finding a pericardial friction rub in a patient with chest pain is highly suggestive of the diagnosis.

Treatment

Treatment of dialysis-associated pericarditis is controversial, but the most accepted stepwise approach is outlined below:

The first step is intensive dialysis (for hemodynamically insignificant effusion), consisting of five to seven sessions per week for 2 weeks. The benefits are questionable in dialysis-associated pericarditis. The response rate is variable in different series and ranges from 10 to 56%. This is in contrast to uremic pericarditis, in which the majority of patients improve rapidly with initiation of dialysis (90%).

Carefully decrease estimated dry weight, avoiding hypotension, which may acutely decrease venous return and cardiac output.

Provide adequate nutrition.

Use tight heparin or citrate anticoagulation.

Administer indomethacin (25 to 50 mg PO t.i.d.) or prednisone (10 mg) for a few days to alleviate symptoms, particularly chest pain.

Hemodynamic parameters of patients treated by intensive dialysis should be closely observed. Repeat echocardiograms every 3 days or more frequently are necessary, particularly if the intensity of friction rub decreases, because this may herald further fluid accumulation. **If hemodynamic evidence of pretamponade or tamponade appears, if the pericardial effusion progressively increases in size, or if a large pericardial effusion persists after 7 to 10 days of intensive dialysis, then the pericardial effusion should be drained.** If the echocardiogram is inadequate for interpretation but evidence of tamponade is physiologically present, the presence of tamponade should ideally be confirmed by cardiac catheterization before attempting surgical drainage. The choice of pericardial drainage procedure depends on local experience.

Pericardiectomy is the definitive procedure. Surgical mortality is <1%, recurrence is <1%, and success is 97%. It can be done by left thoracoctomy or median sternotomy but carries significant morbidity.

Subxiphoid pericardiotomy with surgical placement of an intrapericardial catheter with or without intrapericardial steroid instillation has the advantages of low surgical mortality, a high success rate, and few complications. Intrapericardial triamcinolone is given (50 mg every 6 hours for 2 to 3 days). There is an increased risk of infection. The advantage of this procedure is avoidance of thoracotomy and general anesthesia. The drainage tube is left in place for few days until drainage ceases.

Pericardiocentesis should be resorted to only in patients with life-threatening tamponade. Its complications include myocardial and coronary lacerations and arrhythmias. Pericardiocentesis is not effective for the treatment of pericarditis. Once the patient is stable, the ultimate surgical procedure should be performed.

Chest Pain on Dialysis

Differential diagnosis includes angina, myocardial infarction, first-use syndrome (often associated with backache), acute hemolysis, pericarditis, and a myriad of other causes.

Treatment

Treatment of anginal episodes during dialysis includes nasal oxygen at 2 to 3 L; support of blood pressure if hypotension is present; stopping ultrafiltration until hypotension subsides in this setting; nitroglycerin is given only after blood pressure is stable (otherwise nitroglycerin may produce more hypotension and worsen the angina); transfusion if anemia is present; and using bicarbonate bath to avoid hypotension-induced myocardial ischemia. Dialysis should be stopped, and the patient hospitalized, if the angina is unstable or the history and EKG are suggestive of a myocardial infarction.

Cardiac Arrhythmias in End-Stage Renal Disease and in Patients on Dialysis

Patients on hemodialysis are at special risk for arrhythmias due to factors unique to dialysis. Hypotension during hemodialysis may impair coronary perfusion and predispose to ischemia-induced arrythmia. Other factors that predispose to increased risk of arrhythmias include acute shifts in electrolytes during the procedure (sodium, potassium, calcium, bicarbonate, and magnesium) and cardiovascular instability during acetate dialysis (hypoxia, hypotension). **Electrolyte changes are particularly arrhythmogenic in patients on digitalis preparations (because of the transient hypokalemia, hypomagnesemia, and metabolic alkalosis).** Ischemic and hypertensive cardiovascular disease, pericarditis, and conduction system calcifications frequently underlie recurrent and sustained arrhythmias.

Dialysis may also provide a protective effect against ventricular arrhythmias by decreasing left ventricular failure volume and improving myocardial performance.

Arrhythmias Associated with the Use of Digitalis

Dialysis patients on digitalis preparations are particularly prone to arrythmias because of possible coexisting hypokalemia that results from low dialysate potassium concentration, intracellular movement of potassium from administered glucose (via dialysate or intravenously) or from metabolic alkalosis. In addition, hypercalcemia and hypomagnesemia may enhance the predilection to digitalis toxicity.

> Digitalis cardiotoxicity is prevented by avoidance of the drug.

Many patients are placed on digitalis for symptoms of congestive heart failure before initiation of maintenance hemodialysis. When dialysis is begun, most of the congestive symptoms can be relieved by reduction of volume overload. Reduction of cardiac size can also be achieved, thereby eliminating the need for digoxin, unless digoxin was given for control of ventricular rate in recurrent or persistent atrial fibrillation. Regardless, special caution is required when therapy is undertaken, because of metabolic alterations and drug interactions that can make antiarrhythmic therapy more risky than in the general population. Specifically, dietary counseling is of utmost importance to avoid predialysis hyperkalemia and to obviate the need for rapid rates of decrease of serum potassium on dialysis (Table 18–9).

Arrhythmias Unrelated to Digitalis

Arrhythmias often occur in patients with underlying cardiac disease. Patients with coronary artery disease are at greatest risk. Acetate dialysis in these patients may increase myocardial oxygen consumption (tachycardia and increased contractility). Hypoxemia, hypotension, and anemia are especially detrimental in individuals with fixed coronary stenosis. Hypokalemia does not play the same critical role as in patients with digitalis-induced arrhythmias.

The acute and chronic treatment of asymptomatic and/or life-threatening arrhythmias that

Table 18–9. APPROACH TO DIGITALIS-RELATED ARRHYTHMIAS

Use digoxin only if there is a good reason. Use the lowest dose possible.
Serum potassium level should not be allowed to decrease below 3.5 mEq/L during hemodialysis. Use 3–3.5 mEq/L dialysate potassium concentration.
Avoid excessive reduction of serum K when treating hyperkalemia.
Obtain dietary consultation to avoid predialysis hyperkalemia.
Minimize intracellular potassium shifts.
Avoid IV glucose for cramps or hypotension.
Omit or reduce dialysate glucose if patients are not at risk for hypoglycemia (to 100 mg/dl).
Reduce bicarbonate in dialysate.
If monitoring indicates that arrhythmia occurs mostly or is exacerbated during dialysis, administer a single oral dose of quinidine sulfate, 400 mg, 45 minutes before dialysis, or alternatively, 0.5 g of procainamide 45 minutes before dialysis.

occur during or between hemodialysis treatments is much the same as in nondialyzed patients, execpt that in ESRD the altered pharmacokinetics and protein binding of drugs should be taken into account. A detailed discussion of antiarrhythmic drugs is beyond the scope of this chapter. Important points about some of the common antiarrhythmic drugs are briefly discussed in the paragraphs that follow.

Classes of Antiarrhythmic Drugs

Class I: Sodium channel blockers

Class IA: Quinidine, procainamide, and disopyramide. These agents prolong repolarization and moderately slow conduction. The QT interval is increased. They are useful for atrial and ventricular arrhythmias.

Class IB: Lidocaine, tocainide, and mexiletine. These agents shorten repolarization and minimally slow conduction. The QT interval is unchanged. They are useful only for ventricular arrhythmias.

Class IC: Encainide and flecainide. These agents have little effect on repolarization but markedly slow conduction. The QT interval may be lengthened (↑ QRS but not JT interval). They are useful for atrial and ventricular arrhythmias.

Class II: Beta-adrenergic blockers.

Class III: Amiodarone and *N*-acetylprocainamide (NAPA). These agents primarily prolong repolarization.

Class IV: Calcium channel blockers.

Quinidine

Quinidine is heavily bound to plasma albumin, and binding is not altered by renal failure. Major elimination is by the hepatic route. The kidneys excrete 20 to 50% as unchanged drug. In ESRD, quinidine and active metabolites accumulate, increasing the risk of toxicity. The QT interval should be measured to assess both drug effect and toxicity. Enzyme immunoassay measures only parent quinidine, and a therapeutic level may be misleading because it does not measure the potentially effective active metabolites. A high serum level determined by methods that measure the parent compound and metabolites may be misleading because not all metabolites are active. **Quinidine is dialyzable.** A loading dose = 600 mg PO; the suggested dose in dialysis = 200 mg PO every 8 hours; therapeutic concentration = 2 to 5 mg/L.

Procainamide

Administration of procainamide in patients with renal failure is problematic. The half-life of procainamide is increased from 3 to 5 hours to 5 to 60 hours, and that of its metabolite, NAPA, from 6 to 8 hours to 40 to 70 hours. **NAPA excretion is entirely dependent on the renal route.** Dialysis removes both. Maintaining therapeutic levels is difficult for both, and the need for additional doses after dialysis leads to further variations of blood levels. It is best to avoid procainamide in patients on dialysis. A loading dose = 100 mg IV every 5 minutes (maximum-1000 mg). Maintenance dose = 250 mg PO every 12 hours in patients on dialysis. Therapeutic concentration of procainamide = 4 to 10 μg/ml; NAPA, 10 to 20 μg/ml.

Procainamide intoxications are more effectively treated with hemoperfusion than dialysis.

Disopyramide

Disopyramide poses many problems in patients on dialysis and patients with ESRD. Its anticholinergic activity can cause urinary retention. Dry mouth can lead to increased fluid intake. It has negative inotropic effect and should be given after dialysis. A loading dose (50% reduction) = 150 mg PO. Maintenance dose = 50 mg every 12 hours. Therapeutic concentration = 2 to 5 mg/L.

Digoxin

The half-life of digoxin is prolonged from 40 hours to 80 to 120 hours in ESRD. A loading dose over 24 hours should not exceed 0.325 to

0.5 mg, half the normal loading dose. Maintenance dose is 0.125 mg every other day.

Lidocaine and Phenytoin

These drugs are given in the usual doses: lidocaine, 1 to 3 mg/kg; maximum rate, 7 mg/min (loading dose); 1 to 4 mg/min (maintenance dose).

The loading dose of phenytoin is 1000 mg, given at 50 mg/min. Phenytoin is discussed in detail in the section on seizures.

Calcium Channel Blockers

These drugs can also be given in the usual doses: nifedipine, 30 to 60 mg/day; diltiazem, 120 to 240 mg/day.

Beta Blockers

The majority of beta blockers are degraded in the liver, and dosage and frequency of administration in patients on chronic dialysis are not substantially altered from those in patients with normal renal function. Atenolol in a dose of 50 to 100 mg once daily is recommended for ease of compliance. Propranolol may cause spurious hyperbilirubinemia.

Hemodialysis-Associated Seizures

Several clinical conditions predispose to seizure activity in uremic patients. Table 18–10 lists the causes of seizures in dialyzed patients. The seizure activity associated with uremia or dialysis tends to be generalized. The presence of focal seizure activity often indicates localized neurologic disease. Dialysis-associated seizures can occur during hemodialysis or after temination of the procedure.

Table 18–10. CAUSES OF SEIZURES IN DIALYSIS PATIENTS

Uremic encephalopathy
Disequilibrium syndrome
Hypotension
Hypertensive encephalopathy
Intracranial hemorrhage
Aluminum encephalopathy
Dialysance of anticonvulsant drugs
Epileptogenic drugs (e.g., penicillins)
Arrhythmias
Anaphylaxis
Hypoxemia
Alcohol withdrawal
Hypocalcemia (especially with correction of acidosis)
Hypertonicity (hypernatremia)
Hyponatremia
Hypoglycemia
Hypomagnesemia
Acid-base disturbances
Severe anemia

To lessen the risk of seizure activity during dialysis, particularly in predisposed patients, the following measures are recommended:

Limit osmotic changes during the initial few hemodialyses. Starting with a dialyzer membrane of small surface area, using low blood flow rates initially, and limiting the procedure to a short time are important measures to prevent the disequilibrium syndrome (see below). Some physicians would also use a cocurrent flow of blood and dialysate rather than a countercurrent flow that is routinely applied.

To limit osmotic shifts, use a high dialysate sodium of 140 mEq/L. If BUN is very high (>150 to 200 mg/dl), mannitol infusion (12.5 mg IV in each hour of the initial 2 hours of dialysis) may also be helpful.

Consider prophylactic anticonvulsant therapy if the risk is high, as in patients presenting with mental status changes: phenytoin, 1000 mg PO before dialysis, then 300 to 400 mg every day until the patient is stable. Withdraw medication gradually.

Use a bicarbonate bath instead of acetate to reduce the risk of hypotension.

In diabetic patients, use a dialysate glucose of 200 mg/dl to reduce the risk of hypoglycemia.

In severely hypocalcemic patients, especially in the presence of severe metabolic acidosis, consider calcium treatment even before dialysis if serum phosphorus level is not very high, and use a dialysate calcium of 3.5 mEq/L.

If a patient is known to be on anticonvulsant treatment, give an additional dose if the anticonvulsant is dialyzable (see later discussion).

Avoid rapid correction of uremia and hypertonicity simultaneously. If a patient is hypernatremic, a gradual reduction of serum sodium should be accomplished over 48 hours by dialyzing at dialysate sodium concentrations not much lower than serum sodium.

Check and use appropriate dosing regimens for drugs that may cause untoward central nervous system dysfunction (Table 18–11).

Central Nervous System Complications of Dialysis

The dialysis disequilibrium syndrome is more commonly encountered when a severely uremic patient is dialyzed aggressively. It can occur during dialysis or soon after dialysis.

Table 18–11. DRUGS THAT CAUSE UNEXPECTED NEUROLOGIC DISORDERS IN UREMIA*

Penicillins
Cephalosporins
Phenothiazines
Cimetidine
Meperidine
Morphine
Isoniazid
Reserpine
Anticoagulants
Cyproheptadine
Benzodiazepines
Barbiturates
Nitrofurantoin
Glutethimide
Ethchlorvynol
Meprobamate
Methaqualone
Haloperidol
Methyldopa
Antihistamines
Neuromuscular blocking agents
β-Adrenergic antagonists
Amantadine
Hypoglycemic agents

*Adapted with permission from Stone WJ: Medical complications of end-stage renal disease. In Stone WJ, Rabin PL (eds): End-Stage Renal Disease. New York, Academic Press, 1983, p 77.

Manifestations include nausea, vomiting, blurred vision, headache, muscle twitching, and restlessness. In the severe form, seizures, arrhythmias, and coma occur. The seizures are generalized. The pathogenesis of the disequilibrium syndrome is primarily attributed to cerebral edema. During hemodialysis, the urea concentration and osmolality in cerebrospinal fluid can decrease more slowly than in the blood. In addition, there is a paradoxical acidosis in the cerebrospinal fluid despite correction of severe metabolic acidosis (due to more rapid diffusion of carbon dioxide than bicarbonate across the blood-brain barrier).

Milder forms of the syndrome can also occur in patients on chronic dialysis, manifesting as nausea, vomiting, and headache. **If disequilibrium occurs during dialysis and there are severe manifestations such as seizures, obtundation, or coma, dialysis should be stopped.** Seizures are treated acutely with diazepam and phenytoin loading. Coma is treated supportively and usually subsides within 24 hours when it is due to dialysis disequilibrium syndrome.

Dialysis encephalopathy or dialysis dementia is a neurologic disease occurring primarily in patients on chronic maintenance hemodialysis for many years. It is largely accepted now that the disease is caused by aluminum intoxication. Its earliest manifestations are stuttering and stammering. Other features include myoclonus, seizures, personality changes, and progressive dementia. The electroencephalogram characteristically shows multiple bursts of delta or theta activity, at times accompanied by spikes, which may precede any clinical features of the disease by 4 to 6 months and may persist through its course. Associated other evidence of aluminum intoxication may be found, such as microcytic hypochromic anemia without iron deficiency and aluminum-associated osteomalacia. Baseline plasma aluminum levels >200 μg/L are strongly suspicious of high aluminum burden. A plasma aluminum level <100 μg/L does not rule out the diagnosis. It is uncommon, however, when baseline levels are <50 μg/L. A rise in plasma aluminum of 200 μg/L after deferoxamine challenge test is very suggestive of increased tissue burden of aluminum, and a rise >400 μg/L is very highly predictive of the diagnosis. If the baseline aluminum level is ≥150 μg/L, the deferoxamine challenge should be done with caution and a lower challenge dose used (500 mg to 1 g) because of the risk of precipitating encephalopathy. The high-risk patient should be admitted to the hospital; the test dose given at night, and 12 hours later (next morning) dialysis is performed. A bone biopsy from the iliac crest for aluminum stain is diagnostic. Dialysis frequently exacerbates the symptoms of dialysis dementia, especially seizures. When seizures occur, they respond well to diazepam. The disease is no longer necessarily debilitating and fatal if early diagnosis is made and chelation therapy with defroxamine is initiated. The best treatment of the disease is preventive. **Substituting calcium carbonate or calcium citrate for aluminum-containing phosphate binders and ensuring aluminum-free dialysate are the most important preventive aspects.** Chelation therapy should be continued until basal plasma aluminum levels are only slightly elevated and there is only a small increase in serum aluminum (20 to 30 μg/L) following deferoxamine challenge. One gram of deferoxamine is given twice weekly in the last ½ hour of hemodialysis in an infusion over 1 hour, and the infusion rate is slowed if hypotension occurs.

Anticonvulsant Drug Therapy

General guidelines for anticonvulsant drug therapy on dialysis follow:

Nondialyzable drugs include phenytoin and

carbamazepine. Valproic acid may be removed by hemodialysis.

Dialyzable drugs (need supplemental dose after dialysis) include phenobarbital, ethosuximide, trimethadione, paraldehyde, and primidone. Primidone should be used with extreme caution.

Carbamazepine, ethosuximide, valproic acid, and phenobarbital can be given in 75 to 100% of the usual dose to dialysis patients.

With phenytoin, normally 90% is protein bound and the volume of distribution is 0.6 L/kg. Its half-life is 24 hours. In ESRD, protein binding decreases and half-life decreases to 8 hours. The normal therapeutic range of total drug is 10 to 20 μg/ml. If the fraction unbound is 0.1 (normally), then the free (unbound) fraction that is associated with optimal treatment is 1 to 2 μg/ml. Drugs known to displace phenytoin from plasma protein-binding sites include valproic acid, nonsteroidal antiinflammatory drugs, and salicylic acid. In uremia, the unbound protein fraction can increase up to 0.3. Thus, the concentration of the *total* drug recommended for the patient with ESRD is 5 to 10 μg/ml.

Phenytoin follows dose-dependent kinetics. Any increase in dosing should be small, and sufficient time should be allowed for patients to achieve a new steady state. The altered protein binding and shortened half-life necessitate two adjustments in the dosage schedules of phenytoin in uremia. Give the drug in divided dosage (t.i.d. schedule). If the unbound fraction determinations are not available, then one half to one third of normal range total blood levels should be sufficiently therapeutic.

Hemolysis

Acute hemolysis during dialysis most often is caused by metals or other organic or inorganic substances in the water used for preparation of the dialysate. These include zinc and copper (piping), nitrates and nitrites (water), and chloramine (water purification). Formaldehyde, a disinfectant used to cleanse dialyzers and water and dialysate pipes for reuse, can cause an immunologically mediated hemolysis in addition to being a potent reducing agent. Other causes include overheated dialysate and hypotonic dialysate.

Acute hemolysis is a medical emergency. It may present as chest pain, shortness of breath, or back pain; a port wine appearance of blood in the venous line and pink discoloration of plasma together with an acute decline in hematocrit are clues to the diagnosis. Its most dangerous complication is hyperkalemia, which might lead to cardiac arrest.

Treatment

To treat acute hemolysis, stop the blood pump immediately and clamp the lines. Do not return the blood to the patient. Treat the hyperkalemia. Be aware that delayed hemolysis may occur.

Other causes of hemolysis in dialyzed patients include hypersplenism, infections such as hepatitis and pneumonia, and medications. Drugs causing hemolysis include penicillins, cephalosporins, sulfonamides, phenacetin, hydralazine, alpha-methyldopa, and antimalarials.

Air Embolism

Fortunately, the risk of this catastrophic complication of hemodialysis is small. Air usually enters through the venous end of the extracorporeal circuit. The signs and symptoms of air embolism depend on a patient's position. In patients who are seated or whose head is elevated, air passes up the jugular vein into the cerebral venous system, resulting in loss of consciousness, convulsions, or death. Classically, the patient cries out in alarm because of the sound of air rushing through the venous system. When a patient is lying flat, air forms foam in the right ventricle, interfering with its pumping ability. In patients lying on their right side, air may go to the pulmonary arteries, resulting in acute pulmonary hypertension. Some air may pass to the left ventricle, with resulting arterial embolization, cardiac arrhythmias, and neurologic deficits, and patients may experience sudden dyspnea, agitation, cyanosis, respiratory arrest, and loss of consciousness. Auscultation of the heart reveals a churning sound caused by the air foam in the heart. In patients in Trendelenburg's position, air will pass to the lower extremities, resulting in patchy cyanosis. If air remains entrapped in leg veins, there may be no catastrophic consequences.

Treatment

To treat air embolism, clamp the venous line immediately. Place patients in Trendelenburg's position on their left side. This traps air into the right ventricle, away from the pulmonary valve. Intubate patients if they are unconscious; use 100% mask oxygen if conscious. Attempt intracardiac needle aspiration if foam is detected in the right side of the heart. Defer cardiac massage until foam is evacuated. Administer corticosteroids to reduce cerebral edema. Use a decompression chamber if it is available.

Fever and Endotoxemia

Febrile reactions during dialysis are either the result of endotoxemia causing a pyrogenic reaction (leaching of endotoxin from the membrane) or are due to an infection (an infected access site or an unrelated infection). Rarely they are due to overheated dialysate. Fever due to infection most likely occurs at the start of dialysis or shortly after its end. Fever at the start of dialysis usually is due to contaminated equipment. Fever and chills during the course of dialysis are more likely due to pyrogen reaction. Fever developing within an hour or so of the end of dialysis suggests that infection has occurred during the termination procedure.

To prevent febrile reactions, dialysis equipment should be effectively disinfected, particularly for home dialysis patients and high-flux dialyzers that are more porous. Bicarbonate should not be stored too long because it can support rapid bacterial growth. Solutions prepared from concentrate should be mixed immediately before dialysis.

In undiagnosed febrile reactions, start empiric treatment with vancomycin and an aminoglycoside until culture results are returned.

Overheated dialysis solution can cause severe hemolysis and lethal hyperkalemia. Patients feel an increasing sensation of warmth, and overheating will usually be detected before temperature rise is extreme. Dialysate temperature >51°C causes immediate massive hemolysis and hyperkalemia. Temperature between 47 and 51°C can cause delayed hemolysis (up to 48 hours).

HIGH-EFFICIENCY AND HIGH-FLUX HEMODIALYSIS

Advances in dialysis technology as well as strong patient preference for shorter treatments have recently led to successful implementations of "short dialysis" to treat uremic patients. Dialysis time with such therapy has been reduced to between 6 and 9 hours per week. Short dialysis may ultimately relieve the economic constraints imposed on dialysis units and allow enrollment of more patients dialyzing at a unit.

To achieve a high rate of solute removal during ultrashort dialysis, two approaches have been used. In the first, using high-efficiency dialyzers with a high permeability for small solutes with molecular weight of less than 1000, diffusion across a concentration gradient is the primary mode of solute transport. In the second approach, described as "high flux," dialyzers that have ultrafiltration coefficients of 25 to 60 ml/hr/mm Hg are used. With such dialyzers, the convective contribution to the removal of middle- and high-molecular-weight solutes is significant; hence, much higher clearances of large solutes such as β_2-microglobulin can be achieved. However, the ability to remove large solutes from blood also poses the potential problem of convective transport of large solutes from dialysate to blood. Clinical experience with high-flux dialysis is still limited.

In high-efficiency dialysis, technical requirements for rapid high-efficiency therapies include high blood flow rates, ultrafiltration control systems, bicarbonate as the buffer source, and higher-efficiency dialyzers.

The achievement of adequate fluid removal depends not only on the ability to achieve the desired rate of fluid removal in a reliable and predictable manner, but also on a patient's ability to tolerate the desired rate of fluid removal without untoward symptoms. The use of a direct ultrafiltration control system rather than the indirect control of TMP greatly facilitates fluid removal with high-efficiency dialysis. One of the principal causes of dialysis-induced hypotension is hypovolemia, which results from imbalance between the rate of ultrafiltration and the rate of vascular refilling. Modeling studies of the dynamics of vascular refilling showed large interpatient differences in the hydraulic capillary endothelium permeability. Patients with low permeability will be prone to hypovolemia, and such interpatient variability may pose a limiting factor to shortening treatment time.

Intradialytic complications related to high-efficiency dialysis may relate also to high rates of acetate influx from dialysate to blood, and this, coupled with high rates of osmolality changes, can lead to marked cardiovascular instability. Using a bicarbonate buffer instead allows achievement of desirable dry weight as well as reduction in intradialytic symptoms such as nausea, vomiting, headaches, and hypotension. Bicarbonate dialysis is more complex than acetate dialysis and requires appropriate monitoring and proportioning systems for mixing the acid and bicarbonate concentrates. Bicarbonate concentrates in addition have been shown to support growth of gram-negative organisms that produce significant amounts of endotoxins, and appropriate culture techniques are required to monitor bacterial contamination. Fortunately, such monitoring techniques are available. Avoidance of prolonged storage of bicarbonate concentrates is essential.

Using the urea kinetic modeling, the Regional Kidney Disease Program in Minneapolis reported its experience in more than 300 patients on high-efficiency dialysis. Their target KT/V was 1.3. Blood flow rates were 380 ml/min. Dialysate flow rates were 700 ml/min. Cellulose acetate membranes were used. Treatment time was 165 minutes. Bicarbonate at 35 mEq/L was used as the buffer. The dialysate sodium was 142 mEq/L. Urea clearance of 300 ml/minute was achieved. It is of note that 30% of their patients were diabetic, and the mean age was 59 years.

High-efficiency dialysis requires a blood access to deliver blood flows of 300 to 400 ml/minute. Weight gain in excess of 5 to 6 kg in the interdialytic period and a high incidence of hypotension on standard bicarbonate dialysis excluded patients from enrollment into the study. The incidence of intradialytic complications in this group of patients on high-efficiency dialysis was not different when compared with the incidence on standard dialysis from the large data base of the French Registry. Hypotension was defined as blood pressure less than 90 mm Hg. As assessed by the incidence and duration of hospitalizations, morbidity during high-efficiency dialysis was not different from that during standard dialysis. During an observation period of 12 months, 73% of patients remained on high-efficiency dialysis, 12% died, and 2.4% failed therapy. Causes of death were similar to those observed in patients on standard dialysis. Causes of failure included blood access problems and excessive weight gain, and some patients also had a high incidence of complications on both standard and high-efficiency dialysis.

Although long-term dialysis has given rise to the fear of development of hemodialysis-related amyloidosis, the impact of high-efficiency dialysis on β_2-microglobulin removal is undetermined. The long-term effects of this mode of therapy on patient survival is also unknown.

Selected Readings

Abreo K: Use of deferoxamine in the treatment of aluminum overload in dialysis patients. Semin Dial 1:55, 1988.

Campese VM: Cardiovascular instability during hemodialysis. Kidney Int 33 (Suppl 24):S186, 1988.

Collins AJ, Keshaviah P: "Short dialysis." High efficiency and high flux hemodialysis. AKF Nephrology Letter 5:21, 1988.

Daugirdas JT, Ing TS: First use reactions during hemodialysis: A definition of subtypes. Kidney Int 33 (Suppl 24):S37, 1988.

Dinarello CA, Kochk KM, Shaldon S: IL-1 and its relevance in patients treated with hemodialysis. *Kidney Int* 33(Suppl 24):S21, 1988.

Eiser AR: Gastrointestinal bleeding in maintenance dialysis patients. Semin Dial 1:198, 1988.

Francos GC: Uremic pruritus. Semin Dial 1:209, 1988.

Gotch FA, Sargent JA: A mechanistic analysis of the National Cooperative Dialysis Study (NCDS). Kidney Int 28:526, 1985.

Hakim RM, Lazarus JM: Complications during hemodialysis. *In* Nissenson AR, Fine RN, Gentile DE (eds): Clinical Dialysis. Norwalk, Appleton-Century-Crofts, 1984, pp 179–221.

Hakim RM, Lowrie EG: Hemodialysis-associated neutropenia and hypoxemia. The effects of dialyzer membrane materials. Nephron 32:32, 1982.

Jindal KK, Goldstein MB: Urea kinetic modeling in chronic hemodialysis: Benefits, problems, and practical solutions. Semin Dial 1:82, 1988.

Kleinman KS, Coburn JW: Amyloid syndromes associated with hemodialysis. Kidney Int 35:567, 1989.

Lynn RI, Feinfeld DA: Importance of residual renal function in end-stage renal disease. Semin Dial 2:1, 1989.

Milliner DS, Nebecker HG, Ott SM, et al: Use of the deferoxamine infusion test in the diagnosis of aluminum-related osteodystrophy. Ann Intern Med 101:775, 1984.

Nissenson AR, Ross EA: Dialysis-associated hypoxemia: Insights into pathophysiology and prevention. Semin Dial 1:33, 1988.

O'Hare JA, Collaghan NM, Murnaghan DJ: Dialysis encephalopathy. Medicine 62:129, 1983.

Parker TF, Laird NM, Lowrie EG: Comparison of the study groups in the National Cooperative Dialysis Study. A description of morbidity, mortality, and patient survival. Kidney Int 23(Suppl 13):S42, 1983.

Remuzzi G: Bleeding in renal failure. Lancet, May 28, 1988, pp 1205–1208.

Rutsky EA, Rostand SG: Pericarditis in end-stage renal disease: Clinical characteristics and management. Semin Dial 2:25, 1989.

Sherman RA: The pathophysiologic basis for hemodialysis related hypotension. Semin Dial 1:136, 1988.

Suki WN: Pericarditis. Kidney Int 33(Suppl 24):S10, 1988.

Tilney NL, Kirkman RL, Whittemore AD, et al: Vascular Access for Dialysis and Cancer Chemotherapy. Chicago, Yearbook Medical Publishers, 1986, pp 221–270.

Ullian ME, Hammond WS, Alfrey AC, et al: β_2-microglobulin-associated amyloidosis in chronic hemodialysis patients with carpal tunnel syndrome. Medicine 68:107, 1989.

vonBrecht JH, Flanigan MJ, Feeman RM, et al: Regional anticoagulation: Hemodialysis with hypertonic trisodium citrate. Am J Kidney Dis 8:196, 1986.

CHAPTER 19

RENAL TRANSPLANTATION

Douglas J. Norman

BASIC CONCEPTS/MECHANISMS

Components of a Transplant Program

Renal transplantation requires a multidisciplinary approach consisting of five major components: transplantation surgery, transplantation medicine, patient care nurse coordinators, a histocompatibility/transplantation laboratory, and an organ procurement agency.

Transplantation surgery encompasses organ procurement, the transplant surgery, and postoperative and outpatient surgical care. Transplant medicine comprises pretransplant patient evaluation, postoperative medical care including dialysis and the delivery of immunosuppression, and outpatient medical care.

The nurse coordinators organize and run the transplant office and clinics, coordinate the pretransplant workup of patients, maintain the transplant waiting lists, manage and monitor the data on the patients including laboratory studies and medications, and maintain the integrity of patients' records.

The histocompatibility/transplant laboratory is responsible for screening prospective transplant patients for the presence of anti-HLA antibodies, tissue typing the donors and recipients, crossmatching a recipient's sera with prospective donor cells, and providing the focal point for research and development into advanced techniques of tissue typing, immunomonitoring, and immunosuppression.

The organ procurement agency is responsible for procuring donor organs for patients on the kidney transplant waiting list, assuring the quality of these organs, educating the public about the need for donated organs, educating professionals in the hospitals regarding their responsibility for identifying potential organ donors, and providing a focal point for research and development into the areas of organ preservation and transportation.

Immunology and Immunogenetics

Basic Immunology

The immune system can be divided into two components: nonspecific immunity and specific immunity. The nonspecific immune system, the more primitive of the two, provides the initial barrier to invasion by microorganisms into the body. Its components are polymorphonuclear cells, basophils, eosinophils, platelets, fibrin, and other elements responsible for the inflammatory response. The principal functions of the nonspecific immune system are phagocytosis of invading microorganisms, presentation of these organisms to components of the specific immune system, and mediation of the inflammatory response.

The specific immune system is notable for its specificity and memory. Its components are lymphocytes and their subsets, T cells and B cells. There are three types of T cells: helper cells, suppressor cells, and cytolytic cells, each with its own function. Helper cells initiate the immune response and provide stimulation and growth factors (lymphokines) to other cells including cytolytic T cells, suppressor T cells, B cells, and macrophages. Suppressor cells regulate and turn off an immune response. Cytolytic cells destroy target cells. B cells differentiate into antibody-producing plasma cells. T and B memory cells are quickly reactivated and proliferate on reexposure to an antigen.

Highly variable regions of the T-cell antigen receptor molecule and of the immunoglobulin molecule provide the specificity for this system; each unique region links specifically to only one of millions of potential antigens. Diversity among these variable regions results from random rearrangement of many closely approximated genes in T cells and B cells, producing millions of different combinations. The rearrangement of genes and their subsequent decoding to synthesize polypeptides leads to an incredibly diverse repertoire of target binding structures on T cells and antibodies.

Six mechanisms of target cell injury operate in the specific immune system. These include antibody-dependent cell-mediated cytotoxicity (ADCC), antibody-mediated cytotoxicity, antibody-mediated opsonization of target cells and organisms, delayed-type hypersensitivity, direct T-cell-mediated cytotoxicity, and cytotoxicity mediated by natural killer cells. Most of these are probably involved in the immune response directed to a transplanted renal allograft. The initiation of the allorecognition response that eventually leads to the effector mechanisms of immunity just described depends on a number of cell surface molecules (CD2, CD8, CD4, CD3, LFA-3, and others) that function as adhesion and recognition molecules, cytokines (IL-1, IL-2, IL-3, IL-4, IL-5, IL-6, gamma interferon, tumor necrosis factor [TNF], B-cell growth, and differentiation factors) that serve as intercellular signals and mediators, and accessory cells (monocytes, tissue macrophages, dendritic cells, vascular endothelial cells) that present antigen to T cells (Table 19–1).

Table 19–1. INTERRELATED COMPONENTS OF THE SPECIFIC IMMUNE SYSTEM

Accessory Cells
- Macrophages/monocytes
- Dendritic cells
- Vascular endothelial cells

Inducer Cells
- T helper-inducer cells
- T suppressor-inducer cells

Effector Cells
- T cells → Cytotoxicity
- B cells → Antibodies
- NK cells → ADCC
- Macrophages → DTH
- T cells → DTH
- T cells → Suppression

Memory Cells
- T memory cells
- B memory cells

Cytokines

Lymphokines	*Monokines*
IL-2	IL-1
IL-3	IL-6
IL-4	TNF
IL-5	
Gamma interferon	
LT/TNF	
GM-CSF	
BCGF	

Adhesion/Recognition Molecules

Adhesion	*Recognition*
ICAM	Class I
LFA-1	Class II
CD2	CD4
LFA-3	CD8
	T-cell receptor
	Hypervariable region of immunoglobulin

ADCC, Antibody-dependent cell-mediated cytotoxicity
DTH, Delayed-type hypersensitivity
TNF, Tumor necrosis factor
GM-CSF, Granulocyte-monocyte colony stimulation factor
LT/TNF, Lymphotoxin/tumor necrosis factor
BCGF, B-cell growth factor
ICAM, Intercellular adhesion molecule
LFA, Leukocyte function accessory molecule
CD, Cluster of differentiation

Immunogenetics

Basic Immunogenetics

The major histocompatibility complex (MHC) in humans is found in a small region on the short arm of the sixth chromosome. This region codes for the histocompatibility antigens that are known to be the strongest and that therefore elicit strong immune responses after organ transplantation. Matching for these antigens can reduce the strength of the immune response to a transplanted organ. The gene products of the major histocompatibility region are known as HLA (human leukocyte antigens) molecules or antigens. Every person has two sets (one on each chromosome) of major histocompatibility genes or haplotypes that are codominant—that is, the HLA gene products of each region are expressed equally on body tissues. Because we inherit one haplotype from each parent, we always share one haplotype with a parent, both haplotypes with 25% of our siblings, one haplotype with 50% of our siblings, and neither haplotype with 25% of our siblings. The expected matches among our relatives are shown in Table 19–2.

The genes of the MHC are divided into three classes: class I, class II, and class III. Class I genes code for HLA-A, -B, and -C antigens. Class II genes code for HLA-DP, -DQ, and -DR antigens (DN and DO do not have known products). Class III genes code for the complement components C2, C4, and Factor B. The location of these genes on the sixth chromosome can be seen in Figure 19–1. The tissue distribution of these molecular products of these genes is outlined in Table 19–3. Class I mole-

Table 19–2. FREQUENCY OF HAPLOTYPE MATCHES AMONG FAMILY MEMBERS FOR A PATIENT NEEDING A KIDNEY TRANSPLANT

	Two Haplotype Match	One Haplotype Match	Zero Haplotype Match
Parent	0%	100%	0%
Sibling	25%	50%	25%
Grandparent	0%	50%	50%
Aunt, uncle	0%	50%	50%
Cousin	0%	25%	75%

cules consist of a highly polymorphic glycoprotein heavy chain (approximately 44 kilodaltons) and a noncovalently bound monomorphic light chain, β_2-microglobulin (approximately 12 kilodaltons). The gene for the light chain is not found in the MHC. Class II molecules consist of two polymorphic glycoprotein chains, alpha and beta (approximately 45 kilodaltons each) that are noncovalently linked. Genes for both chains are located in the MHC.

The normal function of class I and II molecules is presumed to be the presentation of processed polypeptide products of a foreign material (antigen) such as a virus to the cells of the specific immune system. All T-cell-mediated specific immune responses are directed to foreign peptides presented in the context of self class I or II molecules. Class I-presented peptides interact with the T-cell receptor on CD8-bearing T cells (cytotoxic cells), and class II-presented peptides interact with the T-cell receptor on CD4-bearing T cells (helper/inducer cells). The exact mechanism by which foreign class I and II molecules on a renal allograft become the target for an immune response is not fully understood. However, it is likely that the foreign HLA molecules are perceived to be self plus a foreign peptide.

The HLA genes are the most polymorphic (many forms or alleles) of all of the genes in the human genome; Table 19–4 shows all of the recognized HLA-A, -B, -C, -D, -DR, -DQ, and -DP molecules. The methods used to detect specific HLA molecules on cells rely on the use of human alloantisera made as a normal result of pregnancy, blood transfusions, or transplantation. It is probable that these allosera are unable to detect small differences between the molecules with which they react; therefore, the number of different alleles at each of the MHC class I heavy chain and class II alpha and beta chain loci is probably much greater than currently recognized. Use of molecular genetic techniques has begun to support this viewpoint.

It is likely that minor histocompatibility genes exist on other human chromosomes. For example, minor histocompatibility genes are known to exist in mice, the species whose genome has been studied the most extensively. Like the HLA antigens, minor histocompatibility gene products probably perform a function other than determining histocompatibility. In humans, these functions are now completely unknown. The presence of minor histocompatibility genes and their products in humans is thought to explain the rare cases of graft loss among recipients of kidneys from HLA-identical (two haplotype matched) siblings.

The gene region for the T-cell antigen receptor consists of numerous V genes (variable), fewer J genes (junctional), fewer D genes (diversity), and one C gene (constant). The enormous diversity of antigen receptors required to recognize the millions of foreign antigens that humans can encounter during their lifetime is made possible by the propensity of this region

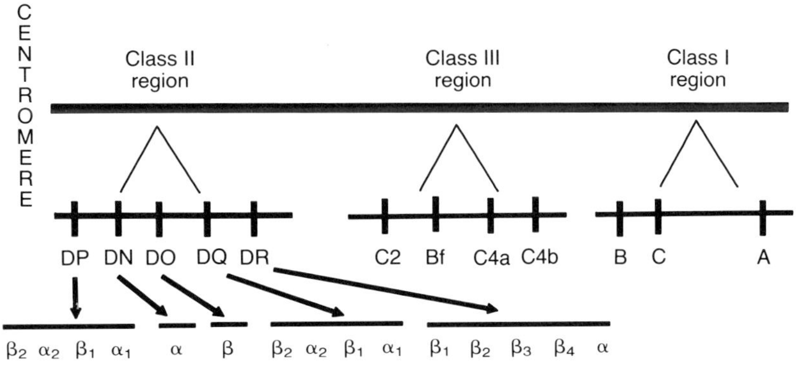

Figure 19–1. The major histocompatibility complex in humans. Genes coding for three classes of molecules are shown: class I, class II, and class III.

to rearrange its genes during an early phase of T-cell development to align one V, D, and J gene with the C gene. Some unused genes are cut out of the genome, and all of the offspring (clones) of a T cell with a rearranged antigen receptor gene will display the identical antigen receptor.

The gene region coding for the immunoglobulin molecules consists of numerous V genes, J genes, D genes, and one C gene for each immunoglobulin isotype (IgM, IgG, IgA, IgE, IgD and their subclasses). Like the T-cell antigen receptor genes, the immunoglobulin genes are rearranged during early differentiation to align one V, J, D, and C gene, and some unused genes are deleted. All offspring (clones) of a B cell with rearranged immunoglobulin genes make identical immunoglobulins (same isotype and same specificity).

The genes that code for class I and II molecules, the T-cell antigen receptor, immunoglobulin molecules, CD2, CD4, and CD8 molecules, and others collectively make up what is called the immunoglobulin supergene family because their molecular products consist of similar repeating glycoprotein domains.

Clinical Immunogenetics/Tissue Typing

The role of the tissue-typing laboratory in transplantation is to determine the tissue type of all prospective recipients and organ donors and to perform a crossmatch before transplantation so that no recipient with antibodies directed to donor HLA antigens will be chosen for transplantation.

Because many recipients still require blood transfusions, the crossmatch assay is perhaps the most important test performed by the laboratory. The basic ingredients for this assay are a current serum specimen plus the past serum that demonstrated peak lymphocyte-panel reactivity (see below) from the patient, donor cells (usually separated into T cells, B cells, and sometimes monocytes), and a method for determining whether or not antibodies in the sera react specifically with the donor's cells.

Table 19–3. TISSUE DISTRIBUTION OF MAJOR HISTOCOMPATIBILITY COMPLEX GENE PRODUCTS

Class I	Class II	Class III
Surface membrane of cells	Surface membrane of cells	Serum
All nucleated cells	B cells, macrophages, dendritic cells	
	Sperm	
	Activated cells including T cells, endothelial cells, and organ parenchymal cells	

Antibodies that can be detected in a crossmatch assay are either cytotoxic or noncytotoxic. Cytotoxic antibodies are capable of binding to and killing cells by a complement-mediated mechanism. Noncytotoxic antibodies are capable of binding to a cell and perhaps initiating inflammatory mechanisms *in vivo*, but they do not bind complement so cannot be detected using standard *in vitro* cytotoxicity assays (see below). Antibody specificities that can be detected in a crossmatch assay are (1) anti-class I and class II HLA antibodies, (2) autoantibodies, and (3) antibodies against antigens that are present on lymphocytes but may or may not be present on organ cells, so may not be important for transplantation.

The common tests that are used for the crossmatch include (1) a standard microlymphocytotoxic assay using a patient's serum, rabbit serum as a source of complement, a vital dye (such as eosin) and donor T cells or B cells, and (2) an enhanced or more sensitive assay. One enhanced assay uses all of the above plus an agent such as a goat antihuman kappa chain antibody that can either (1) convert noncytotoxic antibodies to cytotoxic antibodies or (2) enhance cytotoxicity of antibodies that are present in a low concentration. A second enhancing technique uses prolonged (twice as long) incubation of a patient's serum and complement with a donor's cells. Such a prolonged incubation crossmatch technique results in reactions that do not normally occur with the standard technique. A third even more sensitive technique uses a flow cytometer. Flow cytometry can detect all antibodies (cytotoxic or noncytotoxic) that bind to donor T or B cells. Recipient IgG antibodies can be differentiated from IgM antibodies by using either a goat anti-IgG or anti-IgM antibody as a developing reagent (the significance of IgM vs. IgG antibodies is discussed later). A fourth more sensitive technique that is rarely used today is one using antithymocyte globulin (ATG). A subcytotoxic concentration of ATG will enhance the cytotoxicity of a low-titer antibody that by itself cannot lyse a cell.

One can differentiate autoantibodies from alloantibodies by making several observations. A patient's serum that reacts with his or her own cells contains autoantibodies with or without alloantibodies. Chronic lymphocytic leukemia

Table 19–4. A COMPLETE LISTING OF RECOGNIZED HLA SPECIFICITIES

A	B	C	D	DR	DQ	DP
A1	B5	Cw1	Dw1	DR1	DQw1	DPw1
A2	B7	Cw2	Dw2	DR2	DQw2	DPw2
A3	B8	Cw3	Dw3	DR3	DQw3	DPw3
A9	B12	Cw4	Dw4	DR4	DQw4	DPw4
A10	B13	Cw5	Dw5	DR5	DQw5(w1)	DPw5
A11	B14	Cw6	Dw6	DRw6	DQw6(w1)	DPw6
Aw19	B15	Cw7	Dw7	DR7	DQw7(w3)	
A23(9)	B16	Cw8	Dw8	DRw8	DQw8(w3)	
A24(9)	B17	Cw9(w3)	Dw9	DR9	DQw9(w3)	
A25(10)	B18	Cw10(w3)	Dw10	DRw10		
A26(10)	B21	Cw11	Dw11(w7)	DRw11(5)		
A28	Bw22		Dw12	DRw12(5)		
A29(w19)	B27		Dw13	DRw13(w6)		
A30(w19)	B35		Dw14	DRw14(w6)		
A31(w19)	B37		Dw15	DRw15(2)		
A32(w19)	B38(16)		Dw16	DRw16(2)		
Aw33(w19)	B39(16)		Dw17(w7)	DRw17(3)		
Aw34(10)	B40		Dw18(w6)	DRw18(3)		
Aw36	Bw41		Dw19(w6)			
Aw43	Bw42		Dw20	DRw52		
Aw66(10)	B44(12)		Dw21			
Aw68(28)	B45(12)		Dw22	DRw53		
Aw69(28)	Bw46		Dw23			
Aw74(w19)	Bw47		Dw24			
	Bw48		Dw25			
	B49(21)		Dw26			
	Bw50(21)					
	B51(5)					
	Bw52(5)					
	Bw53					
	Bw54(w22)					
	Bw55(w22)					
	Bw56(w22)					
	Bw57(17)					
	Bw58(17)					
	Bw59					
	Bw60(40)					
	Bw61(40)					
	Bw62(15)					
	Bw63(15)					
	Bw64(14)					
	Bw65(14)					
	Bw67					
	Bw71(w70)					
	Bw70					
	Bw72(70)					
	Bw73					
	Bw75(15)					
	Bw76(15)					
	Bw77(15)					
	Bw4					
	Bw6					

(CLL) cells do not express the antigens to which most autoantibodies react. Therefore, sera that react with CLL cells are presumed to be directed to HLA. Further, autoantibodies are mostly IgM and can be differentiated from IgG either by using flow cytometric techniques (see above) or by reacting a serum with dithiothreitol (DTT), which destroys IgM but not IgG.

Donor cells used in the crossmatch generally come from the peripheral blood, lymph nodes, or spleen. A lymph node source is preferable because it contains an equal number of T cells and B cells, and these are uncontaminated by red blood cells (RBCs). B cells and T cells from the spleen are contaminated with RBCs, which can be difficult to remove. The peripheral blood is the most convenient source of cells for the crossmatch; however, only 10% of peripheral blood lymphocytes are B cells, making it difficult to find enough cells for the B-cell crossmatch. The advantage of peripheral blood is that it can be obtained before the donor surgery. Moreover, removal of contaminating RBCs from the lymphocytes is relatively easy.

There is little argument that antibodies that cause a positive standard T-cell crossmatch (anti-class I antibodies) can cause hyperacute or accelerated rejection. The more sensitive techniques detect low-titer or noncytotoxic antibodies that may not cause hyperacute or even accelerated rejection but may cause graft loss earlier than expected. The flow cytometric technique is the most sensitive and perhaps the least specific but has detected antibodies that caused hyperacute and accelerated rejection even when the standard crossmatches were negative. Some subgroups of patients may benefit more from the added sensitivity of a flow crossmatch: patients with a high panel-reactive antibody (PRA) (see below), regraft recipients, and multiparous women. These patients are the most likely to have anti-HLA antibodies. The value of a B-cell crossmatch (detecting anti-class II antibodies) is controversial, but convincing data exist showing that positive B-cell crossmatches (in the absence of a positive T-cell crossmatch) are associated with early graft loss.

There is some debate about which of the sera from a patient should be used in the final crossmatch. Most centers use the most current serum plus the one with the peak PRA. The serum with peak PRA is used because it contains antibodies that a patient made in the past and may be capable of making again. The relevance of the peak PRA serum if the current serum has a very low PRA is debatable; moreover, a crossmatch using the peak PRA serum may never be negative, making it unlikely that a patient will ever be a transplant recipient. If the PRA falls and remains below 5% for at least 6 months and the standard and flow crossmatch using the current serum is negative, the crossmatch result with the peak reactive serum can be disregarded with an acceptable clinical outcome.

The final choice of a recipient for a donor kidney can be made easier by knowing in advance of the crossmatch whether a patient has any anti-HLA antibodies. This is determined by testing a patient's serum for cytotoxicity against the lymphocytes of a panel of 48 individuals; the result is expressed as PRA percent. Individuals on the panel are either chosen at random to represent the usual frequencies of the HLA antigens or are selected so that all known HLA antigens are represented. If a patient has a high PRA, for example 80%, the chances of finding a crossmatch-negative donor for transplantation are low. If the PRA is zero, the chances of finding a donor with whom a recipient will have a negative crossmatch are quite good. **Therefore, knowing the PRA for each patient on the waiting list is important; a patient with a high PRA and a negative crossmatch should always be prioritized above a patient with a lower PRA and a negative crossmatch.**

The other major test that the histocompatibility laboratory performs is tissue typing. HLA antigen typing uses a microlymphocytotoxic assay similar to that for the standard crossmatch and PRA determination. A patient's cells are reacted on a tray containing monospecific alloantisera directed to each of the known HLA-A, -B, and -DR antigens (also, HLA-C and -DQ in many cases). The pattern of reactivity will identify the patient's HLA phenotype. A patient will occasionally be homozygous for an HLA antigen, so only one HLA-A, -B, or -DR antigen may be identified. The alloantisera used to detect HLA-A and -B specificities are well defined and of high quality; the probability that a patient in whom only one A or B antigen is found is homozygous for that antigen is 98%. The probability that a patient who types for only one DR antigen is homozygous is less, because DR alloantisera are less well defined.

Finally, the tissue-typing laboratory is also responsible for identifying the ABO blood group of the donor and the recipient and also for identifying minor RBC antigens such as Lewis that may be important in some cases. Transplantation cannot be performed across an incompatible ABO blood group barrier.

The U.S. Organ Procurement and Transplantation Network (United Network for Organ Sharing [UNOS]) currently mandates that phenotypically HLA-identical kidneys are to be shared. That is, if by using the UNOS computer, on which all patients in the United States awaiting a cadaveric kidney transplant are listed, a recipient is found who is phenotypically identical for the HLA-A, -B, and -DR antigens identified in a cadaveric donor, a kidney must be sent from that donor to that recipient. UNOS also mandates that cadaver kidneys are to be shared on the basis of ABO blood group identity and not compatibility. That is, blood group O kidneys cannot be placed into blood group A or blood group B recipients because an inordinant number of blood group O recipients would be left waiting for transplantation. This situation has occurred in the past.

Pathogenesis of Renal Dysfunction Episodes

Immunopathogenesis of Rejection

Rejection can be antibody mediated or cell mediated.

ANTIBODY MEDIATED

Hyperacute rejection occurs only rarely and results from antidonor antibodies circulating in the recipient at the time of transplantation. Antidonor antibodies in a patient's serum can develop from prior blood transfusions, pregnancies, or transplantation; the target of these antibodies may be donor class I or II antigens. The graft damage of hyperacute rejection begins by antibodies binding to class I or II antigens on endothelial cells. Complement is then activated, polymorphonuclear cells are recruited, platelets and fibrin are deposited, and microcapillary thrombosis and vasculitis occur. Hyperacute rejection usually occurs minutes to hours after transplantation, and the outcome is virtually 100% graft loss.

De novo antibody production can occur after allograft transplantation and can cause an accelerated graft loss. A final form of antibody-mediated rejection is chronic rejection. In the chronic form of rejection, antibodies seldom cause an acute inflammatory reaction but rather by reacting with vascular endothelium cause endothelial and intimal hyperplasia, which leads to vascular luminal narrowing, ischemia, tubular dropout, and interstitial fibrosis. Chronic rejection also eventually leads to 100% graft loss, but this can take from months to years to occur.

CELL MEDIATED

Cell-mediated rejection is the most common type of rejection encountered after transplantation. It has an onset within days to weeks after transplantation and is mediated by (1) direct T-cell killing, (2) T-cell and monocyte cooperation leading to cytokine and inflammatory mediator release, causing delayed-type hypersensitivity, and (3) perhaps cytotoxicity mediated by natural killer cells. Cell-mediated rejection generally causes an interstitial nephritis but can also cause a vasculitis. Acute cell-mediated rejection seldom causes acute graft loss, as lymphocytes are generally sensitive to steroids or to anti-T-cell antibody preparations, which can inactivate or lyse lymphocytes (see below). However, undetected low levels of cell-mediated rejection or repeated or severe cellular rejection can cause permanent tubular cell or endothelial cell damage, leading to interstitial fibrosis via ischemia or tubular cell necrosis. Patients with prior transplants or transfusions and particularly patients who have received donor-specific transfusions can have a "second-set" or accelerated cellular response due to the presence of memory cells that are quickly activated on exposure to the allograft antigens.

It is generally believed that the immune response that is generated to an allograft is initiated by donor leukocytes that accompany the organ as passengers and on connection of the organ with a recipient's circulation are the first to interact with recipient immune cells. Donor accessory cells (antigen-presenting cells) such as dendritic cells, as well as monocytes/macrophages, are able to directly stimulate recipient T helper cells by providing donor antigen and the appropriate monokine second signal.

Pathogenesis of Graft Dysfunction Due to Other Causes

Acute arterial or venous thrombosis can occur as a result of (1) an intimal tear in the artery induced while excising the donor kidney or by placing a clamp over the donor artery, (2) by hypotension, or (3) by a hypercoagulable state. Cyclosporine arteriopathy can lead to early graft loss and is believed to be due to direct endothelial cell damage leading to fibrin activation and capillary thrombosis. Recurrent glomerulonephritis occasionally leads to immediate graft loss. The most common forms are hemolytic-uremic syndrome, focal segmental glomerulosclerosis, and membranoproliferative glomerulonephritis (MPGN). The pathogenesis of these entities in the allograft is no better understood than in native kidneys. *De novo* glomerulonephritis can also occur in a renal allograft, presumably for the same reasons that it occurs in the native kidneys. A ureteral leak usually results from a failure of the ureteral neocystostomy or distal ureteral necrosis from an inadequate blood supply. Obstruction of urinary flow can result from distal ureteral fibrosis caused

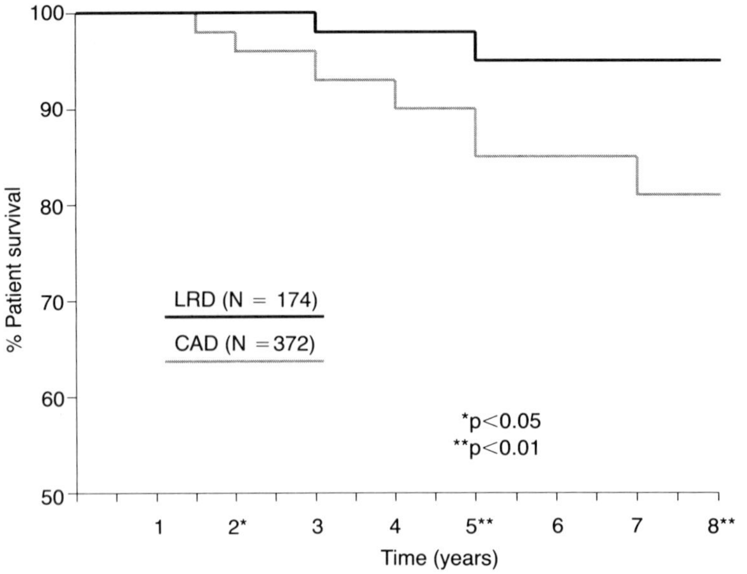

Figure 19–2. Actuarial patient survival among recipients of living related donor (LRD) or cadaveric donor (CAD) kidneys that functioned for at least 1 year. The source of the donor kidney is significantly correlated with outcome. (Oregon Health Sciences University.)

by rejection and a decreased blood supply, by a stone, by a blood clot, or by external compression from a lymphocele or hematoma. Drugs can cause renal dysfunction by directly damaging renal tissue, by inducing a hypersensitivity or allergic reaction in the kidney (in which case the kidney is an innocent bystander), by interfering with the normal function of the kidney without causing kidney damage, or by interfering with the tests that measure kidney function. Infection can cause renal dysfunction in two ways. The renal parenchyma itself can become infected, or infection can rarely trigger a rejection episode. The mechanism for this is not fully understood, but infection can increase the expression of class I and class II antigens on allograft cells. An increased expression of the target antigens might stimulate a rejection response. Renal artery stenosis occurs at the anastomosis site in almost all cases. It is presumed that the anastomosis is a target for platelet and fibrin deposition and atherosclerotic plaque formation.

Expected Clinical Outcomes

Patient Survival

Only rarely does a patient die as a result of a kidney transplantation; when death does occur, it usually is caused by the transplant surgery or the immunosuppressive drugs. However, as can be seen in Figure 19–2, the source of the organ

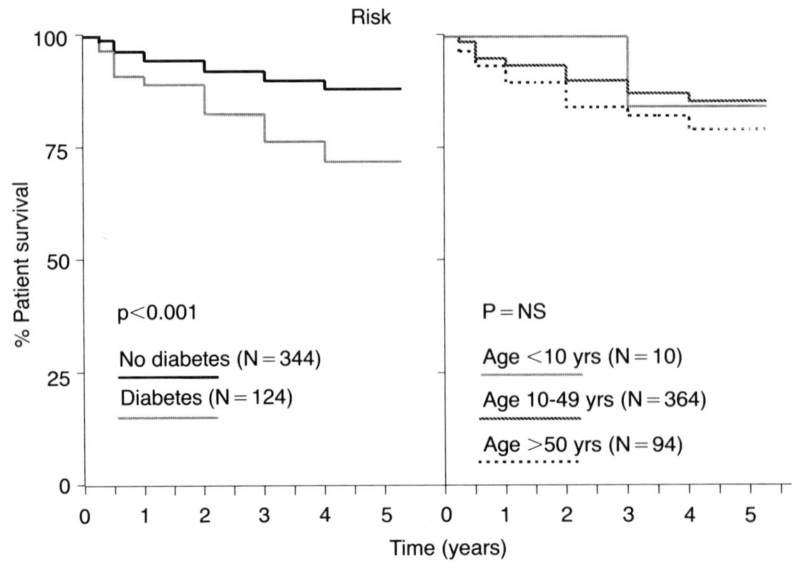

Figure 19–3. Actuarial patient survival according to risk category. The left panel shows that patient survival is significantly poorer among diabetic than among nondiabetic patients. The right panel shows that age does not correlate significantly with patient survival. (Oregon Health Sciences University.)

affects long-term survival of patients. Among recipients whose grafts functioned for at least 1 year, 5-year patient survival was 93% for recipients of living related donor kidneys compared with 85% for recipients of cadaveric donor kidneys. Among the reasons for this difference are that family donors donate to healthy recipients only, and that cadaveric donor kidney recipients receive more immunosuppression. The extrarenal health of recipients is also important. Figure 19–3 shows that survival among diabetic patients is clearly much poorer than among nondiabetics. This presumably is because of the higher incidence of cerebrovascular and coronary vascular disease among diabetics. However, the same figure indicates that age by itself is not a major determinant of survival.

Graft Survival

As is shown in Figure 19–4, graft survival is highly dependent on the antigen match between the donor and recipient. The half-life of a kidney that is an HLA-identical match with the recipient is 20 to 25 years. The half-life of a kidney that is a one-haplotype match is approximately 11 years, and the half-life of a cadaver donor kidney is approximately 7 years. Figure 19–5 shows that long-term graft survival is dependent on the source of the donor kidney even among patients whose kidneys functioned for at least 1 year. Although the subject is still controversial in 1990, the antigen match clearly does play a role in long-term graft survival even among cadaveric donor recipients. Recent data from UNOS (Table 19–5) indicate that the 12-month survival for a kidney with a six-antigen (2A, 2B, 2DR = 6) match is 88% and that there is a stepwise reduction in graft survival with lesser matches, the worst 12-month survival occurring with a zero-antigen match, 73%.

Second grafts do poorer than first grafts; the survival of a second graft is dependent on the survival of the first graft in the same patient. Patients who lose a first graft to accelerated rejection tend to have the same outcome with a second graft. The value of antigen matching among regrafted recipients and recipients with a high PRA is even more obvious than among first-graft and unsensitized recipients.

Graft survival for diabetic patients is poorer than for nondiabetics. In large part, this is the result of a higher death rate. No other systemic disease has either a positive or negative impact on outcome. Age has no major impact on graft survival except when accompanied by cardiovascular disease; the results of pediatric transplantation are somewhat inferior to adult transplantation.

Advances in immunosuppression have improved clinical outcomes. Both cyclosporine and anti-T-cell antibodies used for induction therapy have improved graft survival. Figure 19–6 shows the gradual improvement in graft survival encountered during the 1980s in relation to the immunosuppression used (Table 19–6). Patients who receive blood transfusions before transplantation have better graft survival;

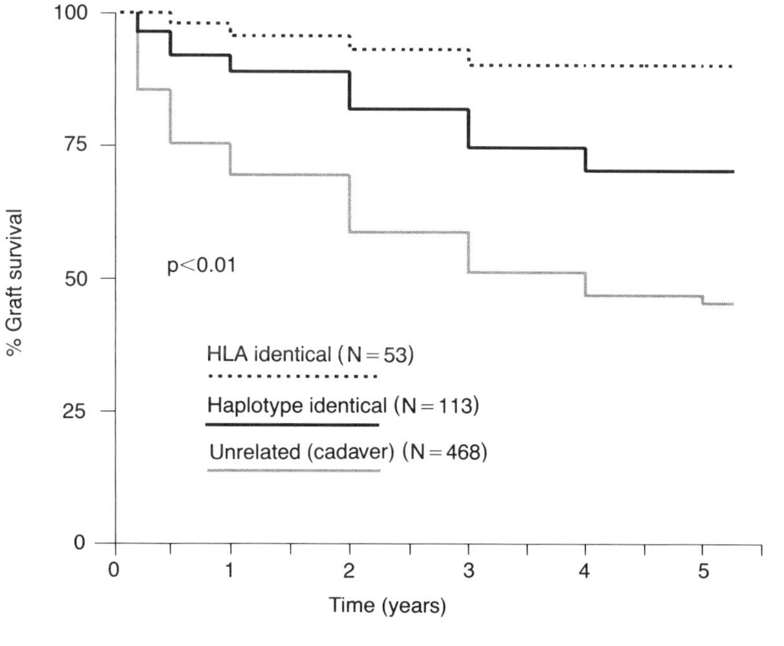

Figure 19–4. Actuarial kidney graft survival according to the source of the donor kidney. The best graft survival is among recipients of HLA identical kidneys, followed by recipients of haplo-identical kidneys, and finally unrelated (cadaveric) donor kidneys. (Oregon Health Sciences University.)

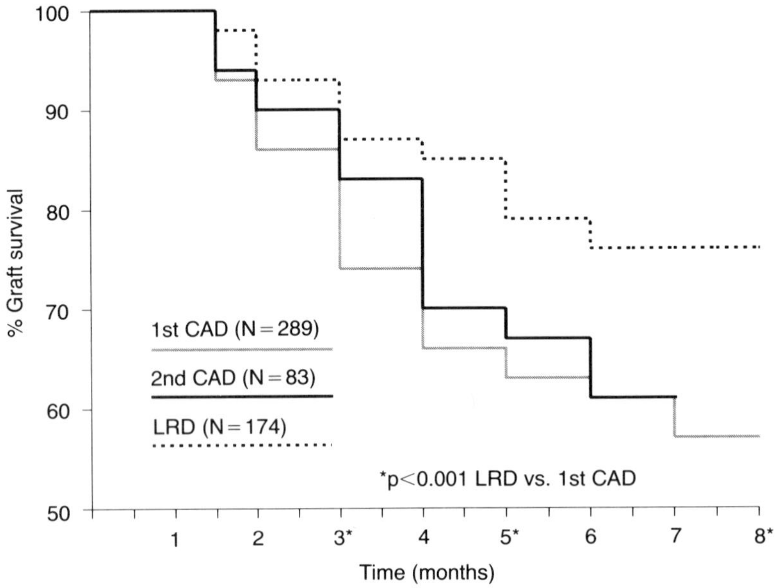

Figure 19–5. Actuarial kidney graft survival among patients whose kidney functioned for at least 1 year. Patients are grouped according to the donor source. Recipients of kidneys from living related donors (LRD) had significantly better graft survival than recipients of either first or second cadaver (CAD) grafts. (Oregon Health Sciences University.)

however, this has become much less obvious since immunosuppression has improved.

PRETRANSPLANT PREPARATION

Donor and recipient factors must be considered in pretransplant preparation.

The Donor and Donor Organ

Donor Selection Criteria and Management

Issues in kidney donation are extremely important for (1) protecting recipients from receiving an organ that may transmit disease or otherwise be damaged, (2) protecting living donors from losing a kidney that they might otherwise need, and (3) protecting living donors from unnecessary morbidity associated with the donation procedure.

Table 19–5. UNITED NETWORK FOR ORGAN SHARING 12-MONTH CADAVERIC KIDNEY GRAFT SURVIVAL

Antigen Match	Number of Patients	Percent Survival
6	89	88 ± 3.2
5	73	84 ± 3.9
4	257	81 ± 2.2
3	1170	81 ± 1.3
2	1562	79 ± 1.3
1	1383	76 ± 1.1
0	714	73 ± 1.7

From Terasaki PI: Clinical Transplants 1989. Los Angeles, UCLA Tissue Typing Laboratory, 1989, p. 3.

Living Donors

Living donors are a valuable resource for patients with end-stage renal disease (ESRD); the best long-term graft and patient survival occurs with a living related donor organ. Accordingly, families may attempt to coerce a sibling or child to be a kidney donor. This situation must be avoided, and all potential donors must be interviewed carefully by a trained social worker or the equivalent before they are accepted.

The standard living donor workup includes renal function tests, urinalysis and culture, intravenous pyelogram and arteriogram, as well as tests to rule out transmissible diseases such as infection and cancer. Donors must be able to survive on one kidney only; therefore, they must not have any evidence of kidney disease or of any systemic illness that predisposes to kidney disease. The long-term consequences of being left with a solitary kidney are unknown, although up to 25 years after donation there appears to be no adverse effect. The left kidney is preferred because of its longer renal vein; however, the smaller of the two kidneys or a kidney with unusual anatomy should always be used so that donors are left with the best kidney.

Cadaver Donors

The acceptable medical and legal criteria for declaring a patient dead vary from state to state

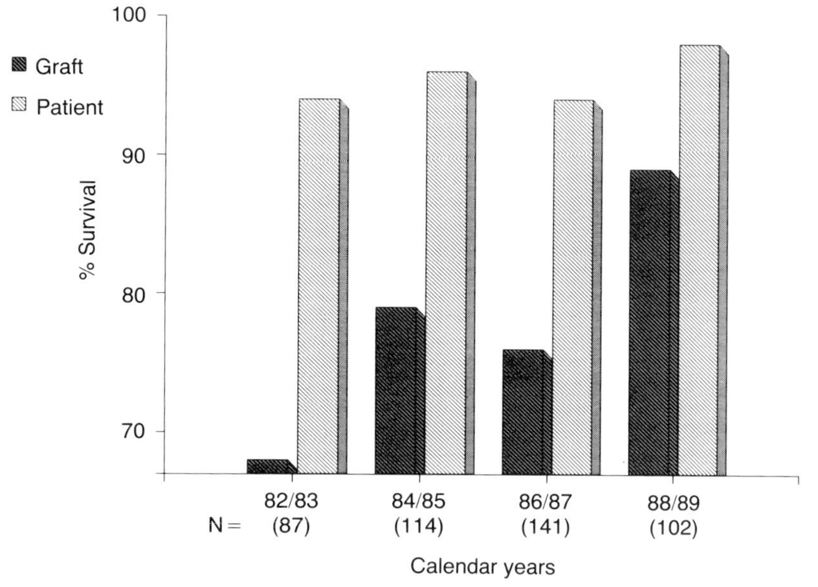

Figure 19–6. Six-month patient and graft survival among actual recipients of cadaveric kidneys according to the calendar years in which they were transplanted. Patients are grouped in 2-year periods. The immunosuppression used during these periods is shown in Table 19–6. Graft survival improved as newer immunosuppressive drugs were introduced (cyclosporine and OKT3). The best survival was seen when OKT3 was used for induction and cyclosporine, azathioprine, and prednisone were used for maintenance immunosuppression. (Oregon Health Sciences University.)

and country to country. Most states in the United States have adopted the uniform anatomic gift act, in which brain death is accepted as death of a patient. Accepted criteria for brain death are listed in Table 19–7. In general, two physicians must declare a patient brain dead, and neither of these should be among the primary transplant physicians or surgeons.

Contraindications for use of cadaveric kidneys vary from center to center. The age limits generally are 6 to 60 years. Donors with renal diseases (including long-standing uncontrolled hypertension) or transmissible diseases such as cancer or infection cannot be used for kidney donation. Kidneys from type 1 and 2 diabetic donors can be used if the renal function is normal and there is no proteinuria; however, these kidneys should not be used for diabetic recipients. The renal function of a cadaveric donor need not be normal; if the serum creatinine level became elevated after the mortal event, then it should be less than 2.5 mg/dl or declining steadily if above 2.5. Individuals with primary brain tumors are acceptable as donors, as are individuals with cured skin cancer or cervical cancer *in situ*. Patients with bacteremia are not acceptable as kidney donors, but patients with treated pneumonia or meningitis are acceptable.

Disseminated intravascular coagulation (DIC) is not uncommon among donors. Mild DIC is probably acceptable in the absence of a rising serum creatinine level or hemoglobinuria. If a patient with DIC is being considered for use as a donor, visual observation of the kidney and perhaps a biopsy at the time of explant is important to rule out severe kidney damage.

The cause of death should always be known in potential donors. If a potential donor dies mysteriously, an undiagnosed infection such as rabies may have been the cause.

According to the University of California, Los Angeles transplant registry, the ideal kidney donor is a male who suffered a traumatic death and the worst donor is a female who suffered a

Table 19–6. IMMUNOSUPPRESSION USED DURING THE 1980S

Year	Immunosuppression Used
1982–1983	Azathioprine and prednisone OKT3 for rejection
1984–1985	Azathioprine and prednisone Cyclosporine and prednisone OKT3 for rejection
1986–1987	Cyclosporine, azathioprine, and prednisone Steroids for rejection OKT3 for rescue and occasionally for prophylaxis
1988–1989	Cyclosporine, azathioprine, and prednisone OKT3 for prophylaxis Steroids for rejection

Table 19–7. BRAIN DEATH CRITERIA

1. A person is dead if he or she has sustained either
   a. irreversible cessation of circulation and respiratory function or
   b. irreversible cessation of all functions of the entire brain including the brain stem.
2. A determination of whether the combination described in paragraph a or b of section 1 has occurred must be made in accordance with accepted medical standards.

nontraumatic death and is over the age of 40. In general, any chronic systemic disease would be considered acceptable if the renal function is normal and the disease is not transmissible.

Most anatomic variations of the kidney are acceptable, including multiple arteries and veins, horseshoe kidneys, dysplastic kidneys, and kidneys with duplicated collecting systems. All anatomically abnormal kidneys should be considered because of the shortage of donor organs. Table 19–8 summarizes the criteria for kidney donation.

Donor Management

Management of a donor once brain death has been declared is an important responsibility of the donor team; it most often falls to the procurement nurse coordinator. The systolic blood pressure should be maintained above 90 mm Hg, and this can be achieved by using saline or, if the hematocrit is less than 30, blood products. Vasopressors are acceptable when necessary. Dopamine is the drug of choice, but dobutamine and isoproterenol have also been used. During surgery for excising the organs, a second- or third-generation cephalosporin is often used for prophylaxis.

Diagnostic Workup

The list of diagnostic studies to be performed in prospective donors includes tests for hepatitis B and C, human immunodeficiency virus (HIV), human T-cell lymphotrophic virus type 1 (HTLV-1), and syphilis (Table 19–9). These tests should be performed both before transfusions to reflect the state of donors themselves and after transfusions to reflect the status of the blood donors. Blood transfused from an infected blood donor to a kidney donor can potentially cause an infection in the kidney recipient. Tests to rule out transmissible disease should include a urinalysis and a chest radiograph. Kidney function tests and electrolytes should be evaluated every 3 hours.

Tissue typing of abdominal lymph nodes should be performed by the histocompatibility laboratory if possible. Peripheral blood can be used occasionally, but because of the problem with obtaining B cells from peripheral blood and the possible contamination of a donor's blood by blood transfusions, lymph nodes are always preferable. However, if adequate B cells can be obtained either from the peripheral blood or from an inguinal lymph node, a prospective crossmatch (performed before excision of a donor organ) and tissue type evaluation are preferred. If the tissue type of the donor and the crossmatch results are known before excision of the organs, ischemia time for the kidneys can be reduced.

Acceptable cold ischemia time for a cadaveric donor kidney is less than 48 hours. The preferred time is less than 36 hours. The warm time (time without perfusion with oxygenated blood or cold preservation solution) should be less than 1 minute when *in situ* flushing (the organs are flushed with the preservation fluids and rendered bloodless before being explanted) is performed.

Organ Preservation and Procurement

The preservation fluids that are most commonly used are Collins II and more recently the Wisconsin (Belzer) solution. The predominant form of preservation is an *in situ* flush with one of these solutions and then placement of

Table 19–8. CRITERIA FOR KIDNEY DONATION

Contraindications	Acceptable Complications
Bacteremia	Primary brain tumor
Other untreated infection	Treated pneumonia
Cancer	Treated meningitis
Recent history of IV drug use	Cured skin cancer
High-risk behavior for acquired immunodeficiency syndrome	Cured cervical cancer
	Mild disseminated intravascular coagulation
Age >60	Acute tubular necrosis if renal function improving
Age <6	Treated urinary tract infections
Unknown cause of death	Type 1 or 2 diabetes with normal renal function
Chronic severe and uncontrolled hypertension	Multiple renal arteries, veins, or ureters
Chronic renal disease	Horseshoe kidney
Cold ischemia time >48 hours	Recurrent herpes simplex infections if inactive
	Hypertension if mild
	Cardiac arrest if the renal function remained stable or is improving

Table 19–9. THE DONOR WORKUP

Transmissible Disease	Renal Function	Histocompatibility
Human immunodeficiency virus (HIV) Syphilis Hepatitis B Hepatitis C Human T-cell lymphotrophic virus type 1 (HTLV-1) Urine culture Chest radiograph	BUN, creatinine, electrolytes every 3 hours Urinalysis	HLA-A, -B, -DR typing Crossmatch

the kidney on ice. Some centers still perfuse kidneys, and although there is very little difference between a perfused and a cold-stored kidney for ischemia times less than 48 hours, there is some experimental evidence that perfusion is superior for kidneys preserved for more than 48 hours.

The Recipient

Transplant Recipient Selection

Medical Evaluation

The main purposes for medical evaluation of potential transplant recipients are (1) to rule out underlying diseases that may be exacerbated by surgery or immunosuppressive drugs, (2) to rule out renal diseases that may recur in a transplanted kidney, and (3) to rule out sociopathic behavior such as noncompliance or drug abuse. Any of these factors may hinder a patient's ability to carry out activities that are known to be absolutely necessary for the long-term success of a kidney transplant. The recipient evaluation is summarized in Table 19–10.

Infections. Chronic infections may not be manifest in an otherwise healthy dialysis patient but can become life-threatening infections in an immunosuppressed patient. Infection with human immunodeficiency virus is probably exacerbated by immunosuppressive drugs, and its presence should be ruled out. Active hepatitis B, manifest by surface antigenemia, is probably a contraindication to transplantation. Tuberculosis, syphilis, diabetic ulcers, and fungal skin infections must be identified and treated before transplantation. Patients with a history of herpes simplex infections should be given acyclovir prophylaxis with each outbreak before transplantation and should be given acyclovir prophylactically for up to a month after transplantation and with each antirejection drug treatment. The cytomegalovirus (CMV) status of the recipient should be identified, because it may be inadvisable to transplant a CMV-negative diabetic or older patient with a CMV-positive kidney. Depending on the part of the country, it may also be useful to screen for coccidioidomycosis, toxoplasmosis, and histoplasmosis.

In addition to these considerations, any patient with an active infection immediately before a scheduled transplantation should not undergo surgery. A bladder infection without pyelonephritis is not an absolute contraindication to transplantation, because nearly 100% of these can be treated successfully with perioperative antibiotics.

Tumors. Patients should be screened carefully for the presence of neoplasia. **The minimum workup for this is a mammogram and Pap smear in all women and a stool sample for occult blood in all patients.** Cytologic study of the bladder should be performed in patients

Table 19–10. THE RECIPIENT MEDICAL EVALUATION

Infections That Must be Identified Before Transplantation
Human immunodeficiency virus (HIV)
Syphilis
Tuberculosis
Hepatitis B
Diabetic ulcers
Fungal skin infections
Herpes simplex
Cytomegalovirus (CMV)
Tumor-Screening Evaluation
Mammogram
Pap smear
Stool for occult blood
Chest film
Bladder wash for cytology if a patient has been on cytoxin or long-standing (>5 years) immunosuppression
Ultrasonography or computed tomography of kidneys looking for neoplasia in acquired cysts
Other
Endoscopy in patients with symptoms of peptic ulcer disease
Stress thallium tests in diabetic, older patients (>50), symptomatic patients, patients with an abnormal electrocardiogram, or patients with risk factors
Pelvic angiography for patients with two prior allografts
Clotting tests to rule out hypercoagulable state
Pulmonary function testing in heavy smokers

who have been on cyclophosphamide or who have been on any immunosuppression for more than 5 years. **Any patient with a history of cancer should be completely free of recurrences 2 years after cessation of all chemotherapy** before consideration for transplantation. Patients should be informed of the potential risk of immunosuppression even if there has been no cancer recurrence. Breast cancer has been known to recur many years after an initial treatment, so for this entity the period of observation should be longer than 2 years before transplantation.

Peptic Ulcer Disease. Peptic ulcer disease has caused serious morbidity and death following organ transplantation. The stress associated with the surgical procedure and early postoperative management is thought to be the cause, as well as perhaps the high doses of steroids that can be necessary for treatment of rejection. Therefore, endoscopy is warranted in any patient who has symptoms of peptic ulcer disease and in any patient who previously had had an upper gastrointestinal bleed resulting from ulcer disease, even if he or she is not symptomatic at the time.

Cardiovascular Disease. Because the most common causes of death following kidney transplantation are myocardial infarction and stroke, the presence of significant cardiovascular disease should be sought before transplantation. All symptomatic patients, diabetic patients, patients over the age of 50, patients with an abnormal electrocardiogram, and patients with a combination of risk factors for cardiovascular disease such as hypercholesterolemia, hypertension, and smoking should have a stress thallium and treadmill test as part of the recipient evaluation. A thallium test when coupled with a treadmill test is 85 to 90% sensitive for detecting the presence of significant coronary disease. If these tests yield positive results, the patient needs to have coronary angiography; lesions should be treated with angioplasty or coronary artery bypass surgery. After such therapy, a repeat thallium test should no longer show reversible ischemia. **Patients who are found to have significant coronary disease that is untreatable should be advised to remain on dialysis and not undergo the risks of transplantation.**

Noninvasive vascular studies of the carotids and peripheral vessels should be performed in any patient with claudication, a history of transient ischemic attacks, or carotid or femoral artery bruits. Lower limb ulcers in diabetic patients should be evaluated by a vascular surgeon and must be healed before transplantation. In some patients, arteriography may be necessary to delineate the pelvic vessels; it must be performed in anyone with two prior kidney transplants, and it may be advisable for some diabetics, elderly patients, and patients with known vascular disease.

Original Cause of Renal Disease. The underlying cause of the original kidney disease must be identified in all cases when possible. Patients who have a history of **Goodpasture's syndrome** and have high-titer antiglomerular basement membrane antibodies should not undergo transplantation until the antibodies are no longer present or are present only in very low titer. Patients with active **lupus** should not receive a transplant because of the possibility of recurrence of lupus in the allograft. Unfortunately, lupus serologies are not always reliable in hemodialysis patients; patients without a history of lupus can develop a positive antinuclear antibody and hypocomplementemia as a result of interactions between their blood and dialysis membranes. Patients with a history of **Wegener's disease** should not undergo transplantation until there is evidence that this disease is quiescent. Certain forms of glomerular disease can recur in transplanted kidneys; most important among these are **focal glomerulosclerosis and membranoproliferative disease type II.** Both of these diseases can recur relatively soon after transplantation and can lead to immediate graft loss. Patients who lose their native kidneys rather quickly from either of these two disorders are at the highest risk for recurrence in the allograft if they undergo transplantation soon after the onset of renal failure; strong consideration should be given to avoiding the use of a living donor. **IgA nephropathy** and diabetes can recur in the allograft but rarely if ever lead to allograft failure. **Oxalosis** with evidence of ongoing peripheral vascular ischemia should be considered a contraindication to transplantation.

A hypercoagulable state should be ruled out in all prospective transplant recipients. If it is present, a patient will require postoperative anticoagulation with heparin initially and warfarin chronically. There is a small incidence of arterial or venous clotting immediately after transplantation; it most frequently occurs in patients with a hypercoagulable state or vascular disease, or following trauma to the donor organ vessels. Table 19–11 shows the typical screening battery that should be performed on all prospective transplant recipients to look for hypercoagulability.

Table 19–11. EVALUATION OF COAGULATION

Prothrombin time
Partial thromboplastin time (PTT)
Protein C activation
Protein S antigen
Anticardiolipin GMA
Kaolin clotting time

Pulmonary. All smokers should be advised to discontinue smoking before transplantation. Pulmonary function testing should be performed in heavy smokers. Patients with severe obstructive or restrictive airways disease should be counseled to avoid transplantation because of their high risk for pulmonary infections coupled with a low functional reserve.

Diabetes. The status of the common end-organ diseases should be assessed in all patients with diabetes. Vascular disease advances in diabetic patients at a higher rate than in nondiabetics after transplantation, presumably as a result of immunosuppressive therapy. Patients with severe vascular disease should be advised to avoid corticosteroids specifically and perhaps to avoid transplantation. **Both diabetic gastroparesis and diabetic enteropathy can impair normal absorption of immunosuppressive drugs and should be considered a relative contraindication to transplantation when present in an advanced form.** All diabetic ulcers must be healed before transplantation, because the institution of immunosuppressive therapy further worsens wound healing and makes patients highly susceptible to infections. A high percentage of diabetic patients with vascular disease will require limb amputation.

Compliance. Controlled substance abuse must be ruled out in renal transplant candidates because of the probability of poor compliance with medications. All patients who have had a history of drug use must have their urine screened for drugs. In addition, monthly unannounced drug screens of the urine or dialysate should be performed for 3 months. **If patients refuse to comply with this, then they should be denied the opportunity for transplantation.**

Each patient should have an interview with a trained social worker who is capable of ascertaining the probability of compliance with medications, laboratory tests, and clinic visits. In pursuit of this, the transplant program social worker should contact the social worker assigned to a patient's home dialysis unit to discuss issues of compliance with the hemodialysis regimen. The nurses and dietitian from the referring hemodialysis unit should also be interviewed in this regard. Specific issues that should be addressed are intradialytic weight gains; history of skipped dialysis sessions; diabetes control; calcium, phosphorus, and potassium control; blood pressure control; compliance with medications; and the presence of any medical condition due to neglect by the patient. Examples of the latter are untreated infections and skin disorders.

UROLOGIC EVALUATION

The purpose of a urologic workup is to assess the competency of the bladder and urethra and the possible need for native nephrectomy before transplantation (Table 19–12). All patients should have a voiding cystourethrogram. If significant urinary retention is present, a patient may have to perform clean intermittent self-catheterization after transplantation. Patients should be advised of this possibility and should be allowed to make a decision about whether they would prefer not to undergo transplantation if self-catheterization were to be required. If the bladder is small and nonfunctional, a urinary pouch made from a piece of bowel may be required, and it must be created and allowed to heal before transplantation. Any patient with a history of recurrent urinary tract infections and ureteral reflux to the native kidneys or kidney stones probably will require bilateral native nephrectomies before transplantation. Patients with long-standing chronic renal failure may acquire cysts in their failing kidneys, and the cyst epithelium may degenerate into a tumor. Abdominal ultrasonography of the native kidneys should always be performed as a screening test, and in the case of an abnormality, the native kidney should be evaluated for possible tumor. Questionable lesions should lead to a nephrectomy.

GENERAL SURGICAL EVALUATION

Because the circulation can be easily accessed by a subclavian or internal jugular vein catheter

Table 19–12. THE RECIPIENT SURGICAL EVALUATION

Urologic
Voiding cystourethrogram
Abdominal ultrasonography to assess for the presence of neoplasia in renal cysts
Urine culture
General
Abdominal ultrasonography for detection of gallstones

for dialysis, it is not required that patients have a permanent access for dialysis before transplantation. However, it should be known whether or not and what kind of access a patient has for dialysis. Dialysis accesses should be assessed for any evidence of a chronic infection. Abdominal ultrasonography should assess the gallbladder for the presence of stones. If stones are present, the current dogma is that a cholecystectomy should be performed before transplantation. An obstructed common duct with ascending cholangitis is associated with a high mortality rate in immunosuppressed patients. Alternatively, stones eroding through the gallbladder in a patient on steroids can lead to a catastrophic abdominal event. The adequacy of the pelvic vessels for vascular anastomosis should always be assessed in diabetics, older patients, and retransplanted patients. In most patients, palpation of the arterial pulses is sufficient. However, in some patients, pelvic arteriography may be necessary. The accessibility of the lower quadrants for surgery should be assessed. The location of the catheter for continuous ambulatory peritoneal dialysis (CAPD) and the presence of prior abdominal surgery should be noted. In general, left kidneys should be placed in the right lower quadrant and right kidneys in the left lower quadrant. Knowledge of prior abdominal surgery can help the procurement coordinators decide which of two kidneys should be assigned to an individual recipient. **If a patient has had significant diverticular bleeding, diverticulitis, or diverticular pain in the past, strong consideration should be given to partial colectomy before transplantation.**

Dental Evaluation

The teeth should be cleaned, all bad teeth should be removed, gum disease must be treated, and dental caries must be repaired. Patients should learn to practice meticulous oral hygiene, because the mouth is a frequent source of infectious complications after transplantation.

Social Service Evaluation

This evaluation should rule out psychiatric disease, assess patients' compliance, and, importantly, assess their financial capabilities. Posttransplantation follow-up and medications can be very expensive, and patients must have resources for these to ensure that the necessary laboratory and clinic follow-up are obtained and, most importantly, that the proper doses of medications will be taken. Patients also must have adequate transportation to and from the laboratory and the clinic.

Nutrition Evaluation

A renal dietitian should assess the dietary compliance as well as the current nutritional status.

Case Review

Following this extensive recipient evaluation, each patient's case must be presented to the Transplant Selection Committee. At this meeting, a report from Transplant Medicine, Urology, General Surgery, Dental Medicine, Social Service, Renal Nutrition, and the Nurse Transplant Coordinator should be presented. The advisability of transplantation should be established, and follow-up tests necessary because of findings during the evaluation should be recorded and forwarded to the nurse coordinator's office, the referring nephrologist, and the dialysis unit.

The final criteria for acceptance of a patient for transplantation will depend on a patient's compliance, the presence of systemic disease that would be made worse by immunosuppression and that would lead to a shortened survival, and financial resources available. All patients who have a potential living related donor then must wait for the donor evaluation. Patients who will be placed on the cadaver kidney waiting list must be registered on the UNOS computer if in the United States.

Pretransplant Patient Management

Immunologic Preparation

Many patients are still given blood transfusions for their immunosuppressive effect. At the Oregon Health Sciences University, all recipients require one unit of packed blood cells from an unrelated donor 6 weeks or more before transplantation. The American Red Cross allows the use of a designated donor, so a donor may be chosen by the recipient for this purpose. We have never seen recipients become sensitized to their HLA-identical donor as a result of blood transfusions. Transfused recipients of HLA-identical kidneys have fewer rejection episodes after transplantation.

Donor-specific transfusions (DST) for haploidentical recipients, although very successful in the era before the advent of cyclosporine, have been abandoned by many centers in the cyclosporine/OKT3 era because of the risk of sensitization, the logistical problems and expense associated with arranging them, and the hope that improved immunosuppression can substitute for the DST effect.

Each month a serum sample should be sent to the histocompatibility laboratory for assessment of anti-HLA antibodies and to provide a current serum sample to be used for the crossmatch. The histocompatibility laboratory must be notified each time a patient has a blood transfusion, and a current serum sample must be sent to the laboratory 2 weeks after this transfusion. If this is not done, a patient will have to have a repeat crossmatch with a fresh serum sample before transplantation.

There has been some experimentation with removal of anti-HLA antibodies using plasmapheresis or columns that are capable of removing immunoglobulin from a patient's blood. These techniques are still investigational, but in at least one report several patients with a high level of anti-HLA antibodies successfully underwent transplantation after use of such an antibody-removing column.

In the case of a living related donor transplant, immunosuppression with azathioprine is begun 1 week before transplantation. For patients who have demonstrated leukopenia or borderline leukopenia, prednisone should be begun with the azathioprine.

Notification of New Illnesses

Each time a patient develops an illness that contraindicates transplantation, the transplant unit must be notified and the patient will be temporarily placed in an off-the-waiting-list status. In general, this does not affect patients' priority on the waiting list once they are reinstated. High-risk (diabetic and older) patients should be reevaluated by the transplant program every 6 to 12 months, as they often develop progressive vascular disease that may contraindicate transplantation.

Patient Education

Educating patients about transplantation should begin before transplantation. Patients need to know the side effects of the immunosuppressive drugs and should be willing to sign a contract indicating that they will take the drugs as prescribed by the transplant physicians. If patients are made aware before transplantation of the importance of being compliant with the posttransplant routine of clinics, laboratories, and medications, they are more likely to be compliant with such a regimen. Patients should be made aware of all study protocols that may be ongoing at the transplant center, and sample consent forms should be sent to patients and their referring physicians.

Dialysis

Some centers promote so-called preemptive transplantation—that is, a patient does not undergo dialytic therapy before transplantation. This is an acceptable approach if it is clear that a patient will require treatment for ESRD within 6 months. Preemptive transplantation is a reasonable policy in the case of living related or living unrelated donor transplantation. If a patient has not yet begun dialysis, he or she must have acceptable nutritional status. Patients with chronic renal failure are often malnourished as a result of a loss of appetite and/or restricted protein intake. However, malnutrition can also be a problem in patients on dialysis, and this problem should be addressed carefully and treated appropriately.

POSTTRANSPLANT MANAGEMENT

The patient is managed first in the hospital, then in the clinic as an outpatient.

The Hospital (Inpatient)

Various procedures and medications are needed after transplantation.

Routine Postoperative Management

Surgical Management

Bladder Catheter. All patients have a bladder catheter after transplantation. The catheter prevents pressure on the ureteroneocystostomy anastomosis and is important for preventing urinary leaks postoperatively. In some centers where end-to-side allograft native pyeloureterostomies are performed, the catheter can be removed as soon as the patient is awake and able to urinate or within 24 to 48 hours. In all other cases, the catheter should be left for 5 to

7 days. The catheter remains in place for 7 days in diabetic patients and in any patient with a thin-walled bladder or difficult anastomosis. Patients who require an indwelling catheter for 5 to 7 days have a relatively high incidence of cystitis and should be carefully evaluated weekly after the catheter is removed for the onset of such infections. Alternatively, they may be given prophylactic antibiotics to prevent infections. Before the catheter is removed, a urine culture and a cystogram to rule out an anastomotic leak should be obtained. While in place, bladder catheters can cause pain and bladder spasms. In the event of a bladder spasm, an anticholinergic drug can be used. Catheters frequently become obstructed by blood clots in the bladder. To prevent this, any patient with gross hematuria should have a catheter irrigated regularly until the urine clears of blood. In males, the catheter should always be taped to the abdomen to avoid unnecessary pressure on the bladder neck.

Drains. When blood oozes from the operative site at the time of wound closure, drains are often left in place so that hematomas that may potentially become infected are not formed. Jackson-Pratt and Hemovac drains, which are closed and under vacuum pressure, are usually used for this purpose. They should be removed when drainage is less than 30 ml/24 hr.

Intravenous Lines. All patients return from the operating room with intravenous lines. Most patients also have a central line for administration of polyclonal antilymphocyte globulins and/or monitoring of central venous pressure. If polyclonal preparations are not being used, the central line should be removed within 24 hours if an adequate peripheral venous access is present. The number of venous access sites should be minimized, and arm veins that may be necessary for dialysis in the future should never be compromised. All venous accesses should be removed as soon as possible to avoid infection.

Nasogastric Tubes. Nasogastric (NG) tubes are usually unnecessary but are indicated for patients who are vomiting as a result of poor gastric emptying or poor bowel motility or for patients with severe pain because of bowel distention. Because NG tubes are supremely uncomfortable, they should be clamped to determine if gastric contents can procede antegrade through the bowel and should be removed as soon as possible.

Endotracheal Tube. Patients usually can be extubated in the recovery room within hours of finishing an operation, and it is rare that a patient will require intensive care after leaving the recovery room and before being transferred to the ward.

Surgical Wound. The surgical wound can become infected, can dehisce, can cause pain and discomfort, and should be watched carefully. Staples can be removed after 7 to 10 days in nondiabetic patients with good skin tone and in diabetic patients between 10 and 14 days after surgery. The surgical wound needs to be dressed only for 48 hours after transplant. After that time, it should be left uncovered unless there is a leak of serous fluid, in which case it should be dressed three times a day with sterile gauze. The wound should be kept clean at all times; povidone-iodine and other antiseptic washings are usually unnecessary.

Ambulation. All patients should be up and out of bed on the first postoperative day, and ambulation and exercise should be advanced quickly. Nothing should be done to put stress on the wound, however. Patients should be allowed maximum sleep to help in their recovery.

Dietary Management. Patients' dietary needs should be assessed daily. The diet should be advanced as quickly as possible according to the status of the gastrointestinal tract. Nothing other than medication should be given by mouth until a patient is passing flatus. Clear liquids should be advanced to full liquids when it is known that a patient can tolerate the liquids without abdominal distention, vomiting, and pain. Patients who have a functioning kidney can be given a regular diet or a diabetic diet if they have diabetes. Patients who have delayed graft function and remain on dialysis should be given a 60-g protein, 2-g sodium, and 2-g potassium diet. All oral intake should be discontinued if it becomes clear that there are gastrointestinal motility problems. High colonic enemas should be avoided because of the potential for bowel perforation and bacteremia. Fleet enemas and rectal suppositories are acceptable for use in these patients.

Routine Daily Surgical Examination. The routine daily examination should include evaluation of the bladder catheter, drains, all intravenous lines, NG tube if present, and the wound. In addition, the kidney should be palpated for the presence of swelling and tenderness, and the flank should be observed for the presence of an ecchymosis that may indicate hemorrhage from the artery or vein. The scrotum and penis should be checked for the presence of edema. If a patient has been on CAPD, it is common for the peritoneum to make a large volume of ascitic fluid. If there has been any interruption of the peritoneum at the time of transplant surgery, it is possible for this fluid to leak through the surgical wound and prevent normal healing; this fluid may also prevent normal recovery of bowel continuity. Therefore, the abdomen should be evaluated for ascites in a patient on CAPD; if a large amount of ascites is present, it should be drained through the CAPD catheter daily or twice daily. The vital signs should be checked on daily rounds, and all vegetative functions such as breathing, bowel continuity, urinary flow, and dietary needs should be checked.

Medical Management

Dialysis. The indications for dialysis following transplantation are the same as those for a patient who has not undergone transplantation and include hyperkalemia, volume overload, acidosis, pericarditis, and symptomatic uremia. After transplantation, early signs of delayed graft function may exist, and a renal scan may demonstrate acute tubular necrosis. However, dialysis should not be initiated without an indication because dialysis might compromise renal function by decreasing blood pressure, and within 48 hours the kidney may be working well. In general it is useful to have generous intravascular volume after transplantation. However, when using the monoclonal antibody OKT3, very high volume must be avoided. The decision about the route for dialysis should be based on the presence of bleeding (*i.e.*, a desire not to use heparin) and the presence of an access. In general, the same type of dialysis is used after transplantation as was used before transplantation.

Hyperkalemia can often be managed with glucose, insulin, and bicarbonate. A very high potassium level often results from hemolysis, hematomas, or the intracellular electrolyte solution used for preservation of the donor kidney. If delayed graft function does occur and a patient is in need of dialysis, then it is easiest to put the patient on a regular thrice-weekly dialysis schedule until the urinary output improves. At this time, the laboratory data can be scrutinized on a daily basis to determine the need for dialysis.

Anticoagulation during hemodialysis should be minimized. Very low doses of heparin, 1000 units or less, are often enough. In some cases of bleeding, it may be possible to hemodialyze a patient without the use of heparin, but there is a small risk of blood loss if the artificial kidney becomes clotted. In these cases, it is best not to use a hollow-fiber kidney but instead to use a plate dialyzer. Other techniques that can be used to avoid heparin include citrate administration or hemofiltration.

Hemodialysis is probably the wisest choice in the event of delayed graft function; if a fistula is present, it should be used. Dialysis fistulas often clot after transplantation because of intraoperative hypotension, inadvertent pressure being placed on the arm during surgery, or reversal of the platelet defect that accompanies chronic renal failure. If no fistula is available, a subclavian or internal jugular access approach is best. These accesses can be inserted in the operating room if the surgeons believe that delayed graft function is probable based on prolonged cold ischemia or the appearance of the kidney in the operating room. Femoral catheters are not recommended because they decrease patients' mobility, they need to be changed frequently because the groin is difficult to keep sterile, and they tend to be more uncomfortable for patients. **When femoral catheters are used, they should not be placed on the side of the allograft because of the remote possibility that the catheter might disrupt the end-to-side venous anastomosis of the allograft vein onto the iliac vein.**

When peritoneal dialysis is being used, it is recommended that small volumes, one-half or less than the usual amount, be used initially; larger volumes are uncomfortable, can prolong postoperative ileus, and can put pressure on the suture line. **Peritoneal dialysis should not be used if the peritoneum was penetrated during the transplant surgery.** If dialysate passes through the wound, then peritoneal dialysis should be discontinued. Peritoneal dialysis is useful if anticoagulation must be avoided, but in general it is less effective than hemodialysis for the rapid removal of potassium or volume. Any of the standard forms of peritoneal dialysis including CAPD, continuous cycled peritoneal dialysis, and intermittent peritoneal dialysis all can be used after transplantation.

Fluid/Electrolyte/Metabolic Management. An insulin drip protocol should be used for all diabetic patients after transplantation (Table 19–13). A sliding scale for insulin use is usually satisfactory for the hyperglycemia that occasionally ensues after transplantation in nondiabetic patients who are given high doses of steroids. All patients should be given the basic nutritional needs intravenously until they begin eating. Hyperalimentation should begin if a patient has not begun eating by the third postoperative day. Hypophosphatemia is common and occurs

Table 19–13. POSTTRANSPLANT INSULIN TREATMENT FOR DIABETIC PATIENTS (CONSTANT IV INFUSION)

Goal: Maintain serum glucose at a level between 150 and 250 mg/dl.

Procedure:

1. Mix 100 units regular insulin in 500 ml D_5W (0.2 units/ml) and infuse via an IVAC pump, along with the regular replacement.
2. From end of surgery, draw blood glucose every 2 hr for 8 hours to establish trend and stability.
3. Draw blood every 6 hr for 3 days when stability is reached.
4. Infuse insulin via the following scale for the first 3 postoperative days:

If glucose—	give insulin—	via ml fluid/hr
>500	6 U/hr	30
>400	5 U/hr	25
>300	4 U/hr	20
>250	3 U/hr	15
>200	2 U/hr	10
<200	1 U/hr	5

5. Exceptions to above insulin scale:
   a. Raise insulin to 10 U/hr for 2 hr if blood glucose has risen or if maintenance of glucose over 500 mg/dl.
   b. Lower next dosage scheduled by 1 U/hr if rate of decline in serum glucose is >200 mg/dl/2 hr (e.g., 570 mg/dl to 350 mg/dl dosage is 6 U to 3 U, not the prior 4 U usually given for >300 mg/dl). Lower next dosage by 2 U/hr if rate of decline >300 mg/dl.
   c. If glucose stabilizes between 250 mg/dl and 500 mg/dl, add 1 U/hr to the scheduled dose to get level between 150 mg/dl and 250 mg/dl.
6. Any fraction of scheduled dosage may be used in an insulin-sensitive patient.

early after successful transplantation; it is due to both phosphate wasting and the transit of phosphorus into cells. K-Phos Neutral is more easily tolerated than Neutra-Phos. Bicarbonate wasting and acidosis are also frequently encountered after kidney transplantation and especially after combined kidney/pancreas transplantation. Bicarbonate wasting occurs as a result of cyclosporine use and secondary to bicarbonate secretion into the bladder or bowel after pancreas transplantation. Bicarbonate should be replaced with either intravenous or oral preparations when the serum carbon dioxide decreases below 15 mEq/L. Magnesium wasting can occur with cyclosporine therapy, and magnesium should be replaced when it is low. A daily measurement of fluid intake and output should be recorded in the chart. Fluid output includes urine output, NG tube drainage, diarrhea fluid, and the output of all of the drains.

Respiratory Management. All patients must have adequate pulmonary function after transplantation to avoid bacterial pneumonia. Patients should be given an incentive spirometer for use and should be encouraged to cough.

Blood Pressure Control. Hypertension following renal transplantation can be due to a number of causes: cyclosporine-induced hypertension, volume overload, transplant renal artery stenosis, a compressed kidney due to perinephritic bleeding or fluid collections, and essential hypertension. Renal artery stenosis is rare immediately after transplantation but should be considered at a later time if renal dysfunction and hypertension coexist. Cyclosporine causes high blood pressure in approximately three fourths of patients who receive it. Which class of antihypertensive agent best treats the hypertension caused by cyclosporine remains controversial. We have found the calcium channel blockers to be useful, but it should be remembered that both verapamil and diltiazem can increase cyclosporine blood levels. **In general, most of the antihypertensive drugs with which a transplant physician is familiar can be used to treat posttransplant hypertension. However, a multidrug approach is often necessary.** Considerations such as coexistent heart failure and diabetes will limit the use of certain drugs. Hypotension also can follow organ transplantation and usually is due to drugs such as OKT3, antihypertensives, or antidepressants, or it can be secondary to volume depletion from bleeding, diarrhea, vomiting, or, rarely, urinary output.

Infection Surveillance. Intraoperative cultures of the bladder and kidney should be obtained. A chest radiograph should be obtained after surgery, and urine cultures should be obtained routinely before the catheter is removed and when needed for symptoms.

Renal Function Surveillance. After kidney transplantation, it is important to anticipate all problems that may occur. Rejection usually occurs in the first 2 weeks, but this event depends on the type of immunosuppression protocol used. For example, when an antilymphocyte antibody is used, the onset of rejection is usually delayed, and rejection frequently does not occur. After donor-specific transfusions, rejections often occur in the first week. Urinary leaks are usually evident in the first week or at the time that the bladder catheter is removed. In general, urinary leaks occurring within the first week are treatable by continued bladder catheter drainage. Urinary leaks occurring after 2 weeks often require surgery and a neoureteroneocystostomy. Obstruction to urinary flow can occur early after transplantation but in general occurs late when there is distal ureteral ischemia and fibrosis. Hemorrhage into the bladder can lead to blood clots, which can block the normal drainage through a bladder catheter.

Daily Medical Examination. The daily medical examination should include an assessment of the need for dialysis, an evaluation of the fluid electrolyte and metabolic status, an evaluation of the blood pressure, inspection of all of the cultures, an appropriate physical examination and mental status examination, and a review of the laboratory values regarding renal function and immunologic monitoring.

Diagnostic Studies. Daily laboratory values should be obtained to monitor renal function tests, the immunosuppressive drugs, the metabolic status of a patient, and the possibility of bleeding. Blood urea nitrogen (BUN) and creatinine levels should be obtained daily.

For patients on cyclosporine, a daily cyclosporine level during the first week after initiating therapy is useful. After this the frequency can be decreased, but surveillance should always be increased whenever a drug that interferes with cyclosporine metabolism is introduced (see below). Many assays for measuring cyclosporine are available, and there are no exact formulas available to convert the results from one assay to that of another assay. The majority opinion currently is that an assay that measures parent compound and not any of the many cyclosporine metabolites is most accurate. It is extremely important to know the target ranges for the assay used in the laboratory of the transplant program. In general, the levels are measured 12 to 24 hours after the previous dose. **Whenever interpreting a cyclosporine level, it must be known how many hours after the dose was taken that the level was measured.** Patient compliance on this issue is very important. It takes three to five doses to achieve a steady state after initiation of cyclosporine therapy, so doses should not be adjusted after the first three to five doses unless the level is extremely low.

The white blood cell (WBC) count and platelet count should be measured daily because both azathioprine and ATG can lower the WBC count and platelet count and steroids and infections can elevate the WBC count. The WBC count should be kept above 3000.

If a patient is receiving OKT3, another monoclonal antibody, or a polyclonal antilymphocyte preparation, T-cell analysis should be performed daily or every other day. When using OKT3, it is necessary to have the laboratory assess the approximate number or percent of T cells that express the target molecule CD3 and, if possible, the approximate amount of target molecule on those cells. Table 19–14 shows one method of monitoring patients who are receiving OKT3. When using ATG, many centers monitor sheep RBC rosettes and attempt to keep the percent of lymphocytes forming rosettes under 10%.

When attempting to differentiate between rejection and infection, it can be useful to measure the helper:suppressor T-cell ratio. The normal T4:T8 ratio is approximately 2; in rejection it remains approximately 2 or higher, and with CMV infection it can be either normal or very low. A combination of fever, renal dysfunction, and a T4:T8 ratio of less than 1 can be interpreted as a viral infection, and in such a case it is unwise to treat for rejection.

Both azathioprine and cyclosporine can cause hepatic dysfunction. Therefore, liver function tests should be obtained at least three times each week. Serum glucose, electrolytes, magnesium, calcium, and phosphorus levels should be measured daily during the first week following transplantation.

A daily hematocrit should be obtained in addition to the WBC count and platelet count to monitor possible blood loss or hemolysis after transplant surgery.

Renal Scan. A renal scan should be obtained on the first postoperative day to assess the renal blood flow and to determine whether there is an intrarenal infarction, obstruction, or urinary leak. The initial renal scan can often predict the dialysis requirement. Two substances are generally used for the renal scan. Diethylenetriaminepentaacetic acid (DTPA) measures renal blood flow and glomerular func-

Table 19–14. DOSE ADJUSTMENT FOR OKT3 ADMINISTRATION

Daily or every other day monitoring of T cells is useful.
- Percent CD3 positive cells
- CD3 antigen density on T cells

Dose adjustment:
- Days 0–4 of therapy: Do not adjust the dose.
- Thereafter, adjust the dose as follows:
  1. If one of the below parameters is *not* present, increase the dose:
     a. Percent CD3-positive cells (excluding dim cells) <10%
     b. Mean CD3 antigen density on all CD3-positive cells <20,000
  2. Increase the dose as follows:
     a. Dose <5 mg/day = increase by 1 mg
     b. Dose >5 mg/day = increase by 2.5 mg

tion, and hippurate measures tubular extraction and excretion. The glomerular filtration rate (GFR) is assessed by measuring the amount of isotope in the bladder after an injection of DTPA. If a catheter is in place in the bladder, this test is invalid. If a patient has delayed graft function, it is useful to obtain a renal scan twice a week, because monitoring of BUN and creatinine levels will not be useful until dialysis is no longer required. The renal scan can be useful for any episodes of renal dysfunction occurring after transplantation. However, it is important to understand that the scan is unable to distinguish between cyclosporine nephrotoxicity, rejection, and acute interstitial nephritis. In general, any intrarenal cause of a rising serum creatinine level will affect the renal scan in about the same way.

Ultrasonography. An ultrasonogram should be obtained on the second postoperative day to assess the presence of a perinephric fluid collection such as a hematoma, urinoma, or lymphocele. Ultrasonography can evaluate kidney size, the collecting system, and blood flow if Doppler is used. It is also used for localizing the kidney to obtain a renal biopsy specimen.

Discharge Planning

Patient Education. All patients should begin learning to take their own medications as soon as they have recovered from transplant surgery. The medications must be known and understood before the patient is discharged. The pharmacy, along with the ward nurses, should be responsible for beginning this education. The outpatient transplant nurse coordinators also must be involved with this educational process, but their responsibilities encompass more than just the medications and also include issues of diagnostic tests and clinic visits. It is useful for physicians to reinforce on daily rounds the notion that the immunosuppressive medications are required for life and to discuss the consequences of discontinuing them.

Timing of Discharge. Most patients can be discharged from the hospital within 7 to 10 days of transplant unless complications occur. Before patients can be discharged they must be afebrile, ambulating, and eating and their bowels must be working. It is useful to have stable or improving renal function, although most patients can be discharged from the hospital even if they have delayed graft function and require dialysis; they can be seen and evaluated three times a week in the inpatient hemodialysis unit. Patients must also be psychologically and socially ready to be discharged. There should always be a caretaker, the home environment must be ready to accept a patient, there must be transportation to and from the clinic and laboratory, and, as previously mentioned, patients must be able to understand and take their medications.

Routine Postoperative Medications

Immunosuppressive Drugs

Unequivocally, the enormous success of renal transplantation is due to the immunosuppressive drugs used. A brief discussion of the pharmacology and mechanisms of action of these drugs follows. The toxicities of these drugs are summarized in Table 19–15.

Maintenance Immunosuppression

Azathioprine. Azathioprine, a purine antimetabolite, is an imidazole derivative of 6-mercaptopurine and can be given both orally and intravenously. The biologic effects of azathioprine are thought to be due to metabolism of this drug to 6-mercaptopurine in the liver. In fact, azathioprine is extensively metabolized, and very little of the parent compound remains after a few passes through the liver. The half-life of all of the metabolites of azathioprine is approximately 5 hours. Azathioprine and its metabolites are usually undetectable in the urine after approximately 8 hours. Because the metabolites are eliminated from the blood so quickly, tissue levels rather than plasma levels are better at predicting a clinical response. Metabolism of the derivatives of azathioprine to an inactive 6-thiouric acid via xanthine oxidase is an important metabolic pathway. Patients who are receiving the xanthine oxidase inhibitor allopurinol must have their azathioprine dose reduced by approximately two thirds.

The principal pharmacologic activities of azathioprine and its metabolites result from a competitive inhibition of enzymes concerned with the new production of purine bases. Azathioprine appears to work best on rapidly dividing cells by preventing normal synthesis of RNA and DNA. Its major effect appears to be on T cells, but patients receiving azathioprine are also noted to have poor antibody response to injected antigens; therefore, in humans there may be some effect on B cells as well. Azathioprine is most effective as a maintenance immunosuppressive drug and should be started at

Table 19–15. TOXICITIES OF IMMUNOSUPPRESSIVE DRUGS

Side Effects	*Rare Side Effects*
Cyclosporine (Sandimmune)	
Kidney damage (nephrotoxicity)	Liver damage (hepatotoxicity)
High blood pressure	Seizures
New hair growth	Decreased or abnormal sensation (neuropathy)
Abnormal growth of gums (gingival hyperplasia)	Destruction of red blood cells (hemolytic anemia)
Tremors	Damage to blood vessel linings causing small blood clots
Azathioprine (Imuran)	
Reduced white blood cell count	Bone marrow failure (aplastic anemia)
Reduced platelet count	Liver damage (hepatotoxicity)
	Inflammation of the pancreas (pancreatitis)
	Hair loss
Prednisone (Deltasone)	
Weight gain	Damaged bone tissue in hips, knees, and shoulders (osteonecrosis)
Distribution of fat to stomach, neck, and face	Worsening of atherosclerosis (hardening of the arteries)
Softening of bones (osteoporosis)	Diabetes
Thinning of skin	Cataract formation (eye damage)
Weakening of muscles and other tissues	
Delayed wound healing	
Increased cholesterol	
Fluid retention and edema	
Mood swings	
OKT3	
Fever and chills	Skin rash
Low blood pressure	Stiff neck
Nausea and vomiting	Weakness
Diarrhea	Brain swelling
Headache	Hallucinations
Anti-OKT3 antibody production	Loss of consciousness
	Shortness of breath
	Water on the lungs (pulmonary edema)

the time of transplantation or before. It has very little effect on ongoing rejection episodes or secondary immune responses.

The major toxicity of azathioprine appears to be bone marrow depression leading to leukopenia, thrombocytopenia, and a macrocytic anemia. Isolated leukopenia and anemia have occurred. These toxicities are mostly dose related and will reverse on a reduction in the amount of drug given. However, the effect of azathioprine may last beyond its discontinuation. The leukopenia does not correlate with the therapeutic effect, so the dose of the drug should not be increased to tolerance of the WBC count. Infections and neoplasia are other complications of azathioprine therapy. Many women receiving azathioprine have had successful pregnancies, but they must be advised of possible complications such as low birth weight, prematurity, and spontaneous abortion.

Of the immunosuppressive drugs used, azathioprine probably has the fewest troublesome side effects. However, occasional hypersensitivity reactions to azathioprine can result in pancreatitis. If this occurs, the azathioprine should be discontinued and probably not reintroduced. Occasional patients have developed severe abdominal pain not due to pancreatitis. This can often be reduced by either giving azathioprine in a divided dose or by giving it with food. If neither of these interventions is effective, the drug should be discontinued. Rarely, alopecia has occurred, but the hair frequently grows back even if azathioprine is continued. Veno-occlusive disease of the liver is a serious but extremely rare complication of azathioprine use. When it is encountered, azathioprine must be discontinued. The diagnosis of veno-occlusive disease is a difficult one but should be considered whenever marked hepatic dysfunction occurs.

The initial dose of azathioprine is usually 5 mg/kg IV given just before transplantation. In live donor transplantation, azathioprine can be begun 5 to 7 days before transplantation. The usual maintenance dose of azathioprine is 2.5 mg/kg/day when given with prednisone only or 2 mg/kg/day when given in combination with cyclosporine and prednisone. In general, azathioprine doses are not tapered unless leukopenia or anemia supervenes. Tables 19–16, 19–17, and 19–18 show the immunosuppressive regimens for drugs including azathioprine that have proved effective for kidney transplantation at Oregon Health Sciences University.

Cyclosporine. Cyclosporine is the first example of a fungal metabolite that can modulate the immune response. The fungi that produce cyclosporine are *Cylindrocarpon lucidum Booth* and *Tolypocladium inflatum Gams* (both strains of fungi imperfecti). Cyclosporine is a hydrophobic cyclic peptide composed of 11 amino acids. One of the amino acids is unique and previously was unknown to exist. Cyclosporine is insoluble in water but is soluble in many organic reagents, for instance ethanol.

Cyclosporine is used as a maintenance immunosuppressive drug and not for treatment of rejection episodes. However, it does appear to have some effect on ongoing rejection episodes, and in this way it is different from azathioprine.

Cyclosporine is available in both oral (liquid and capsules) and intravenous preparations. In general, the oral preparation is preferred because of the increased hepatic and renal toxicities associated with the intravenous preparation. However, during the early postoperative period, at a time when bowel motility is poor, the intravenous preparation often has to be used.

The major mechanism of action of cyclosporine is thought to be prevention of cytokine production, specifically interleukin-2, by helper T cells. In *in vitro* assays, cyclosporine can prevent the activation of T cells and generation of cytotoxic T cells but cannot impair the function of already committed T cells. Cyclosporine appears to have very little direct effect on B cells. Its effect is thought to occur in the cytoplasm: By binding to calmodulin and cyclophilin, it blocks normal cytosolic calcium activity and blocks normal RNA transcription.

Cyclosporine is one of the most difficult

Table 19–16. IMMUNOSUPPRESSION FOR HLA-IDENTICAL LIVING RELATED DONOR RENAL TRANSPLANTATION

Pretransplant Transfusions

- For patients with ≥1 unit of packed red cells or ≥5 units leukopoor cells: No further transfusions required.
- For patients without the above: 1 unit packed cells required.
- Clinically necessary transfusions beyond required units: Leukocyte filter, DG cells or leukocyte-poor-washed packed cells only.

Maintenance Immunosuppression

- Azathioprine
  - Dose schedule:
  - Day minus 6 and thereafter = 2.5 mg/kg/day
  - Dose reduction
    - 50% drop in WBC = 50% reduction in dose
    - WBC <3000 = discontinue
    - Concomitant allopurinal = 67% reduction in dose
  - If azathioprine cannot be tolerated initially because of leukopenia, cyclosporine (7 mg/kg/day) should be substituted.
- Solu-Medrol dose schedule:
  - Day 0: = 500 mg IV on call to operating room
  - Day 1: = 125 mg IV b.i.d.
- Prednisone:
  - Days 2–30: 0.5 mg/kg/day
  - Month 2: 0.4 mg/kg/day
  - Month 3: 0.3 mg/kg/day
  - Month 4: 0.2 mg/kg/day
  - Month 5: 0.15 mg/kg/day
  - Months 6–18: 0.1 mg/kg/day
  - Begin further taper to discontinue only after 6 months of rejection-free status. If rejection occurs during or after taper, return to 0.1 mg/kg/day dose permanently.
  - Months 19, 20: 0.075 mg/kg/day
  - Months 21, 22: 0.05 mg/kg/day
  - Months 23, 24: 0.025 mg/kg/day
  - Thereafter: discontinue

Table 19–17. IMMUNOSUPPRESSION FOR ONE- AND ZERO-HAPLOTYPE-MATCHED LIVING RELATED DONOR TRANSPLANTATION

Pretransplant Transfusions

- For patients with ≥ 1 unit of packed red blood cells or ≥5 units leukopoor cells: No further transfusions required.
- For patients without the above: 1 unit packed cells required.
- Clinically necessary transfusions beyond required units: Leukocyte filter, DG cells or leukocyte-poor-washed packed cells only.

Maintenance Immunosuppression

- Azathioprine
  - Dose schedule:
    - Day minus 6–month 3: 2 mg/kg/day
    - Thereafter: 2.5 mg/kg/day
  - Dose reduction:
    - 50% drop in WBC = 50% reduction in dose
    - WBC <3000 = discontinue
    - Concomitant allopurinol = 67% reduction in dose
- Cyclosporine
  - Dose schedule:
    - Day 0–4: none
    - Day 5–month 3: 7 mg/kg/day as a single evening dose.
    - Months 4, 5, 6: 25% reduction in current dose per month.*
    - Month 7: discontinue†
  - Intravenous dose equals ⅓ oral dose (give as continuous 24 hr infusion).
  - Adjust dose according to target levels.
  - If a drug affecting the metabolism of cyclosporine cannot be avoided, the cyclosporine dose should be increased or reduced for drugs that increase or decrease the metabolism of cyclosporine, respectively.
- Solu-Medrol
  - Day 0: 500 mg IV on call to operating room
  - Day 1: 125 mg IV b.i.d.
- Prednisone
  - First week:
    - Day 2: 1 mg/kg
    - Day 3: 0.9 mg/kg
    - Day 4: 0.8 mg/kg
    - Day 5: 0.7 mg/kg
    - Day 6: 0.6 mg/kg
    - Day 7–30: 0.5 mg/kg/day
  - Month 2: 0.4 mg/kg/day
  - Month 3: 0.3 mg/kg/day
  - Month 4: 0.2 mg/kg/day
  - Month 5: 0.15 mg/kg/day
  - Thereafter: 0.1 mg/kg/day
- OKT3
  - Days 0–11: 1–5 mg IV bolus injection beginning in the operating room.
  - or
- Antithymocyte globulin (equine)
  - Days 0–11: 15 mg/kg/day

*Begin taper only after 2 months of rejection-free status.

†Discontinue only after biopsy specimen shows no rejection.

Table 19–18. IMMUNOSUPPRESSION FOR CADAVERIC AND LIVING UNRELATED DONOR TRANSPLANTATION

Pretransplant Transfusions
- For patients with ≥1 unit of packed red blood cells or ≥5 units leukopoor cells: No further transfusions required.
- For patients without the above: 1 unit packed cells required.
- Clinically necessary transfusions beyond required units: Leukocyte filter, DG cells or leukocyte-poor-washed packed cells only.

Maintenance Immunosuppression

Azathioprine
- Dose schedule:
  - Day 0: 5 mg/kg IV on call to operating room
  - Thereafter: 2 mg/kg/day (IV or PO)
- Dose reduction:
  - 50% drop in WBCs = 50% reduction in dose
  - WBC <3000 = discontinue
  - Concomitant allopurinol = 67% reduction in dose

Cyclosporine
- Dose schedule:
  - Day 0–4: None
  - Thereafter: 7 mg/kg/day given as a single daily evening dose.
- Intravenous dose equals ⅓ oral dose (give as continuous 24 hr infusion).
- Adjust dose according to target levels.
- If a drug affecting the metabolism of cyclosporine cannot be avoided, the cyclosporine dose should be increased or decreased for drugs that increase or decrease the metabolism of cyclosporine, respectively.

Solu-Medrol:
- Day 0 = 500 mg IV on call to operating room
- Day 1 = 125 mg IV b.i.d.

Prednisone:
- First week:
  - Day 2: 1 mg/kg
  - Day 3: 0.9 mg/kg
  - Day 4: 0.8 mg/kg
  - Day 5: 0.7 mg/kg
  - Day 6: 0.6 mg/kg
- Days 7–30 = 0.5 mg/kg/day
- Month 2: 0.4 mg/kg
- Month 3: 0.3 mg/kg
- Month 4: 0.2 mg/kg
- Month 5: 0.15 mg/kg
- Month 6: 0.1 mg/kg
- Months 7, 8: 0.075 mg/kg
- Months 9, 10: 0.05 mg/kg
- Months 11, 12: 0.025 mg/kg
- Thereafter: None
- Do not taper prednisone if a patient is having frequent rejection episodes.

OKT3:
- Days 0–11: 1–5 mg/day bolus injection beginning in the operating room

or

Antithymocyte globulin (equine):
- Days 0–11: 15 mg/kg/day

drugs to use clinically because of its variable absorption from the gastrointestinal tract; additionally, many drugs affect its metabolism (see Table 19–19). As a result, drug level monitoring has become common at most transplant centers. The monitoring of cyclosporine levels is also problematic because of the myriad different assays available and because the substrate in which the cyclosporine level is measured can be either whole blood, serum, or plasma (Table 19–20). There is no single universally used assay or target level for cyclosporine.

It appears that cyclosporine can be given either once a day or twice a day with little difference in either its immunosuppressive or toxic side effects. When first used for human organ transplantation, recommended doses were 17 to 18 mg/kg/day. It soon became apparent that these doses were much too high and quite nephrotoxic. It is now known that much lower doses are still immunosuppressive and less nephrotoxic. Typical initial doses of cyclosporine currently being used range between 5 and 10 mg/kg/day.

The major toxicity of cyclosporine is renal (Table 19–21), which can be either a reversible vascular or tubular dysfunction or can be a more serious vasculopathy or tubulopathy. The latter may not be reversible with discontinuation or lowering of the cyclosporine dose. Vascular dysfunction can probably occur in the absence of the vasculopathy and is primarily a manifestation of vasoconstriction leading to depressed renal plasma flow and GFR. The vasculopathy associated with cyclosporine is manifest by damaged endothelium, expansion of the arteriolar intima by eosinophilic material, and occasional capillary thrombosis. The latter is thought to be induced by endothelial cell injury and a reduced ability to produce prostacycline (a potent inhibitor of platelet adhesiveness), leading to fibrin and platelet deposition. Vasculopathy can lead to ischemia and interstitial fibrosis. Tubular dysfunction can probably occur in the absence of tubulopathy and is manifest as magnesium and bicarbonate wasting and impaired secretion of potassium. The tubulopathy of cyclosporine is manifest by vacuolization of renal tubular cells, occasional tubular necrosis, and fibrosis.

It is possible that cyclosporine toxicity and

Table 19–19. DRUGS THAT INTERFERE WITH CYCLOSPORINE METABOLISM

Increase Metabolism	Decrease Metabolism
Dilantin	Verapamil
Phenobarbital	Diltiazem
Tegretol	Ketaconazole
Sulfamethoxazole given intravenously	Erythromycin
	IV Solu-Medrol
Rifampin	Cimetidine
Isoniazid	Amphotericin B

Table 19–20. ASSAYS FOR CYCLOSPORINE MEASUREMENT

Method	Matrices	Reagents
Immunoassays	Blood	Anticyclosporine antibodies:
Radioimmunoassay (RIA)	Serum	Polyclonal antibody
Fluorescence polarization immunoassay (FPIA)	Plasma	Specific monoclonal antibody
		Nonspecific monoclonal antibody
High-pressure liquid chromatography (HPLC)	Blood	
	Serum	
	Plasma	

rejection can coexist. Low normal cyclosporine levels do not rule out the existence of cyclosporine nephrotoxicity. However, high cyclosporine levels generally are not associated with rejection. It seems reasonable to assume that chronic tubulopathy and perhaps even vasculopathy can occur in the absence of vascular dysfunction (detected by a rise in BUN and creatinine levels); it is probably appropriate to reduce cyclosporine doses in patients who have high levels despite low doses and unimpaired renal function.

Other troublesome dose-dependent side effects of cyclosporine are new hair growth, gum hypertrophy, and neuropathy. The principal manifestations of the neuropathy are tremor, a burning pain on the bottoms of the feet, and muscle cramps. Attentive oral hygiene may prevent the gum disease, the muscle cramps can be treated successfully in most cases with quinine, and the hair growth can be managed by depilatory agents. Most side effects can be managed by reducing the cyclosporine dose.

A few centers have found that cyclosporine can be safely tapered from a patient's regimen 12 months after transplantation; others have found that withdrawal is difficult at any time but definitely inadvisable before 3 months. When cyclosporine is discontinued, it should be done gradually over a 4-month period by reducing the level 25% each month. At the same time, the azathioprine dose should be increased to 2.5 to 3 mg/kg. At a later date, the azathioprine dose can be reduced to 2 to 2.5 mg/kg. Renal function should be monitored

Table 19–21. RENAL TOXICITIES OF CYCLOSPORINE

Vasculopathy	Tubulopathy
Microthrombi	Tubular necrosis
Vascular intimal eosinophilic deposits	Tubular cell vacuolation
Interstitial fibrosis	Interstitial fibrosis
Vascular Dysfunction	**Tubular Dysfunction**
Decreased GFR	Magnesium wasting
Decreased renal plasma flow	Bicarbonate wasting
	Potassium retention

frequently during cyclosporine withdrawal. If possible, a low dose of cyclosporine should be continued indefinitely in cadaver transplant recipients.

A major problem with cyclosporine is its cost. Cyclosporine can cost between $5,000 and $10,000 per year. For patients who are on phenytoin or equivalent drugs that increase cytochrome P-450 activity and therefore cyclosporine metabolism, the cost of cyclosporine can be enormous. Some centers have used drugs such as verapamil, diltiazem, erythromycin, or ketoconazole, which reduce cytochrome P-450 activity, to increase cyclosporine levels and therefore reduce its cost. Such an approach may not be advisable, because reducing cytochrome P-450 activity might also affect the metabolism of other substances, which may rise to toxic levels. However, it certainly seems reasonable to use verapamil or diltiazem in patients who require antihypertensive medications.

Corticosteroids. **Steroids remain the mainstay of drugs used for reversal of rejection episodes, but they also play an important role in maintenance immunosuppression regimens.** They are also the most broadly reactive of all of the immunosuppressive drugs, having effects on leukocytes as well as many other cells in the body. Their main mechanism of action is blocking the transcription of DNA to messenger RNA; this is accomplished via a cytoplasmic steroid receptor. In *in vitro* assays, steroids block release of interleukin-1 and reduce class II antigen expression on macrophages. Through this mechanism and also perhaps by a direct effect on T cells, steroids reduce the alloactivation of T cells and the release of interleukin-2 and gamma interferon. They have a marked effect on migration and function of effector T cells.

Clinically, steroids produce two effects on the WBCs. In high doses, they cause a marked leukocytosis, predominantly by demarginating polymorphonuclear cells. Steroids also cause lymphopenia, predominantly of the CD4-positive lymphocytes. Impaired transit of lymphocytes through the bone marrow and lymphoid tissue is thought to be the mechanism. Steroids can directly lyse immature thymocytes, but mature circulating lymphocytes are less likely to be affected. Steroids appear to block or reduce azathioprine-induced leukopenia. Several patients have developed azathioprine-induced leukopenia while tapering to discontinue prednisone.

Table 19–15 shows the common steroid-induced toxicities. **The most troublesome of the steroid toxicities are the bone diseases; osteoporosis leading to vertebral fractures and avascular hip necrosis leading to the need for bilateral hip replacements are particularly malignant side effects of steroids.** Many other side effects are mostly cosmetic and less intolerable. Patients receiving steroids initially may have steroid-induced psychosis or other central nervous system manifestations such as euphoria or depression. These effects should be observed and treated by a psychiatrist if necessary.

Steroids are necessary early after transplantation; without them there may be a higher incidence of rejection episodes. It has become evident, however, that most recipients of HLA-identical grafts can be safely tapered from their steroids 1 to 2 years after transplantation. Moreover, many recipients of haploidentical and cadaveric transplants can be tapered from steroids after 1 or 2 years if cyclosporine alone or cyclosporine and azathioprine together are used. It would be inadvisable to discontinue steroids in a cadaveric kidney recipient who is on azathioprine alone.

Antilymphocyte Antibodies

Monoclonal Antibodies. Monoclonal antibodies are unique drugs derived from hybridoma cells that are made by fusing an antibody-producing B cell from a mouse, which has been repeatedly injected with an immunogen such as human thymocytes, with a long-lived and rapidly dividing myeloma cell. A single hybridoma cell can be stimulated to proliferate, yielding a clone of cells that make antibodies of a single immunoglobulin isotype directed to a single antigen.

OKT3 is an example of a monoclonal antibody that reacts with T cells and has been used for therapy in transplantation. It is a murine monoclonal IgG 2a antibody directed to CD3, a molecule that is found only on circulating T cells and thymocytes. CD3 is closely associated with the T-cell receptor for antigen on the T-cell surface. The mechanisms of action of OKT3 are (1) opsonization and removal of T cells from the circulation by mononuclear phagocytes after the initial doses and (2) removal (modulation) of the CD3 target molecule and, by association, the T-cell receptor for antigen from the T-cell surface. While OKT3 is being given, T cells found in the circulation have a very low level of CD3 and the T-cell antigen receptor; these cells are thought to be incapable of mediating an immune response. The half-life of OKT3 is approximately 18 hours. Other than anti-OKT3 antibodies, no other drugs are known to affect its metabolism.

The density of CD3 molecules on T cells and the number of circulating T cells varies among individuals. Therefore, the amount of OKT3 required for a desired effect also varies from patient to patient. Effective doses of OKT3 range between 2 and 5 mg/day initially, but in some patients, such as those who develop antibodies to OKT3, much higher doses may be required. OKT3 can be safely given after induction of anesthesia in the operating room. It can be given by an intravenous bolus injection (30 to 60 seconds) in a peripheral hand vein. During treatment, it is important to monitor T cells for the presence of the target CD3 molecule. If CD3 begins to appear on T cells, the dose of OKT3 must be increased according to the guidelines in Table 19–14. The ideal treatment period for rejection or prophylaxis is 10 to 14 days.

OKT3 generally causes a flulike symptom complex consisting of fever, chills, nausea, and fatigue. These symptoms, which can be severe, are thought to be due to cytokines released from activated T cells and monocytes. The cytokines IL-1, IL-2, γ-interferon, IL-6, and tumor necrosis factor have all been found to be released following the first dose of OKT3. Cytokines are probably responsible for the additional signs and symptoms of pulmonary capillary leak, meningitis-like syndrome, and transient renal dysfunction.

Polyclonal Antilymphocyte Antibodies. Polyclonal antilymphocyte antibodies are made by repeatedly injecting a horse, rabbit, or goat with human lymphocytes and harvesting the animal's serum after several weeks. As is the case with OKT3, the prophylactic use of polyclonal preparations is primarily to avoid early cyclosporine use and to delay or prevent the need for steroid use for rejection treatment. Polyclonal preparations that have been used in the United States are predominantly ATGam, produced by the Upjohn Company, and Minnesota Anti-Lymphoblast Globulin (MALG), produced by the University of Minnesota. Both of these preparations are equine based and are recommended to be used in a dose of approximately 15 mg/kg/day. These preparations must be given by a central intravenous line over a 4- to 6-hour infusion. Common side effects of the polyclonal antibody preparations are leukopenia, thrombocytopenia, and serum sickness.

Total Lymphoid Irradiation. The technique of irradiating the lymph nodes in a pattern identical to that used for treatment of Hodgkin's disease has been used on an investigational basis in South Africa, Israel, and the United States (Stanford-Pacific Medical Center). Early reports of the results of this technique indicate that in a small subset of patients, tolerance to graft antigens has been achieved. This technique still requires refinement before it can be widely used in kidney transplant centers.

Treatment of Rejection (see Table 19–22)

***Corticosteroids.* Corticosteroids are highly effective for reversing acute rejection episodes. Steroids can be given either as the intravenous preparation methylprednisolone or as oral prednisone.** A 1-g dose of methylprednisolone given daily or every other day for three doses can reverse most rejection episodes. However, the use of such megadoses of steroids is usually unwarranted, and it is known that oral prednisone given in a dosage of 5 mg/kg for 5 days is effective for reversing most acute rejection episodes. Later acute rejection episodes may even be reversible by using 3 mg/kg of prednisone for 5 days (Table 19–22).

Some patients on high doses of steroids become emotionally labile. It is useful to warn family members as well as patients that they may be moody or perhaps may even hallucinate. For patients who have a history of herpes simplex infections, it is always useful to give prophylactic acyclovir whenever treating a rejection episode. Corticosteroids are more effective if given in two daily doses; therefore, if a severe rejection is encountered, the daily dose should be divided and given at 12-hour intervals.

Antilymphocyte Antibodies. If corticosteroids are ineffective at reversing a rejection episode after 5 days, antilymphocyte antibody preparations, either OKT3 or polyclonal ATG, should be used (see Table 19–22). Steroids alone are successful in about 75% of acute rejection episodes. Of those rejections that are unresponsive to steroids in the first 3 months after transplantation, greater than 90% will be susceptible to OKT3 reversal. OKT3 may be more effective than ATG for this purpose, and it is easier to administer.

Biopsy specimens obtained at the end of OKT3 therapy can be misleading. In many cases, the kidney is not completely cleared of lymphocytes and yet the renal function continues to improve and there may be no subsequent rejection. Approximately half of the patients will have a subsequent rejection within 1 month after successful reversal of rejection with OKT3.

If a patient has previously received OKT3, it is unwise to give a second course if the patient made antibodies in a titer of 1:1000 or greater after the first course. Rejections are usually not successfully reversed in this setting, even if the antibodies developed after the first course have disappeared before the second course. When OKT3 is being given a second time, it is important to monitor CD3 daily. When there is

Table 19–22. TREATMENT OF ACUTE REJECTION

Treatment Protocols	Protocol Use
1. Micropulse = prednisone, 2 mg/kg/day × 5 days; taper by 30% of peak dose per day to maintenance prednisone dose.	1. With initial acute rejection occurring in the first 3 postoperative months: use maxipulse.
2. Minipulse = 3 mg/kg/day × 5 days; taper by 30% of peak dose per day to maintenance prednisone dose.	2. With subsequent acute rejections occurring in the first 3 postoperative months or initial rejections occurring 3 or more months after transplant: use minipulse.
3. Maxipulse = prednisone, 5 mg/kg/day × 5 days; taper by 30% of peak dose per day to maintenance prednisone dose.	3. With persistent (steroid resistant) renal dysfunction: Obtain renal biopsy; if marked cellular rejection is present, upgrade to next treatment protocol (minipulse → maxipulse; maxipulse → OKT3 or ATG). If minimal cellular rejection is present, continued renal dysfunction may be due to edema or vasospasm. In this case, give a micropulse and follow renal function closely (three times a week).
4. OKT3: OKT3, 5 mg per day × 10 days. A biopsy must be obtained prior to OKT3 use. Give micropulse (see above) and reduce cyclosporine by 50% while awaiting biopsy results. Cyclosporine must be maintained at the reduced dose until the next to last dose of OKT3.	4. With early recurrent (<7 days after returning to maintenance dose after steroid pulse) rejection: upgrade to the next treatment protocol.
5. ATG: ATGam or MALG 15 mg/kg/day × 10 days. A biopsy must be obtained prior to ATG use. Give micropulse (see above) and reduce cyclosporine by 50% while awaiting biopsy results. Cyclosporine must be maintained at the reduced dose until the next to last dose of ATG.	5. With late recurrent (>7 days after returning to maintenance dose after steroid pulse) rejection: begin with minipulse.

Table 19–23. GUIDELINES FOR PROPHYLAXIS OF CYTOMEGALOVIRUS INFECTIONS

Definition:	Any renal transplant recipient who is known to be CMV antibody negative and is receiving an organ from a CMV antibody positive donor.
Exclusions:	History of acyclovir intolerance or allergy. Women of childbearing potential who are unwilling to use effective contraception.
Guidelines:	One 800-mg acyclovir tablet 8 hours or less pretransplant. One 800-mg acyclovir tablet 24 hours posttransplant. Frequency of subsequent doses depends on creatinine clearance rate or serum creatinine level as follows: 1. Less than 0.167 ml/sec or serum creatinine level greater than or equal to 3.5 mg/dl: 800 mg daily 2. 0.167 to 0.417 ml/sec or serum creatinine level less than 3.5 and greater than or equal to 2 mg/dl: 800 mg t.i.d. 3. Greater than 0.417 ml/sec or serum creatinine less than 2 mg/dl: 800 mg q.i.d. 4. Dialysis dependent: 800 mg b.i.d.
Continue for 12 weeks	

Balfour HH Jr, Chase BA, Stapleton JT, et al: A randomized, placebo-controlled trial of oral acyclovir for the prevention of cytomegalovirus disease in recipients of renal allografts. N Engl J Med 320:1381, 1989.

evidence of inadequate CD3 removal from T cells, the OKT3 dose should be increased in 2.5-mg increments (see Table 19–14). A dose as high as 15 mg has been successful when lesser amounts were not.

Graft Irradiation and Plasmapheresis. Graft irradiation has no proven place in the treatment of ongoing rejection. There is no proven benefit of the use of plasmapheresis to treat ongoing rejections.

OTHER MEDICATIONS

Antibiotics. All patients who have a history of herpes simplex infections should be given acyclovir, 200 mg PO b.i.d. for 7 to 14 days, with immunosuppression induction and with each treatment for a rejection episode. A second-generation cephalosporin with antistaphylococcal activity such as cefazolin is sufficient for antibacterial prophylaxis; it should be continued until negative results of the intraoperative cultures are obtained (usually 48 hours). If the intraoperative cultures are positive, the appropriate antibiotic should be continued for 7 days. An oral antifungal agent such as clotrimazole or nystatin should be used in all cases of antibiotic use. In women, a vaginal antifungal suppository should also be employed.

The use of prophylactic antibiotics to prevent *Pneumocystis* and urinary tract infections may be effective, although their use is not universal and may not be necessary. CMV-negative recipients of kidneys from CMV-seropositive donors should be given prophylactic hyperimmune anti-CMV globulin if available. In the absence of an available preparation, acyclovir, 800 mg one to four times a day, may be given for 3 months after transplantation (Table 19–23); however, its efficacy for this purpose is controversial. Tinea versicolor infections are very common after transplantation, especially in diabetic patients, and are easily treated with Selsun Lotion. Patients should be reminded to wash and change their underclothes frequently to prevent these skin infections.

Others. Diabetic patients should be given a continuous insulin infusion immediately after transplantation (see Table 19–13); it should continue until they begin eating, at which time subcutaneous insulin can be reinstituted. Patients with a prior history of peptic ulcer disease should be given ranitidine in the appropriate dose. Antihypertensive medications should be used as necessary; calcium channel blockers, especially long-acting nifedipine, are particularly effective for cyclosporine-induced hypertension.

Anticoagulation with subcutaneous heparin should be administered to all patients with a hypercoagulable state. In addition, any patient with a history of a prior thrombosis, systemic lupus erythematosus with or without a lupus anticoagulant, a damaged or atherosclerotic donor or recipient artery, or a donor with mild DIC should also be anticoagulated. Anticoagulation can be discontinued when the patient is discharged from the hospital, except for patients with a hypercoagulable state, who should be given warfarin indefinitely. Enough subcutaneous heparin should be given every 8 hours to cause the activated partial thromboplastin time to remain at the upper limits of normal (Table 19–24). Using such a protocol, the risk of bleeding is minimal and anticoagulation is sufficient.

Bicarbonate should be given to patients whose carbon dioxide decreases below 15, and K-Phos Neutral should be given to patients whose phosphorus level declines below 2.

Routine postoperative medications are summarized in Table 19–25.

Table 19–24. ADJUSTED-DOSE PROPHYLACTIC HEPARIN PROTOCOL

Purpose: Adjust APTT to be in upper normal range (34–37 seconds) 6 hours after each dose.
Method: Give heparin subcutaneously every 8 hours. Measure APTT 6 hours after the dose.
Dose: Begin with 3500 units heparin.
Adjustment of heparin dose:
APTT <28 seconds: add 1000 units to each dose.
APTT 28–31 seconds: add 500 units to each dose.
APTT 31.5–36: none.
APTT 36.5–39: reduce each dose by 500 units.
APTT >39 seconds: reduce each dose by 1000 units.

APTT, activated partial thromboplastin time.

The Clinic (Outpatient)

Routine Management/Preventive Care

Clinic Visits. Patients should return to the clinic weekly for two to three visits after discharge from the hospital. The staples are usually removed from the surgical wound at the time of the first clinic visit (7 to 10 days after transplant); during this visit, special attention should be given to the wound, looking for evidence of infection, dehiscence, hemorrhage, and other problems. Clinic visits should be extended to 2 weeks for two visits, to 1 month for two visits, and then to 2 months for the remainder of the first year.

Renal Function and Immunologic Monitoring. An SMA-18 and CBC count should be obtained three times a week for the first 2 months after transplantation, twice a week for the next 4 months, and then once a week until the end of a year. Cyclosporine levels should be assessed three times a week for the first month, once a week for the next 2 months, every other week for 3 months, and once a month until the end of a year. A urinalysis and culture should be performed weekly for the first month, every other week for the next 2 months, then once a month until the end of the year.

Table 19–25. ROUTINE POSTOPERATIVE MEDICATIONS

Immunosuppression
Prednisone
Azathioprine
Cyclosporine
OKT3 or antithymocyte globulin
Antibiotics/antivirals/antifungals
Acyclovir*
Oral/vaginal nystatin or clotrimazole
Urinary tract prophylaxis†
Cytomegalovirus hyperimmune globulin
H_2 blocker
Phosphorus replacement
HCO_3 replacement
Heparin
Insulin drip
Antihypertensives

*For patients with a history of herpes simplex; for patients at risk for a primary CMV infection.

†Controversial.

Patient Notebook. Every patient should be given a notebook into which he or she can record medications and the laboratory test results. This becomes a permanent record that patients can take on vacation and when seen by physicians outside the transplant center. It also encourages the patients to become involved with their own care; the notebook will have a positive long-term effect on outcome.

Complications After Transplantation

RENAL DYSFUNCTION EPISODES

Definition. Because of laboratory variation, one can expect that the BUN and creatinine levels will vary by 10 to 15% on routine determinations. A renal dysfunction episode is defined as a sustained rise in the serum creatinine level by greater than 25% or in the BUN by greater than 40%. This degree of elevation generally is not due to laboratory variation.

Differential Diagnosis. The many causes of renal dysfunction following renal transplantation are summarized in Table 19–26.

Rejection. **Acute rejection episodes in the first month after transplantation can be associated with the typical signs of rejection such as fever, graft tenderness, graft swelling, oliguria, high blood pressure, ileus, and lymphocyturia.** Typical symptoms such as graft pain, abdominal pain, nausea, and malaise also accompany these signs of acute rejection. It is important to note that acute rejection later than 1 month after transplantation and occasionally within the first month can occur in the absence of any of the previously mentioned "classic" signs and symptoms.

Diagnostic tests should always be performed to confirm the presence of rejection. If all of the classic signs and symptoms occur in the absence of bacterial pyelonephritis, then it is safe to assume that the renal dysfunction episode is due to rejection. The BUN usually increases first and decreases last in rejection episodes. **A rise in the creatinine level alone without an increase in BUN is not consistent with acute rejection.** A rapid rise in the serum creatinine and BUN levels is usually due to rejection or other catastrophic event such as

Table 19–26. CAUSES OF RENAL DYSFUNCTION FOLLOWING TRANSPLANTATION

Acute rejection
Chronic rejection
Drugs
Diuretics (volume depletion)
Acyclovir
Nonsteroidal antiinflammatory drugs
Trimethoprim
Cimetidine
Amphotericin
Cyclosporine
Verapamil
Diltiazem
Ketoconazole
Erythromycin
Hyperglycemia/ketoacidosis
Infection
Allograft
Other
De novo intrinsic renal disease
Recurrent renal disease
Renal artery stenosis
Renal artery/vein thrombosis
Obstruction of urinary flow
Lymphocoele
Ureteral stenosis
Gross hematuria
Ureteral leak

venous or arterial thrombosis, obstruction, or a leak. Examination of the urinary findings is rarely useful, but lymphocytes can often be seen in acute rejection. A renal scan will show decreased tubular function; decreased blood flow; and the absence of urinary leak of isotope into the pelvis, complete cessation of blood flow, and an infarct. Ultrasonography will reveal swelling of the kidney and the absence of a perinephric collection causing obstruction.

If the diagnosis of rejection cannot be made on the basis of signs, symptoms, biochemical tests, the scan, or ultrasonography, a renal biopsy should be performed. The biopsy can be helpful in determining the type of antirejection therapy to use as well. A number of events must occur before a biopsy, an invasive test that must be performed with caution, can be performed. First it must be ascertained that a patient is not taking antiplatelet medications such as aspirin or other nonsteroidal antiinflammatory agents and that the prothrombin time and partial thromboplastin time are normal. Patients must sign a consent form; a parent or guardian must give consent for a minor. The biopsy is performed under ultrasonographic guidance using a Tru-Cut needle or Biopty gun. A dissecting microscope should always be available in the ultrasonography suite so that the tissue obtained can be observed for glomeruli. Only cortex is useful for diagnosing the cause of renal dysfunction episodes; the medulla is generally useless in making a diagnosis unless infection is present.

After the biopsy, patients should lie on a rolled-up towel that is placed directly under the biopsy site for 6 hours; alternatively, a 10-pound sandbag should be placed directly over the biopsy site while the patient is supine. Vital signs should be obtained every 15 minutes for 1 hour, then every 30 minutes for 3 hours after the biopsy. A repeat hematocrit should be obtained 8 hours after the biopsy, and a nurse should observe the urine for the presence of hematuria. If there is some worry about perinephric bleeding, ultrasonography can be repeated.

Chronic Rejection. **Chronic rejection is seldom associated with symptoms unless renal dysfunction is so severe as to cause uremia.** Chronic rejection can cause a sudden increase in the serum creatinine level as progressive vascular disease causes intrarenal ischemia. More commonly there is a gradual elevation in the serum creatinine level. To establish the diagnosis of chronic rejection, a biopsy is usually required.

Drugs. Volume depletion or electrolyte disturbances resulting from diuretic use are a common cause of renal dysfunction episodes. Trimethoprim inhibits the secretion of creatinine from the renal tubules, leading to an elevation in serum creatinine level. Cyclosporine is a frequent cause of renal dysfunction episodes. Cimetidine interferes with the assay that measures creatinine and causes an elevation in its level. Amphotericin B is a tubular toxin and, like cyclosporine, can cause significant and sometimes irreversible renal dysfunction. Nonsteroidal antiinflammatory agents can cause tubulointerstitial disease or a glomerulopathy that can lead to a renal dysfunction episode. Acyclovir can cause renal dysfunction when given intravenously. In general, this does not occur when given by mouth, even in very high doses such as are required for prophylaxis against CMV. A number of drugs impair the metabolism of cyclosporine and, in a patient who has an acceptable cyclosporine level the addition of these drugs (see Table 19–19), can elevate the serum level of cyclosporine and lead to a renal dysfunction episode.

Hyperglycemia and Ketoacidosis. Both hyperglycemia and ketoacidosis interfere with the measurement of the serum creatinine level, and hyperglycemia can cause an osmotic diuresis and lead to volume depletion, which can also lead to a renal dysfunction episode.

Infection. Acute pyelonephritis can cause renal dysfunction. If rejection is mistakenly diagnosed, grave harm can result from antirejection treatment. Some viral infections, specifically CMV, can cause an episode of renal dysfunction; antirejection therapy should be avoided. Viral infections can also stimulate rejection episodes by causing the increased expression of histocompatibility antigens on donor tissues. In this case, once the viral infection is under control, antirejection therapy can be instituted.

De Novo *Intrinsic Renal Disease.* Membranous nephropathy is a frequent cause of *de novo* renal disease, and the first manifestation can be an episode of renal dysfunction. More commonly, this entity presents as proteinuria in the absence of renal dysfunction. Any disease that develops in native kidneys can develop in an allograft.

Recurrent Renal Disease. Focal glomerulosclerosis, MPGN type II, hemolytic-uremic syndrome, and membranous nephropathy are four diseases that can recur rather quickly in a transplanted kidney and can lead to renal dysfunction episodes. These can only be diagnosed by obtaining an allograft biopsy specimen.

Renal Artery Stenosis. Renal artery stenosis occurs most commonly at the site of anastomosis but might also occur more distally in the donor artery, where the intima might have been damaged during the retrieval process. Renal artery stenosis is rare early after transplantation; when a late renal dysfunction episode is accompanied by high blood pressure, this entity should be considered. The diagnosis can be suggested by a Doppler-echo study of the renal arteries, but the only definitive study is a renal arteriogram. Whenever arteriography is performed, one must be certain that the patient is well hydrated. In addition, furosemide should be given to enhance clearance of the contrast agent. A simple and effective protocol is to give a liter of normal saline over 4 hours before the test, 40 mg of furosemide IV at the time of the arteriogram, then match the urinary output with intravenous input over the subsequent 4 hours.

Renal Artery Thrombosis and Renal Vein Thrombosis. Both of these entities occur rarely after transplantation and often result in a sudden deterioration of renal function. The diagnosis can be confirmed with a venogram or arteriogram.

Obstruction. Obstruction must always be considered in an asymptomatic patient with an episode of renal dysfunction. The diagnosis can be made either with ultrasonography or with a renal scan. Stones, blood clots, external ureteral pressure from a lymphocele or hematoma, and most commonly a distal ureteral fibrotic scar can cause obstruction. Distal ureteral ischemia can be caused by poor blood supply to the distal ureter or by rejection.

Urinary Leak. A ureteral leak can occasionally occur at the ureteroneocystostomy anastomosis, especially in diabetic patients, resulting in rising BUN and creatinine levels and oliguria.

Workup of Renal Dysfunction Episodes

History Taking. Because many of the causes of renal dysfunction are due to entities other than rejection, a careful history must be taken. One must focus carefully on new drugs, episodes of dehydration, symptoms of urinary tract infections, and diabetic control. In addition, symptoms that can rule in rejection such as fever, graft pain, nausea, and oliguria should be sought.

Physical Examination. In general, the physical examination is not very useful for diagnosis of acute renal dysfunction episodes. However, a tender and swollen graft is consistent with either rejection or graft pyelonephritis. High blood pressure is consistent with rejection and renal artery stenosis. A new allograft arterial bruit or the disappearance of one that was present can herald renal artery stenosis. Low blood pressure and orthostatic changes would be consistent with volume depletion due to diuretics or hyperglycemia. Congestive heart failure is a rare cause of renal dysfunction but can be diagnosed by a physical examination.

Diagnostic Tests. If the history and physical examination do not reveal the cause of the renal dysfunction episode, diagnostic tests should be used. A renal scan can disclose information regarding blood flow, tubular function, obstruction, and leakage. Ultrasonography can disclose the presence of obstruction either from a lymphocele that surrounds the kidney or from ureteral obstruction. A urine culture can disclose the presence of infection. An SMA-18 can reveal information such as elevated uric acid and carbon dioxide levels, which may support the diagnosis of volume depletion. It may also reveal hypokalemia, which suggests the overuse of diuretics, or hyperglycemia, which by itself can cause a false elevation in creatinine level or can lead to an osmotic diuresis and subsequent volume depletion. It is often necessary to perform a renal biopsy to diagnose the cause of renal dysfunction. The workup and treatment of renal dysfunction are summarized in Table 19–27.

Table 19–27. WORKUP AND TREATMENT OF ACUTE RENAL DYSFUNCTION

Repeat BUN and creatinine determinations if in doubt.
Obtain a detailed history regarding:
1. Diuretic use and weight loss (volume depletion)
2. Use of nephrotoxic drugs (nonsteroidal antiinflammatory drugs, gentamicin, tobramycin, amphotericin B, contrast agents, penicillins)
3. Use of drugs that affect the creatinine measurement (trimethoprim, cimetidine, *etc.*)
4. Current immunosuppression (are these appropriate; have they been discontinued?)
5. Symptoms of a urinary tract infection or pyelonephritis
6. Any other unusual symptoms including non-urinary tract infections and CMV
7. Recent dietary changes (increased protein)
8. Change in laboratory performing tests
9. New onset of high or more difficult to control blood pressure
10. Presence of fever and kidney pain or tenderness

Check other pertinent laboratory results:
1. Cyclosporine level (nephrotoxicity)
2. Glucose (increased glucose can cause increased creatinine and/or osmotic diuresis)
3. Potassium (decreased K^+ may reflect diuretic abuse)
4. CO_2 (increased CO_2 indicates diuretic abuse and volume contraction)
5. Albumin (decreased albumin may indicate nephrotic syndrome)
6. Hematocrit (increased hematocrit may reflect volume contraction and vice versa).
7. Urinalysis (pyuria means infection, not rejection)
8. Uric acid (uric acid can cause renal dysfunction by a variety of mechanisms)
9. Calcium (increased calcium can decrease GFR)

Treat all nonrejection causes of acute renal dysfunction listed above. If none are present, then take the next step:

Obtain an ultrasonogram and renal scan to rule out ureteral obstruction, urinary leak, lymphocoele, infarction, and renal artery stenosis. If these have been done recently (within 3 months), take the next step:

If no nonrejection cause of renal dysfunction is found, treat for rejection.

Histopathologic Diagnosis of Causes of Renal Dysfunction

Rejection. The elements involved in hyperacute rejection are antibodies, polymorphonuclear cells, platelets, and thrombin. The micropathologic patterns include glomerular capillary thrombosis, fibrin thrombi in the glomerular capillaries and small vessels, a vasculitis, and capillary fragility leading to interstitial hemorrhage and necrosis.

The cells involved with acute rejection include lymphoblasts, both helper cells (CD4) and cytolytic cells (CD8), plasma cells, macrophages, and eosinophils. Patterns of response include a diffuse interstitial nephritis, invasion of renal tubular cells by lymphocytes, necrosis, hemorrhage, and a cell-mediated vasculitis.

Pathologic findings in chronic rejection include mesangial thickening with interposition of mesangium into the basement membrane of the capillary loops, interstitial fibrosis, loss of renal tubules, and intimal hyperplasia of the intrarenal arteries. Interstitial fibrosis and vasculopathy can occur in the absence of the glomerulopathy.

Acute Tubular Necrosis. ATN has a characteristic pattern that includes loss of the epithelial border and necrosis of tubular cells, a polymorphonuclear cell infiltrate, calcium deposition, and sometimes interstitial edema.

Thrombosis. Arterial thrombosis is usually bloodless, leading to ischemic necrosis. In renal vein thrombosis there is often interstitial hemorrhage, dilation of the venules, and edema.

Infection. The pathologic findings of interstitial infection are classic and include the findings of polymorphonuclear cells in an interstitial pattern and occasionally tubular necrosis.

Hypersensitivity. Certain drugs can cause a hypersensitivity interstitial nephritis, and this is usually manifest by the finding of multiple eosinophils as well as lymphocytes and monocytes. OKT3 has been reported to cause this pathologic picture.

Cyclosporine. Cyclosporine can cause a characteristic vasculopathy in which intimal deposits of an eosinophilic material, thought perhaps to be due to necrosis, can be noted. In addition, capillary microthrombi can occasionally be seen in the glomerular vessels. The tubulopathy of cyclosporine is manifest by tubular vacuolation and necrosis. A striped interstitial fibrosis, presumably due to ischemia from the vasculopathy, has also been described.

Recurrent Renal Diseases. Hemolytic-uremic syndrome, focal glomerulosclerosis, MPGN type II, and membranous nephropathy all have classic findings that are easily diagnosed on renal biopsy.

SURGICAL COMPLICATIONS

Allograft

Urinary Drainage. Immediately after transplantation, ureteral leaks, ureteral obstruction, urinary tract infections, and stones can complicate the postoperative course.

Vascular. Venous thrombosis, arterial thrombosis, and arteriovenous malformations from allograft biopsies can occur in the immediate postoperative period.

Other. Lymphoceles are a relatively uncommon occurrence after renal transplantation but when present can cause recurrent collections and obstruction of normal urinary flow. These must be drained initially and if recurrent must be treated by opening the peritoneum so that they can drain into the abdominal cavity. Capsular ruptures can occasionally occur, but in the cyclosporine era, severe rejections such as are required to cause a capsular rupture are extremely rare.

The Wound. In older, diabetic, and obese patients, the wound can dehisce. Bacterial wound infections are more common in diabetic patients. Incisional hernias are rare but have occasionally occurred. A stitch abscess should be dealt with by incision and drainage and removal of the stitch.

Vascular. In patients who have had two renal transplants, if both the right and left hypogastric arteries are used, a male patient will become impotent. In diabetic patients, a vascular steal can sometimes occur and will lead to claudication of the buttocks and occasionally of a leg. Femoral nerve palsies can also occur at times as a result of vascular insufficiency.

Genital. Hydrocele, varicocele, and penile edema can occasionally occur after transplantation. These should be evaluated by a urologist.

Abdominal. An acute abdomen can occur in renal transplant recipients. When this occurs, one must first think of a bowel rupture due to a diverticulum, *Clostridium difficile* enteritis, or ischemic bowel. Cholecystitis and pancreatitis as well as peptic ulcer disease can be the cause. An acute abdomen can have a high mortality rate and therefore should be acted on immediately. A general surgery consultation should be obtained early in all cases of abdominal pain.

EXTRARENAL COMPLICATIONS

Infection. The most common infections in the first month after transplantation are bacterial infections including urinary tract infections, wound infections, pneumonia, sepsis, and endocarditis. Infections occurring in the first month are due to either endogeneous causes such as a preexisting pneumonia, urinary tract infection, hepatitis, or herpes simplex; to infections transmitted by the graft such as hepatitis B, human immunodeficiency virus, CMV, or bacterial infection; or exogenous causes such as those infections introduced by a bladder catheter, endotracheal tube, intravenous lines, or a surgical wound.

During the second month after transplantation, opportunistic infections are more common, and these include CMV, *Pneumocystis*, fungal infections, and the bacterial infections caused by *Listeria*, *Nocardia*, and tuberculosis. The most common and serious among these is CMV. The primary disease that can occur in a seronegative recipient of a seropositive organ can range between mild, in which the only manifestation of infection is evidence for seroconversion, to a serious illness that may include life-threatening pneumonia, hepatitis, or ulcerative intestinal disease. A blinding retinitis can also occur. Approximately half of the general population has never been exposed to CMV and therefore is CMV seronegative (no detectable IgG antibodies to CMV-associated proteins). Unless an attempt is made to match CMV-positive donors with CMV-positive recipients, approximately 25% of recipients will be at risk for a primary CMV infection. Until better therapy is available for CMV, it is prudent to avoid placing diabetic and older patients at risk for primary CMV disease. Secondary or recurrent CMV infections can also occur, but these are uncommonly life-threatening. Possible preventive measures for CMV include the use of a hyperimmune CMV globulin or acyclovir in high doses (see Table 19–22). Gancyclovir has proved effective in many cases of CMV disease.

CMV disease can lead to depressed cell-mediated immunity, which can make a patient further susceptible to opportunistic infections with *Pneumocystis* and *Aspergillus*. It is always wise to lower immunosuppression doses during a CMV infection and to discontinue these during a life-threatening infection. A combination of leukopenia, fever, and a reversed T-cell subset ratio (CD4:CD8 <1) is highly suggestive of CMV disease. Late infections after transplantation also tend to result from opportunistic organisms, and common viral infections also occur. The incidence of late infections correlates with the success of the transplant. Patients who have adequate renal function and who are on minimal immunosuppression have a very slight risk of an opportunistic infection. Patients who have chronic rejection or who are on high doses of immunosuppression are at high risk of opportunistic infections. Table 19–28 summarizes the serious infections encountered by transplant patients and the suggested preventive measures.

Tumor. The incidence of all tumors appears to be increased in renal transplant recipients. The most common tumors encountered are skin cancer, cancer of the cervix, and lymphomas. All of these should be anticipated. Women should have a Pap smear at least annually, patients should avoid being in the sun except

Table 19–28. SERIOUS INFECTIONS AND PREVENTIVE MEASURES

	Infection	Prevention
Month 1:		
	Bacterial pneumonia	All patients should discontinue smoking before transplant. Transplant should be postponed if respiratory symptoms are present. Incentive spirometer should be used after transplant. Pneumovax vaccination.
	Urinary tract infections	Minimize bladder catheter dwell time. Culture urine routinely for a month after transplant. Consider prophylactic antibiotics.
	Wound infections	Culture donor organs and treat positive cultures for 7–10 days. Do not perform transplant on malnourished patients. Change dressings frequently if wound is leaking serous material. Evacuate *large* perinephric hematoma or fluid collections. Use prophylactic antibiotics.
Month 2:		
	Cytomegalovirus	Avoid potential primary infections by matching donors/recipients by serologic testing. Use prophylactic hyperimmune globulin or acyclovir in at-risk patients (donor positive, recipient negative). Minimize immunosuppression when infection occurs.
	Pneumocystis	Consider prophylaxis during severe CMV disease.
	Tuberculosis	Screen all patients before transplantation and treat a positive PPD test result.
Thereafter:		
	Bacterial, viral, fungal illnesses	Annual flu shot. Do not overtreat chronic rejection with immunosuppression. Encourage patients to quit smoking. Use prophylactic antibiotic for all dental procedures and surgeries. Give Heptavax before transplantation.

when using a sun screen, and all abnormal lymph node findings should be evaluated for possible lymphoma. A finding of occult blood in the stools should be evaluated with endoscopy, and hematuria should be evaluated with cystoscopy.

Lipid Abnormalities. Transplant recipients are prone to develop severe lipid disorders after transplantation, especially if they have a preexistent lipid disorder. The hyperlipidemia usually involves an increase in very low-density lipoprotein and low-density lipoprotein (LDL) particles and a decrease in high-density lipoprotein cholesterol. Of the immunosuppressive drugs used, prednisone is the most serious offender as it increases hepatic lipoprotein production. Moreover, other drugs such as thiazide diuretics, cyclosporine, and beta blockers adversely affect plasma lipid concentrations. Azathioprine has no known effect on lipids. Treatments of hyperlipidemia should begin with dietary management, which can often have a significant impact on serum lipid levels. Excessive alcohol consumption should be avoided. **If the LDL is particularly high (100 to 190 mg/dl), drug therapy should be begun.** Lovastatin is a particularly effective drug for reducing cholesterol levels. However, muscle lysis and acute renal failure can occur in some patients if high doses of lovastatin are given. It appears that cyclosporine might be a cofactor in this problem. A 20-mg dose of lovastatin given each day is both safe and effective. In patients given higher doses, creatine kinase levels should be monitored closely. If hypertriglyceridemia is a coexisting problem, gemfibrozil can be used with good success.

Patients with elevated serum cholesterol levels should be evaluated by the lipid clinic, and dietary measures and lipid-lowering medications should be used. Therapy is aimed at reducing atherogenic lipoproteins to reduce the risk of accelerated atherosclerosis and to prevent hypertriglyceridemia, which can lead to pancreatitis.

Bone Disease. Avascular necrosis is a rare occurrence after transplantation; it is related to steroid use and is probably exacerbated by alcohol abuse. Once it occurs, there is very little that can be done short of total hip replacement. In general, orthopedic surgeons are unwilling to replace a hip until it causes disabling pain.

Hypertension. Hypertension occurs commonly after organ transplantation. The most common cause is cyclosporine. Renal artery stenosis must also be considered. The native kidneys are occasionally the cause of posttransplant hypertension and can be removed. Many drugs are effective for treating posttransplant hypertension. Calcium channel blockers appear to be the most useful drugs for treating cyclosporine-induced hypertension.

Liver Disease. Abnormal liver function test results are very common after kidney transplantation. The reported incidence ranges between 6 and 60%. In most cases, the hepatic dysfunction first appears during the first few postoperative months. The majority of patients have chronic liver disease of unclear cause, which may be hepatitis C (formerly known as non-A, non-B). Other patients have acute infectious hepatitis caused by hepatitis A or B viruses or by CMV. Drug-induced liver dysfunction can be caused by azathioprine, cyclosporine, and many other drugs. Azathioprine in particular has been reported to cause a cholestatic or mixed hepatocellular and cholestatic hepatitis, veno-occlusive disease, sinusoidal dilation and peliosis hepatis, nodular regenerative hyperplasia, or portal hypertension. Coincidental liver disease not associated with the transplant or immunosuppressive drugs include that associated with alcoholism, biliary tract disease, iron overload, and tumors. All patients with abnormal results of liver function tests should be evaluated by a liver specialist.

Vascular Disease. Corticosteroids accelerate vascular disease. Vascular disease is extremely common among diabetics and is progressive after transplantation. Many diabetic patients develop ischemic ulcers and may require digit or limb amputation. All diabetics with lower limb ischemic disease should be monitored by a knowledgeable physician to minimize the need for amputation. Symptomatic coronary disease must be identified early before a catastrophic event. It is important to remember that asymptomatic coronary disease is present in most diabetic patients.

Eye Disease. Cataracts, glaucoma, and CMV retinitis are three diseases of the eye that can occur after transplantation.

SUMMARY

Renal transplantation is a life-saving procedure that can also significantly improve a patient's rehabilitation potential. It also must be recognized as a chronic condition that can be life-threatening. Caring for a renal transplant recipient begins with the appropriate screening evaluation long before the actual transplant procedure and ends only after a kidney has failed and immunosuppression has been withdrawn. Care of a renal transplant recipient requires familiarity with a significant body of knowledge that is unique to transplantation and an ability to apply that knowledge to an individual patient. A great deal of medical art is required in managing transplant patients. Experience and an ability to anticipate problems are essential to properly practice transplant medicine and surgery.

CASE SUMMARY 1: ACUTE REJECTION

The patient is a 21-year-old Caucasian woman with cerebral palsy and ESRD secondary to dysplastic kidneys. She began hemodialysis 8 years previously. Two prior cadaver kidney transplants, 7 and 6 years previously, failed as a result of rejection. She was put back on the cadaver kidney waiting list 3 years previously and had a peak PRA of 100%. She received her third cadaveric transplant from a donor with whom she was a four-antigen HLA-A, -B, -DR match (one antigen mismatch) and with whom the T-cell standard, antiglobulin, and B-cell crossmatches were negative with both the current and peak PRA sera. In addition, a retrospective flow crossmatch was negative against T cells and B cells. Because she had previously received both OKT3 and equine ATG, her initial maintenance immunosuppression was with cyclosporine, azathioprine, and prednisone. On admission, her serum creatinine level was 15.2 mg/dl. She achieved immediate graft function, and by the fifth postoperative day her serum creatinine level was 1.7 mg/dl. The routine postoperative renal scan and ultrasonogram were unremarkable. On the sixth postoperative day, her creatinine level rose to 2.7 mg/dl. She felt tired and nauseated and was febrile (39°C), and her kidney felt swollen on examination but was nontender. Her cyclosporine level was markedly subtherapeutic. Prednisone therapy was started in large doses (5 mg/kg/day for 5 days). Her creatinine level peaked at 3.5 mg/dl and began to decline but leveled off at 3 mg/dl on the 11th postoperative day. Her symptoms improved. A renal biopsy specimen showed continued moderate rejection. There were no anti-OKT3 antibodies present in her serum from the treatment 6 years previously. A course of OKT3 was begun on the 13th postoperative day. The creatinine level increased briskly to 4.7 mg/dl on the 15th postoperative day and decreased progressively to 1.4 mg/dl on the 20th postoperative day. She was discharged to complete a 10-day course of OKT3 as an outpatient.

CASE SUMMARY 2: CHRONIC REJECTION

The patient is a 34-year-old man who had previously received two cadaveric kidney grafts. He received his third cadaveric kidney graft and was immunosuppressed with quadruple immunosuppression including OKT3 initially, azathioprine, prednisone, and, beginning on the sixth postoperative day, cyclosporine. His peak PRA was 31%, and the latest PRA was 11%. Crossmatches with both of these sera were negative in the T-cell standard and antiglobulin and B-cell crossmatches. A flow crossmatch was not performed. He had delayed graft function requiring hemodialysis until the 49th postoperative day. Two allograft biopsies during this time showed no evidence of acute cellular rejection. The lowest serum creatinine level achieved was 2.6 during the fourth postoperative month. However, the lowest BUN achieved was 78 mg/dl. A biopsy specimen obtained during the fourth postoperative month showed marked ischemic changes consisting of interstitial fibrosis but no evidence of a cell-mediated rejection. Cyclosporine levels were therapeutic. Thereafter, there was a progressive deterioration in his renal function, requiring reinstitution of hemodialysis 7 months after transplantation.

CASE SUMMARY 3: DRUG-INDUCED RENAL DYSFUNCTION

The patient is a 38-year-old Caucasian man who underwent his first cadaveric kidney transplant. Under quadruple therapy using OKT3, azathioprine, and prednisone initially with cyclosporine beginning on the sixth postoperative day, he achieved immediate graft function. On the ninth postoperative day, his serum creatinine level was 1.7 mg/dl. After transplantation, he gained excessive weight. The patient lived at great distance from the transplant center, was a nurse by profession, and stated that his weight gain was in part due to fluid retention. A combination of furosemide and metolazone was prescribed approximately 2 weeks before admission. At that time, the creatinine and BUN levels were 1.9 and 45 mg/dl, respectively. Because of an increase in his BUN to more than 100 mg/dl and in his serum creatinine to 3.4 mg/dl, he was admitted to the hospital for an allograft biopsy. The patient noted that he had lost approximately 17 pounds during the previous 2 weeks, and this represented approximately 7% of his body weight. However, he was asymptomatic. There was no evidence of volume depletion on examination. Of note was a serum potassium level of 2.8 mEq/L. The biopsy specimen showed only a mild interstitial infiltrate of questionable importance. The diuretics were discontinued, and the potassium was repleted. Five days later, his creatinine level had fallen to 2.1 and his BUN to 69 mg/dl. Two weeks later, his creatinine level was 1.7 mg/dl and his BUN 41 mg/dl.

CASE SUMMARY 4: GRAFT PYELONEPHRITIS

The patient is a 35-year-old Hispanic woman who underwent primary cadaveric kidney transplantation 2 years previously. She was treated with triple immunosuppression consisting of cyclosporine, azathioprine, and prednisone. She had one acute rejection episode on the sixth postoperative day; it was treated successfully with high-dose prednisone therapy, 5 mg/kg/day for 5 days. One year after transplantation, her serum creatinine and BUN levels were 1.1 and 19 mg/dl, respectively. Because of financial reasons, an attempt was made to discontinue her cyclosporine. However, a month later she had an acute rejection episode, which responded to steroid pulse therapy and reinstitution of the cyclosporine. After this she had a new baseline of renal function. Her serum creatinine and BUN levels were 1.5 and 29 mg/dl, respectively. Eight days before admission, she developed a flulike illness with headaches, neck and shoulder stiffness, diarrhea, fevers, chills, sweats, arthralgias, anorexia, and nausea. She denied a decrease in her urine output, vomiting, or pain in her allograft. These symptoms resolved 3 days before admission. Two days before admission she noted an outbreak of recurrent oral herpes simplex lesions.

Because of an acute rise in her serum creatinine level to 3.6 mg/dl and in her BUN to 70 mg/dl, she was admitted to the hospital for evaluation. She denied symptoms of a urinary tract infection. A physical examination revealed no signs of acute rejection. Her cyclosporine level was within the therapeutic range. The laboratory data were remarkable for a urinalysis showing 30 to 50 WBCs in clumps and occasional bacteria. A subsequent culture grew greater than 10^5 colonies of *Escherichia coli*. She was begun on intravenous ampicillin and acyclovir. Blood cultures demonstrated no evidence of bacteremia. At the time of discharge 5 days later, her serum creatinine level had fallen to 2 mg/dl and her BUN to 51 mg/dl. Ten days later her serum creatinine level was 1.6 mg/dl and her BUN 26 mg/dl.

CASE SUMMARY 5: URINARY TRACT OBSTRUCTION

The patient is a 36-year-old Caucasian woman who underwent her second cadaveric kidney transplant 3 months previously. Using triple immunosuppression therapy with cyclosporine, azathioprine, and prednisone, she achieved immediate graft function; however, on the 10th postoperative day she had an acute rejection episode, which was treated successfully with steroid pulse therapy. Three weeks after transplantation, her serum creatinine and BUN levels were 1.7 and 30 mg/dl, respectively. Approximately 2 months after transplantation, her serum creatinine level gradually increased over a 1-week period from 1.7 to 2.7 mg/dl. A renal scan and ultrasonogram were obtained. The renal scan showed slight deterioration in both blood flow and tubular function. The ultrasonogram showed a large perinephric fluid collection and mild hydronephrosis. The fluid was drained and was determined to be a lymphocele. After drainage of approximately 500 ml, the serum creatinine level fell to 2.1 mg/dl. On two subsequent occasions, her serum creatinine level increased by approximately 0.5 mg/dl, coincident with reaccumulation of the lymphocele. On both occasions the fluid was drained. Three months after transplantation, the patient was admitted to the hospital for marsupialization of a reaccumulated lymphocele into the peritoneum. Subsequent to this there has been no evidence of a lymphocele on ultrasonography. Ten months after transplantation, her serum creatinine and BUN levels were 1.6 and 35 mg/dl, respectively.

CASE SUMMARY 6: SYSTEMIC INFECTION AND RENAL DYSFUNCTION

The patient is a 39-year-old Caucasian man who underwent primary cadaveric kidney transplantation. Using triple immunosuppression therapy with cyclosporine, azathioprine, and prednisone, he achieved immediate graft function but had an acute rejection episode approximately 1 month after transplantation. This was treated successfully with steroid pulse therapy. After this, his baseline serum creatinine and BUN levels were 2.1 and 39 mg/dl, respectively. Approximately 9 weeks after transplantation, he developed an illness consisting of high spiking fevers, profound fatigue, and diffuse aches. There was no evidence of pneumonia or hepatitis. He was admitted to the hospital for observation. His serum creatinine level rose to 5.5 and his BUN to 78 mg/dl. A renal scan showed a deterioration in tubular function, and an ultrasonogram showed no evidence of obstruction or perinephric fluid collections. A renal biopsy was not performed. His WBC count declined to 3800. The azathioprine was temporarily discontinued. Both buffy coat and urine cultures grew CMV. All other cultures were negative, and the patient was discharged from the hospital. His renal function gradually improved, and approximately 30 days after this illness his serum creatinine and BUN levels had decreased to 1.7 and 34 mg/dl, respectively. The azathioprine was reinstituted gradually to a full therapeutic dose.

CASE SUMMARY 7: GROSS HEMATURIA AND RENAL DYSFUNCTION

The patient is a 22-year-old woman who underwent her second cadaveric kidney transplantation. Under triple therapy coverage with cyclosporine, azathioprine, and prednisone, she achieved immediate graft function, but on the fourth postoperative day developed acute rejection. She was treated with steroid pulse therapy. Her serum creatinine level fell from 2.5 mg/dl to 1.5 mg/dl 3 days after beginning the steroid pulse. Her serum creatinine level subsequently rose to 2.6 mg/dl, and a renal biopsy was performed. The biopsy showed resolving rejection and possible evidence of pyelonephritis. The urinalysis and culture demonstrated a urinary tract infection, for which antibiotics were begun. Her serum creatinine level subsequently fell to 1.3 mg/dl and her BUN to 40 mg/dl on the 11th postoperative day. On the 13th postoperative day, she suddenly developed gross hematuria. A Foley bladder catheter was reinserted. A renal scan showed a wedge-shaped defect in the area where the allograft biopsy specimen was obtained. A renal ultrasonogram showed no evidence of obstruction or perinephric fluid collections. The following day, her serum creatinine level increased suddenly to 3.7 mg/dl. A repeat ultrasonogram was interpreted as showing no significant evidence of obstruction. However, the clinicians taking care of the patient interpreted the film as showing a very mild increase in the intrarenal collecting system. The gross hematuria persisted, but there was no evidence of blood clots. The next day, her serum creatinine level had decreased slightly to 3.5 mg/dl, and 2 days later the creatinine level had fallen to 1.7 mg/dl. A repeat renal scan showed no evidence of the wedge-shaped defect. The serum creatinine level continued to decline, and the gross hematuria gradually disappeared.

CASE SUMMARY 8: CYTOKINE NEPHROPATHY

The patient is a 44-year-old woman who underwent a cadaveric kidney transplant. She had previously had a living unrelated transplant that failed as a result of recurrent lupus nephritis. Her pretransplant creatinine and BUN levels were 13 and 105 mg/dl, respectively. She was treated with quadruple immunosuppression consisting of OKT3, azathioprine, and prednisone, and she achieved immediate graft function. The routine renal scan on the first postoperative day showed excellent perfusion and tubular function. Her serum creatinine level on the second postoperative day was 6.4 and her BUN 68 mg/dl. On the third postoperative day, her serum creatinine and BUN levels increased to 6.5 and 82 mg/dl, respectively, and on the fourth postoperative day to 6.6 and 96 mg/dl. The renal scan showed both decreased perfusion and tubular function. An allograft biopsy on the third postoperative day showed no evidence of acute rejection but did show marked generalized glomerular basement membrane thickening. The OKT3, azathioprine, and prednisone were continued, and on the fifth postoperative day cyclosporine was begun. Her renal function subsequently improved rapidly, and on the 12th postoperative day her serum creatinine and BUN levels were 1.1 and 19 mg/dl, respectively. Twelve months after transplantation, her serum creatinine and BUN levels were 1.2 and 25 mg/dl, respectively. Biopsy was not repeated.

CASE SUMMARY 9: RENAL ARTERY STENOSIS

The patient is a 27-year-old Caucasian man who underwent his second cadaver kidney transplantation. The kidney donor was an 18-month-old child. Triple immunosuppression with cyclosporine, azathioprine, and prednisone were used. The patient had delayed graft function and required hemodialysis until the 16th postoperative day. On the 11th postoperative day, acute rejection was diagnosed on the renal scan, and a course of OKT3 was begun. Five weeks after transplantation, his serum creatinine and BUN levels had fallen to 2.5 and 39 mg/dl, respectively. After transplantation, the patient had increasing difficulties with blood pressure control. Six weeks after transplantation, his serum creatinine level increased from 2.5 to 3.3 mg/dl. A renal scan showed decreased perfusion, and the patient was treated with a steroid pulse. His serum creatinine level reached a peak of 5.6 mg/dl but gradually fell, although it never declined below 2.5 mg/dl. Because of increasing difficulties with high blood pressure and the lack of continued improvement in renal function, approximately 4 months after transplantation the cyclosporine was gradually discontinued. Following this, his serum creatinine and BUN levels progressively fell to 1.8 and 17 mg/dl, respectively. However, 5 months after transplantation, his serum creatinine level again increased to 2.5 mg/dl and high blood pressure again became a problem. A Doppler study of the allograft indicated the possibility of renal artery stenosis. Arteriography confirmed the presence of a high-grade stenosis at the anastomosis. Because of the smallness of the vessels, the radiologist believed that this lesion was not treatable with angioplasty. During the next 12 months, his creatinine level remained stable, ranging between 1.9 and 2.2 mg/dl.

However, the patient was having severe episodic high blood pressure, which was becoming increasingly difficult to control. Approximately 18 months after transplantation, the patient was admitted to the intensive care unit with malignant hypertension. He had a seizure and became stuporous. His blood pressure rose to 250/160 mm Hg. His serum creatinine level concomitantly increased to 8.5 mg/dl. He was treated with intravenous antihypertensive medications, with subsequent excellent control of his blood pressure. His serum creatinine level gradually declined to approximately 1.9 mg/dl. Because of continued recurrent episodic hypertensive crises, the allograft was removed approximately 20 months after transplantation.

CASE SUMMARY 10: *DE NOVO* RENAL DISEASE

The patient is a 38-year-old man who received a kidney from his HLA-identical sister. He had developed ESRD secondary to MPGN. Because he had demonstrated an intolerance to azathioprine in the past, his immunosuppression was with cyclosporine and prednisone. He did very well until approximately 1 month after transplantation, when he had a minor rejection episode. His baseline creatinine and BUN levels were 1.5 and 23 mg/dl, respectively. Two years after transplantation, he was noted to have proteinuria. A 24-hour urine collection demonstrated 8 g of protein. A renal biopsy demonstrated membranous nephropathy. A 2-month course of high-dose prednisone every other day had no effect on the proteinuria. He developed all of the signs and symptoms of nephrotic syndrome including hypercholesterolemia, hypoalbuminemia, and peripheral edema. At the time of diagnosis of the membranous nephropathy, his serum creatinine and BUN levels were 1.5 and 23, respectively. During the third year after transplantation, his creatinine level gradually increased to 2.9 mg/dl. His nephrotic syndrome persisted, but his symptoms were only minimal on appropriate drug therapy. His maintenance immunosuppression continued with cyclosporine and prednisone.

CASE SUMMARY 11: HYPERCOAGULABILITY AND IMMEDIATE GRAFT LOSS

The patient is a 29-year-old woman who received a kidney from her haploidentical sister after donor-specific transfusions 5 years previously. The surgical procedures for both the donor and recipient were unremarkable, and the kidney initially made urine. On the second postoperative day, urine output fell precipitously, and a renal scan showed no flow to the kidney. On the third postoperative day, the allograft was surgically removed, and intra- and extrarenal venous thrombosis was noted. Two months later, the patient received a transplanted cadaveric kidney. Intraoperative heparin was given because of the prior history. The kidney functioned immediately, and her creatinine level 1 week after transplant was 1 mg/dl. Chronic rejection intervened, and the patient was reinstated on the cadaveric kidney transplant list 36 months after transplant, when the creatinine clearance declined below 10 ml/min. Two months later, a second cadaveric kidney transplant (third transplant) was performed. Intraoperative heparin was used initially, but because of the presence of gross hematuria was discontinued 3 days after transplantation. Four days postoperatively, the renal scan showed no blood flow to the recently transplanted kidney. The next day, the allograft was removed, and it again showed intra- and extrarenal vein thrombosis. The previous cadaveric kidney transplant continued to function; thus dialysis was not required. The patient was thoroughly evaluated by the hematology coagulation service. It was determined that she had a hypercoagulable state. Ten months later, 4 years after her first transplant, the patient received her third cadaveric kidney (her fourth transplant). She was treated with low-dose heparin given every 8 hours to maintain the partial thromboplastin time at the upper limits of the normal range. The kidney functioned immediately, and her serum creatinine level 1 week after transplant was 1.5 mg/dl on triple immunosuppression using cyclosporine, azathioprine, and prednisone. Before discharge from the hospital, she was converted to oral anticoagulation therapy with warfarin. The kidney continued to function well 6 months after transplantation.

Suggested Readings

Abramowicz M: Antimicrobial prophylaxis in surgery. Med Lett Drugs Ther 31:105–108, 1989.

Castaneda-Zuniga WR (ed): Radiologic Diagnosis of Renal Transplant Complications. Minneapolis, University of Minnesota Press, 1986.

Flye MW (ed): Principles of Organ Transplantation. Philadelphia, WB Saunders, 1989.
Garvoy MR, Guttman RD (eds): Renal Transplantation. New York, Churchill Livingstone, 1986.
Milford EL, Brenner BM, Stein JH (eds): Renal Transplantation. Contemporary Issues in Nephrology. New York, Churchill Livingstone, 1989.
Rubin RH, Young LS: Clinical Approach to Infection in the Compromised Host, 2nd ed. New York, Plenum Publishing, 1988.
Terasaki PI (ed): Clinical Transplants 1988. Los Angeles, UCLA Typing Laboratory, 1989.
Williams G, Burdick JF, Solez K (eds): Kidney Transplant Rejection. Diagnosis and Treatment. New York, Marcel Dekker, 1986.

CHAPTER 20

URGENT PROBLEMS IN THE RENAL PATIENT

Kevin D. Burns, Nuhad Ismail, J. Harold Helderman, and Raymond Hakim

This chapter focuses on problems in renal patients that require urgent decision-making. The emphasis is on rapid recognition of these situations and initial therapy, rather than on detailed pathophysiology or differential diagnosis. Fluid and electrolyte disorders are discussed first, followed by hypertensive crises, dialysis emergencies, and urgent problems in the patient who underwent renal transplant.

FLUID AND ELECTROLYTE DISORDERS

Hyponatremia

Definition. Hyponatremia occurs when the serum sodium concentration is less than 135 mEq/L. Hypotonicity of body fluids is *not* always present. Isotonic "pseudo" hyponatremia occurs in states of hyperlipidemia or hyperproteinemia, whereas hypertonic hyponatremia occurs in hyperglycemia.

Clinical Features. The severity of symptoms is related to both the degree of reduction of serum sodium concentration and the rate at which it has been lowered. Most serious abnormalities (ranging from lethargy, to confusion, to seizures, to coma) occur with serum sodium concentration less than 120 mEq/L.

States of excess sodium loss (volume depletion) must be distinguished from those of water excess (such as syndrome of inappropriate antidiuretic hormone) to determine appropriate therapy.

Treatment. The goals of therapy are to correct the serum sodium concentration to a safe level—125 mEq/L—and to reduce free H_2O intake. The hypovolemic patient should receive IV isotonic saline and should have albumin infusion if hypoalbuminemia exists. The presence of neurologic symptoms merits aggressive therapy (increase serum sodium concentration by 1 to 2 mEq/L/hr).* If the patient has a water excess type of hyponatremia, hypertonic (5%) saline (50 mm Na/hr IV) should be infused. In cases of preexisting volume expansion or risk of pulmonary edema, furosemide should be added. The physician should beware of overrapid correction of hyponatremia and risk of central pontine myelinolysis.

Hypernatremia

Definition. Hypernatremia occurs when serum sodium concentration is greater than 145 mEq/L. Total body sodium may be normal (with pure H_2O loss), decreased (with H_2O loss greater than sodium loss), or increased (with sodium gain).

Clinical Features. Neurologic impairment owing to brain cell shrinkage occurs in proportion to the degree of hypernatremia. Progressively severe symptoms usually occur beyond a serum sodium concentration of 155 mEq/L.

The expected normal renal response is the excretion of a *minimal* volume of *maximally* concentrated urine. Excretion of hypotonic urine implies renal H_2O loss owing to diabetes insipidus (central or nephrogenic) or use of diuretics.

Treatment. In acute conditions, the physician must end the ongoing H_2O loss: for example, by using replacement therapy in ADH deficiency, and by eliminating the cause of osmotic diuresis, if present. Also, the H_2O

*If the hyponatremia is chronic (lasting >48 hours), it is advisable to increase the serum sodium concentration at a rate up to 0.6 mEq/L/hr.

deficit must be replaced, avoiding too-rapid correction (aim for 1 mEq/hr fall in serum sodium concentration). Oral H_2O is preferred. Free H_2O can also be replaced with hypotonic saline infusion and 5% dextrose in water (rate not >300 ml/hr to avoid severe hyperglycemia). If the patient is severely hypovolemic from excess sodium and water loss, isotonic saline should be given until the patient is hemodynamically stable. Pure sodium gain is a rare cause of hypernatremia. In these cases, a diuretic may be necessary in addition to free H_2O replacement.

Hypokalemia

Definition. Hypokalemia occurs when serum potassium concentration is less than 3.5 mEq/L; it is severe if the serum potassium concentration is less than 3.0 mEq/L.

Clinical Features. The most important consequences of hypokalemia are impaired neuromuscular transmission (flaccid paralysis is possible) and susceptibility to cardiac arrhythmias. Severe hypokalemia may induce rhabdomyolysis.

Clinical severity is increased if the fall in serum potassium concentration is sudden and marked, or if the patient is on digitalis therapy.

Treatment. Urgent treatment is indicated if the patient is symptomatic, on digitalis therapy, in diabetic ketoacidosis, or if the serum potassium concentration is less than 3.0 mEq/L.

Several hundred mEq of potassium are generally required to correct severe hypokalemia, unless an intracellular shift of potassium is responsible.

For urgent correction, potassium may be infused (usually in the form of KCl) at no greater than 40 to 60 mEq/hr, to avoid a large bolus to the heart. Electrocardiogram (ECG) monitoring is indicated, and serum potassium concentration should be determined frequently.

Hyperkalemia

Definition. Hyperkalemia is present when the serum potassium concentration is greater than 5.5 mEq/L. The physician must rule out factitious hyperkalemia due to hemolysis, thrombocytosis, or leukocytosis. Hyperkalemia is considered severe if the serum potassium concentration is greater than 6.0 mEq/L.

Clinical Features. ECG changes dictate the urgency of therapy (progressing from peaked T waves, to widening of QRS, to loss of P wave and sine wave formation). Flaccid paralysis may also occur.

Treatment. In acute hyperkalemia, the physician must stop all potassium intake. If ECG changes are present, give calcium gluconate 10%, 10 ml IV to stabilize the patient's myocardium.

Shifting of potassium into cells can be achieved with IV $NaHCO_3$ (50 to 100 mEq) or glucose and insulin (infused as 500 ml 10% glucose with 10 units regular insulin).

Potassium should be removed from the body with potassium binding resins (a 100 g enema has a more rapid effect than oral resins) or with diuretics. If renal failure is present, initiate hemodialysis with low potassium dialysate.

Hypocalcemia

Definition. Acute hypocalcemia occurs when the serum calcium concentration is less than 2.25 mmol/L (4.5 mEq/L or 9 mg/dl). It must be distinguished from the decrease in protein-bound calcium occurring secondary to hypoalbuminemia. Acute hypocalcemia commonly occurs following surgical correction of primary hyperparathyroidism.

Clinical Features. The severity depends on the rapidity of the decrease in calcium, and not necessarily on the level (patients with renal failure may tolerate profound hypocalcemia). Neuromuscular symptoms (paresthesias, tetany) dominate in true hypocalcemia. The physician should attempt to elicit Chvostek's sign (facial twitching on tapping the facial nerve) and Trousseau's sign (carpal spasm after 3 minutes of inflation of a blood pressure cuff to above systolic pressure). Cardiac arrhythmias may occur (ECG may show a prolonged Q-T interval).

Treatment. Urgent treatment is required to relieve tetany and prevent cardiac arrhythmias and seizures.

The physician should give IV calcium 10 to 15 mEq immediately, either as 10% calcium gluconate (4.5 mEq/10 ml) or 10% calcium chloride (18 mEq/10 ml). Follow this with infusion of calcium, 0.75 mEq/kg over 4 to 6 hours.

Hypomagnesemia must be ruled out as a cause of hypocalcemia (serum magnesium concentration is less than 0.8 mEq/L [1 mg/dl]). If hypomagnesemia is present, treat with parenteral magnesium (8 to 16 mEq 10% $MgSO_4$ IV over 10 to 15 minutes).

Hypercalcemia

Definition. Hypercalcemia is present when the serum calcium concentration is greater than 2.60 mmol/L (5.2 mEq/L, or 10.5 mg/dl). Severe hypercalcemia is present if the serum calcium concentration exceeds 3.0 mmol/L (12 mg/dl).

Clinical Features. In severe hypercalcemia, the most common symptoms are nausea and vomiting, confusion, somnolence, polyuria, and polydipsia. There is increased risk of nephrocalcinosis, metastatic calcification, and even cardiac arrest. Most patients are volume contracted and have a decreased glomerular filtration rate.

Treatment. For severe hypercalcemia, the physician must expand extracellular fluid volume with IV isotonic saline, 1 to 2 L over 1 hour, then 200 to 300 ml/hr (increases urinary calcium excretion). Furosemide 40 to 120 mg p.o. or IV every 4 to 6 hours is needed once the patient is volume replete.

Strictly monitor input and output and serum and urine electrolytes, and replace potassium losses. Monitoring of central venous pressure is recommended in patients with a history of cardiac disease.

Control of hypercalcemia by extracellular fluid volume expansion is temporary—other measures are required to both decrease calcium efflux from bone (*e.g.*, calcitonin, or chemotherapy for malignancies) and decrease gut calcium absorption (*e.g.*, corticosteroids).

If severe renal failure is present, hemodialysis with low dialysate calcium is effective.

Hypophosphatemia

Definition. Hypophosphatemia is present when the serum inorganic phosphorus concentration is less than 0.8 mmol/L (2.5 mg/dl). Hypophosphatemia is severe when the phosphorus concentration is less than 0.5 mM (1.5 mg/dl). It may be associated with normal total body phosphate or with phosphate deficiency.

Clinical Features. Severe hypophosphatemia is associated with skeletal muscle weakness and cardiomyopathy. Rhabdomyolysis has been reported. Hemolysis may occur. Severe hypophosphatemia is most frequently observed in alcoholics, during the recovery phase of diabetic ketoacidosis, with excessive use of phosphate binders, and with hyperalimentation.

Treatment. For acute severe hypophosphatemia, the physician should administer phosphate 1 mmol/L/kg IV over 24 hours (as potassium phosphate), if phosphate depletion is present.

Monitor serum calcium, phosphorus, and potassium during therapy. Beware of hyperphosphatemia. Stop parenteral treatment when serum phosphorus concentration exceeds 0.5 mmol/L.

Hypophosphatemia caused by acute respiratory alkalosis or carbohydrate infusions does not require replacement therapy.

Hyperphosphatemia

Definition. Hyperphosphatemia is present when serum inorganic phosphorus concentration is greater than 1.7 mmol/L (5 mg/dl).

Clinical Features. Hyperphosphatemia most commonly results from decreased urinary excretion of phosphorus (as in renal failure). It can also be induced by IV phosphate infusion, and it is observed in states of increased catabolism and tissue breakdown.

Hyperphosphatemia can cause hypocalcemia and tetany. Ectopic calcification may occur.

Treatment. The physician should decrease gut phosphate absorption with phosphate binding agents and should expand extracellular fluid volume to increase urinary phosphate excretion, if renal function is adequate. In cases of severe renal failure or tissue breakdown, peritoneal or hemodialysis may be necessary to remove phosphorus.

Acid-Base Disorders

Metabolic Acidosis

Definition. Metabolic acidosis exists when there is a primary reduction in the plasma $[HCO_3^-]$ below 24 mEq/L. Severe metabolic acidosis exists when the plasma $[HCO_3^-]$ is <10 mEq/L. Below this level, blood pH is sensitive to small changes in $paCO_2$ and $[HCO_3^-]$.

Clinical Features. The physician can expect that for every 1 mEq decrease in plasma $[HCO_3^-]$ below 24 mEq/L, $paCO_2$ will decrease by 1 mm Hg below 40 mm Hg.

Calculation of the plasma anion gap ($[Na^+] - ([HCO_3^-] + [Cl^-])$) is essential to determine the cause of the acidosis. Acidemia impairs myocardial contractility and enhances venoconstriction. Patients may therefore have signs of congestive heart failure. Otherwise, the etiology of the acidosis determines the clinical features. For example, in type A lactic acidosis, signs of poor tissue perfusion and low paO_2 are usually present.

Treatment. The physician should ensure that there is adequate oxygenation and hemodynamic support. If combined severe metabolic and respiratory acidosis are present, immediate ventilation is indicated.

The physician must treat the underlying cause (for example, provide insulin in diabetic ketoacidosis) to arrest ongoing H^+ production.

HCO_3^- therapy is indicated to correct plasma $[HCO_3^-]$ to >10 mEq/L or blood pH >7.20 in the following formula:

Amount of $NaHCO_3$ to administer (mEq) = (desired plasma $[HCO_3^-]$ − actual plasma $[HCO_3^-]$) × 50% body weight in kilograms.

The physician should administer $NaHCO_3$ IV, paying attention to the following potential complications: sodium overload; overshoot alkalosis (especially in patients with organic acidoses in which the salts are potential HCO_3^- sources); hypokalemia (give potassium supplements if serum potassium concentration is less than 4 mEq/L at the start of therapy); and rising $paCO_2$ in mechanically ventilated patients ($NaHCO_3$ is a source of CO_2).

In patients with severe metabolic acidosis and pulmonary edema, consider phlebotomy (in addition to O_2, morphine, diuretics) to permit IV $NaHCO_3$. If severe renal failure is present, initiate dialysis.

Metabolic Alkalosis

Definition. A primary increase in the plasma $[HCO_3^-]$ greater than 25 mEq/L in association with an elevation in blood pH (>7.40) signifies metabolic alkalosis.

Clinical Features. For every 1 mEq rise in $[HCO_3^-]$ above 25 mEq/L, the physician can expect a 0.7 mm Hg increase in $paCO_2$ above 40 mm Hg.

With severe metabolic alkalosis (blood pH >7.60), the patient may present with mental confusion, paresthesias, cramping, tetany, or seizures. Cardiac arrhythmias may occur. Severe hypokalemia may be present.

To determine the cause of the alkalosis, the source of alkali *generating* the disorder (endogenous or exogenous) must be known. Also, one of three renal mechanisms must be responsible for *maintaining* the alkalosis: 1) severely decreased glomerular filtration rate (inability to excrete excess HCO_3^-); 2) extracellular fluid volume contraction (enhanced proximal HCO_3^- reabsorption and secondary hyperaldosteronism); or 3) hypermineralocorticoidism (stimulation of distal H^+ secretion—saline-resistant alkalosis).

Treatment. The physician should remove the underlying stimulus to HCO_3^- generation; for example, discontinue diuretics or prevent vomiting.

Also, he or she should remove factors sustaining alkalosis. NaCl and KCl will correct saline-responsive alkalosis, whereas saline-resistant forms require therapy directed at the specific cause.

In severe alkalemia, dilute HCl or NH_4Cl infusion can be used to reduce plasma $[HCO_3^-]$. Acetazolamide can be given to increase renal HCO_3^- excretion. If severe renal dysfunction exists, dialysis with a low bath $[HCO_3^-]$ is preferred.

Respiratory Acidosis

Definition. Increased $paCO_2$ (>40 mm Hg) and blood pH <7.40 signify respiratory acidosis. With metabolic acidosis, if $paCO_2$ is not appropriately reduced, respiratory acidosis coexists.

Clinical Features. In acute respiratory acidosis, the physician can expect a 1 mEq/L increase in plasma $[HCO_3^-]$ for every 10 mm Hg increase in $paCO_2$. In chronic respiratory acidosis, expect a 3 mEq/L increase in plasma $[HCO_3^-]$ for every 10 mm Hg increase in $paCO_2$.

Acute hypercapnia is associated with CNS dysfunction (anxiety, confusion, or coma). Chronic respiratory acidosis may be well tolerated. The absence of a history of chronic lung disease or illness causing chronic CNS depression suggests that the respiratory acidosis is acute.

Treatment. Therapy includes improved ventilation. When ventilating patients with chronic respiratory acidosis, the $paCO_2$ should be corrected to the known chronic $paCO_2$.

Respiratory Alkalosis

Definition. A low $paCO_2$ (<40 mm Hg) and high blood pH (>7.40) signify a respiratory alkalosis.

Clinical Features. In acute respiratory alkalosis, the physician can expect a 2 mEq/L decrease in plasma $[HCO_3^-]$ for every 10 mm Hg decrease in $paCO_2$. In chronic respiratory alkalosis, expect a 5 mEq/L decrease in plasma $[HCO_3^-]$ for every 10 mm Hg drop in $paCO_2$.

Symptoms of alkalemia may be present. Acute hypocapnia reduces cerebral blood flow and may cause light-headedness or even seizures.

Treatment. Treatment should focus on the underlying cause of respiratory alkalosis. In acute respiratory alkalosis due to anxiety states, air rebreathing may be useful to relieve symptoms.

HYPERTENSIVE EMERGENCIES AND URGENCIES (THE HYPERTENSIVE CRISES)

Rotating housestaff in nephrology are often called on to assess patients with severe elevation in blood pressure. The appropriate initial management of these patients requires 1) a knowledge of the distinction between a hypertensive emergency and urgency; 2) an ability to assess the patient for acute end-organ damage by history, physical examination, and initial laboratory work; and 3) sound knowledge of the pharmacology of antihypertensive drugs.

Definitions. *Hypertensive emergency* is defined as a clinical situation in which the patient's blood pressure must be lowered within 1 hour (Table 20–1). In all cases, there is evidence of ongoing acute end-organ damage. *Hypertensive urgency* is present when there is marked elevation of blood pressure (diastolic pressure >115 to 120 mm Hg) without signs of acute end-organ dysfunction or hypertensive neuroretinopathy. Blood pressure should be lowered within 24 hours in these situations.

Clinical Features. The patient with hypertensive crisis may have a history of difficult-to-control blood pressure, or recent change or cessation of antihypertensive therapy. A history of underlying illness (such as angina or heart failure) that may affect the choice of initial antihypertensive therapy should be elicited. In malignant accelerated hypertension, headache and blurred vision are common presenting symptoms.

Hypertensive emergencies are not defined solely by the degree of elevation of blood pressure. The physical examination should determine the degree of target organ involvement by hypertension, with attention to the optic fundi, cardiovascular status, and central nervous system. In malignant hypertension, the optic fundi reveal papilledema, flame-shaped hemorrhages, and cotton-wool exudates (grade IV hypertensive neuroretinopathy).

The initial laboratory evaluation of the patient with severe hypertension is shown in Table 20–2.

Treatment (Table 20–3). Hypertensive emergencies generally warrant IV antihypertensive therapy and admission to an intensive care unit. Treatment should be initiated prior to return of laboratory results.

For hypertensive urgencies, the blood pressure can be lowered more gradually. It is sometimes helpful to place the patient in a quiet, dark room for 30 to 60 minutes while awaiting laboratory results, prior to starting therapy.

MEDICAL EMERGENCIES DURING HEMODIALYSIS

Medical emergencies arising during hemodialysis, although rare, can be lethal. These in-

Table 20–1. THE HYPERTENSIVE CRISES

Hypertensive Emergencies	Hypertensive Urgencies
Malignant/accelerated hypertension	Severe elevation in blood pressure (≥120 diastolic) without hypertensive neuroretinopathy or acute end-organ dysfunction
Hypertensive encephalopathy	Severe hypertension in patients with a history of congestive heart failure, stable angina, chronic renal failure, or transient ischemic attacks
Severe hypertension accompanied by Acute pulmonary edema Angina or myocardial infarction Dissecting aortic aneurysm Progressing renal failure Postoperative bleeding CNS catastrophes (subarachnoid hemorrhage, intracerebral bleeding, head trauma) Extensive burns	Pre- and postoperative hypertension
Preeclampsia/eclampsia	
Catecholamine excess states with severe hypertension —Pheochromocytoma —MAO inhibitor interactions —Antihypertensive drug withdrawal syndromes	

Table 20–2. INITIAL LABORATORY EVALUATION OF SEVERE HYPERTENSION

Test	Significance
Complete blood count	Rule out microangiopathic hemolytic anemia (in malignant/accelerated hypertension)
Electrolytes	Rule out hypokalemic metabolic alkalosis (occurs in malignant/accelerated hypertension due to hyperreninemic hyperaldosteronism)
BUN, creatinine	Helpful to know previous values. If creatinine is elevated and anemia is present (Hb <12.5 g/dl) without microangiopathy, chronic renal disease may be the cause of the hypertensive crisis
Urinalysis	Proteinuria, micro/macroscopic hematuria (+/− RBC casts) in malignant/accelerated hypertension
ECG	Left ventricular hypertrophy suggests longstanding hypertension Rule out acute myocardial ischemia
Chest radiograph	Rule out heart failure Check for widened mediastinum (aortic dissection)

clude acute hemolysis, air embolism, hyperthermia, and cardiac tamponade. The more common complications are generally not lethal. These include seizures, cardiac arrhythmias, anaphylactic reactions, hemorrhage, angina pectoris, hypotension, and endotoxemia. Finally, unique fluid, electrolyte, and acid-base emergencies arise that can require particular caution in management and dialysis prescription.

The discussion that follows is aimed at defining the first few interventions that should be followed during these emergencies. The reader is referred to other chapters for a discussion of pathophysiology.

Potentially or Immediately Lethal Emergencies

Acute Hemolysis (Hypotonic Dialysate)

This complication usually requires two simultaneous failures: failure to fill the delivery system with concentrate, and incorrect setting of the conductivity alarm limits or malfunction of the conductivity monitors.

Acute hemolysis is an extreme emergency that produces abrupt onset of hemolysis, transient marked hyperkalemia that may lead to cardiac arrest, and acute water intoxication and cerebral edema.

> A port-wine appearance of blood in the venous line and pink discoloration of plasma, together with an acute fall in hematocrit, are clues to the diagnosis of acute hypotonic hemolysis.

Clinical Features. Manifestations include burning pain in the venous return site, restlessness and headache, chest pain, dyspnea, arrhythmias, acute lumbar pain, abdominal cramps, confusion, seizures, coma, and death. Arterial and venous lines will differ in appearance. There is a decrease in pulse rate initially and, later, tachycardia with cold and clammy skin. Sodium concentration in hemolyzed blood in venous lines is very low. A sample should be saved for subsequent analysis if possible.

Treatment. The treatment of a patient with acute hemolysis includes immediately clamping return blood lines and stopping the blood pump. Hemolyzed blood should not be returned. The patient should be placed on cardiac monitor and should receive oxygen. Use a high transmembrane pressure to remove excess water. Blood type and crossmatch should be performed, and transfusion if hematocrit is lowered severely. Dialysate concentrate should be changed and dialysis restarted as soon as possible with a new dialyzer. The patient should be hospitalized and myocardial injury ruled out; caregivers should watch for hyperkalemia.

Air Embolism

The risk of this catastrophic complication of hemodialysis is rare. Causes are usually retention of air in the dialyzer, leaks in blood lines or loose connections, errors during air rinse, or attachment of an empty saline or albumin bottle with failure to clamp infusion lines or failure of the clamp on an infusion line.

Although 50 to 100 ml of air may be tolerated, as low as 5 ml may be lethal if it is sequestered in a strategic location.

Clinical Features. The symptoms and signs of air embolism depend on the position of the patient. If the patient is sitting with the head elevated, air will go up in the jugular vein with resultant loss of consciousness, hemiparesis, seizures, or death. The patient classically cries out in alarm as the sound of air rushes through

Table 20–3. DRUG THERAPY FOR HYPERTENSIVE CRISES

Drugs	Route	Dose	Onset	Comments
		Emergencies		
Nitroprusside	IV	0.5–10 μg/kg/min	instantaneous	Direct arteriolar and venous dilator. ICU monitoring needed. Thiocyanate toxicity may ocur in patients with renal insufficiency.
Nitroglycerin	IV	3–5 μg/min initially	minutes	Use in ICU setting. Advantageous in myocardial ischemia.
Diazoxide	IV	Minibolus 50–100 mg over 5–10 min	minutes	Reflex tachycardia, sustained hypotension may occur.
Labetalol	IV	Minibolus 20 mg, then 40–80 mg over 10 min	minutes	α_1 and β blocker. Contraindicated in heart block, asthma, congestive heart failure, pheochromocytoma.
Trimethaphan	IV	0.5–5.0 mg/min	minutes	Ganglionic blocker.
Phentolamine	IV	1–5 mg bolus	minutes	Useful in catecholamine crises.
Hydralazine	IM	10–50 mg	30 min	Safe in pregnancy.
	IV	5–10 mg bolus or continuous infusion 50–150 μg/min, after loading dose of 200–300 μg/min for 30–60 min		Avoid in angina, aortic dissection, stroke.
		Urgencies		
Nifedipine	Oral	10–20 mg	20 min	Has been used effectively in hypertensive emergencies.
	Sublingual	10–20 mg	5 min	
Clonidine	Oral	0.2 mg, then 0.1 mg QIH	30 min	No reflex tachycardia. May cause sedation.
Captopril	Oral	10–50 mg	30 min	Treatment of choice in scleroderma renal crisis. Hypovolemia leads to increased hypotensive effect.
Minoxidil	Oral	5–20 mg	1–4 hours	Requires use of diuretic and adrenergic blocker.

the venous system. Visual problems include "seeing stars," diplopia, or blindness. If the patient is flat when embolism occurs, air may form a "foam" in the right ventricle and interfere with the pumping action of the heart; air may go to the pulmonary circulation if the patient is lying on the right side, resulting in acute pulmonary hypertension; heart auscultation reveals a "churning sound." Finally, if the patient is in Trendelenburg's position, air may go to the lower extremities, with resulting cyanosis.

Treatment. The physician must clamp the venous line immediately and place the patient in Trendelenburg's position on the *left* side (to trap air in the right ventricle away from the pulmonary valve).

The physician should give 100% oxygen and intubate the unconscious patient. The patient should be placed on a cardiac monitor. Cardiac massage is deferred until air foam is evacuated by intracardiac needle aspiration. Corticosteroids are administered to reduce cerebral edema. The patient should be placed in a decompression chamber, if one is available.

Hyperthermia (Overheated Dialysate)

Overheated dialysate can cause severe hemolysis and lethal hyperkalemia. Dialysate temperature > 51° C causes immediate massive hemolysis, and temperatures between 47 and 51° C may cause delayed hemolysis (up to 48 hours).

Clinical Features. If conscious, the patient complains of feeling hot. However, often hyperthermia occurs in an otherwise comatose or intubated patient. Coma and death may ensue if not already present.

Treatment. Dialysis should be stopped immediately, and heat-damaged blood should not be returned. The physician should determine hematocrit and electrolytes immediately and serially monitor for delayed hemolysis. The patient should be redialyzed with new equipment and new concentrate, and transfusion should be performed, as necessary. External cooling should be applied to lower a temperature >107° F.

Cardiac Tamponade

The major concern of pericarditis in the patient on hemodialysis is that it may lead to cardiac tamponade. Cardiac tamponade that is incipient or that has not reached a critically severe stage frequently may be missed. Diagnosing early cardiac tamponade is vital, as it may progress to life-threatening cardiac tamponade quickly (within hours sometimes).

Finding a pericardial friction rub in a dialysis patient with chest pain (often worse when supine) or dyspnea is highly suggestive of pericarditis. Although pericarditis does not by itself cause acute cardiac embarrassment, at times it heralds the development of hemorrhagic pericarditis and tamponade. One of the characteristic signs of this condition is early hypotension during dialysis in a patient who is volume overloaded. It is hazardous to wait for the development of pulsus paradoxus (systolic blood pressure falls more than 10 to 12 mm Hg during inspiration) or for a large increase in central venous pressure or severe symptoms before making the diagnosis of cardiac tamponade. Instead, uremic patients with pericarditis should be hospitalized, with close monitoring of hemodynamic parameters and serial echocardiograms. If indicated and if the patient's condition is deteriorating, cardiac catheterization should be performed to prove the diagnosis.

The treatment of pericarditis in the hemodialysis patient is outlined in the chapter on hemodialysis. Note, however, that unless the patient has an acute hemodynamic collapse from severe cardiac tamponade, pericardiocentesis should not be performed in the hemodialysis unit or at the bedside. Instead, the patient should always be transferred to the cardiac catheterization unit and the procedure performed by an experienced cardiologist under adequate hemodynamic and arrhythmia monitoring.

Often Serious and Possibly Lethal Complications of Hemodialysis

Seizures

Clinical conditions that predispose the uremic patient to seizure activity have been discussed in Chapter 18. Hypotension is a frequent cause of seizures and should be avoided. Seizure is often generalized, and the presence of focal seizures often indicates localized neurologic disease.

In the emergency treatment of a convulsion, the physician must stop dialysis, assure a patent airway and give oxygen, and treat hypoglycemia and hypotension. Diazepam 5 to 10 mg IV every 5 minutes to a maximal total dose of 30 mg should be administered to terminate seizure. Also needed is a loading dose of phenytoin (10 to 15 mg/kg) by slow IV infusion, no greater than 50 mg/minute, with constant ECG monitoring.

Important in the management of dialysis-associated seizures is adjusting for changes in drug metabolism in uremia. When an anticonvulsant drug is administered to the dialysis patient, remember that diphenylhydantoin, carbamazepine, and valproic acid are not dialyzable, whereas phenobarbital, ethosuximide, trimethadione, and paraldehyde are dialyzable, and a supplemental dose postdialysis needs to be given.

Cardiac Arrhythmias

Patients on hemodialysis are at a special risk for arrhythmias owing to factors unique to dialysis. These factors include hypotension, which may impair coronary perfusion, acute shifts in electrolytes (particularly potassium), and cardiovascular instability during acetate dialysis. Patients on digitalis preparations are particularly at risk. Frequently, ischemic and hypertensive cardiovascular disease, pericarditis, and conduction system calcifications are present in the dialysis patient and underlie recurrent and sustained arrhythmias.

Treatment of arrhythmias during the hemodialysis session is much the same as in nondialysis situations, except that in end-stage renal disease the altered pharmacokinetics and protein binding of drugs should be taken into account.

In the event of a serious arrhythmia (paroxysmal atrial tachycardia with block or ventricular tachycardia), the physician should stop hemodialysis and return blood to the patient, though dialysis needles should be kept patent for emergency drug use. Blood pressure should be supported with colloids or crystalloids. The physician should proceed with pharmacologic or electrical treatment of the arrhythmia.

The patient should be hospitalized. If the patient is volume overloaded, further isolated ultrafiltration can be resumed, preferably in the intensive care unit or in the hospital dialysis unit under continuous ECG monitoring.

If a critical coronary perfusion underlies the

arrhythmia, transfusion to maintain hematocrit close to 30% is important.

Patients on digitalis should have a dialysate potassium concentration between 2 and 3 mEq/L, and the serum potassium concentration should not be allowed to drop below 3.0 to 3.5 mEq/L.

First-Use Reactions During Hemodialysis

Severe reactions during hemodialysis are uncommon but can be life-threatening. Mild reactions, however, are common and can pose a diagnostic challenge. Reactions to dialyzers occur with first use. Reactions during reuse are distinctly uncommon.

There are two types of first-use reactions. Type A is characterized by anaphylactic signs and symptoms. Manifestations begin to appear within 20 minutes of the start of dialysis (usually within the first few minutes) and include dyspnea, a burning sensation throughout the body, angioedema, urticaria, rhinorrhea, abdominal cramps, and itching. Cardiac arrest may occur. Differential diagnoses include myocardial infarction, air embolism, acute hemolysis, pulmonary embolism, or pyrogen reactions.

To treat type A reaction, the physician should stop dialysis immediately and clamp tubing. The blood in the dialyzer and tubing should be discarded. Anaphylaxis is treated with antihistamines, glucocorticoids, or epinephrine as appropriate for the severity of the reaction. Oxygen is administered. Consider using dialyzers that are not cuprophane or not sterilized with ethylene oxide.

Type B reactions manifest primarily as chest pain and back pain. Symptoms are usually observed in the first hour of dialysis and characteristically disappear or lessen dramatically during the subsequent hours of dialysis. Type B reactions must be differentiated from angina pectoris and pericarditis or musculoskeletal symptoms. Treatment of type B reactions is supportive and the dialysis procedure can continue, but at low blood flow rates for the first 1/2 hour. Predialysis administration of antihistamines may be effective for patients with mild dialyzer reactions.

Angina Pectoris During Dialysis

Important differential diagnoses to be excluded are myocardial infarction, pericarditis, first-use syndrome, and acute hemolysis.

If the angina is not unstable, dialysis may be continued. Management of the simple anginal episode includes administering nasal oxygen; supporting blood pressure if hypotension is present; stopping ultrafiltration until hypotension subsides; giving sublingual nitroglycerin only after blood pressure is stabilized; transfusing if anemia is present; placing the patient on cardiac monitor; giving sedation, if the patient is anxious and blood pressure is stable; and stopping dialysis and hospitalizing the patient if angina is severe or is unstable.

Hemorrhage

Hemorrhagic episodes in dialysis patients may be dramatic. Bleeding may be obvious (*e.g.*, gastrointestinal bleeding) or overt, as with retroperitoneal bleeding, subdural hematoma, epidural hematoma, subcapsular liver hematoma, or hemopericardium. These overt hemorrhages require a high index of suspicion for early and proper diagnosis. Dramatic exsanguination may also occur in the dialysis patient owing to tubing disconnections or tubing or dialyzer rupture. The bleeding tendency of uremia appears to be most directly related to a functional platelet disorder and abnormal platelet–vessel wall interaction. This bleeding tendency is also influenced by the presence of anemia and anticoagulation. Obviously and most importantly, uremic patients should be "adequately" dialyzed.

Treatment of an acute bleeding episode includes blood transfusion to keep hematocrit at >30%; DDAVP (0.3 mg/kg) in 50 to 100 ml 0.9% saline solution over 15 to 30 minutes; and cryoprecipitate of 10 units IV every 12 to 24 hours.

Conjugated estrogens (0.6 mg/kg IV daily for 5 days) are not useful for the acute bleeding episode but are useful adjuncts in the patient who continues to bleed when the other agents (DDAVP and cryoprecipitate) have been used.

Hypotension

The sequelae of hemodialysis-associated hypotension are protean. When severe, particularly in the elderly, hypotension may cause a decrease in mental status, seizures, cardiac ischemia, arrhythmias, and vascular access clotting. Frequent blood pressure monitoring during hemodialysis is the most important factor to prevent severe hypotension.

Treatment of the acute hypotensive episode includes putting the patient in Trendelenburg's position; reducing transmembrane pressure and blood flow rates; administering 100 to 200 ml IV boluses of normal saline; and, if serum albumin is low, administering 12.5 to 25 g of hyperoncotic albumin. (Do not administer albumin in the last 45 minutes to 1 hour of dialysis.)

Fever and Endotoxemia

Febrile reactions during dialysis are the result of either endotoxemia or infection. Very rarely, they are caused by an overheated dialysate. Pyrogenic reactions are treated with acetaminophen or acetylsalicylic acid. If the patient is clinically septic, the physician should start empiric antimicrobial coverage with vancomycin and an aminoglycoside (give a loading dose after blood cultures are drawn).

Altered Mental Status

Causes of alteration in mental status during hemodialysis are varied. Treatment depends on the underlying cause. Always consider drugs (narcotics, sedatives), hypotension, hypo- and hyperglycemia, and electrolyte disorders (hypercalcemia, hypermagnesemia, and hypo- and hypernatremia) and treat these conditions.

Fluid and Electrolyte Emergencies

Hyponatremia

Hyponatremia and hypo-osmolality secondary to a hypotonic dialysate is a major emergency and can lead to massive, severe hemolysis. This condition is extremely rare because of multiple safety devices in the dialysis delivery machine. More commonly, hyponatremia is present in an acutely ill patient in the intensive care unit or may be associated with severe hyperglycemia in a dialysis patient. (For every 100 mg/dl increase in serum glucose, there is a corresponding decrease of 1.6 mEq/L in serum sodium concentration due to osmotic shifts.)

When plasma osmolality is corrected rapidly, cerebral dehydration may ensue, triggering the osmotic demyelination syndrome. A similar phenomenon, the dialysis disequilibrium syndrome, may follow if severe azotemia is corrected rapidly with hemodialysis. It is prudent to correct severe symptomatic hyponatremia (>48 hours' duration) at a slow, gradual rate, as is recommended for patients with normal renal function. To achieve this gradual correction, it is advisable that the dialysate sodium concentration be no higher than 15 mEq/L above the plasma levels, and that a shorter dialysis session at low blood-flow rates be used. The latter will ensure that the cerebral edema of hyponatremia is not exacerbated by disequilibrium and that hyponatremia is corrected during multiple dialysis treatments performed over several days.

The maximum safe rate of correction of serum sodium concentration in severe hyponatremia is controversial. At present, it is safe to raise serum sodium concentration no faster than 0.6 mEq/L/hr, particularly if the hyponatremia is chronic (>48 hours).

Hypernatremia

Hypernatremia is less common than hyponatremia in hemodialysis. Like hyponatremia, it usually occurs secondary to an error in the preparation of the dialysate solution or may be due to dehydration. The consequences of hypernatremia are intracellular water depletion and hyperosmolarity. The patient complains of profound thirst and headache, nausea, vomiting, and convulsions. Coma and death may supervene.

The physician should avoid correcting the hypernatremia using too low a dialysate sodium concentration. Use of such a solution may precipitate hypotension or exacerbate the disequilibrium syndrome by inducing cerebral edema. One should particularly avoid a low dialysate sodium if the blood urea nitrogen is high (>100 mg/dl). If the patient has volume depletion and hypotension, normal saline solution is given. If there is no hypotension, half normal saline or one quarter normal saline may be administered. The aim is to correct the hypernatremia slowly, at a rate not to exceed 1 mEq/L/hr.

Hyperkalemia

There is about 10% incidence of severe predialysis hyperkalemia (serum potassium concentration >6 mEq/L) in outpatients on chronic hemodialysis. It may be the result of dietary indiscretions or underdialysis, and it commonly occurs in the patient who misses one or several dialysis sessions. It may also develop in association with acute hemolysis or severe hyperglycemia. During hemodialysis, a dialysate potassium between 1 and 3 mEq/L results in net removal of potassium.

> A potassium-free dialysis solution should be avoided particularly in a patient with left ventricular hypertrophy or in a patient on digoxin.

Rapid lowering of serum potassium concentration may precipitate cardiac arrhythmias. If a zero potassium bath is used, follow-up of serum potassium should be checked in 30 to 45 minutes. In the patient with hyperkalemia who is weak or lethargic, an immediate ECG should be obtained, and if electrocardiographic signs of potassium toxicity are evident (peaked T waves, low or absent P waves, widened QRS complexes), the patient should immediately receive IV calcium chloride (1 ampule), IV glucose + insulin and IV sodium bicarbonate, together with emergency hemodialysis.

Hypokalemia

Hypokalemia is usually a threat to the hemodialysis patient who is on digitalis glycosides or has left ventricular hypertrophy. Management of the patient who has chronic predialysis hypokalemia requires a dialysate potassium concentration of 3 mEq/L. In a patient on digoxin, a dialysate potassium of 3 to 3.5 mEq/L is recommended, and if a dialysate bath containing 4 mEq/L is used, the serum potassium concentration should be carefully followed, as sudden hyperkalemia may appear if the patient has dietary indiscretions.

Alkalemia and Acidemia

When arterial pH is >7.55, dangers of cardiac arrhythmias exist. Dialysis patients with respiratory alkalosis cannot have a compensatory metabolic acidosis. In this situation, standard acetate or bicarbonate solutions (35 mEq/L of HCO_3) should be avoided even if the plasma bicarbonate is near normal or slightly reduced. In the patient with sepsis or pulmonary edema in the setting of acute dialysis, the dialysate acetate or bicarbonate should be reduced to normalize the arterial pH and keep the serum bicarbonate at 18 to 20 mEq/L.

Severe metabolic acidosis should not be corrected rapidly but rather should initially be partially corrected to a plasma bicarbonate level of 15 to 20 mEq/L, preferably with a bicarbonate dialysate rather than acetate, because such patients may be hemodynamically unstable.

Patients with severe respiratory acidosis, particularly if they have associated hypoxemia, should be treated with a bicarbonate bath at a concentration of 35 to 40 mEq/L, rather than with an acetate bath, to avoid exacerbation of the hypoxemia in the initial phase of hemodialysis.

Hypophosphatemia

When severe, hypophosphatemia can cause respiratory arrest. Patients with poor nutritional intake and those on total parenteral nutrition should have their serum phosphorus closely followed, particularly if they are on phosphate binders.

Hypermagnesemia

Most dialysis centers use deionization or reverse osmosis to control divalent-ion levels in water used to prepare dialysate. If water treatment fails, the combination of hypermagnesemia and hypercalcemia may precipitate an acute syndrome called the hard-water syndrome, though this occurs very rarely. Hypermagnesemia nowadays is most often seen secondary to use of magnesium-containing laxatives or antacids. Severe hypermagnesemia may cause clinical and electrocardiographic findings similar to hyperkalemia and should be treated similarly, with urgent dialysis and reversal of the cardiotoxic effects of magnesium on the myocardium.

Hypercalcemia

In the dialysis patient, hypercalcemia is often due to calcium supplements or vitamin D treatment. These should be stopped when serum calcium rises above 2.75 mM (or 11 mg/dl). Hypercalcemia may also be secondary to severe hyperparathyroidism, aluminum-related bone disease, or an associated medical illness (cancer, tuberculosis, sarcoidosis). When hypercalcemia is severe, salmon-calcitonin (4 to 8 IU/kg subcutaneous or IM every 8 to 12 hrs) can be used. A low calcium dialysate bath (2.5 mEq/L) can also be used with careful monitoring of serum calcium and blood pressure. Saline diuresis and fluids are contraindicated in the hemodialysis patient.

EMERGENCIES IN THE RENAL TRANSPLANT PATIENT

Perioperative Emergencies

Hyperacute Rejection

The patient with hyperacute rejection presents with sudden cessation of urine output and with inflammatory diathesis hours to within the first 24 hours after surgery. The diagnosis is presumptive because pathologic alterations exist at the level of the larger arteries in the kidney and because a biopsy can be normal; IgG and complement appear in biopsy of vessels on occasion.

Preventive therapy relies on sensitive cross-matching to avoid cytotoxic anti-HLA IgG. Urgent nephrectomy is needed in hyperacute rejection to prevent rupture.

Anastamotic Hemorrhage

The patient presents with hypertension, shock, and low central venous or wedge pressure. These features appear later in slower bleeding. Falling hematocrit and perigraft pain radiating to the back and flank are other manifestations.

Diagnosis is based on difficulty maintaining blood pressure, central venous pressure, or PCW with fluid resuscitation. Ultrasound reveals perigraft fluid collection.

Treatment involves immediate exploration toward possible repair of the anastamosis, and massive early fluid resuscitative measures, especially administration of blood.

Urinary Leak

The patient with urinary leak presents with a fall in urine flow. The patient's creatinine level falls slowly, less than would be expected from preleak experience. Later in the course, a slow rise in creatinine occurs. The patient also has perigraft tenderness and unilateral edema of labia, scrotum, or ipsilateral thigh. The patient occasionally has fever if a secondary infection is present.

In the diagnosis of urinary leak, ultrasound examination detects extrarenal collections (sensitivity, $\geq$2 cm). A nuclide scan reveals isotope in extrarenal sites. A fluid sample reveals chemistries similar to the composition of urine. Retrograde pyelogram reveals the leak. Another diagnostic measure is the indigo carmine test, in which dye instilled in the bladder found later in the fluid collected reveals a ureterovesicular leak. Also, dye given intravenously is found in the fluid collected and identifies a proximal ureteric leak.

A ureteric leak requires surgical repair if possible—a native ureterovesiculostomy. For bladder leak, prolonged Foley drainage often is adequate; surgical repair is needed if drainage fails. To treat pelvic leak, the physician must seal the pelvis and drain the transplant with an intracalyceal catheter exiting the skin. One can later attempt native ureterovesiculostomy.

Postsurgical Acute Renal Failure

The patient with postsurgical acute renal failure presents with lack of excretory clearance with or without urine flow.

Clinical features often help make this diagnosis. The disorder can be suspected in kidneys harvested from older donors; in patients who had prolonged warm ischemia time, prolonged preservation time, or difficult harvest surgery; in a donor or recipient with hypotension; or with use of pressor agents in the donor.

Other procedures also can identify postsurgical acute renal failure. A nuclide scan shows delayed initial uptake. Biopsy or early fine-needle aspiration shows no evidence of immune cell activation within the graft. Tubular changes indicative of ischemia may be found. A core biopsy in the perioperative period is generally not necessary. However, if primary nonfunction persists 10 to 14 days postoperatively, a core biopsy may be indicated.

Early Transplant Course (Days to Several Months)

Acute Renal Dysfunction

Acute Rejection. In the patient with acute rejection, inflammatory symptoms may be found but are less common when cyclosporine is used. Symptoms such as fever, myalgias, arthralgia, perigraft tenderness, and hypertension may be present.

The patient has reduced urine flow. Chemical abnormalities include a reduced glomerular filtration rate, elevated serum creatinine, acidosis, hyperkalemia, proteinuria, and lymphocytosis. Special laboratory measurements including elevated β_2-microglobulin, neopterin, and lysozyme may be found.

A nuclide scan may reveal nonfunction of the allograft. An ultrasound revealing no evidence of mechanical problems can implicate rejection. Sometimes edema, graft swelling, and increased echogenicity may be part of rejection. Doppler ultrasound reveals a high resistive index, the result of hemorrhage and edema. Also revealing is classical core or fine-needle biopsy.

Treatment can include pulse steroids, using dosages ranging from 100 mg methylprednisolone orally for 5 days to 1 g methylprednisolone IV for 3 to 5 days.

Other treatments include a course of polyclonal anti–T cell antibodies, and use of monoclonal antibodies (*e.g.*, anti CD3).

Acute Cyclosporine Toxicity. The patient with acute cyclosporine toxicity presents with reduced urine flow, reduced glomerular filtration rates, increased serum creatinine, hyperkalemia, and elevated blood levels.

Diagnosis can be made based on the absence of a classic presentation for acute cellular rejection and on absence of elements of classic rejection seen on radiographic and biopsy studies. Also useful in diagnosis is the finding of isometric vacuoles in renal parenchymal cells by core or fine-needle aspiration biopsy. More difficult to appreciate are the changes described on biopsy relating to pericapillary congestion.

Treatment requires reducing or ceasing cyclosporine administration. Amelioration in renal function must be seen in 2 to 3 days to sustain the diagnosis.

Other Nephrotoxins. Patients present with impaired renal function. Diagnosis is based on a history of the use of agents such as aminoglycosides, nonsteroidal antiinflammatory drugs, angiotensin-converting enzyme inhibitors in the presence of transplant artery stenosis, and drugs that increase cyclosporine levels, leading to cyclosporine toxicity (*e.g.*, ketoconazole, rifampin, and erythromycin). To treat nephrotoxicity, the physician should stop the drug and reevaluate the patient.

Lymphocele. The patient's presentation may differ depending on the site of obstruction and the size of the lymphocele. The patient can have a detectable mass, unilateral and ipsilateral swelling of the lower extremity, or reduced urine flow or renal function associated with increasing serum creatinine in the absence of signs and symptoms of rejection.

Ultrasound reveals fluid collection and obstruction of the renal transplant. Nuclide scan shows a flow indicative of obstruction. Magnetic resonance imaging (MRI) also can show an obstructive pattern. Finally, the composition of the fluid in the extrarenal collection has the features of serum.

Late Reduction in Renal Function

Chronic Rejection. A patient with chronic rejection demonstrates the staircase phenomenon—episodic elevation in serum creatinine followed by stable periods. With progressive dysfunction, slow rise in serum creatinine occurs. With abrupt dysfunction, a sudden increase in serum creatinine occurs.

Diagnosis is based on elimination of mechanical possibilities, absence of other diagnostic possibilities, and core biopsy revealing progressive interstitial fibrosis or bland arteriolosclerosis.

Because the immunologic etiology of this dysfunction is unknown, little treatment is possible. Therapies directed against acute rejection generally fail.

Chronic Cyclosporine Nephrotoxicity. The patient presents with a slow, steady rise in serum creatinine and no other symptoms.

The toxicity is generally unrelated to cyclosporine levels. Although a common finding in long-term use of cyclosporine for immunologic disease other than transplant or for nonrenal organ transplantation, chronic cyclosporine nephrotoxicity is uncommon in the renal transplant recipient. Diagnosis by biopsy is difficult; some researchers have felt that striped fibrosis, areas of scar interspersed with normal areas, is indicative of this form of drug reaction.

Once chronic cyclosporine nephrotoxicity ensues, withdrawal from cyclosporine or reduction in dose generally affords no benefit. Some have argued that conversion to precyclosporine immunosuppression can prevent this problem. In the renal transplant recipient, conversion is generally met with acute rejections in otherwise stable patients and is, therefore, generally unwise.

Nephrotic Syndrome. The affected patient may present with heavy proteinuria, the full-blown nephrotic syndrome with edema, or a nephritic urine, depending on etiology.

For diagnosis, a renal biopsy is mandatory and generally undertaken when the nephrotic syndrome is accompanied by reduction in renal function. One may see recurrence of an original glomerulonephritis, *de novo* glomerulonephritis, or glomeular changes of chronic rejection.

If the biopsy demonstrates a treatable form of glomerulonephritis (a rarity), the physician may undertake approaches similar to that in primary glomerular disease in native kidneys.

Fever in the Transplant Recipient

Perioperative fever is generally related to surgery; the physician should evaluate atelectasis, potential wound infection, and catheter-induced infections.

Fever in the first several months can result

from viral infection, particularly by the DNA viral groups such as herpes and cytomegalovirus. Cultures negative for bacteria, leukopenia, fourfold increases in IgG, twofold increases in IgM, or recovery of virus from the buffy coat or urine is helpful in making this diagnosis. In cases of systemic infection, acyclovir for herpes and gancyclovir for cytomegalovirus are helpful.

Fever after the first several months is usually the result of opportunistic infections. Distinct syndromes demand diagnostic and therapeutic strategies. In a patient with fever and headache, *Listeria* and fungal infections are most common. Immediate lumbar puncture with Gram's stain, India ink analysis, and serologies are mandatory. Early definitive therapy is a must. In a patient with pneumonia, pneumocystis and legionella are the most important causes to be considered. Very early bronchoscopy with cultures, washings, and immunologic diagnostic techniques is mandatory. If the diagnosis is not rendered by bronchoscopy, more invasive diagnostic techniques, such as open lung biopsy, must be considered.

Suggested Readings

1. Halperin ML, Goldstein MB (eds): Fluid, Electrolyte and Acid-Base Emergencies. Philadelphia, WB Saunders Company, 1988.
2. Helderman JH: Principles of rejection. *In* Jacobson HR, Striker GE, and Klahr S (eds): Principles and Practice of Nephrology. Philadelphia, BC Decker. (in press)
3. Reuler JB and Magarian GJ: Hypertensive Emergencies and Urgencies: Definition, Recognition and Management. J Gen Intern Med 3:64, 1988.
4. Wolfson AB and Singer I: Hemodialysis-related emergencies, Part I. J Emerg Med 5:533, 1987.
5. Wolfson AB and Singer I: Hemodialysis-related emergencies, Part II. J Emerg Med 6:61, 1988.

INDEX

Page numbers in *italics* refer to illustrations; page numbers followed by t indicate tables.